SURGICAL COMPLICATIONS

Diagnosis & Treatment

SURGICAL COMPLICATIONS

Diagnosis & Treatment

COMPLICATIONS

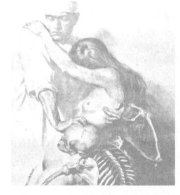

EDITORS **NADEY S. HAKIM   VASSILIOS E. PAPALOIS**

Hammersmith Hospital, London, UK

Imperial College Press

Published by

Imperial College Press
57 Shelton Street
Covent Garden
London WC2H 9HE

Distributed by

World Scientific Publishing Co. Pte. Ltd.
5 Toh Tuck Link, Singapore 596224
USA office: 27 Warren Street, Suite 401-402, Hackensack, NJ 07601
UK office: 57 Shelton Street, Covent Garden, London WC2H 9HE

British Library Cataloguing-in-Publication Data
A catalogue record for this book is available from the British Library.

ISBN-13 978-1-86094-692-9
ISBN-10 1-86094-692-5

Typeset by Stallion Press
Email: enquiries@stallionpress.com

Printed by FuIsland Offset Printing (S) Pte Ltd, Singapore

To my wife, Nicole, and children
Alexandra, David, Andrea and Gabriella, NH

To my wife, Vana, and children
Timos, Sundy, Zoe and Pavlos, VP

CONTENTS

CONTRIBUTORS

Editors:

Nadey S. Hakim, KCSJ, MD, PhD, FRCS, FRCSI, FACS, FICS
World President, International College of Surgeons
Surgical Director, West London Renal and Transplant Centre
Hammersmith Hospital, Imperial College London
Du Cane Road, London W12 0HS, UK

Vassilios E. Papalois, KSJ, MD, PhD, FRCS, FICS
Consultant Transplant and General Surgeon, Honorary Senior Lecturer
West London Renal and Transplant Centre
Hammersmith Hospital, Imperial College London
Du Cane Road, London W12 0HS, UK

Rajesh Aggarwal, MA, MRCS
Specialist Registrar in Surgery
Department of Biosurgery and
    Surgical Technology
St. Mary's NHS Trust
St. Mary's Hospital
Praed Street, Paddington
London W2 1NY, UK

Nicholas Alexakis, MD
Department of General Surgery,
    Medical School
University of Athens
Hippocration Hospital
V Sofias 114
Athens 11527, Greece

Thanos Athanasiou,
    MD, PhD, FETCS
Consultant Cardiothoracic
    Surgeon-Senior Lecturer
Department of Biosurgery and
    Surgical Technology
Imperial College London
10th Floor, QEQM Building
Department of
    Cardiothoracic Surgery
St. Mary's NHS Trust
St. Mary's Hospital
Praed Street, Paddington
London W2 1NY, UK

Paul B. Boulos, MS, FRCS,
    FRCS Ed, FCSHK(Hon)
Professor of Colorectal Surgery
Department of Surgery
University College London
74 Huntley Street
London WC1E 6AU, UK

Patrick J. Bradley, MBA, FRCS
Consultant Head and Neck
    Oncologic Surgeon
Nottingham University Hospitals
Queens Medical Centre Campus
Nottingham NG7 2UH, UK

Allan Chapman, MA, DPhil,
    DUniv, FRAS
Member
Modern History Faculty Office
Wadham College University
    of Oxford
Broad Street
Oxford OX1 3BD, UK

Joanna Chikwe, FRCS
Specialist Registrar,
    Cardiothoracic Surgery
Royal Brompton and
    Harefield Hospitals
Sydney Street
London SW3 6AH, UK

Justin P. Cobb, MBBS, MCh, FRCS
Professor and Chair
  Department of Orthopaedic
Surgery Imperial College London
Charing Cross Campus
7th Floor, East Wing
Fulham Palace Road
London W6 8RF, UK

Christopher N. Compton, MD
Staff Vascular Surgeon
Arizona EndoVascular
6565 E. Carondelet Drive
Suite 235, Tucson
AZ 85710, USA

Gabriel Conder, MBBS,
  MRCP, FRCR
Research Fellow
Magnetic Resonance Unit
Department of Radiology
St. Mary's NHS Trust
St Mary's Hospital
Praed Street
London W2 1NY, UK

Saxon Connor, FRACS
Department of Surgery
Christchurch Hospital
Riccarton Avenue
Private Bag 4710
Christchurch
New Zealand

John M. Daly, MD
Dean, Temple University
  School of Medicine
Harry C. Donahoo Professor
  of Surgery
3420 N. Broad Street
  MRB 102, Philadelphia
PA 19140, USA

Wael Dandachli, BSc, MBBCh, MRCS
Orthopaedic Specialist Registrar
Charing Cross Hospital
Fulham Palace Road
London W6 8RF, UK

Ara Darzi, KBE, MD, FRCSI
Professor of Surgery
Department of Biosurgery
  and Surgical Technology
Division of Surgery, Oncology,
  Reproductive Biology
  and Anaesthetics
Faculty of Medicine, Imperial College
  London, 10th Floor, QEQM
  Building, St. Mary's NHS Trust
St. Mary's Hospital, Praed Street
Paddington, London W2 1NY, UK

Lloyd Dayes, MD, FACS, FICS
Professor of Neurosurgery
Loma Linda University
  School of Medicine
CA 92350, USA

**Natale Ferreira Gontijo
    De Amorim**, MD
Assistant Professor
    of Plastic Surgery
The Pontifical Catholic
    University of Rio de Janeiro
    and the Carlos Chagas
    Postgraduate Medical
    Institute, Rua Dona
    Mariana 65
Rio de Janeiro 22280-020
Brazil

Muhammad Tariq Dosani,
    MRCSEd, FICS
Clinical Fellow
West London Renal and
    Transplant Centre
Hammersmith Hospital
Honorary Clinical Fellow
Imperial College London
Du Cane Road
London W12 0HS, UK

Justin L. Dwyer, MBBS
Senior Registrar in Psychiatry
North Western Mental Health
The Royal Melbourne Hospital
Parkville 3050, Victoria
Australia

Jonathan C. Evans, FRCR
Department of Radiology
Royal Liverpool University
Prescot Street
Liverpool L7 8XP, UK

William R. Fleming, FRACS, FRCS
Consultant Surgeon
Endocrine Surgery Unit
Hammersmith Hospital
Imperial College London
Du Cane Road
London W12 0HS, UK

Colleen B. Gaughan, MD
Thoracic and Foregut Surgery
    Fellow, University of Southern
    California, 1510 San Pablo St.
Suite 514, Los Angeles
CA 90033, USA

Wady Gedroyc, MBBS, MRCP, FRCR
Professor of Radiology
Head of Magnetic Resonance Unit
Department of Radiology
St. Mary's NHS Trust
St Mary's Hospital
Praed Street, London W2 1NY, UK

Paula Ghaneh, FRCS
Division of Surgery and Oncology
University of Liverpool
5th Floor UCD Block — RLUH
The Duncan Building, Daulby Street
Liverpool L69 3GA, UK

Basil Ch. Golematis,
    MD, PhD, FRCS, FACS
Professor of General Surgery
First Department of
    Propaedeutic Surgery
Hippocration Hospital of Athens
Athens Medical School
Athens, Greece

Carlos M. H. Gómez,
LMS, FRCA, MD
Consultant in Intensive Care
  Medicine and Anaesthesia
St. Mary's NHS Trust
St. Mary's Hospital
Praed Street, Paddington
London W2 1NY, UK

Ilias P. Gomatos, MD
First Department of Propaedeutic
  Surgery
Hippocration Hospital of Athens
Athens Medical School
Athens, Greece

Tamsin J. Greenwell,
MD, FRCS(Urol)
Consultant Urological Surgeon
  and Honorary Senior Lecturer
Institute of Urology
University College London and
  University College London
  Hospital
235 Euston Road
London NW1 2BU, UK

Navyash Gupta, MD, FACS
Assistant Professor
Division of Vascular Surgery
Department of Surgery
University of Pittsburgh
  Medical Center, and
Presbyterian University Hospital

200 Lothrop Street
A1010 PUH, Pittsburgh
PA 15213, USA

Hoonbae Jeon, MD
Assistant Professor of Surgery
Transplant Section
University of Kentucky
  College of Medicine
800 Rose Street
C-447, Lexington
Kentucky 40536, USA

Christopher Johnstone,
MB, ChB, FRCA
Consultant Anaesthetist
Department of Anaesthesia
Crosshouse Hospital
Kilmarnock
Ayrshire KA2 0BE, UK

Panagiotis B. Kekis, MD, PhD
Clinical Fellow
Endocrine Surgery Unit
Hammersmith Hospital
Imperial College London
Du Cane Road
London W12 0HS, UK

Umraz Khan, MBBS, BSc, FRCS,
FRCS(plast)
Consultant in Plastic and
  Reconstructive Surgery
The Frenchay Hospital
Beckspool Road Frenchay
Bristol BS16 1LE, UK

Wolff M. Kirsch, MD, FACS
Professor of Neurosurgery
    and Biochemistry
Director of Neurosurgical
Center for Research,
    Training, and Education
Loma Linda University
    School of Medicine
CA 92350, USA

Manousos M. Konstadoulakis,
    MD, PhD
Assistant Professor
    of General Surgery
Department of Propaedeutic
    Surgery
Hippocration Hospital of Athens
Athens Medical School
Athens, Greece

John A. Lynn, MS, FRCS
Consultant Surgeon
Endocrine Surgery Unit
Hammersmith Hospital
Imperial College London
Du Cane Road
London W12 0HS, UK

Michel S. Makaroun,
    MD, FACS
Professor and Chief
Division of Vascular Surgery
Department of Surgery
University of Pittsburgh
    Medical Center, and
Presbyterian University Hospital

200 Lothrop Street
A1010 PUH, Pittsburgh
PA 15213, USA

Martin A. Mansell, MD FRCP
Consultant Nephrologist
Royal Free and University
    College London Hospitals
13 Ashbourne Ave
London NW11 0DP, UK

Victoria J. Mansell, BA, LLM
Medico-Legal Ethicist
Royal Free and University
    College London Hospitals
13 Ashbourne Avenue
London NW11 0DP, UK

Cosme Manzarbeitia, MD, FACS
Chairman, Division of Transplantation
Albert Einstein Medical Center
5401 Old York Road
Klein Building, Suite 509
Philadelphia, PA 19141, USA

Sir Peter J. Morris, AC, FRS, FRCS
Emeritus Nuffield Professor and
    Chairman of Surgery
University of Oxford
Honorary Consultant
Oxford NHS Trust Hospital
Honorary Professor
University of London
Past President, Royal College of
    Surgeons of England

Anthony R. Mundy
MS, FRCP, FRCS
Professor of Urology and
 Honorary Consultant
 Urological Surgeon
Institute of Urology
University College London and
 University College
London Hospital
235 Euston Road
London NW1 2BU, UK

Nazar A. Mustafa, MD, FRCSI,
 FEBU, FICS
Urology and Transplant Fellow
West London Renal and
 Transplant Centre
Hammersmith Hospital
Imperial College London
Du Cane Road
London W12 0HS, UK

Antony A. Narula, MA, FRCS,
Consultant Otolaryngologist
St. Mary's NHS Trust
St Mary's Hospital
Praed Street, Paddington
London W2 1NY, UK

John P. Neoptolemos, FRCS
Head of School of Cancer Studies
Division of Surgery and Oncology
University of Liverpool
5th Floor UCD Block - RLUH
The Duncan Building

Daulby Street
Liverpool L69 3GA, UK

Lisa A. Newman, MD, MPH, FACS
Director, Breast Care Center
Associate Professor of Surgery
University of Michigan
 Comprehensive Cancer Center
1500 E. Medical Center Drive
3308 Cancer Center
Ann Arbor, MI 48109-0932, USA

Enrico Nicolo, MD, FACS, FICS
Assistant Clinical Professor
 of Surgery
Department of Surgery
University of Pittsburgh
 Medical Center
200 Lothrop Street
Pittsburgh, PA 15213-2582, USA

Austin O'Bichere, MD, FRCS
Consultant Colorectal Surgeon
University College Hospital
235 Euston Road
London NW1 2BU, UK

Jorge A. Ortiz, MD
Associate Director
Clinical Operations for Liver
 and Kidney Transplantation
Texas Transplant Institute
Methodist Specialty and
 Transplant Hospital
8201 Ewing Halsell Drive, #280
San Antonio, Texas 78229, USA

Earl Owen, AO, MD, DSc,
FRACS, FRCS, FICS, FRCSE
Medical Director of The
Microsearch Institute
of Australia
Suite 303, Level 3
121 Walker Street
North Sydney, NSW 2060
Australia

Nick Pace,
MBChB, FRCA, FRCP, PhD
Position Consultant Anaesthetist
Western Infirmary
Dumbarton Rd.
Glasgow G12, Scotland, UK

Alexander A. Parikh, MD
Assistant Professor of Surgery
Division of Surgical Oncology
Vanderbilt University
Medical Center
597 Preston Building
2220 Pierce Avenue
Nashville, TN 37232-6860, USA

Ivo Pitanguy, MD
Head Professor of the
Postgraduate Courses
in Plastic Surgery
The Pontifical Catholic
University of Rio de Janeiro
and the Carlos Chagas
Postgraduate Medical Institute
Rua Dona Mariana 65
Rio de Janeiro 22280-020, Brazil

Henrique N. Radwanski, MD
Assistant Professor
of Plastic Surgery
The Pontifical Catholic University
of Rio de Janeiro
and the Carlos Chagas
Postgraduate Medical Institute
Rua Dona Mariana 65
Rio de Janeiro 22280-020, Brazil

David J. Reich, MD, FACS
Associate Director
Liver Transplantation and
Hepatobiliary Surgery Program
Albert Einstein Medical Center
Associate Professor of Surgery
Jefferson Medical College
Thomas Jefferson University
5401 Old York Road
Klein Building, Suite 509
Philadelphia, PA 19141, USA

Steven Reid, MBBS, PhD, MRCPsych
Consultant Liaison Psychiatrist
St. Mary's NHS Trust
St. Mary's Hospital
20, South Wharf Road
London W2 1PD, UK

Krishen Sieunarine, MRCOG
Special Registrar in Obstetrics
and Gynaecology
North Thames (West) Deanery
Honorary Research Fellow
Imperial College School of
Medicine at Chelsea and
Westminster Hospital

19 Oxford Court, Wellesley Road
London W4 4DJ, UK

J. Richard Smith, MD, FRCOG
Consultant Gynaecologist
West London Gynaecological
    Cancer Centre
Hammersmith Hospital
Imperial College London
Du Cane Road
London W12 0HS, UK

Simon G. T. Smith, BSc, MS, FRCS
Senior Registrar
Endocrine Surgery Unit
Hammersmith Hospital
Imperial College London
Du Cane Road
London W12 0HS, UK

Vernon K. Sondak, MD, FACS
Chief, Division of Cutaneous
    Oncology Director of Surgical
    Education
H. Lee Moffitt Cancer Center
    and Research Institute
Professor, Departments of
    Interdisciplinary Oncology
    and Surgery
University of South Florida
    College of Medicine
Tampa, FL 33612, USA
Stabile Research Building
Rm 23031

12902 Magnolia Drive
Tampa FL 33612

Robert Sutton, FRCS
Division of Surgery and Oncology
University of Liverpool
5th Floor UCD Block - RLUH
The Duncan Building
Daulby Street
Liverpool L69 3GA, UK

Shabnam Undre, FRCSEd
Specialist Registrar in Surgery
Department of Biosurgery
    and Surgical Technology
Division of Surgery, Oncology,
    Reproductive Biology
    and Anaesthetics
Faculty of Medicine
Imperial College London
10th Floor, QEQM Building
St. Mary's NHS Trust
St. Mary's Hospital
Praed Street, Paddington
London W2 1NY, UK

Konstantinos Vlachos,
    MD, PhD, FICS
Hellenic Army Medical Officer
Surgical Research Fellow
Transplant Unit
St. Mary's NHS Trust
St Mary's Hospital
Praed Street, Paddington
London W2 1NY, UK

Panagiotis Vlavianos, MD
Consultant Physician
  and Gastroenterologist
Department of Gastroenterology
Hammersmith Hospital
Imperial College London
Du Cane Road
London W12 0HS, UK

David Westaby, MD, FRCP
Consultant Physician
  and Gastroenterologist
Department of Gastroenterology
Hammersmith Hospital
Imperial College London
Du Cane Road
London W12 0HS, UK

FOREWORD

The editors have done an excellent job in compiling a series of contributions on complications after surgery. The contributors are from the UK in addition to a substantial number of contributions from other countries.

The book opens with a fascinating chapter on the history of surgical complications. The author concludes by pointing out that complications in surgery today vastly exceed those encountered in the past, but hastens to add that this is because of the complexity and variety of operative procedures performed today compared with the past. Furthermore, the advances in surgery allow contemporary surgeons to deal with these complications more satisfactorily than was the case previously. The next few chapters deal with generic complications in surgery and include contributions on anaesthetic complications, cardiopulmonary complications, surgical infection and surgical wound complications. The majority of the remaining chapters are anatomically based ranging again from complications of breast surgery to complications of abdominal surgery. In addition, there are contributions on the complications of gynaecological surgery, neurological surgery, orthopaedic surgery, plastic and reconstructive surgery and minimally invasive surgery as well as transplant surgery. Later chapters deal with complications following gastrointestinal endoscopic procedures and interventional radiological procedure, while the two final chapters deal with psychiatric complications related to surgery and the medico-legal issues raised by complications occurring after surgery. These two chapters provide a fitting finale to this book.

In every case, each chapter deals with diagnosis and management of the various complications that may occur after the various types of surgery in different organ systems. The value of this book will not only be that it describes complications after surgery as a fact of life in modern surgery, but that it helps the young surgeon to be more knowledgeable about surgical complications. The more knowledgeable surgeons are about the complications that they may encounter the better they are able to inform their patients of the risks associated with a particular procedure and also the more likely they are to take steps to prevent such complications occurring. All in all this is a very valuable text and will be particularly useful to surgeons in training, to consultant surgeons and to physicians and specialists in the medico-legal field.

Sir Peter J. Morris, AC, FRS, FRCS
Emeritus Nuffield Professor and Chairman of Surgery
University of Oxford
Honorary Consultant, Oxford NHS Trust Hospital
Honorary Professor, University of London
Past President, Royal College of Surgeons of England

PREFACE

As Professor Owen H. Wangensteen, one of the greatest academic surgeons of the 20th century, said: "You are a true surgeon from the moment you are able to deal with your complications." Prompt and accurate diagnosis, as well as effective treatment of surgical complications, is one of the most important elements of surgical practice. This is today more important than any other time since, over the last 20 years, we have observed the development of new surgical subspecialties, the performance of very complicated operations in very challenging patients, the introduction of new surgical technologies and, last but not least, an increasing interest in monitoring the quality, the medico-legal implications and the ethical dimensions of surgical practice and malpractice. However, the issue of surgical complications has been presented briefly and sporadically in various textbooks and only as a small part of chapters dealing with surgical techniques. Therefore, this book aims to present the surgical complications of all specialties in a systematic way and with emphasis on what is happening in real life and in everyday practice.

We are truly grateful to all the authors for contributing their expertise in a sound, smooth and elegant way. We would also like to express our sincere gratitude to Professor Sir Peter Morris for his inspiring Foreword and to all our colleagues at Imperial College Press for their outstanding work. Finally, we would like to say how fortunate we feel to discover the painting on the cover of the book, which was created by an anonymous artist as if he/she had in mind the context of this book! It demonstrates in the best possible way our everlasting, tough and, sometimes, desperate battle to save our patient's life. In order to fight and, even more, win this battle, we need once again to prove right what Hippocrates said 2,500 years ago, "... a great doctor has the value and the strength of many other people together ..." and we hope that this book will serve as a wise companion and loyal ally to surgeons at all levels in their noble effort to do so.

Nadey S. Hakim & Vassilios E. Papalois
London, January 2007

Chapter 1

A HISTORY OF SURGICAL COMPLICATIONS

Allan Chapman

"Why is my pain perpetual, and my wound incurable, which refuseth to be healed?"

Jeremiah XV:18

Defining a surgical complication before the latter part of the 18th century is not as straightforward a thing as it might appear at first sight. For one might argue that not until after John Hunter's monumental study of pathological processes in his *Treatise on the Blood, Inflammation and Gun-shot Wounds* (1794) did surgeons really come to develop a concept of surgical healing that, by definition, did not assume complications as part of the course of nature, a thing that had to be managed and nursed around, if the strength of the patient allowed, rather than something that could be avoided altogether. For by definition, a *complication*, in any sphere of endeavour, is something out of the norm, and the product of extraneous and unexpected factors. Yet since time immemorial, pain, trauma, haemorrhage, inflammation, fever and infection in all their complex forms had been reckoned as normal in surgery, along with the acceptance of a very high death rate amongst surgical patients.

The Roman medical writer, Aulus Cornelius Celsus, summed up the four characteristic signs of inflammation in more clinically explicit terms, as "rubor et tumor cum calore et dolore" ("redness and swelling with heat and pain"), in Book III.10 of his encyclopaedic treatise *De Medicina* (*c*. AD 30). However, the symptoms that Celsus rounded up into a enduring pithy dictum had been familiar to earlier classical medical writers. For Greek writers such as Hippocrates already had a practised familiarity with these and other aspects of surgical and other types of complications, as would Claudius Galen of Pergamum a century after Celsus in the second century AD.

Indeed, 2000 years before Celsus, the compilers of the Law Code of the Babylonian king Hammurabi (*c*. 1700 BC) were familiar with surgical complication, at least as a category of professional mishap, for the Code stated that if a surgeon took a bronze lancet to a patient who was of high status, and the patient died, then the surgeon's hand had to be cut off! Considering the prevalence of serious infection and postoperative inflammation in any pre-late-19th-century AD surgical environment, however, one wonders who would have been foolhardy enough to have trained as a surgeon in ancient Mesopotamia in the first place. The *Edwin Smith* and *Ebers* Egyptian medical papyri from *c*. 1700–1600 and 1550 BC, respectively (though probably deriving from much earlier originals) display a familiarity with certain surgical procedures. The *Edwin Smith* papyrus in particular deals with no less than 48 specifically surgical conditions, including the setting of broken bones, the treatment of spinal damage, and the diagnosis and treatment of no less than 27 cases of head injury, as well as making reference to various healing salves and religious ceremonies, which were clearly intended to facilitate a speedy and uncomplicated recovery; while at the same time Egyptian operators do not seem to have lived under the fear of dire legal retribution if their cases went wrong. One would, however, like to know what became of the medical practitioners who attended the 18-year-old king Tutankhamun in his final illness. For a recent (2005) CT scan of his mummy, conducted by Egyptian scientists in Cairo, revealed that the Pharaoh seems to have suffered multiple and unhealed fractures of both legs immediately prior to his death, which could well have actually occasioned his death. Did the Egyptian physicians and surgeons attempt to reduce these fractures — the scan showed the presence of embalming materials inside the post-mortem injury, suggesting an open wound — and the Pharaoh die from a subsequent bacterial infection?

It was not uncommon amongst classical and later writers on surgery to associate certain types of complications with the incompetence of the operator, and thereby see a complicated operation as the logical outcome of botching. Hippocrates around 420 BC was very much of this way of thinking, and set a precedent which was to be followed by many surgical writers down the ensuing centuries. In his elaborate discussion of bandaging for orthopaedic cases, for instance, in Book XXXV of *On Joints*, which formed one of the surgical books in his *Corpus*, Hippocrates warned against seeking treatment from surgeons who boasted of their operative dexterity, yet who were really foolish fellows in so far as they did not understand the broader problems involved in surgery or place their procedures within the wider regimen of healing the sick. When attempting to re-set a broken nose, for instance, these practitioners "delighted" in the chance of showing off their skills and made a great display of their elaborate bandaging technique, yet applied too much pressure, in consequence of which the re-set nose dipped down in the middle rather than healed straight. Hippocrates gave similar warnings (*On Joints* XXXIII) against the over-enthusiastic bandaging of a broken jaw, when the two halves of the fracture are not re-set evenly, and the patient ends up with a kink in his jaw-line.

Yet these are not complications in a scientific sense, but the results of incompetence. And as Hippocrates in his practice, teachings and extensive writings did more than any other early Greek to define and professionalise the medical arts, he was at obvious pains to separate the true healers — who were also wise philosophers and religious men — from the empirics and quacks who would have a go at any disease or injury given half the chance.

Incompetence on the part of the operator, moreover, was also alleged by Hippocrates as the reason for complications arising from a trephination of the skull (in *On Wounds in the Head* XV). To ensure healing in such cases, observed Hippocrates, it was essential to ensure complete dryness around the site of the operation. For moisture would attract excess heat to the wound, and this in turn would result in a suppuration. This association of proliferating moisture, usually in the form of pus, heat and discomfort with a suppurating surgical wound would survive as a perceived corollary of surgery down to the great teaching hospitals in the young Queen Victoria's London, and Celsus' "rubor et tumor cum calore et dolore" would ring down the centuries with the inevitability of sunrise.

But what seems to have separated the surgical sheep from the goats over the centuries, as it were, was the possession of not only humane, but also scientific instincts. For when one reads Hippocrates' *On Joints, Fractures, On Wounds in the Head* and *In the Surgery*, Celsus on surgical procedures, or what Claudius Galen had learned from the management of wounded gladiators, one is immediately struck by what one might call a scientific instinct. For the injury was not just a thing to put right in a purely topical sense, but something to be studied, compared, and seen in a wider context of health. And details concerning the success or failure of the treatment, moreover, should also be remembered, or written in a case book, to act as a guide to the treatment of future patients.

But one major factor separated all pre-19th-century surgeons from their latter-day colleagues, and this was the relative infrequency and sheer diversity in their practice. For even in a large city, such as ancient Rome or medieval Cairo, the number of persons willing to submit themselves to surgical procedures of any kind would have been relatively small at any one time. For all the premodern writers on surgery ultimately saw it as the forlorn hope of the medical arts, and a thing to be resorted to when all gentler methods had failed, or else — as in the case of battle and other injuries — a sudden and drastic intervention which offered the only possibility of survival. This must have meant that even the most subtle of hands got out of practice in a way that would be unimaginable to a modern surgeon, who would probably operate several times a week on one specific part of the body; one can only marvel at those men who would amputate an arm, "tap" a dropsical abdomen, and couch a cataract in June, cut for the stone, treat a fistula, and reduce a compound fracture in July, and then drain a dental abscess, struggle with a hernia, and trephine a skull in August! For this was the traditional surgeon's art: operations performed occasionally, diversely and reluctantly, and, in that noble tradition that ran from Hippocrates to University College, London, and Dr Robert Liston, performed *scientifically*. And if a man could not hope to make a consistent livelihood from such occasional heroics, then one must not forget that many surgeons made a bread-and-butter living from phlebotomising the generally unwell who wished to have their humoral balances altered, and from dispensing *materia medica*, especially if they did not hold some salaried appointment.

Yet what was a *scientific* operation? Generally speaking, it was an operation performed by a man who not only had a good eye and an experienced hand, but also worked within an extensive framework of prior anatomical and medical knowledge. A man, moreover, who, in the tradition of Hippocrates, kept a detailed case book, and who passed on his knowledge to capable pupils. For if certain types of complication arose out of ignorance and inexperience, then they might be avoided if the practitioner had a sound understanding of the body's structure and function. And herein lies surgery's long-standing and intimate relationship with academic anatomy. For while a pre-modern surgeon had no reliable way of preventing gangrene or other infections, nonetheless if he possessed a thorough knowledge of what lay below the skin in the region of the body on which he was operating, he *might* be able to contain excessive blood loss, prevent unnecessary muscular laceration, avoid splitting a bone, and inflict minimal collateral damage on the operative site.

Yet why did scientific anatomy only begin with the Greeks? For the Egyptians, after all, had been eviscerating and embalming their dead for over 3,000 years before Herophilus and Erasistratus in Greek-occupied Alexandria began to cut up humans and animals in the fourth century BC. The answer lies, I would suggest, in the nature of curiosity itself. For though the Egyptians did compile books of practical medical and surgical procedures, drugs, prayers and incantations, such as in the *Ebers* and *Edwin Smith* papyri mentioned at the start of this chapter (though it is true that the *Edwin Smith* papyrus contained some astonishingly perceptive one-off diagnoses), there is no real evidence, in the vast surviving literature of their culture, that they thought of the body in what we might recognise as anatomical and physiological terms. The brain, liver, lungs and other organs so carefully removed after death by the low-status embalmers, to be preserved in their correct Canopic jars, were simply seen as being *there*, inside a body. Their precise functions or physiological interrela-tionships in life were simply not part of Egyptian medical consciousness. For while external injury, poisoning and blindness brought on by accidents, wind-blown sand and snake-bites were recognised as having a physical basis, most illnesses were generally ascribed to divine or spiritual agencies. So while an eye salve, a purge or a bandage for a broken arm might be prescribed because of its predictable physical effect, most remedies were expected to work because the rituals and sacrifices which they entailed were thought to please the rele-vant deities. In consequence, and in the absence of an organ-based concept of disease, anatomy was an irrelevance, and the embalming of millions of corpses across 40 centuries produced no contribution whatsoever to the advancement of medicine as a physical, scientific discipline.

Why the Alexandrian Greeks of the fourth century BC began to cut up human and animal carcasses is a good question, but one could perhaps connect it with that wider intellectual curiosity which so characterised the rise of early modern science in Greece. For the Greeks certainly showed a driving concern with getting below the surface appearance of nature, and explaining its innermost connections. Thales, Pythagoras, Euclid and several others had already done this for the great truths of geometry. Anaximander, Heraclitus and Anaximenes did the same for cosmology, while a whole succession of Greek physical scientists from Anaximander's own teacher, Thales around 590 BC to Claudius Ptolemy in the second century AD would do it for mathematical astronomy. As we have seen, Hippocrates pioneered an observational and taxonomic approach to the practice of medicine, while Aristotle, in the half century down to his death in 322 BC, sought out the rational foundations of perhaps a dozen sciences comprising physiology, embryology, meteorology, cosmology and optics, and the human sciences of politics, grammar and logic.

For what fascinated the Greeks was the inner logic of the whole of nature. And while they preserved a deep reverence for the divine order and wonder that ran through nature, they nonetheless de-mythologised the details of its regular workings, seeing *action* and *agency* in nature — be it a solar eclipse or a suppurating wound — not as the consequences of spiritual squabbles, but as the implicit expressions of wider regularities or laws. These regularities or laws, moreover, were amenable to the study of the disciplined, inquiring human intellect, and could, within given limits, be harnessed or predicted. Thus, a combination of prior observation and mathematical analysis could enable Thales to predict the eclipse of 585 BC, and Aristotle's theory of cardiac heat could provide a form of rational explanation of why bloodletting could cool and ease a paralysed patient.

It was this wider context of naturalistic explanation which enabled dissection to make sense to Herophilus, Erasistratus and others. And while Aristotle's extensive writings in many branches of the life sciences contain few examples of regular dissection *per se*, they nonetheless include numerous brilliant examples of careful description: of the scales of fishes, of human and animal teeth, limbs and skeleton bones, and details of the external anatomy of many creatures. Even genetics can trace its first scientific utterances to Aristotle where, in *De Generatione Animalium* (Book IV, 3, 767a), he looks at examples of heredity: how children can resemble one parent more than the other, how it is that a man who has lost a limb in battle can later father children with all of their limbs present as normal, and why parents sometimes produce "monsters," or creatures which resemble neither their parents nor their ancestors. Of course, none of these observations were especially original when Aristotle was conducting his researches around 350 BC, yet he was certainly the first person to discuss them in the wider context of what might be called scientific medicine. He was, perhaps, the first to see structural and functional parallels between humans and animals, as well as being one of the first to develop an integrated and encompassing model for the disease process in a way that amplified Hippocrates' earlier studies of fever types and the association of specific diseases and human temperaments with given geographical and climatic locations, dealt with in *On Fevers* and *Airs, Waters, and Places*.

Indeed, one tends to find that explanations of why wounds go wrong and complicated have always hinged on broader theories of health and disease. And just as the post-Pasteurian explanation for surgical infection has hinged predominantly on the action of microbes, and later viruses, so that of the writers of the classical period turned upon their wider views concerning health. For when reading the classical medical writers, one invariably encounters a set of assumptions about the innate healthiness of the human body. Quite simply, it is *natural* be healthy, for functional efficiency is the teleological end of a body's existence. And when illness in any form supervenes, then it must be caused by some sort of invasion or upset. This model is implicit in the balance theory of health encountered in all the writings of Hippocrates, and given its definitive clinical expression in the four humours — Yellow Bile, Black Bile, Blood and Phlegm — of Aristotle. For in these humours, the four great qualities of nature, the hot, the cold, the moist and the dry, are built up into an over-arching clinical scheme. In a healthy body, all are in their correct balance, but in disease, one or the other predominates over the rest. And humours could be put out of balance by a variety of external factors, including drastic changes of domicile, diet or climate, or an encounter with foul airs, injury or surgical intervention. And in the way that a penetrating wound of any kind, be it a battle injury or the Hippocratic case of a complicating scalp wound following trephination, would invariably upset the body's natural balance, so it would often lead to the generation of excess heat. "Rubor et tumor cum calore et dolore" would set in, and one hoped that, if the surgeon had nourished and nursed his patient gently and well, the superfluous heat would be eased away, and the patient would recover. As the author of the Biblical book *Proverbs* (20:30) wisely summed up, "the blueness of a wound cleanseth away evil", the colour-change indicating that the infected state is passing.

But this balance theory of health, and the heat-attracting concept of surgical infection, paid no more than lip-service to anatomy as such. For it was the classical Greek doctor's self-perceived task to chase imbalances around and out of the body, rather than to associate specific diseases with specific organs. Yes, it is true that Greek doctors had progressed streets ahead of their Egyptian and Mesopotamian predecessors and colleagues in the way they saw the disease process in terms of naturalistic rather than occult agencies, but their knowledge of the operations and functions of the body's interior remained rudimentary. On the other hand, it was the Greeks who developed the first "approximately true" theory of physiology. For did not food ingested by the mouth produce juices in the stomach that somehow led to the liver becoming engorged with blood? And did not this blood, in its heaviest and crudest form, get sucked up into the heart via the vena cava? In the heart, according to Aristotle, it was heated up due to the innate crucible-like nature of that organ, and refined. The lungs then acted like bellows, blowing life-giving *pneuma*, or air imbued with spirit, into the blood, after which the refined and vital juice entered the *veins*, where, after a series of pulsating motions, it arrived at the extremities of the body. Here it not only congealed to become new flesh, but also carried the innate heat of the heart and its very life-force to every part of the living creature. Some blood was even believed to pass through the thick septal wall of the heart into the left chamber, and up through the two carotids in the neck, to refine yet further into those salty-tasting animal spirits which were found in the lateral ventricles and cortical mass of freshly-removed brains.

But this concept of the interior of mammalian bodies was essentially didactic rather than therapeutic in character, for the functions ascribed to organs such as the stomach, liver, heart, brain or veins were either vague or else plainly wrong. And it is no doubt for this reason that anatomy played a relatively minor part in classical medicine — in spite of its otherwise scientific status. It is true that the importance of these organs to the continuance of life had probably been known from time immemorial, and Homer and Old Testament Biblical writers of around 1000 BC had been all too well aware of the incurable nature of spear or arrow wounds that penetrated the liver, spleen or thoracic cavity, even though the precise physiological roles of these organs were not understood. In a running fight described in the Old Testament, for instance (*II Samuel* 2:23 and 3:27), Abner inflicted instant death on his pursuer Asahel by striking him with a spear under the fifth rib, and with such force that the weapon emerged from Asahel's back, before Abner got his just deserts by receiving Joab's avenging spear in exactly the same place. So while none of these men were anatomists, they certainly knew where to direct a weapon if it were intended to strike a fatal blow through a major organ!

On the other hand, and bearing in mind the caveats outlined above, we do know quite a lot about surgery in the ancient world, especially from the time of the Romans. Claudius Galen, for instance, was not only an accomplished operator, but also a flamboyant anatomical demonstrator, especially when working on live animals. One of Galen's party-piece demonstrations showed the central importance of the spinal nervous system. Galen would make a series of decisive severances of the spinal nerves of a well-secured pig, starting from the tail and working towards the head. The still living yet progressively paralysed animal suddenly stopped squealing when its laryngeal nerves were severed, to be eventually despatched when the brain was reached, thereby showing the importance of the spinal cord and the nervous branches which came from it, to the motor functions of different regions of the body. Likewise, tradition has it that Galen got his first main job as surgeon to the gladiators at the amphitheatre at Pergamum in Asia Minor (now Bergama, Turkey), by demonstrating his skill at re-assembling a previously disembowelled monkey. It appears that candidates for the surgeon's job were presented with a specially-eviscerated living primate, and the surgeon had to demonstrate his skill in putting the animal back together again. Galen's monkey lived — presumably making a relatively uncomplicated recovery — and thus began one of the most illustrious surgical careers of all time! It is not for nothing that our internationally-used word for the place where surgical procedures are performed derives from the Latin *theatrum*: a place of public display and ceremonies!

In addition to textual sources, archaeology has added considerably to our knowledge of the sophistication of Roman surgery from the instrumental point of view. There is the beautifully-carved votive relief of a Roman surgeon from the Asklepeion, Athens, showing his folding instrument case, containing scalpels, probes and other instruments. And our knowledge of Roman surgery has been greatly amplified following the discovery of large collections of bronze and steel instruments in archaeological digs in Bingen, Germany, and especially at what has come to be known as the "House of the Surgeon" at Pompeii. Dating from some time before AD 79, when the Roman town was destroyed in the eruption of Vesuvius, these Pompeian instruments include trephines, probes, bone levers, obstetrical instruments, and various types of forceps and scalpels. They are beautifully-made instruments, some containing screw-operated and detachable parts, while a circular trephination saw has a central point (probably detachable before it partly corroded away) of a similar type to the "crown trephine" or *modiolus* described in Celsus' *De Medicina* Book VIII.3. In using this type of instrument to perform a trephination, Celsus recommends, the operator should, upon commencing the operation, place the central pin in a small chiselled nick in the skull to act as a central point for the rotation of the "crown trephine." Once the teeth of the strap- or belt-actuated trephine had begun to bite into the skull, the surgeon would remove the centre pin, and then spin the trephine on its own. In this way, he produced an exact and controlled circular hole in the desired part of the skull, and avoided damaging the pia mater dura mater or meninges which lay beneath.

Although it has been pointed out that classical medical writers thought of the wider disease process *not* in terms of systemic organic malfunctions but in terms of humoral imbalances, it is clear from the writings of Celsus and Galen in particular that they had a good knowledge of the inner layout of the interiors of bodies. It is true that this may have derived from veterinary rather than from human dissections — Galen especially conducting most of his anatomical researches on the carcasses of Barbary apes, Rhesus monkeys and pigs — but in their scientific spirit, they deemed such knowledge essential to a learned medical man.

Book IV, 1 of Celsus' *De Medicina* consists of a carefully-conducted tour of the body's interior, the topic details of which have a strong ring of direct hands-on familiarity. We are told, for instance, that the windpipe is a thick pipe with strong external ridges, rather like vertebrae, though smooth on the inside; that the interior chambers of the lungs are "spongy"; and that descending from the two kidneys are two tubes — called *ureters* by the Greeks — which lead to the bladder. Celsus also speaks of the healthy and diseased appearances of organs, and the special infirmities to which they were prone, in what was a remarkable essay on descriptive anatomy. But it is in Celsus' *De Medicina* Book VII, which deals with surgical procedures, that we first encounter the range and ingenuity of Roman surgery. The causes and treatment of abscesses and fistulae, for example, are discussed with remarkable insight and accuracy of detail. He tells us how to read the stages through which an abscess can pass, and whether to use medical or surgical procedures in its treatment. Celsus also tells us that, while all surgery upon the abdomen is likely to be fatal, it can sometimes succeed: fistulae of the stomach *can* be healed with the right cutting and stitching, while the guts can even be forced back through an aperture in the abdomen wall, and stitched in. A patient who has been thus operated upon, moreover, should lie on his back so that the intestines can re-seat themselves in their natural place. Various types of hernias are also described, along with their prosthetic or surgical treatment.

Yet while Celsus is only too well aware of how gangrene, putrefaction and complication can set in in any wound, he has no coherent idea of what their causes could be, or how they might be prevented. They are simply part of the risks involved in surgery. On the other hand, we today, with hindsight, can see the clinical sense of some of the surgical procedures which he mentions as one of several options. When discussing the detailed technique for "tapping" a dropsical patient to draw off water from the abdomen, for instance, he mentions the especial benefit of using a hot cautery scalpel. For unbeknown to Celsus or to anyone else in that pre-bacterial age, a cautery scalpel killed bacteria and allowed the wound to heal by first intention, without needing to suppurate.

In many ways, however, the final and most enduring opinion, as far as wound treatment, infection and suppuration were concerned, came from Galen. His monumental anatomical and clinical studies, including *On the Use of Body Parts*, *Commentaries on the Hippocratic Oath*, *Aphorisms* and *On the Natural Faculties*, to name but four titles, contain such a wealth of medical observation and insight as to cause their author to become the great authority on matters anatomical for the next 1300 years. And as far as Galen was concerned, any surgeon who operated upon a patient, or attempted to cure a battle or other wound, must take steps to enable the wound to slowly excrete its poisons, from the bottom upwards, during a process of slow closure. For to Galen suppuration was natural and the pus generated "laudable". The ensuing Galenic doctrine of "laudable pus" was to constitute something of a surgical orthodoxy down to the late 18th century, with what we would recognise as a *complicated* wound being seen as a naturally healing wound. One suspects that the gladiators of Pergamum may not have complained, however, as their lengthy convalescences under this regime inevitably kept them out of the arena for a few months, and thereby extended their lives!

In spite of the Roman love of bathing and general cleanliness, at least amongst the comfortably-off classes, one must never lose sight of the fact that Galen, Celsus and their colleagues would have worked in highly septic professional environments. For as they had no knowledge of bacteria, and lacked a coherent theory of inflammation and suppuration, their instruments and dressings must have been just as contagious as those of their Victorian successors who complained about the omnipresence of gangrene in their hospitals. After all, "healing salves" of egg-white, wine and aromatics did not kill germs. So while classical culture gave birth to many of the concepts and intellectual ideals of humane scientific medicine, while it invented the basis of rational medical nomenclature, and developed the necessary relationship between anatomy and physiology and surgery, it nonetheless contributed very little to our modern knowledge of surgical complications as such.

It was in the medieval Arab world that surgery began to develop a scientific medical literature that really took up where the classical writers had left off. And while the greater part of Arabic literature in the healing arts was devoted to medicine, especially disease and drug taxonomies, with figures such as al-Razi [Rhazes], Abu Ali al-Husayn Ibn Aballah Ibn Sina [Avicenna], and Ibn al-Haytham [Alhazen] leading the way, there were some surgical commentators. Indeed, the word "commentator" is a significant one when dealing with early medieval science in either the Muslim or the Christian world, for it was from the translated works — into either Arabic or Latin — of the classical writers that medieval scientific culture sprang. Hippocrates, Diosciorides, Galen and quite a few others became current medical sources to Christians and Muslims alike (though Celsus' works were lost, and not re-discovered until the Renaissance), as these foundation works were first commented upon and *glossed*, and then used as patterns in accordance with which fresh researches could be conducted.

In surgery, however, it was Abul Qasim uz-Zahrawi [Albucasis], living in Spain between AD 936 and 1013, who became the overwhelmingly important Arabic surgical writer. Albucasis pays his intellectual debts to Hippocrates, Galen and Celsus, in whose tradition he saw himself, and in his *magnum opus*, entitled *Altasrif* (known in the West as *On Surgery and Instruments*), he discussed a wide range of surgical conditions and instruments from his own practice. Particularly fascinating is his detailed treatment of eye surgery, where his meticulous accounts of how to operate for *ungula* (*pterygium* to the Greeks) eye growths, and for cataract, carry strong resonances of the descriptions of Celsus and other Western classical authors, whose works he would have known in Arabic translations. His *Altasrif* also discussed most of the other conditions deemed operable by ancient and medieval surgeons, including treatments for wounds and fractures, abscesses and fistulae. It is very clear, moreover, that Albucasis was all too familiar with operations that went wrong, yet, like the figures we have seen already, he seemed to have no consistent concept of a complication as such. His account of the procedure for eye cataract, for instance, contains a meticulous postoperative regimen: the bandages must not be touched until the third day, and after an examination of the eyes by the surgeon, rebound until the seventh day. Without such binding, complications will follow, in the form of the depressed or "couched" lens (or "humour") ascending from the vitreous humour and returning to block out the light. But total immobility of the patient's head on a specially-devised bed could prevent this from happening. Likewise, bad after-care could lead to an abscess forming, and destroying the patient's vision altogether.

Yet what we find here is that long-familiar resonance going back to Hippocrates: surgical complications are a product of professional incompetence. A good surgeon does not overreach himself, does not leap at the chance of showing off his skill, is wise and learned, and imposes a meticulously-supervised postoperative regime. Always willing to see off quacks and incompetents, Albucasis hammers the point home when describing the treatment for fistula, a condition which he ascribes to the poor quality of the patient's blood. But in this case, that of a young man, which he describes in detail, instead of the blood being strengthened, the treatment had been botched. For this man had developed a discharging leg ulcer which became a major fistula. Sinking more and more, as one quack after another poked around in his wound, Albucasis tells us plainly: "Eventually he sought me". At this juncture, Albucasis found that the fistula led down to the necrotic bone. But after two operations, during which the necrotic matter was cut away, the wound healed, and the patient enjoyed a perfect cure. The message was clear: a master surgeon was reversing the complications which the botching of lesser men had occasioned.

Likewise, in skilled hands, even gangrene, a "creeping corruption of a limb, consuming it as a fire consumes dry wood" could be cured, so Albucasis tells us. This will come about by the judicious application of the red-hot cautery iron to the affected part, followed three days later by soothing salves of sulphur and oil. Indeed, the cautery was one of Albucasis' favourite therapeutic devices when treating infection or even cutting the flesh, for (as Celsus had noted) such surgical wounds, while especially painful at the time, stood the best chance of healing by first intention, though no one at the time knew why.

Popular medical mythology tells us that the European middle ages were a period of ignorance and butchery in surgery. But like so many myths, this one vanishes into smoke upon careful examination. And while it is true that high-quality surgical writing does not go back quite so early in Western Europe as did that of Albucasis, one must not forget that Arabic medical and scientific writings, along with Greek books from the Byzantine world, began to be translated into medieval Latin by the late 11th century. Indeed, the arrival of these books — translated from classical Greek writers via Arabic intermediaries, in many cases — became a mighty flood by the 12th and 13th centuries. They provided the vigorous intellectual soil out of which medieval Europe's great universities — Bologna, Paris, Oxford, Cambridge, Padua and Montpellier — sprang. And Latin translations of the great Arab scientists themselves came to be studied in Europe. Alhazen's optical and ophthalmological researches were studied and developed by Roger Bacon in 13th-century Oxford, Rhazes' medical ideas were discussed in Paris, while Avicenna's encyclopaedic *Canon*, or Rule of Medicine, was even referred to by Geoffrey Chaucer in *The Pardoner's Tale* (l. 890).

By the late 12th century, Hugo of Lucca was both practising and teaching sophisticated surgery, while his pupil Theodoric's *Chirugia* (1267) dealt with the nature of infection. Indeed, in "high medieval" Europe, after about 1180, a remarkable level of sophisticated discussion took place on medical and surgical topics. And just like the Arab medical writers before them, they looked for fundamental guidance back to Hippocrates, Galen and the great classical physicians, seeing healing in all its branches as an essentially conservative art. Yet in this medieval world, one finds active, fresh discussion of how best to treat wounds and manage surgical cases. How should one best treat perforative wounds inflicted by arrows or crossbow bolts? Or, outside the theatre of war, how should one treat nasal polyps, haemorrhoids, accidental wounds, bad burns, compound fractures, cataract, tumours of various kinds, and dental complications leading to jaw abscesses?

Especially relevant, moreover, from our present point of view, was the medieval surgical debate about pus. Was it a natural part of healing or was it a poison, and should a surgeon try to eliminate it altogether? The ancient medical community of Salerno, on the Bay of Naples, arguably the first hospital and medical school in Europe, pre-dating Bologna, Paris and Oxford by the best part of a century, tended to follow a conservative line. Being a major conduit of classical Greek medicine into the West that was in itself fairly independent of the abovementioned Arabic tradition, while at the same time being familiar with Arab work, the Salernitian School followed the precepts of Hippocrates and Galen in particular. Galen's doctrine of "laudable pus" was an orthodoxy, and argued that after the treatment of wounds or the performing of surgical operations, pus formation was a natural part of healing. Wounds should therefore be left open, with drains to enable the pus to rise out, and only closed by degrees as everything became progressively dry.

By the 13th century, however, active medical and surgical teaching, including the dissection of *human* corpses (spasmodic in antiquity and probably non-existent in the Arab world) was under way in Bologna, Montpellier and Paris. Figures such as the abovementioned Hugo of Lucca and Theodoric, then William of Saliceto, his own pupil the Frenchman Lanfranc, and the Norman Henri de Mondeville, were all asking what happened when the skin of the body was broken. And *contra* Galen, they were coming to see pus as *not necessary* for the healthy healing of a wound. For observation showed that a well-managed wound *could* heal aseptically or by first intention. And while none of these men had any coherent idea of infection or surgical complication, beyond the caveats against bad air, putrid blood and incompetent colleagues noted by their ancient predecessors, it is nonetheless strange that the historical period so associated in the popular mind with backwardness should have done so much to advance surgery. For while the Arab world had had brilliant and inspired medical teachers and taxonomists, the peculiar and enduring achievement of medieval Europe lay in its invention of the university as an enduring corporate institution by 1180. What is more, the medical faculties of these universities not only taught and set standards — inventing the Doctorate in Medicine as an internationally recognised benchmark of excellence for a medical practitioner — but also pioneered the scientific study of the human body. In the Italian universities, such as the Papal University at Bologna (but not in the north European schools), surgery was included as a curricular subject, being studied as a branch of medicine.

One of the decisive turning-points in the history of surgery, which was to lead by the late 18th century to the recognition of surgical complication as a clinical and pathological condition within the wider healing process, was the introduction of firearms in warfare. This took place in the early to middle parts of the 14th century, and by 1420 European military surgeons were having to come to terms with battle wounds that were fundamentally different from the relatively clean puncture, slash and contusion wounds which had predominated since the most ancient times. For cannon shot shattered human bodies in a myriad of different ways, while the soft lead musket ball produced wounds of the most frightful complexity. And by the time that Hieronymus Brunschwig wrote his vernacular treatise *Buch der Wund-Artzney* (1497) ("Book of Wound Dressing"), which was one of the first of many treatises that described treatments for gunshot wounds, it had come to be accepted that gunshot wounds were unlike all others in so far as they were automatically taken to be poisoned. The gunpowder, and the lead of the balls themselves, were thought to be highly toxic, and the radical opening up of such wounds to enable the surgeon to remove such projectiles and debridement was taken to be *de rigueur*. And when soldiers on campaign were likely to have been long unwashed, and wearing filthy clothes, and a musket ball likely to carry a trail of garment fabric deep into the wound behind it, we today realise from our modern clinical perspective that such wounds must have been extremely complicated. It is hardly surprising, therefore, that contemporary surgeons regarded gunshot wounds as being poisoned by definition.

These wounds, moreover, led to the writing of a great many books on surgery after 1497, often recording the experiences and practices of individual military and naval surgeons. They represent the first books aimed at a readership of surgeons who were *not* learned university physicians (as had been the case with most Western medieval writers), but were hands-on practical surgeons who had learned their art from vernacular sources and come up through the channel of apprenticeship. The books are not in Latin, but in German, French and English, and while often translated between vernacular languages, rarely had Latin intermediaries.

Giovanni de Vigo laid down what would become an enduring procedure in 1514, when he recommended that debrided gunshot wounds should be cauterised by pouring in boiling Oil of Elder. This would neutralise the poisons, and while the collateral damage inflicted by such an invasive treatment might lead to a slow and painful convalescence, it nonetheless seemed to give the best chance of survival. For while we now know that chemical poisoning was not in reality as great a problem as 16th-century surgeons feared, it was well known by ancient empirical practice that cauterisation seemed to clear away infection. To modern-day understanding, it killed germs. And while de Vigo's method was challenged by Ambrose Paré after 1536, when he discovered, on running out of boiling oil during the siege of Turin, that a mixture of rose water, egg yolks and turpentine had a cleansing without a secondary traumatising effect when treating gunshot wounds, it is not clear whether his patients had a better long-term postoperative survival. Sadly, Renaissance doctors and surgeons invariably spoke of individual cases, and were innocent of longer-term statistical analyses.

Indeed, the English surgeon William Clowes devised an ingenious experiment to test the "poisoned bullet" idea of gunshot wound complication around 1580. Clowes asked a soldier to fire a military arrow out of his musket at a gate post, working on the idea that if the discharge explosion was going to poison the projectile, then it should also burn or singe the arrow. Upon inspecting the embedded arrow, however, he found it quite undamaged and even its feathers unsinged-presumably, so he argued, because the arrow left the gun barrel *before* the flames and noxious sulphurous fumes! I suspect this was probably the first controlled experiment in scientific history to investigate the possible cause of a wound complication.

In addition to the new surgical techniques necessary to treat debrided gunshot wounds, 16th- and 17th-century surgeons made fundamental improvements to amputation techniques. References to major amputations are relatively rare in classical and medieval surgical practice, though they had become commonplace by 1700. What made these operations *technically* possible, however, were the massive advances in *human* (as opposed to monkey) anatomy that began with the public dissections of medieval Bologna, Padua and Montpellier, and which raced ahead after the publication of Andreas Vesalius's monumental *De Fabrica Humani Corporis* (1543). By 1640, in fact, no surgeon would have been able to go through his apprenticeship and — in London — pass the Worshipful Company of Surgeons qualifying examination unless he had attended lectures in anatomy and partaken, if only as an observer, in full-scale human dissections, starting with the subcutaneous muscles and finishing with the details of the skeleton.

For radical amputations of the knee-joint, thigh and shoulder, in particular, demanded a sound knowledge of the whereabouts of the veins and arteries, which would be encountered during the course of the operation, if the patient was going to survive. Amputation "above the knee" or of the thigh, for instance, does not seem to have been known before William Clowes successfully performed one some time before 1588, writing up the case on page 33 of his *A prooved practice for all chirugians*. For the massive blood loss implicit in such an operation meant that the operator not only had to be swift and resolute with his knife, but also fully prepared to ligature or cauterise the large number of blood vessels which he would encounter. Clowes's case was not a victim of war, however, but a "mayde" of "Hygate", London, and a charity patient. We are not told how her leg had become "so greevously corrupted, that we were driven upon necessitie to cut it off above the knee", but Clowes and his colleagues did a thoroughly professional job, with relatively little blood loss, "and so cured her after within a very short time". By first intention, one presumes. Yet the new, radical amputations of the post-gunshot-wound era — even when performed on civilians who had fallen from roofs or been run over by wagons — presented a whole new series of complications for the surgeon: massive haemorrhages, enormous postoperative scars which were prime sites for complex infections, and, of course, appalling trauma. Clowes's "mayde of Highgate" was very lucky indeed to survive. A surgeon facing cases such as these would not only have to be a highly-skilled and versatile anatomist, but also a careful planner, and the head of a well-drilled team of five or so assistants. Men who would know exactly how to hold and restrain the fully-conscious patient, set out the instruments in likely order of use, and have the pre-threaded ligatures or cauteries ready at hand, along with several dozen carefully-rolled absorbent "buttons," "dossils", bandages, blood bowls and finally a bed especially prepared to place the postoperative patient at his maximum ease.

There were many master-surgeons who published their experiences for the guidance of others, especially in England. William Clowes' *A Profitable and Necessaire Booke of Observation* (1596), John Woodall's *The Surgeon's Mate* (1617), Richard Wiseman's *Several Chirurgical Treatises* (1676), a work based upon no less than 600 of his own personal cases, and his earlier *Treatise of Wounds* (1672), which came to be popularly nicknamed "Wiseman's Book of

Martyrs", were four of the most outstanding. It was Wiseman who — without properly understanding its cause — was the first to describe a joint swollen and damaged by tuberculosis: he referred to the lesions as "white swellings". Woodall, moreover, who was writing particularly for sea surgeons, set his surgical knowledge within the wider context of a total medical practice, as was necessary for a man working in the isolation of a warship. Yet what shines through all of these men's writings, in addition to their measured confidence and thoroughgoing professionalism, was their caution. For no surgeon worth his name by the 17th century took up his knife easily, being all too aware of the dangers involved. "For", as John Woodall aptly put it when contemplating a major leg amputation, "it is no small presumption to Dismember the Image of God". And the relative rarity with which even a surgeon of Woodall's standing — being senior surgeon at St. Bartholomew's Hospital, London — exercised that "presumption" is brought home in the 1639 edition of the *Surgeon's Mate*. For in this work, Woodall tells us that he had performed a little over 100 amputations in 24 years. On the other hand, his success rate could have been the envy of many senior surgeons of two centuries later, for out of the 100 add amputations, he had only 20 fatalities.

Yet one still looks in vain in the writings of these men, and of their contemporaries, for any coherent sense of a "surgical complication" as we think of them today. For as in the days of Hippocrates and Celsus, there were good, bad and bogus surgeons who cured, mauled or killed their patients; there were great wounds that could go wrong because of the patient's unique humoral imbalance; Divine Providence might cause a ligatured artery to burst and kill the patient; while, as Woodall reminds us, gangrene might proceed "by reason of an inward cause" to necessitate a second operation or else kill the patient. And as Woodall further reminds his reader, when dealing in particular with ulcers and fistulae — which only serves to emphasise the fundamentally unknowable nature of illness and wound complication, in his mind — "the malignity of the humour or other evill disposition of the body changeth itselfe into a rebellious *Ulcer, concavous, fistuleas*, or unto any the like height of malignity". One might almost draw the rule: very sick people develop complications which kill them; less sick people get better!

But in spite of very high and generally accepted death rates, especially in major surgery, it is clear that the repertoire and frequency of operations was increasing by 1700. And some highly-skilled surgeons, who liked to specialise in a particular procedure wherever possible, could achieve remarkable success rates. Thomas Hollier, the lithotomist of St. Thomas's and St. Bartholomew's Hospitals, London, who removed a stone the size of tennis ball from the bladder of the fully-conscious Samuel Pepys on 26 March 1658, was one of them. Hollier (who operated on Pepys not in hospital but privately in the house of a relative) prepared for the ordeal like a general preparing for battle, with every contingency covered, and had the stone out within a few minutes after the first incision. The cleansed wound healed by something approaching first intention, and the 25-year-old Pepys was on his feet again within 35 days and lived another 45 years. Indeed, Hollier must have been a truly virtuosic operator, for an oft-repeated story, passed down through the 18th, 19th and 20th centuries in various narratives, and appearing in Thomas Hollier's entry in *New Dictionary of National Biography* (Oxford, 2004), has it that in one single year he performed no less than 30 lithotomies without a single fatality. On the other hand, Hollier did have his fatalities, for in a letter to his patron, Lord Montagu, dated 3 December 1659, Pepys mentioned a visit to the Jewish Synagogue in London, where he heard "many lamentations made by Portugall Jewes for the death of fferdinando the merchant, who was lately cutt (by the same hand with myselfe) of the stone".

Indeed, by the 18th century, feats of prodigious surgery came to be reported on a fairly regular basis, often in the pages of the *Philosophical Trans-actions* of the Royal Society. The rapid burgeoning of London's private medical schools and great public and teaching hospitals, and abundant wars to act as "nurseries" for up-and-coming surgeons, and the growth of scientific societies and a scientific press, all colluded to produce that proliferation of surgeons, students and learned audiences keen to witness the dissection of corpses. Even Samuel Pepys, the scientifically-minded senior civil servant who would be elected F.R.S. in 1665, attended on 27 February 1663 the dissection at Surgeons' Hall, London, of one Dillon, a sailor who had just been hanged.

In his detailed *Diary* entry recording the event, Pepys says how he was hosted at the dissection by Dr Charles Scarborough and other medical friends. A sumptuous dinner for the doctors and their friends was laid on as part of this conspicuous piece of medical theatre, and then, after the meal was over, Pepys was taken for a private view of the cadaver, where he saw "the Kidneys, Ureters, yard [penis], stones [testicles] and semenary vessels" laid out for his inspection, so as to "show very clearly the manner of the disease of the stone and the cutting and all other Questions that I could think of". Indeed, Pepys's own ordeal of five years earlier had given him a lifelong fascination with diseases of the urinary tract! The *Diary* entry does not record whether Thomas Hollier was present at this somewhat macabre feast, for the lithotomist who had saved Pepys's life also went on to become the Pepys's family doctor and a good personal friend.

A good example of this proliferation of learned medical and surgical culture, with its combined surgeon, hospital and fascinating case write-up format, came in 1735 when Claudius Amyand F.R.S., the eminent Huguenot surgeon at St. George's Hospital and Serjeant Surgeon to King George II, treated an 11-year-old boy with a hernia complicated by the presence of a scrotal fistula. When Amyand and his colleagues decided to operate on 8 December, they got more than they bargained for in so far as one complication now followed upon another. In the process of trying to relocate the falling gut, for instance, they found that not only had the *Appendix Coeci* descended into the scrotum, but that a "Pin incrusted with Stone" which the boy must have swallowed was poking through it. The attempt to replace the gut and close the fistula eventually resulted in a complex "Dissection" of the intestines of the courageous 11-year-old Hanvil Anderson who "bore … with great Courage" his fully-conscious half-hour ordeal. As Amyand had placed a ligature around the inflamed appendix before excising it, he became the first surgeon to perform, albeit inadvertently, an appendectomy. What is more, young Hanvil Anderson made a spectacular recovery, being discharged a month later simply wearing a "Truss, which he was ordered to wear some Time, to confirm the Cure".

Claudius Amyand later spoke of the operation as "the most complicated and perplexing I ever met with, many unsuspected Oddities and Events concurring to make it as intricate as it proved laborious and difficult". Of course, he is using the term "complicated" to indicate the sheer range of problems that descended one after the other as he tried to "Dissect" his way through the mess of living intestines, and close the fistula. But very clearly, as indicated by the patient's well-nigh miraculous recovery, no postoperative complications could have arisen. Amyand wrote up the case for the *Philosophical Transactions* of the Royal Society in 1736, along with several related ones, including a case where he had operated on and cured a soldier with a gunshot wound in the abdomen.

Eighteenth-century Britain — London, Edinburgh and Glasgow — along with Paris, became the world centres of excellence in anatomy, diagnostics and surgery, with figures like William Cheselden, Percival Pott, Alexander Monro (primus), Louis Petit and others winning enduring fame as medical scientists. It was Pott in particular who showed that a surgeon could not simply look at a surgical case in isolation, but must do so in the wider context of the environment, occupation and underlying disease conditions. It was Pott, for instance, who in 1775 first recognised the connection between high levels of scrotal cancer amongst chimney sweeps and the particular circumstances of their occupation. And more significant was his recognition in 1779 that hunchbacks with suppurating vertebral abscesses displayed a syndrome of complications that appeared to have links with tuberculosis — Pott's Disease, in fact. And while none of these conditions were specifically surgical complications in themselves, they were recognised as being the products of wider complicating conditions that the surgeon was called upon to treat.

But it was one man, a Scotsman brought up in Glasgow, yet whose surgical training and creative career was entirely based in London, who was to take the medical sciences down a new road, and was to become, in many respects, the first person to study surgical and wound complications as a branch of science in their own right. This was John Hunter.

Though he never ceased to be an active operating surgeon, John Hunter's contemporary and enduring fame rested on his scientific studies of bodily growth, change, decay, putrescence and response to invasion by foreign bodies. He was a brilliant and inspiring teacher who built up a very substantial income from pupil fees drawn from his successive domestic and teaching establishments in Golden Square and Jermyn Street, in addition to St. George's Hospital, and from the 1760s down to his death in 1793, Hunter shaped the careers and attitudes of hundreds of young men who would go on to become the medical and surgical élite of the late Georgian and early Victorian periods in England.

Hunter was an astute observer and a natural diagnostician, who saw connections which other men had missed. His independent scientific career began after working for several years as his older but less famous brother's assistant in London. Then during the Seven Years War in the early 1760s, John Hunter became a surgeon in the British Army, and was struck by the way in which untreated bullet wounds in soft tissue healed faster and more naturally than those which had been enlarged and probed by the surgeons. His later studies of teeth transplantation, platelet bone growth in piglets, fractures, and the nourishing role of a healthy blood supply, enabled him to draw profound conclusions about the life process. And much of this, passed on in papers or taught to students, was set out systematically in his monumental yet sadly posthumous *Treatise on the Blood, Inflammation and Gun-shot Wounds* (1794). For while Hunter died still innocent of any knowledge of the role of either cells or bacteria to the life process, he was the first surgical scientist to explore the process of *complication*, and see it not as an Act of God, an accident, or a result of incompetence, but as the product of a very specific set of biological factors. And at the heart of these studies was Hunter's work on inflammation. From scores of meticulous case studies, he concluded that suppuration is not a natural or necessary part of the healing process, and abandoned the still prevalent doctrine of "laudable pus" and bodily balances. Suppuration, rather, is the result of some prior inflammation, and the way to resolve it is to prevent or remove the source of inflammation. Hunter later specified three main types of inflammationary reactions: adhesive inflammation between parts; suppuration with pus formation; and ulceration, where tissue is lost through absorption. And in the Second Section of his monumental *Treatise*, moreover, he not only saw blood as conveying nutrition around the living body, but noted that when that blood was somehow defective or inadequate in supply or systolic force, its deficiency allowed inflammations to take told. Hunter perceived a connection, for instance, between valvular defects of the heart and the weakening of blood supply to the extremities, which could result in leg ulcers.

Injuries which did not break the skin, however, such as simple fractures or simple contusions, seemed to heal more directly, without inflammation setting in if the patients were vigorous and had efficient hearts. Hunter also recognised the natural therapeutic importance of scab formation, and came to see scabs as natural protective layers that facilitated the repair process, and protected that process from interference from outside. To remove such natural scabs and insert irritant powders as a way of bringing about suppuration came to be seen by Hunter as inducing complications where they did not naturally exist. In some ways, one might say, Hunter realised that the less the surgeon interfered with a wound of any kind, the fewer the complications that occurred. And all of these results, moreover, came not from the application of one of those all-embracing theoretically-based medical "systems" so beloved by 18th-century physicians, but from meticulously-conducted experimental investigations.

Hunter's colossal legacy to medicine was the bringing about of a sea-change in what surgeons did. More than any other single individual, he broke down many ancient and enduring "truisms" of medicine, and did this on the back of meticulously-recorded experimental researches, and that vast collection of specimens which was later bought for the nation and lodged at the Royal College of Surgeons as the Hunterian Museum.

Hunter's scientific legacy was international. Henry Clift, John Abernethy, Robert Knox, Charles Bell and Sir Astley Cooper were amongst some of his greatest British disciples. Men who, even if not studying under him directly, modelled their approach to their profession in accordance with Hunter's teachings and principles. Hunter's experimental approach to the study of life and decay processes further influenced the researches in continental Europe and America. John Collins Warren, for instance, who performed the world's first scientifically-monitored operation to use an anaesthetic at Boston, Massachusetts, in 1846, had been a "grand pupil", as it were, of Hunter, having studied at Guy's and St. Thomas's in the late 1790s, where the Hunterians Henry Cline and Astley Cooper ruled the roost. Warren, indeed, was one of several American medical men who took the Hunterian approach to the New World at the outset of what would turn out to be a distinguished surgical and medical career.

By 1846, Warren was Professor of Surgery at Harvard, and Surgeon to the Massachusetts General Hospital, when, on 16 October, he became the principal player at one of the greatest discoveries in the history of surgery. For on that day, in the Massachusetts General Hospital, he operated on a man who had been rendered insensible by sulphuric ether, administered to him by the dentist Dr William Morton. The success of that operation had reverberated around the world by Christmas 1846, for the mercy of anaesthesia promised to remove a set of problems from surgery which hardly anyone had thought of as a complication before they were removed, for their very presence had been seen since time immemorial as simply synonymous with the surgeon's art: pain and trauma. By the new year of 1847, in Boston, New York, London, Paris, Berlin, Vienna and the other great medical centres of America and Europe, surgeons found themselves working in a wholly new environment. Patients, knowing of the power of ether, no longer approached surgery as terrified lambs going to the slaughter. Powerful restraining assistants were no longer necessary; the patient's screams no longer drove young medical students out of the profession, as they had done to the medically-aspiring Charles Darwin at Edinburgh in 1827; while the postoperative patient was no longer a traumatised wreck who stood in need of months of convalescence if he survived at all. Surgeons, quite simply, did not fully realise what a major complication pain and fear had been until they vanished. For their sudden disappearance opened up wonderful new therapeutic prospects which would have been unthinkable before October 1846. Speed ceased to be a surgical prerequisite, and more complex operations could be planned and attempted on patients in deep anaesthesia which might even last for 20 or 30 minutes.

Post-1846 surgeons also found that other side effects of surgery which went back centuries could be drastically reduced and controlled. William Clowes, John Woodall, Richard Wiseman, Astley Cooper and Robert Liston (who was the first Briton to operate on an anaesthetised patient) had all been aware of the grave dangers stemming from massive haemorrhages, especially if working on the thigh, for no matter how good the surgeon's anatomical knowledge was or how well-disciplined his assistants were, pints of blood were easily squandered when a patient's convulsions made it impossible to seize and ligature the arteries. Yet when a patient was in deep anaesthesia, haemorrhage control became so much easier, and another complication was greatly reduced.

And once anaesthesia had been demonstrated as a medical reality, the hunt was immediately on for better anaesthetic substances with fewer side effects than ether. Sir James Simpson in Edinburgh, with a group of colleagues, began the systematic inhalation of various new chemical substances, and was delighted to discover the superior anaesthetic properties of chloroform — a new chemical preparation originally isolated by Soubeiran and Liebig in 1832 and already used in pharmacies — in 1847. Then in addition to powerful inhalants intended for operating theatre usage, Victorian chemists and doctors began to search for other types of pain-killing drugs, from those to control severe postoperative pain at one end of the spectrum, to sedatives and relatively mild analgesics at the other. It seemed that once the concept of efficient chemical pain control had sunk into the thinking of the medical and scientific communities, then the race was on. Crude opiates gave way to the power of the new analytical chemistry to produce morphine by 1805 and heroin by 1898. Then there was cocaine after 1885, which opened up entire new vistas for ophthalmic surgery, where the need for patient cooperation during surgery precluded the use of a general anaesthetic. Chloral hydrate became medicine's first "safe" sedative and sleep-inducer after 1871, while 1900 saw the isolation and wholescale manufacture of that drug which would be marketed as Aspirin. The mode of administration of pain-killing drugs also fundamentally changed in the latter half of the 19th century. For half a century after its chemical isolation from poppy juice by Friedrich Sertürner in 1805, morphine had been administered orally, as drugs had been since time immemorial. But in 1855, Alexander Wood of Edinburgh invented intravenous administration by hypodermic syringe, whereby a much more exact and physiologically specific dose of the drug could be given. Likewise, following their entry into medicine, cocaine and heroin came in turn to be delivered by hypodermic. And by the end of the century, the mass manufacture of pure, laboratory-produced pharmaceuticals, by firms such as Bayer and Merck, and the development of machines which could manufacture pills of exact dosage, were essential to the launch of the ubiquitous Aspirin and other tablets by 1900. Pain, one of surgery's most enduring complications, therefore, had been removed on the primary operative level, and rendered controllable at the secondary.

Surgery went through a honeymoon period in the years following 1846. Longer and more complex operations were now being tried, though surgeons were beginning to notice that postoperative infection and inflammation could ruin good work done in theatre.

For centuries surgeons had had their own chosen "antiseptics", without any coherent concept of what sepsis was or how it could be prevented, and long-standing favourites had included vinegar, turpentine and wine (or alcohol distilled from wine). Indeed, the great 14th-century French surgeon Guy de Chauliac had recommended "biting wine" or early brandy for such purposes. Yet none of these substances were used in accordance with any proper system quite simply because no one knew how sepsis occurred in the first place, and empirical attempts to mop up "putrefied blood" and then swill out the wound with turpentine or brandy were hit and miss in the extreme.

The overcoming of the next great surgical complication — gangrenous infection — had to wait until the 1860s. After the introduction of anaesthesia, surgeons, especially when working in hospital theatres as opposed to the homes of private patients, were alarmed to find that gangrenous complications tended to be on the increase. We now recognise, however, that the larger and more complex operative sites made possible by anaesthesia, and the much longer duration of anaesthetic operations, quite simply provided more opportunities for infection to occur. Several solutions to the problem of "hospital gangrene" were being actively sought during the period 1846–1866, and all seemed to offer some kind of success. A drive towards what was considered to be "cleanliness" was one of them, especially in the wake of Florence Nightingale's return from the Crimea in 1856, when it became clear that her nursing regime had undoubtedly improved the survival rates of wounded soldiers. Floors, walls, furniture and fittings were now regularly scrubbed, and the new breed of Nightingale nurses looked smart and well-starched. And because bad air, or "miasmas", were thought to hang around places where the unwashed poor were huddled together — in workhouses, prisons, military barracks and the Charity Wards of great hospitals — the encouragement of a brisk "through ventilation" was deemed necessary to remove them, thereby dictating the high ceilings and lofty architecture of our Victorian hospitals. And as mentioned above, varying degrees of trust were placed in the liberal application of "antiseptics". Turpentine became a favourite in the early 1860s, and was used extensively in the hospitals of the American Civil War. Yet none of these substances or procedures offered real or enduring success.

It was not until Joseph Lister, the young Regius Professor of Surgery at Glasgow, read Louis Pasteur's recent researches into fermentation in 1865 that a solution to the abounding complications of hospital sepsis in its various forms began to take shape. For while the concept of airborne sepsis was implicit in the miasmic theory, Pasteur's researches had shown that it was not the air itself which caused sepsis, but rather the presence of micro-organisms contained in the air, for as the Frenchman had demonstrated, if those micro-organisms were destroyed, such as by heating, then the air would lose its power to turn soup putrid or produce decomposition in meat.

One of Lister's brilliant insights was his recognition of the connection between putrescence and surgical sepsis, and as soon as he had read Pasteur's paper, he began to look for ways of applying its scientific principles to surgery. Though he could not remove bacteria from the air around and inside a wound with heat, he realised that one might be able to do so with chemicals. We have already seen that "antiseptics" had already been around on a hit and miss basis for centuries, but Lister chose a dilute preparation of a relatively new chemical substance which had already proved its worth in the treatment of sewage: carbolic acid, or phenol.

The class of surgical complication on which he began his antiseptic researches was an all too common one at the time: compound fractures. Why did even a bad fracture which did not penetrate the skin heal without septic complications, whereas one which only slightly penetrated the skin often became infected, gangrenous, and finally required amputation? The scenario was not a new one, and clearly harked back to John Hunter's observations concerning the different healing tendencies of punctured and non-punctured wounds. But Joseph Lister came to see that it was not the air itself which was the culprit, but Pasteur's microbes being carried in the air, as well as — as he later realised — microbes on the surgeon's hands and instruments.

His first attempt at antiseptic healing in the light of the Pasteurian discoveries was on a Glasgow road accident victim, a boy named James Greenless who, in August 1865, was run over by a wagon. The reduced fracture was meticulously cleansed with carbolic solution, and the whole wound site wrapped in carbolic-soaked lint. James Greenless's leg healed by first intention, and he walked out of the hospital six weeks later.

Lister began to refine the technique and, crucially, developed a precise antiseptic system for compound fracture cases, often wrapping a treated limb in tinfoil to prevent evaporation from the chemical dressings. Lister's technique was streets ahead of what had been done before, not because phenol was a magic drug in surgery, but because it was used in accordance with a precise method rather than just splashed around a wound site, as had been the case with earlier antiseptic substances. Then in the 16 March 1867 number of *The Lancet*, he published an account of 11 compound fracture cases in which he had used his method, all of which had healed without sepsis: an unprecedented run of success for the time.

But applying the method to elective operative surgery seemed more difficult, and still working with the idea of airborne bacteria, Lister devised a spray machine which would produce a carbolic aerosol atmosphere around the operating site. The ensuing results were decisive. He found that his fatalities for amputation cases fell from 45.7% for 35 persons operated upon without antiseptics between 1864 and 1866, to 15.0% for 40 antiseptic cases for the period 1867–1870.

Yet Lister's results, decisive as they seem to us today, still left many doubting, and the decisive Achilles heel of Lister's method was his inability, at the time, to show which particular microbes caused which complications. Surgery, let us not forget, has always been the most pragmatic of all the healing arts, and tends to attract persons of a pragmatic turn of mind to its practice. And as British science in particular was deeply Baconian in the 19th century, and its practitioners concerned with using experiments to establish precise cause and effect relationships in nature, Lister's theory was easy to shoot down from a cause and effect perspective. Why did wounds sometimes heal by first intention even without "Listerianism", especially if performed upon private patients in their own homes in rooms that had been well scrubbed in advance? Were hospitals dangerous places in which to perform surgery simply because the poor folk who inhabited their wards were less vigorous or fundamentally degenerate?

Although we know that Lister was correct, one must not write off powerful critics of his method, such as Robert Lawson Tait or John Hughes Bennett, as dinosaurs: indeed, the anti-Listerian Lawson Tait — who had, from purely empirical criteria, developed a form of aseptic surgery — was almost a generation younger than Lister himself. For quite simply, if one adhered to the new yet pre-Listerian doctrines of cleanliness, good ventilation and competent nursing, a surgeon stood to have higher survival rates for his patients than a colleague who employed the older and dirtier methods, quite apart from the use or otherwise of Lister's techniques. For to many, there seemed no proven connection between the creatures seen under the microscope in pus or fluid specimens from wounds and the occurrence of surgical gangrene, septicaemia or pyaemia. Indeed, even Robert Hooke and Antoni van Leeuwenhoek, the discoverers of the "animalcules" of bacteria back in the 1660s, 1670s and 1680s, had pointed out that one found them wriggling about everywhere: in plant moulds, teeth scrapings, saliva and blood; and by the age of the high-power compound microscope in the 1860s, it seemed that creepy crawlies were everywhere! So why was Lister's method significant?

In many ways, the turning-point in the intellectual acceptance of antisepsis came from Robert Koch's researches during the 1870s which showed that a specific inflammatory or infectious disease could be connected with a specific bacterium. What mattered, therefore, in the avoidance of inflammatory complications in surgery, was the absence of specific strains of bacteria from the site of the operation, and not necessarily *all* bacteria. Koch's researches, first published in 1879, were to produce the key pieces of Baconian "proof" for the correctness of Lister's idea of protecting the surgical site from microbes, though by the time that Koch's work on the connection between specific bacterial strains and specific diseases was coming to win over doubters to the germ theory in general in the 1880s, surgery itself was going beyond Lister's chemical method. For one thing, Koch demonstrated that heat, rather than chemicals, was more effective in killing bacteria. And while no one suggested that the entire operation had to be performed at sterilising temperatures, it was found that if surgical instruments and dressings could be heat-sterilised before operating, then the wounds stood a good chance of healing by first intention even without Listerianism.

After 1865, surgery forged ahead in a way which would have been unimaginable in 1840, for once the monumental obstacles of operative and postoperative pain had shown themselves to be amenable to control, and Lister had demonstrated the same for septic infections, a foundation had been established upon which one innovation after another would be built. By the 1890s, for instance, many surgeons in Europe and North America had gone beyond Listerian carbolic methods to develop aseptic, as opposed to antiseptic, techniques. Theodor Billroth, William Halstead, the surgeons of the new Johns Hopkins research school, the Minnesota brothers Charles and William Mayo, and others had come to see the operating theatre not as a carbolic-soaked place, but one in which germs were not so much killed as excluded from entry. For aseptic conditions could be achieved if the surgeon and his assistants were well scrubbed, wore the new thin flexible gloves developed by the Dunlop Rubber Company, and were aseptically gowned rather than merely aproned. Their instruments, moreover, were re-designed, losing their traditional black bone handles, and were stripped down to the steel, so as to be capable of sterilisation in high-temperature autoclaves.

The old problem of haemorrhage came to be controlled not just with advancing anatomical knowledge and ligatures, but also with special locking forceps, and with special clips. And then, one might say, the old complication of haemorrhage found its ultimate solution after 1900 when Karl Landsteiner's researches opened up the possibility of using transfusion as a way of replacing lost blood. Landsteiner came to his discovery after studying why previous transfusions had failed, and the patient's and donor's blood had coagulated and produced an allergic reaction, which often resulted in death. Laboratory experiments led Landsteiner to realise that antigen reactions were at work between different groups of red blood cells, and by 1900, he was able to isolate distinct blood groups which he called A, B, O and later AB. When blood from a compatible donor was given to a surgical or accident patient, blood loss caused by haemorrhage could now be replenished. Most of these early transfusions were direct between donor and patient, but the establishment of the first blood banks in the late 1930s opened up all kinds of possibilities for surgeons, and by definition, reduced complication.

Although the number of surgical operations performed increased dramatically after 1846, and they became progressively safer in the wake of Lister's work in the middle and late 1860s, the actual repertoire of operations still remained fairly fixed. Yes, it is true that a military surgeon, working on extreme battlefield injuries and attempting whatever procedure, just might save the patient's life, be it replacing abdominal viscera or trying to remove projectile debridement from the cranial or thoracic cavities — sometimes with success; but what would be considered operable within the context of a hospital theatre remained much more conservative. For elective surgery remained deeply cautious for many years to come after 1865. Joseph Lister's own repertoire of operations, conducted in his capacity as professorial surgeon at three of Europe's greatest university teaching hospitals — Glasgow, Edinburgh and King's College, London, successively — did not change much over the decades. Orthopaedics, attempts at repairing damage occurring in tuberculous joints (especially the wrist), and the excision of external tumours and growths remained his essential stock-in-trade, as they did with scores of his colleagues. What changed drastically were the chances of patient survival, and of wounds healing by first intention.

The abdomen was the first traditional "no go" area of the human body to be worked on electively by surgeons using the new techniques of anaesthesia, antisepsis and asepsis. And while cases were on record of abdominal operations where the patient had survived, these had all been performed in emergency or unexpected contexts — such as Claude Amyand's 1735 hernia operation on the boy who was found to have a pin stuck through his appendix. Quite simply, abdominal operations seemed replete with complications, even after anaesthesia, as infection, muscle damage and blood loss made them too dangerous.

Yet curiously enough, some surgeons had been opening the abdomen with varying degrees of success since 1809, when Ephraim McDowell, an Edinburgh-trained surgeon of Danville, Kentucky, removed an ovarian tumour weighing 23 ½ pounds from one Mrs Jane Todd Crawford. This radical ovariectomy healed by first intention. Mrs Crawford was up and making her own bed five days after surgery, "and in 25 days, she returned home as she came [on horseback] in good health which she continues [1817] to enjoy". Jane Todd Crawford lived for another 31 years, dying in 1842, and outliving her surgeon by 12 years. McDowell performed over eight ovariectomies before he died in 1830, and in most of these cases the patient lived. Of course, while the 1809 operation on Mrs Crawford was elective, it was in reality just like a severe gunshot wound — a forlorn hope, for as McDowell told his courageous patient, she would die if she did not risk it. During her 25-minute, fully-conscious ordeal, Jane Todd Crawford sustained herself by singing *Psalms*. Ovariectomy was also practised with varying degrees of success by surgeons on both sides of the Atlantic, both before and after anaesthesia and antisepsis came on the scene. By 1880 Spencer Wells in London had clocked up his incredible 1000th operation, and while not adopting Lister's techniques until around 1878, his concern with overall cleanliness and exact procedures meant that he had a mortality rate of only 25%.

Crucial to the development of abdominal surgery, however, was the seeming increase of what had once been called the *Illiac Passion*, which by the 1880s had become known as *Typhilitis*, and after Reginald Heber Fitz in Boston in 1886, as *Appendicitis*. John Woodall in 1617 had left a detailed account of this frightful condition, which appeared to be connected with total constipation and blockage of the gut, and which, *in extremis*, led to the voiding of the faeces from the mouth shortly before death. Hunter had done a classic study, in which he noticed massive inflammation of the peritoneum and blockage of the gut by adhesion in *post mortem*. By the 1880s, however, several surgeons were attempting the opening up of the abdomens of living people with this condition, and it is hard to be sure who was first, for Robert Lawson Tait in England, Ulrich Rudolf Krölein in Germany, Reginald Heber Fitz in America, and so on, were all attempting operations for typhilitis in the early 1880s. Generally speaking, they were not trying to remove the whole *veriformis appendix* so much as drain away the infection and separate the adhesions, and even as late as June 1902, when the Prince of Wales, soon to be crowned King Edward VII, went down with appendicitis, his surgeon, Sir Frederick Treeves, only drained the site rather than removing the appendix altogether. For massive septic complications could all too easily set in, and as late as 1907, Mair, the 17-year-old daughter of the future British Prime Minister David Lloyd

George, died from the complications of an appendectomy. However, when [Sir] Winston Churchill went through a similar ordeal on 19 October 1922, he was just about back on his feet, though looking skeletal, within a month. Charles Mayo, of the celebrated clinic which bore the name of that family of surgeons at Rochester, Minnesota, was to develop the appendectomy as well as several other abdominal procedures into something of a routine between 1890 and the 1930s.

Some surgeons, however, in spite of the inherent dangers involved, became so eager to open up the abdomen by the mid-1880s that one almost hears the Hippocratic alarm bells about rash surgery ringing in one's ears. Sir William Arbuthnot Lane, for instance, was so obsessed with the pernicious effects of constipation, and the supposed absorption thereby of "poisons" into the blood-stream, that he became the virtuoso of the radical colotomy, where substantial pieces of the patient's gut would be removed in the hope of speeding up bowel action. Some surgeons were coming to see themselves as heroes of the knife!

Indeed, by the 1880s, surgery was developing rapidly, and the massively influential Theodor Billroth was to train up in Berlin, Zurich and Vienna a whole new generation of surgeons who would establish his methods on both sides of the Atlantic. For Billroth took surgery out of the operating theatre, seeing that it had to be matched by meticulous laboratory work if its full curative effects were to be realised. Pathological specimens had to be examined in the laboratory, and the pre- and post-surgical state of the patient carefully monitored. Carl Wunderlich's mid-19th-century researches into medical thermometry were seen by Billroth as having a direct surgical relevance, as Billroth related degrees of inflammation to thermometric readings, thereby showing how a surgeon might measure the occurrence and response to treatment of a complication. And Billroth's methods were not reserved for surgery on any one part of the body, but could be applied to any kind of procedure: to amputations, tumour, and liver, renal or abdominal surgery, not to mention the first tentative openings of the cranium and the thorax. What mattered was that the practitioner of the new surgery saw his work within a context which included the laboratory, instrumental monitoring and statistical analyses. And of course, the sheer scope for surgical complications was now expanding at an unprecedented rate, for with each new procedure attempted on the human body, the things that could go wrong increased. On the other hand, these complications could be seen as part of a wider biological and pathological whole, with new scientific methods developed for their control and elimination.

At the same time as some surgeons were risking opening up the abdomen, others were taking the ancient procedure of trephination several stages further, and trying to treat conditions of the brain. As early as 1879, Sir William Macewan in Glasgow successfully removed a tumour from the *dura mater* of a patient, while in the 1880s Eugene Hahn in Germany and Sir Rickman Godlee in England successfully removed potentially malignant growths, or else drained abscesses, from the surface coatings of the human brain. Yet the surgery of the brain and its deeper glandular structures really began to take off with Harvey Cushing in America after his successful removal of the pituitary gland from an acromegalic patient in 1909, based as that operation was on a meticulous study of that gland by Cushing over the previous four years.

It was not really until after World War I, however, that a surgical approach to the human heart was made, although there was an abundance of material in the historical medical literature recording chest and even heart injuries from which the patient had sometimes recovered. But it was that Napoleon of abdominal surgery Sir William Arbuthnot Lane, who first resuscitated a heart which had suddenly stopped during surgery. This feat was reported in *The Lancet* in 1902, where it was told how, when he was removing the appendix of a 65-year-old man, the patient's heart stopped beating. Having the patient already open before him on the operating table, however, the redoubtable Arbuthnot Lane simply thrust his arm into the upper abdominal cavity until he could feel the motionless heart through the diaphragm wall. Then "he gave it a squeeze or two and felt it re-start beating". The patient recovered from both his abdominal and his unplanned cardiac surgery!

Of course, as Arbuthnot Lane was all too well aware, he had not actually *entered* the thoracic cavity, so much as used the elasticity of the diaphragm to enable his hand to feel and squeeze the heart. For in 1902 invading the thorax and tampering with the pericardium, heart and other structures was too much of a closed domain to risk entering. Even so, Arbuthnot Lane became the first surgeon to face the complication of death on the operating table with a new and successful solution.

But it was the sheer volume of battle injuries sustained in World War I, assisted by diagnosis with X-ray machines, which really brought home to surgeons what a living human heart could take and survive. In his paper "The

Surgery of the Heart", in the 3 January 1920 number of *The Lancet*, Sir Charles Ballance described the case of a French infantryman who was found, 70 days after his original medical examination, to have a 1.5 cm piece of steel from a German grenade lodged in his right ventricle. It was subsequently removed in a Paris hospital where the operating surgeon found, to his surprise, that "The heart could not be held in the gloved hand, from which it slipped like a live fish". Other World War I surgeons reported embolic rifle bullets lodged in the aorta and carried with the blood current, penetrated chest walls, damaged pericardia and other conditions which the patients sometimes survived. But as Sir Charles Ballance emphasised in his 1920 *Lancet* paper, sepsis was the killer complication of all such surgery.

As far as I am aware, however, the first elective, as opposed to battle wound, surgery to be performed on the heart had to wait until 1925, when Henry Sessions Souttar of the London Hospital attempted a radical procedure on a young woman whom he believed to have mitral stenosis, a case which he reported in the 1925 *British Medical Journal*. Souttar made a large flap in the region of her left breast, cut through three ribs, and entered the ventricle via the mitral valve, and in a couple of minutes seemed to have cleared away some of the stenosed material, so that when his finger was removed, the blood flow seemed better than before. The one-hour-long operation appears to have been complication-free, as "her condition had never caused the slightest anxiety" and she recovered after six weeks of bed rest and rural convalescence, though remaining short of breath upon exertion.

Regular thoracic and cardiac surgery took a long time to develop, however, for the complications involved could be so enormous, with patient mortality rates of over 70%. Drugs and a severe body-cooling regime (surrounding the anaesthetised patient with ice) were tried as ways of reducing the heart-beat rate in surgery to make the organ more amenable to handling, though sepsis still remained the overwhelming problem. It would take a Second World War, and the whole cascade of new surgical and medical techniques which came from that, before cardiac surgery could become remotely safe. By the 1950s, however, cardiac surgery began to advance rapidly, especially with the development of biomedical technology, and extracorporeal circulation machines of the type used for Charles Lillehei's operations at the University of Minnesota, which made possible complex surgical procedures on living human hearts.

Yet the most powerful surgical tool and combater of septic complication derived in fact from an essentially medical discovery: antibiotics. Antibiotics research really began in World War I, when the young [Sir] Alexander Fleming had been studying wounds and resistance to infection. This was at a time when the concept of the body's immune system, and the role played therein by enzymes, were first coming to be explored by medical scientists. Then in 1928, Fleming noticed how a penicillin mould had destroyed a staphylococcus culture in his laboratory at St. Mary's Hospital, London, and published his results a year later. However, it was Howard Florey, Ernst Chain and Norman Heatley at the Oxford University Dunn School of Pathology a decade later who began work on isolating the active ingredient in *penicillium notatum*, and succeeded in 1940. Though much of the research for the mass-production of penicillin was undertaken in the USA after 1941, research also continued in England, and by the D-Day invasion of Europe in June 1944, penicillin was already in such abundant supply as to transform the prospects of the Allied wounded. And after the War, penicillin and other antibiotics made it possible for surgeons to electively open up the abdomen, cranium and thorax with a much higher likelihood of the patient not succumbing to a lethal postoperative septic or pulmonary infection. An assault upon the causes of sepsis which had been begun by Lister in 1865 had developed beyond recognition by 1945, and would continue doing so in a fairly exponential fashion, at least up to the late 1980s, when antibiotic-resistant strains of bacteria began to emerge.

Although surgical complications have no doubt been around since the stone age, when primitive men first used pieces of sharpened flint to chisel holes in injured heads or perhaps to open painful ulcers or tumours, it was really not until the late 18th century that those complex pathological changes which can take place inside wounds, were studied scientifically. For in the last two centuries, surgery and medicine in all of their branches have changed, both conceptually and technically, beyond recognition. Conditions which had hitherto been seen as "natural" — such as inflammation, pus, pain, haemorrhage, fever and high mortality — were increasingly perceived as essentially extraneous factors which could be eradicated from the surgical environment if not yet, at least at some stage in the not too distant future. And while post-Renaissance anatomy and the experiences gained in the treatment of gunshot wounds had made the surgeon much more confident in so far as he now knew exactly what he would encounter beneath the surface whenever he took up his knife to operate, it was really not until after 1846 that this vast treasury of accumulated body knowledge began at last to reap a sweeping therapeutic harvest in terms of new and increasingly safe operations which eventually extended into every cavity area and organ of the human body. And ironically, one might say that nowadays the range of potential surgical complications is greater than ever before; but this is only because the modern surgeon can confidently address problems within the human body which would have been unimaginable 25, 50, 100 or 200 years ago, yet by the judicious use of that vast armamentum of clinical techniques available today, he stands a very good chance of stabilising and overcoming such complications as and when they occur.

BIBLIOGRAPHY

Primary Sources

1. *Albucasis, On Surgery and Instruments*, edited with translation from the Arabic by Spink MS, Lewis GL (Wellcome Inst., London, 1973).
2. Claudius Amyand, F.R.S. (October 1736) "Of an Inguinal Rupture, with a Pin in the *Appendix Coeci*, incrusted with Stone; and some observations on Wounds in the Guts". *Philos Trans* 443: 329–342.
3. Aristotle. (1912) *De Generatione Animalium*. In: *The Works of Aristotle*, translated and edited by Smith JA, Ross WD (Clarendon Press, Oxford).
4. Sir Charles Balance (3 January 1920) "The surgery of the heart." *The Lancet* 1: 1–6.
5. Sir John Bland-Sutton. (10 May 1919) "Missiles as emboli" (a lecture delivered to the Surgical Section, Royal Society of Medicine). *The Lancet*. i: 773–775.
6. William Clowes. (1588) *A prooved practice for all young chirugians, concerning burnings with gunpowder, and wounds made with gunshot* (London), p. 33 for thigh amputation.
7. William Clowes. (1637) *A Profitable and Necessarie Booke of Observations, for all those that are burned with the flame of Gun-powder*, 3rd edn. (London).
8. Harold Ellis. (1994) *Surgical Case Histories from the Past* (Royal Society of Medicine, London). Reprints several key papers in the history of modern surgery, several of which are in relatively obscure journals.
9. *Galen, On Anatomical Procedures*, translated and edited by Singer C (Wellcome Medical Museum and Oxford University Press, 1956). Contains Books I–IX.

10. *Galen, On Anatomical Procedures, The Later Books,* translated by Duckworth WLH, Lyons MC, Towers B (Cambridge University Press, 1962). Contains Books X–XV.

11. Hippocrates, III (1928) *Wounds, Surgery, and Fractures,* translated by Withington ET, Loeb Classical Library (Heinemann, London and Harvard University Press).

12. Robert Hooke. (1665) *Micrographia* (London), Observation XX, for plant mould micro-organisms.

13. John Hunter. (1794, 1812) *A Treatise on the Blood, Inflammation and Gun-Shot Wounds* (London).

14. Joseph Lister. (16 March 1867) "On a new method of treating compound fractures …". *The Lancet* **1**: 326–329. (Reprinted in Ellis, *Surgical Case Histories.*)

15. Ephraim McDowell. (1817) "Three cases of extirpation of diseased ovaria". In: *The Eclectic Repertory*, vii, (Philadelphia), p. 242. (Reprinted in Schachner, *Ephraim McDowell*, and Ellis, *Surgical Case Histories.*)

16. Sir William Macewan. (1879) "Tumour of the dura mater – convulsions – removal of tumours by trephining – recovery". *Glasgow Med J* **12**: 210–212. (Reprinted in Ellis, *Surgical Case Histories.*)

17. *Letters and the Second Diary of Samuel Pepys,* edited with Introduction by Howarth RG. (Dent, London, 1932).

18. August Schachner, M.D. (1921) *Ephraim McDowell, "Father of Ovariotomy" and Founder of Abdominal Surgery* (Lippincott, Philadelphia and London). N.B. This detailed biography re-prints McDowell's ovariotomy papers of 1817 and 1819, and includes correspondence, and other documents.

19. Henry Sessions Souttar. (1925) "The surgical treatment of mitral stenosis". *Br Med J* **2**: 603–606. (Reprinted in Ellis, *Surgical Case Histories.*)

20. Tutankhamun. Details of recent CT scan findings reported: *The Daily Telegraph*, 11 May 2005; *The Guardian* press release, 5 May 2005. Also Internet "News in Science", abc.net.au/science/news, http://abc.net.au/cgi-bin/common/printfriendly (20/07/05).

21. John Collins Warren. (1846) "Inhalation of ethereal vapour for the prevention of pain in surgical cases." *Boston Med Surg J* **35**: 375–379. (Reprinted in Ellis, *Surgical Case Histories.*)

22. Richard Wiseman. (1676) *Severall Chirugicall Treatises* (London).

23. John Woodall. (1617) *The Surgeon's Mate* (London), facsimile edn., with Introduction and Appendix by John Kirkup (Kingsmead Press, Bath, 1978).

24. Leading article "Resuscitation in syncope due to anaesthetics and in other conditions by rhythmical compression of the heart", *The Lancet*, 29 November 1902, p. 1476. N.B. Arbuthnot Lane is not given as the author, but he is named as the

surgeon, and Dr. E. A. Starling as anaesthetist. (Reprinted in Ellis, *Surgical Case Histories.*)

Secondary Sources

25. Allbutt TC. (1905) *The Historical Relations of Medicine and Surgery to the End of the Sixteenth Century* (London).
26. Armstrong Davison MH. (1965) *The Evolution of Anaesthesia* (Altringcham, Great Britain).
27. Bishop WJ. (1960) *The Early History of Surgery* (Robert Hale, London).
28. Brock RC. (1952) *The Life and Work of Astley Cooper* (Livingstone, Edinburgh and London).
29. Brown K. (2004) *Alexander Fleming and the Antibiotic Revolution* (Sutton, Stroud).
30. Cartwright FW. (1967) *The Development of Modern Surgery* (London).
31. Chaucer G. (1957) The pardoner's tale. In: Robinson FN (ed.), *The Works of Geoffrey Chaucer* (Boston, Mass).
32. Walker AE. (1951) *A History of Neurological Surgery* (London).
33. Ellis H. (1983) *Notable Names in Medicine and Surgery*, 4th edn. (Lewis, London).
34. Fisher R. (1977) *Joseph Lister, 1827–1912* (MacDonald and James, London).
35. Fulton JF. (1946) *Harvey Cushing. A Biography* (Blackwell Scientific Publications, Oxford).
36. Gest H. (2004) "The discovery of microorganisms by Robert Hooke and Antoni van Leeuwenhoek, fellows of the Royal Society". *Notes Rec R Soc Lond* **58**(2): 187–201.
37. Gest H. (2004) "The discovery of microorganisms revisited". *Am Soc Microbiol News* **70**: 269–274.
38. Jackson R. (1988) *Doctors and Diseases in the Roman Empire* (British Museum, London).
39. Malgaigne JF. (1965) *Surgery and Ambrose Paré*, translated from French and edited by Hamby WB (University of Oklahoma Press).
40. O'Malley CD. (1964) *Andreas Vesalius of Brussels 1514–1564* (University of California, Berkeley and LA).
41. Morris GCR. (2004) "Thomas Hollier". *New DNB* **27**: 733 (Oxford).
42. D'Arcy Power. (1904) "Who performed lithotomy on Mr Samuel Pepys?" *The Lancet*, 9 April 1904, pp. 1011–1012.
43. Quist G. (1981) *John Hunter, 1728–1793* (Heinemann Medical Books, London).

44. Ruestow EG. (1996) *The Microscope in the Dutch Republic* (Cambridge University Press).
45. Singer C, Underwood EA. (1962) *A Short History of Medicine* (Oxford University Press).
46. Tomalin C. (2003) *Samuel Pepys. The Unequalled Self* (Penguin).
47. Wangensteen OH, Wangensteen SD. (1978) *The Rise of Surgery from Empiric Craft to Scientific Discipline* (Dawson, Folkestone, Kent, and University of Minnesota).
48. Zimmerman LM, Veith I. (1961) *Great Ideas in the History of Surgery* (Baltimore).

Chapter 2

ANAESTHETIC COMPLICATIONS

Christopher Johnstone and Nick Pace

INTRODUCTION

The aim of anaesthesia is to provide optimal operating conditions required for the proposed surgery. This may involve providing a combination of reversible loss of consciousness, pain relief and muscle relaxation. If a regional anaesthetic is chosen then loss of consciousness is usually not required. However, complications or side effects may be more severe than if a general anaesthetic is chosen. The complications arising from anaesthesia, or critical incidents, are events occurring that could or do lead to death, disability or prolongation of hospital stay. Many are detected prior to any actual harm coming to the patient. The anaesthetist and surgeon should work together to this end, as many of the incidents are preventable. It is estimated that a critical incident will occur in 11% of anaesthetics and 70% are related to human error, in association with equipment and monitoring failure, inadequate preoperative preparation of the patient and organisational failure. Complications are more likely to arise at the extremes of age, emergency surgery and intercurrent illness.[1,2]

Strategies for reducing complications have been developed from national audits such as the Confidential Enquiry into Perioperative Death (CEPOD), Scottish Audit of Surgical Mortality (SASM) and critical incident reporting encouraged by the Royal College of Anaesthetists.

In addition, the Association of Anaesthetists of Great Britain and Ireland has produced a number of guidelines that should be adhered to:

- theatre efficiency,
- preoperative assessment, the role of the anaesthetist,
- recommendations for standards of monitoring during anaesthesia and recovery,
- anaesthesia and perioperative care of the elderly,
- immediate postoperative recovery,
- risk management,
- anaphylactic reactions associated with anaesthesia, and
- checking anaesthetic equipment.

preoperative assessment[3,4] allows the anaesthetist to take a history, and examine, assess and discuss the risks of anaesthesia with the patient. In addition, medical and anaesthetic problems that may require further investigation or optimisation prior to the commencement of anaesthesia are identified. For example, this may involve preparation of the patient with a known difficult intubation for an awake fibre optic intubation or an alternative regional technique such as a spinal anaesthetic.

Preoperative fasting times should also be clarified with the nursing staff and the patient. The Association of Anaesthetists of Great Britain and Ireland have recommended the adoption of the fasting guidelines of the American Society of Anaesthesiologists (ASA):

- 6 hours for solid food, infant formula or other milk,
- 4 hours for breast milk, and
- 2 hours for clear non-particulate and non-carbonated fluids.

The chewing of gum is a contentious issue but it is best treated as if it was an oral clear, non-carbonated fluid and therefore prohibited two hours prior to anaesthesia. These guidelines are for patients undergoing elective surgery, the aim of which is to ensure an empty stomach, thereby preventing passive reflux and pulmonary aspiration of gastric contents, which itself has a high morbidity and mortality. Patients undergoing bowel preparation, children, pyrexial patients and breastfeeding mothers should not be left fasting for prolonged periods of time without adequate hydration. They may require intravenous fluids, thereby enhancing patient comfort and reducing preoperative dehydration.

A typed theatre list should be constructed prior to the start of a list. It should be adhered to as this enables premedication to be given at the correct time, prevents prolonged fasting times and reduces the likelihood of patient mix up. The anaesthetic equipment should be checked before the start of each theatre session, by the anaesthetist responsible.[5] The anaesthetic room is a feature of practice in the UK. In most other countries induction of anaesthesia takes place in the operating room. The presence of a separate room for induction reduces the stress of being awake in the operating theatre. This is especially important in paediatrics as it allows parents to remain with their child until he or she is unconscious. Upon arrival of a patient at the anaesthetic room, all documentation for that patient should be present. This includes the consent form, radiographs, notes, medicine prescription chart and any results of investigations that may have been requested. The patent should be clearly identified and monitoring applied. Minimum monitoring should be in place before induction, continued throughout the operation, and may be discontinued following recovery. The Association of Anaesthetists has described minimum monitoring as follows:

- the continued presence of the anaesthetist,
- the anaesthetist must check all equipment prior to use,
- pulse oximetry,
- non-invasive blood pressure (NIBP),
- capnography (carbon dioxide monitoring),
- electrocardiography (ECG),
- vapour analysis, and
- oxygen analysis.

Monitoring of temperature and neuromuscular transmission must be immediately available. Instrumental monitoring will not prevent complications arising but the combination of pulse oximetry, capnography and blood pressure monitoring should detect over 90% of incidents prior to organ damage occurring. Technology will never be a substitute for skill or vigilance. Furthermore, most monitors have technical limitations. For example, non-invasive blood pressure cuffs overestimate low blood pressure and underestimate high blood pressure. Cuff size is also important. Too small a cuff overestimates and too large a cuff underestimates the true blood pressure value. Similarly, the accuracy of pulse oximetry may be limited by hypothermic states, if the patient is vasoconstricted or if diathermy is in use. Also, the presence of carboxyhaemoglobin will result in overreading of the true value.

The patient's state of health may require more invasive monitoring, such as arterial cannulation and central venous pressure monitoring. On occasion, it may be necessary to place these before induction of anaesthesia. The localisation of the internal jugular vein to allow central venous cannulation is currently an area of great debate. Complications may occur in up to 10% of cases and the failure rate may be as high as 35%. There are many important surrounding structures that may be damaged; notably the carotid artery may be punctured and incidences of 1–3% have been reported. Rarely a pneumothorax may occur (although this is more common with the subclavian vein approach). Thus there has been increasing interest in the use of two-dimensional ultrasound as an aid in the placement of central venous catheters and recently the National Institute for Clinical Excellence has recommended this as the preferred method for insertion. Other complications of central venous catheterisation include infection, haematoma formation, thrombosis of the vessel, the creation of an arteriovenous fistula, cardiac tamponade, arrhythmias, brachial plexus damage and air (and catheter) embolism.

It is important to minimise the number of connections in the anaesthetic circuit to limit the risks of disconnection and leaks. Furthermore, the volume of dead space and the resistance to the work of breathing may increase. This may be important in the severely compromised patient and especially so in the paediatric setting.

Different patient positions are indicated to facilitate particular operations. Positioning is the joint responsibility of the anaesthetist and surgeon. Care is required to ensure patient safety. The main areas to be considered are effects on the cardiovascular and respiratory systems; whether the patient has an abnormality of the autonomic nervous system; and limiting the risk to joints and pressure points, especially if movement is restricted. Careful attention is needed to prevent ocular, neural or pressure injury to tissues whilst patient is anaesthetised. In the upper limb, the brachial plexus, ulnar and radial nerves can be overstretched. In the lower limb, the common peroneal and saphenous nerves can be compressed if the lithotomy position is used. There is also the risk of displacing the endotracheal tubes, ECG monitoring or intravenous lines when the patient is positioned.

Induction of anaesthesia produces physiological changes, especially in the cardiovascular and respiratory systems. Many are further altered by the positioning of the patient, especially if also placed head up or down. These changes can induce serious complications.

COMPLICATIONS OF THE AIRWAY AND RESPIRATORY SYSTEM

The complications involving the respiratory system include intubation problems, pulmonary aspiration of gastric contents, respiratory obstruction and hypoxia. Before these are discussed, the effect of anaesthesia on the respiratory system will be reviewed to enable an understanding of the pitfalls that may arise. This can be divided into the effects on the control of breathing, the upper airway, and the mechanics of the lung and respiratory muscles. These factors all have an impact on ventilation and perfusion.

Control of Breathing

Inhalational anaesthetic agents in general cause an increase in the frequency of respiration, a fall in the tidal volume and a reduction in the ventilatory response to $PaCO_2$. Intravenous agents tend to cause an initial increase in the tidal volume followed by a reduction in ventilatory drive until a period of apnoea develops. Opioids prolong the expiratory pause, thereby reducing the frequency of respiration and reduce the response of ventilation to a rising $PaCO_2$.

Upper Airway

The upper airway comprises of two groups of muscles: dilators which maintain patency and constrictors, which are involved in swallowing. Anaesthesia causes a reduction in the tone of these muscles as well as loss of protective airway reflexes. This may result in airway obstruction. Topical local anaesthesia to the upper airway will enhance this, thereby increasing airway obstruction. Therefore care must be taken to ensure that respiratory obstruction does not occur during sedation whilst using topical anaesthesia.

Respiratory Muscles and Lung Mechanics

The distribution of lung perfusion and ventilation is affected by gravity as well as the mechanics of the chest wall and diaphragm. Respiratory muscle tone is reduced during general anaesthesia. This leads to a reduction in overall chest wall tone, and in turn leads to a reduction in functional residual capacity (FRC) which is further exacerbated if there is a reduction in diaphragmatic tone. The FRC may also be reduced by posture. A 70 kg man with an FRC of 3l changing positions from standing to supine reduces his FRC by approximately 700 ml. Anaesthesia and muscle paralysis reduces this by a further 700 ml. FRC is maintained in the prone position but it may be further decreased in obese patients placed in a head-down tilt.

The reduction in lung volumes as a consequence of anaesthesia leads to airway collapse due to a reduction in traction on air passages and therefore narrowing of bronchi and bronchioles. This causes an increase in airway resistance, leading to a reduction in lung compliance and consequently an increase in the work of breathing.

The reduction in lung volumes and airway patency results in ventilation/perfusion mismatching (V/Q), with areas of ventilation with no perfusion (high V/Q ratio, dead space) and areas of perfusion with absent ventilation (shunt).[6]

In the supine, prone and lateral positions, if the patient is breathing spontaneously, the dependent lung is better perfused and ventilated. Paralysing and ventilating the patient leads to a decreased contribution of diaphragmatic excursion to the tidal volume, which in turn leads to a decrease in ventilation of dependent lung regions and thus V/Q mismatching. This is most pronounced if the paralysed ventilated patient is in the lateral position, when the weight of the mediastinum above and the abdominal contents below hinder ventilation of the dependent lung. Hypoxic pulmonary vasoconstriction, a physiological process that reduces blood flow to atelectatic areas of the lung, thereby reducing shunt, is reduced by the action of inhalation anaesthetic agents and thus augments V/Q abnormalities.

Intubation problems

Intubation problems that may occur are:

- oesophageal intubation,
- endobronchial intubation,
- difficult intubation and failed intubation, and will be dealt with sequentially.

Oesophageal intubation is an important and preventable cause of anaesthetic morbidity and mortality. Direct visualisation of the endotracheal tube (ETT) passing through the vocal cords anterior to the arytenoids cartilages is insufficient evidence of correct placement of the tube. The gold standard for confirmation of ETT placement is capnography. In addition to this the chest should be auscultated to confirm bilateral air entry. Preoxygenation ensures that the patient will not become hypoxic for several minutes following incorrect placement and therefore pulse oximetry is an unreliable indicator of such an event. If there is any doubt as to ETT position, the tube should be taken out and the patient reoxygenated by facemask.

Endobronchial intubation occurs when the ETT passes into either the right (more commonly) or left main bronchus, usually if the ETT is uncut or cut too long. The result of undetected endobronchial intubation is that of recurrent desaturation, high peak airway pressures due to a large tidal volume being delivered to only one lung, and atelectasis of the non-ventilated lung. This may be detected on auscultation of the chest, noting that breath sounds are heard in only one lung field. The corrective action is to withdraw the ETT until both lung fields have audible breath sounds.

Difficult intubation has been defined as an intubation that has required more than three attempts or taken longer than 10 minutes to accomplish. Failure to appropriately manage a difficult intubation leads to morbidity, such as dental and airway trauma, pulmonary aspiration and hypoxia, or in extreme cases mortality. The aetiology of difficult intubation is shown in Table 1. The incidence of difficult intubation is approximately 1 in 100 anaesthetics. The incidence of failed intubation is 1 in 2000 in the general population but 1 in 300 in the obstetric population.

preoperative assessment, allows the patient to volunteer or be questioned about any previous difficulties encountered with their airway. Documentation of previous ease of intubations is, however, not a guarantee that the subsequent

Table 1.   The Aetiology of Difficult Intubation

Anaesthetist	Inadequate preoperative assessment		
	Failure to check equipment		
	Inadequate experience		
Equipment	Inexperienced assistant		
	Equipment malfunction		
	Equipment unavailability		
Patient	Congenital	Treacher Collins syndrome	
		Trisomy 21	
		Pierre Robin syndrome	
		Marfans syndrome	
		Achondroplasia	
		Encephalocoele	
	Acquired	Morbid obesity	
		Pregnancy	
		Acromegally	
		Reduced jaw movement	Trismus
			Fibrosis
			Rheumatoid arthritis
			Jaw wiring
			Tumour
		Reduced neck movement	Cervical spine Pathology
		Airway	Oedema
			Extrinsic compression
			Tumour
			Fibrosis

intubation will be easy. A hoarse voice or the presence of stridor should alert the anaesthetist to possible laryngeal problems, such as tumour or vocal cord palsy, which may hinder the passage of an ETT. Examination of the airway can also be undertaken to detect the possibilities of difficult laryngoscopy, i.e. difficulty inserting a laryngoscope to obtain a view of the vocal cords. Examination is quick and easy to perform. Each test by itself, however, is insufficient to predict a difficult laryngoscopy although the sensitivity is increased with multiple tests.

Gross abnormalities of the face, head and neck should be immediately obvious. Many congenital abnormalities are associated with a small mouth, large tongue and cleft palate. Importantly, Down's syndrome or trisomy 21 is associated with atlanto-axial instability. Mouth opening should be examined. This tests temporomandibular joint (TMJ) movement. Mouth opening should normally be between 4–6 cm or allow access of the patient's three middle fingers. If the mouth opening is limited, for example, by spasm of the masseter and medial pterygoid muscles due to dental abscesses or fractures of the mandible, then it may not be possible for the laryngoscope to be inserted. Rheumatoid arthritis may also affect the TMJ.

Mallampatti examination (Fig. 1), takes place with the patient in the sitting position, with the head in a neutral position and the mouth open to allow examination of the pharynx. A score of 1 is associated with a Cormack & Lehane grade 1 view of the larynx (Fig. 2) 99% of the time. Mallampatti

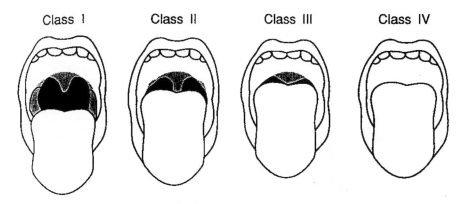

Fig. 1. Mallampatti scoring. Class 1: Pharyngeal pillars, soft palate, uvula visible. Class 2: Soft palate and uvula only visible. Class 3: Soft palate only visible. Class 4: Soft palate not visible.[7]

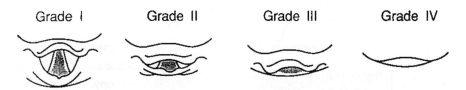

Fig. 2. Cormack & Lehane grades of laryngoscopy. Grade I: Vocal cords visible. Grade II: Posterior vocal cords and arytenoids cartilages visible. Grade III: Epiglottis only visible. Grade IV: Epiglottis not visible.[7]

scoring, however, may fail to predict 50% of difficult intubations. Thyromental distance i.e. the distance between the superior border of the thyroid cartilage and the chin with the neck in full extension, is also measured. A short thyromental distance equates with an "anterior larynx" and less space for tongue compression on insertion of the laryngoscope blade. A thyromental distance of 6.5 cm or greater is associated with easy intubation. Mandibular length may also be measured. A short mandible is associated with difficult intubation, while a length greater than 9 cm is associated with easy laryngoscopy. A short mandible or receding chin occurs in patients who have Pierre Robin syndrome. A patient's dentition may also cause difficulties, e.g. large protuberant or buckteeth may impede laryngoscopy.

The ability to extend the neck at the atlanto-occipital (AO) joint is important for intubation. Delikan (Fig. 3) devised a simple test. With the head in a neutral position whilst sitting, the index finger of the left hand is placed on the patient's jaw whilst the index finger of the right hand is placed on the patient's occiput. The patient is asked to look up (i.e. extend the AO joint) and the movement of the examiner's fingers is assessed. The cervical spine and AO joint may be involved in the disease processes of rheumatoid arthritis,

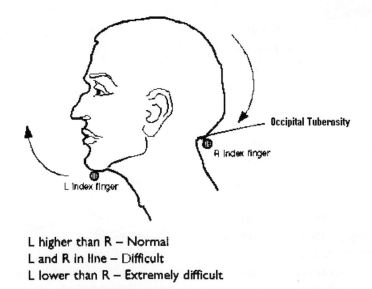

L higher than R — Normal
L and R in line — Difficult
L lower than R — Extremely difficult

Fig. 3.   Testing the movement of the occiput on the atlas. The Delikan warning signs.[8]

Table 2.   Wilson Risk Index

Parameter	Risk	
Weight	0–2	$> 90\,\text{kg} = 1 : \; > 110\,\text{kg} = 2$
Head & Neck movement	0–2	
Jaw movement	0–2	
Receding mandible	0–2	
Buck teeth	0–2	
		Maximum score 10

ankylosing spondylitis and osteoarthritis, making excessive movement of the cervical spine undesirable.

The Wilson risk index, described in 1993, combined the features of airway examination (Table 2). A total of 3 predicts 75% of difficult intubations while a score of 4 predicts 90%. The test, however, has a poor sensitivity and may fail to predict 50% of difficult intubations.

Regional anaesthesia should be used if possible to avoid the risks of a difficult and failed intubation. If general anaesthesia is required, provided the patient is not at risk of gastro-oesophageal reflux, has a full stomach or if muscle relaxation and ventilation are deemed to be necessary, this may be undertaken with a laryngeal mask.

If the patient requires intubation and muscle relaxation then the following plan may be adopted. It is essential that skilled assistance and all difficult airway aids are present prior to the start of the procedure. Skilled assistance includes a second anaesthetist and an anaesthetic assistant.

If limited mouth opening is due to trismus, a sleep dose of induction agent may be given following preoxygenation. An attempt at mask ventilation is made and if the lungs are easily inflated a short acting muscle relaxant such as suxamethonium can be given to facilitate intubation. If not, the patient is allowed to wake up whilst attempting to maintain oxygenation. If any difficulty is encountered, the patient is ventilated with oxygen and a volatile agent until spontaneous respiration commences.

For patients with a known difficult airway or a known airway obstruction, there are two options. These are inhalational induction of anaesthesia followed by the use of a fibreoptic laryngoscope or an awake fibreoptic intubation. Muscle relaxants should not be used until an ETT is secured in place with demonstration that the lungs can be ventilated. Many would argue that the safest technique when encountering a difficult airway is to use an awake fibreoptic intubation.

Failed intubation

The aim of management of a failed intubation is to maintain oxygenation whilst at the same time preventing the aspiration of gastric contents. A failed intubation drill is followed under these circumstances.

pulmonary aspiration of gastric contents

Aspiration is defined as the misdirection of gastric or pharyngeal material into the larynx and lower respiratory tract, resulting in the development of acute lung injury (ALI). Mendelson's syndrome is characterised by a severe chemical pneumonitis, which may progress to ARDS. Unless the patient has been prescribed proton pump inhibitors or H_2 antagonists, the gastric contents are usually sterile. The initial process is therefore purely inflammatory. Bacterial super infection may, however, occur.

Twenty millilitres of gastric fluid at below pH 2.5 is all that is required to develop the syndrome. However, particulate matter such as food may also cause the development of ALI. Steroids and antibiotics are of no value in the initial treatment unless there has been the possibility of regurgitation of small or large bowel contents into the stomach. Treatment is therefore supportive to maintain oxygenation and clearance of excess secretions as a result of the inflammatory process.[9]

Those at risk of regurgitation and pulmonary aspiration are detailed in Table 3. Therefore aspiration of gastric contents is more likely to occur in the pregnant, obese, non-fasted and emergency situations. The risks are also greater if the patient is in the prone position or in a head-down tilt, both due to increased intra-abdominal pressure. Although fasting guidelines exist to try to ensure gastric emptying occurs, this is not guaranteed. Rapid sequence induction of anaesthesia or regional anaesthesia should be employed to prevent this complication from arising should there be any symptoms of gastro-oesophageal reflux or doubt over the degree of gastric emptying despite appropriate fasting.

When performing a rapid sequence induction, preoxygenation with 100% oxygen is mandatory. Following induction, suxamethonium is the muscle relaxant of choice due to its rapid onset and short duration of action. It is

Table 3.   Patients at Risk of Regurgitation and Aspiration

Inadequate lower oesophageal sphincter function	Hiatus hernia
	Pregnancy
Delayed gastric emptying	Pyloric stenosis
	Opiates
	Alcohol
	Pain
	Trauma
Intra-abdominal pathology	Peritonitis
	Bowel obstruction
Increased intra-abdominal pressure	Obesity

contraindicated if there is a history of allergy, suxamethonium apnoea, a risk of malignant hyperpyrexia (see later) or muscular dystrophies. It may also lead to a dangerous rise in potassium in spinal cord injuries or burns.

Respiratory obstruction

The airway is usually maintained by a laryngeal mask (LMA), face mask or endotracheal tube. The use of oropharygeal airways may be complicated by trauma to the soft tissues of the mouth and damage to the teeth. It is also possible to stimulate the gag reflex. Nasopharygeal airways are much softer and better tolerated but may lead to bleeding and trauma to the nasal passages.

Obstruction may occur at any point from the breathing system to the alveolus. Table 4 illustrates the aetiology of obstruction.

Respiratory obstruction can be divided into two categories: complete and partial. Complete obstruction will rapidly lead to hypoxia if not corrected.

In the spontaneously breathing patient, partial respiratory obstruction will present as noisy and laboured respiration, with a poorly moving reservoir bag in the circuit and a slow-rising capnograph trace. Attempts to improve the airway should be undertaken. If an LMA is in place this may need to be repositioned. If not, 100% oxygen should be given while simple manoeuvres such as a chin lift or jaw thrust to elevate the tongue should be undertaken in an effort to open the airway. If this is unsuccessful the oropharynx should be suctioned to remove any secretions or debris and an oral or nasophayngeal airway inserted.

Table 4.   The Aetiology of Respiratory Obstruction

Equipment	Breathing circuit	Kinked Foreign body Valve malfunction	
	ETT	External compression Internal occlusion	Surgical gag Mucus Cuff herniation
Patient	Orophaynx	Loss of muscle tone Soft tissue oedema Secretions Tumour Foreign body	
	Larynx	Laryngospasm Recurrent laryngeal nerve palsy Tumour Foreign body Oedema	
	Trachea	Extrinsic compression	
	Bronchial tree	Secretions Bronchospasm Pneumothorax Tumour	

Complete obstruction presents as silent respiration with no reservoir bag movement and no capnograph trace. The patient will have paradoxical chest and abdominal movement (so-called see-sawing) and a tracheal tug. This is a life-threatening situation and the simple manoeuvres described above should be immediately undertaken. It may, however, quickly become apparent that to overcome the obstruction the patient will require urgent intubation.

In the ventilated patient, complete obstruction will present with high peak airway pressures, an apnoeic capnograph trace and oxygen desaturation. It is usually due to an equipment problem. The breathing system should be examined immediately as this is the commonest location of a complete obstruction. A fine suction catheter may also need to be passed down the ETT to confirm patency. If not patent, the ETT should be removed and the patient reoxygenated prior to reintubation. If no equipment cause is found, medical conditions need to be considered.

Laryngospasm

Laryngospasm is a fairly common complication that occurs during light anaesthesia. If the laryngeal reflexes are not completely suppressed, any foreign body, such as mucus, oropharyngeal airway or intense surgical stimulation such as anal stretching, may lead to reflex closure of the glottis. This is a protective reflex to prevent foreign body aspiration. The treatment of laryngospasm includes administration of 100% oxygen, clearing of any secretions from the pharynx, addition of continuous positive airway pressure (CPAP) and cessation of surgical stimulation. It usually resolves with simple measures. If not, the patient should be intubated using a short-acting muscle relaxant such as suxamethonium.

Bronchospasm

Bronchospasm occurs due to increased reflex activity of the smooth muscle and production of excessive mucus within the bronchial tree. This leads to an increase in the resistance to breathing and airflow obstruction. Bronchospasm may occur in patients who have poorly treated asthma, recent upper or lower respiratory tract infections, anaphylaxis and the administration of drugs such as non-steroidal anti-inflammatories, muscle relaxants and opiates.

The treatment includes confirmation of bronchospasm, the deepening of anaesthesia with an inhalational agent such as Sevoflurane and the administration of 100% oxygen. In severe cases, intravenous bronchodilators such as salbutamol, theophylline and magnesium may be considered. It is also important to exclude the presence of a pneumothorax (see later).

Pneumothorax

Any history of chest wall trauma, rib fracture, traumatic central venous line insertion or chronic lung disease may present as a pneumothorax during anaesthesia. This is potentiated by the use of nitrous oxide because it is insoluble in blood and will diffuse into any air-containing cavity, leading to an increase in the pressure and volume of that cavity. Unrecognised, this may result in a tension pneumothorax leading to hypoxia and ultimately cardiac arrest. Initially there will be uneven air entry with higher peak airway pressures on ventilation, hypoxia, tachyarrhythmias and hypotension.

A pneumothorax should be immediately decompressed. If it is a tension pneumothorax it should be decompressed by a carefully placed canula in the second intercostals space anteriorly in the mid-clavicular line, followed by chest drain insertion. This complication may be prevented by the siting of chest drains in any patient with a preoperative history of chest wall trauma.

Hypoxia during anaesthesia

The aetiology of hypoxia or desaturation during anaesthesia is shown in Table 5. It occurs frequently in the perioperative period and unrecognised, the outcome is disastrous. Hypoxia initially results in sweating, tachycardia and hypertension followed by a terminal bradycardia. The spontaneously breathing patient will be tachypnoeic.

Hypoxia may first be noticed by desaturation monitored by pulse oximetry. Cyanosis is an unreliable sign. The cause should be immediately identified and corrected. Initial ventilation with 100% oxygen, followed by examination of the equipment, circuit and patient should identify the cause.

Table 5.   Hypoxia During Anaesthesia

Hypoxic gas mixture	Equipment	Disconnection circuit Obstruction of circuit Oxygen failure	
Hypoventilation	Equipment Patient	Ventilator failure Slow respiratory rate	
V/Q Mismatch	Patient	Inadequate ventilation	Secretions Endobronchial intubation Atelectasis Bronchospasm Pneumothorax Aspiration Pulmonary oedema
		Inadequate perfusion	Hypotension Low cardiac output Thromboembolism Gas embolism

COMPLICATIONS OF THE CARDIOVASCULAR SYSTEM

The effects of anaesthesia on normal cardiovascular physiology will be briefly discussed prior to the sections on complications of hypotension, hypertension, arrhythmia, ischaemia and embolism.

In general, the use of anaesthetic agents results in a reduction of blood pressure and cardiac output.[10] Table 6 details the physiological effects of the anaesthetic agents currently in use.

Catecholamine sensitivity is most marked with halothane, resulting in an increased incidence of arrhythmias due to myocardial excitability. This is augmented by hypercapnia and hypoxaemia and enhanced by concurrent administration of epinephrine in local anaesthetics. The maximum dose of epinephrine (adrenaline) with concurrent halothane anaesthesia is 1 mg in 10 min, i.e. 10 ml of 1:100,000 adrenaline. Concentrations greater than 1:100,000 should be avoided.

Hypotension

Hypotension is defined as a fall of the systolic blood pressure by 25%. This is especially important in patients with pre-existing hypertension. Postural

Table 6.   Effects of Anaesthetic Agents on Cardiovascular Physiology

Agent	Heart Rate	Cardiac Output	Peripheral Resistance	Blood Pressure	Catecholamine Sensitivity
Thiopentone	↔	↓	↔	↓	↔
Propofol	↔	↓	↓	↓	↔
Etomodate	↔	↔	↔	↔	↔
Ketamine	↑	↑	↑	↑	↔
N$_2$O	↑	↑	↔	↔	↑
Halothane	↓	↓	↓	↓	↑
Enflurane	↑	↓	↓	↓	↑
Isoflurane	↑	↓	↓	↓	↑
Desflurane	↑	↓	↓	↓	↑
Sevoflurane	↔	↓	↓	↓	↑

↑ Increase.
↓ Decrease.
↔ No change.

hypotension is a common consequence of positioning of the patient, especially when tilted or if the extremities are dependent. Mean Arterial Pressure (MAP) is equal to the product of Cardiac Output (CO) and Systemic Vascular Resistance (SVR) [2.1], whilst Cardiac Output is the product of Heart Rate (HR) and Stroke Volume (SV) [2.2]. Therefore any reduction in heart rate, stroke volume and/or systemic vascular resistance will lead to a fall in MAP, i.e. Hypotension.

$$MAP = CO \times SVR \quad [2.1]$$
$$CO = HR \times SV \quad [2.2]$$

Stroke volume is related to pre-load, i.e. venous return, so any obstruction to venous return will ultimately reduce cardiac output and mean arterial pressure. This may, for example, occur during pregnancy when the gravid uterus compresses the aorta and inferior vena cava against the vertebral bodies. A similar problem may be seen with large abdominal tumours. Those at risk require the insertion of a wedge or a left lateral tilt on the operating table. Similarly, when the patient is placed in the prone position, it is important that any supports do not compress the abdomen as this could lead to a decreased venous return.

Adequate preoperative resuscitation with fluids is especially important in patients with pronounced fluid losses such as burns, bowel obstruction, active bleeding and sepsis. A guide to adequate fluid resuscitation should be a urine output greater than 0.5 ml/kg/h and a normal heart rate, MAP and CVP. If the blood pressure drops dramatically intra-operatively, the usual cause is surgical haemorrhage. Whatever the cause, 100% oxygen and intravenous fluids should be immediately administered. At the same time, examination of the patient should be undertaken. This includes a review of the ECG to exclude any obvious myocardial problem, while maintaining a high index of suspicion for anaphylaxis, concealed haemorrhage and pneumothorax.

Hypotension resulting from vasodilation occurring with anaesthetic overdosage or neuraxial blockade usually responds well to the administration of fluids and sympathomimetics such as ephedrine or metaraminol.

Hypertension

The most common causes of hypertension are as follows:

- inadequate anaesthesia/awareness,
- inadequate analgesia,

- inadequately treated hypertension,
- hypoxia,
- hypercapnia,
- undiagnosed pre-existing hypertension,
- drug over-dosage: epinephrine, ephedrine, metaraminol, norepinephrine,
- phaechromocytoma, and
- malignant hyperthermia (see later).

Any obvious underlying problem such as hypoxia, hypercapnia or inadequate analgesia must be rectified.

Arrhythmia

Disturbances of rhythm are the most commonly reported critical incidents. Bradycardia is defined as a heart rate less than 60 beats per minute, and tachy-cardia a heart rate greater than 100 beats per minute.

If a disturbance of rhythm is observed, two questions should be asked:

1. How is the patient?
2. What is the rhythm?

The first question addresses the patient's condition. Do they have a pulse? Do they have any evidence of adverse signs? The presence or absence of adverse signs determines the course of action to be taken.

Adverse signs include evidence of a low cardiac output, tachy- or bradycar-dia and heart failure. Evidence of a low cardiac output includes cold extremities, pallor, diaphoresis (sweat) and hypotension. If the patient is awake following a regional anaesthetic technique, there may be confusion and an impaired level of consciousness as a result of a reduction in cerebral blood flow and cerebral perfusion pressure.

Tachycardia

Myocardial oxygen delivery occurs during the period of diastole in the cardiac cycle. As heart rate increases, the diastolic time gradually decreases, thereby reducing the time available for coronary blood flow. Excessive tachycardia results in impaired oxygen delivery at a time of increasing oxygen demands and may therefore produce myocardial ischaemia. Narrow complex tachycardias are not tolerated above 200 beats per minute whilst broad complex tachycardias are not tolerated above a ventricular rate of 150 beats per minute.

Bradycardia

Patients with a poor cardiac reserve do not tolerate heart rates below 40 beats per minute.

Heart failure

Heart failure may occur with any arrhythmia because the efficiency of the heart as a pump declines in abnormal rhythm states. This may lead to an elevation of left atrial pressure and subsequent pulmonary oedema.

Aetiology

Arrhythmias occur for a variety of reasons. These include electrolyte abnormalities, excessive sympathetic or parasympathetic stimulation, cervical or anal stretch (leading to bradycardia), myocardial ischaemia, use of anti-arrhythmic agents, anaesthetic drugs (halothane) and underlying myocardial abnormalities such as accessory pathways in the Wolf Parkinson White syndrome.

Management

Treatment options for any arrhythmia include the cessation of any surgical activity that may be initiating the rhythm, such as bradycardia occurring at the pneumoperitoneum during laparoscopic surgery, the correction of any underlying electrolyte abnormality, the use of anti-arrhythmic drugs and dc cardioversion and pacing (Figs. 4 and 5).

The failure to manage any arrhythmia appropriately may lead to a loss of cardiac output and subsequent cardiac arrest. The management of cardiac arrest using the universal advanced life support algorithm is shown in Fig. 6.

Myocardial ischaemia

Myocardial ischaemia occurs when there is an imbalance in the myocardial supply/demand ratio, i.e. the supply of oxygen to the myocardium is insufficient for its demands. Episodes of hypertension increase the afterload and therefore the work of the heart, leading to ischaemia, whilst episodes of hypotension reduce coronary perfusion pressure and therefore blood flow. A

Bradycardia Algorithm

(includes rates inappropriately slow for haemodynamic state)

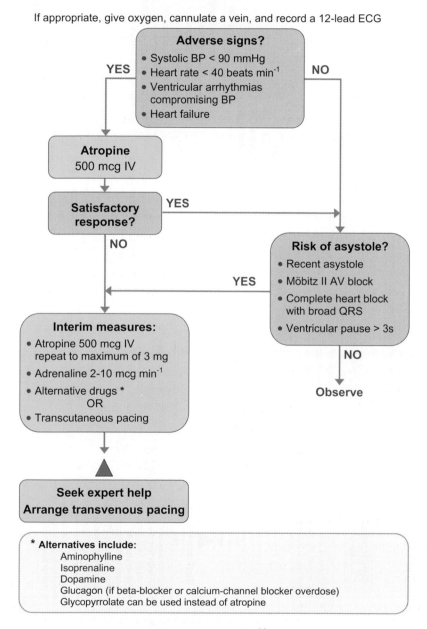

If appropriate, give oxygen, cannulate a vein, and record a 12-lead ECG

Adverse signs?
- Systolic BP < 90 mmHg
- Heart rate < 40 beats min^{-1}
- Ventricular arrhythmias compromising BP
- Heart failure

Atropine
500 mcg IV

Satisfactory response?

Risk of asystole?
- Recent asystole
- Möbitz II AV block
- Complete heart block with broad QRS
- Ventricular pause > 3s

Observe

Interim measures:
- Atropine 500 mcg IV repeat to maximum of 3 mg
- Adrenaline 2-10 mcg min^{-1}
- Alternative drugs *
  OR
- Transcutaneous pacing

Seek expert help
Arrange transvenous pacing

* Alternatives include:
 Aminophylline
 Isoprenaline
 Dopamine
 Glucagon (if beta-blocker or calcium-channel blocker overdose)
 Glycopyrrolate can be used instead of atropine

Fig. 4.   Bradycardia.[11]

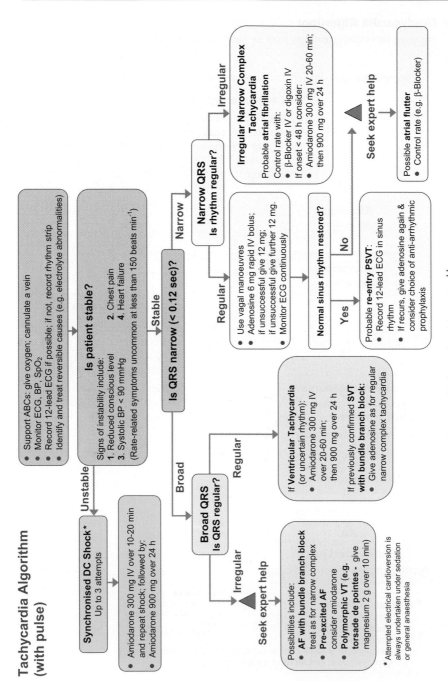

Fig. 5.   Tachycardia with a pulse.[11]

Adult Advanced Life Support Algorithm

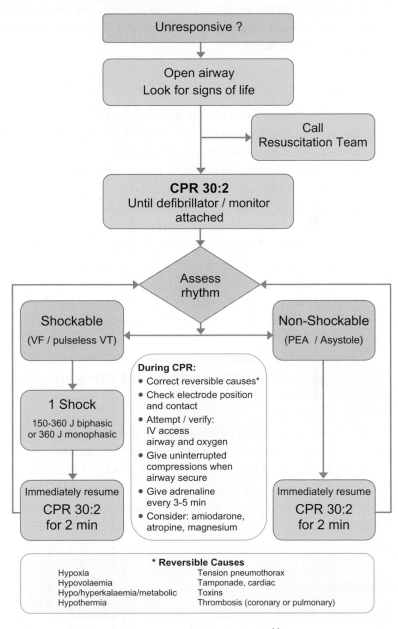

Fig. 6.   The management of cardiac arrest.[11]

tachycardia reduces the diastolic time required for coronary perfusion, therefore reducing the oxygen supply to the myocardium. The sub-endocardial area of the heart is a watershed area of perfusion and is most at risk of ischaemic damage intra-operatively.

Clinical features

Patients with ischaemic heart disease are most at risk. It usually presents as an arrhythmia, ST segment changes, hypotension and pulmonary oedema. There may, however, be no clinical features of ischaemia intra-operatively. The use of the CM5 electrode position for ECG monitoring gives the best indication of left ventricular ischaemia intra-operatively.

The goals of treatment are to reverse and prevent further myocardial ischaemia. This is achieved by improving the myocardial oxygen supply demand ratio, by preventing hypertension, hypotension, hypoxia and hypercapnia, while using an anaesthetic technique appropriate to the patient's state of health.

In 2002, the American College of Cardiology and the American Heart Association published a task force document allowing effective risk stratification for patients.[12]

The patient's history and physical examination are the crux of the strategy. The patient and intervention are classified into different groups of risks. Table 7 shows patient-associated risks while intervention-associated risk factors are shown in Table 8.

The functional capacity of the patient is also taken into account. Patients who can climb two flights of stairs without angina or dyspnoea, i.e. New York Heart Association (NYHA) class II or better, Canadian Cardiovascular Society (CCS) class II or better, are considered to have an acceptable level of function. Table 9 shows the abbreviated synopsis of patient- and intervention-associated risk factors and risk stratification of the American Heart Association task force report.

Embolism

Embolism is defined as the transfer of abnormal material by the circulation. Of particular importance in anaesthesia are those of gas embolism, thromboembolism and amniotic fluid embolism.

Table 7.   Patient-Associated Risks (CCS Canadian Cardiovascular Society)

High Risk	Intermediate Risk	Low Risk
Unstable angina or MI within last 30 days	Stable angina pectoris (CCS class I or II)	Higher age
PCI/stent implantation within last 4 weeks	Compensated heart failure without actual decompensation	Abnormal ECG
Congestive heart failure with actual signs of decompensation	Previous MI > 30 days	No sinus rhythm on ECG
Dysrythmia (2nd or 3rd degree AV block, SVT without uncontrolled ventricular rate, non-sustained or sustained VT)	Serum creatinine > 2.0 mg/dl	History of stroke
Severe valvular dysfunction (aortic or mitral stenosis)	Diabetes mellitus	Sub-optimally treated hypertension
Pulmonary hypertension		
Intra-cardiac shunts with right-left shunt and cyanosis		

Table 8.   Intervention-Associated Risk Factors

High Risk	Intermediate Risk	Low Risk
Emergency operation, specially in older people	Carotid endarterectomy	Endoscopic intervention
Surgery on aorta or other major vessels	Head and neck surgery	Superficial procedures
Peripheral vascular surgery	Intraperitoneal or intra-thoracic surgery	Ophthalmic surgery
Prolonged surgical procedures with large fluid shifts or blood losses	Orthopaedic surgery	Breast surgery
	Prostate surgery	

Table 9.   Patient- and Intervention-Associated Risk Factors and Risk Stratification of the American Heart Association Task Force Report

| | Patient-Associated Risk | | |
Intervention-Associated Risk	Low	Intermediate	High
Low	Surgery ok	Surgery ok	Surgery ok
Medium	Surgery ok	Surgery ok	Further diagnosis
High	Surgery ok	Further diagnosis	Diagnosis + Treatment

Gas embolism

This is the entry of gas, usually air, into the circulatory system and usually occurs from the venous circulation, when the pressure in an open vein is less than atmospheric pressure, thereby permitting gas entry. Procedures at particular risk are: sinus and mastoid surgery, posterior fossa neurosurgery or the sitting position, laparoscopy, hysteroscopy and arthroscopy, hip surgery, caesarean section and the insertion of venous cannulae, especially CVP lines.

The clinical presentation varies with the rate of gas entry. Gas will pass through the venous side of the circulation and collect in the right atrium. If a sufficient volume accumulates there will be obstruction to venous return and subsequent cardiac arrest. If an atrial or ventricular septal defect is present then gas bubbles may cross to the systemic circulation and manifest themselves clinically as myocardial ischaemia, stroke or arterial embolism.

Examination may reveal a mill wheel murmur. There will be a fall in the end tidal CO_2 trace on capnography as cardiac output falls, with gas accumulation in the pulmonary circulation leading to an increase in respiratory dead space.

Initially treatment is to ventilate with 100% oxygen and support the circulation whilst flooding the surgical area with saline to prevent further entrainment of gas. Turning the patient onto the left lateral position allows gas to accumulate in the right atrium whence insertion of a central venous catheter may allow aspiration.

Thromboembolism

Virchow's triad of venous stasis, hypercoagulability of blood and intimal wall trauma predispose to the formation of blood clot within veins. Patients particularly at risk of venous thrombus formation within the deep veins of the pelvis are those with pelvic trauma, immobility, dehydration, malignancy, smoking, on the oral contraceptive pill and those with hereditary deficiencies of protein c and protein s.

Venous thromboembolism is itself rare during the intra-operative period but more common in the postoperative period due to relative immobility of patients and the hypercoagulable state that develops as a stress response to surgery.

The clinical features are those of an initial arrhythmia, with probable cardiovascular collapse with hypotension and desaturation due to an increase in pulmonary dead space and obstruction to venous return. If thromboembolism occurs the patient should be ventilated with 100% oxygen, fluid resuscitated and inotropes commenced to support the circulation. Thrombolytic therapy can be instituted in an attempt to lyse the clot. Prevention is better than cure, however. Prophylactic anti-coagulation with low molecular weight heparin and the use of TED stockings and pneumatic compression stockings intra-operatively all reduce the risk of thrombus formation.

OTHER COMPLICATIONS

Awareness

Very rarely the patient is able to recall events that occurred during general anaesthesia. This can be extremely distressing and worsened by the hospital and its staff denying it occurred. It is most likely to occur during the induction or recovery of anaesthesia, especially if there have been multiple attempts at intubation. Certain techniques, such as the high oxygen and low volatile concentrations employed for caesarean sections or the moribund patient, carry a higher risk. Clinically, the presence of a tachycardia, hypertension, lacrimation, dilated pupils and sweating are indicative of light anaesthesia. The patient may be unable to move because of the use of muscle relaxants. No single measurement is a reliable indicator of the level of consciousness.

Adverse Drug Reactions

Adverse drug reactions are defined as the effects of a drug that are of no therapeutic, diagnostic or prophylactic benefit to the patient. There are two broad categories. Type A are the more common dose-related effects and are an extension of the pharmacological effects of a drug. Type B adverse drug reactions are rare, non-dose related and not related to the usual pharmacological effect of the drug. Type B reactions can be subdivided into anaphylactic reactions and anaphylactoid reactions.

Anaphylactic reactions

These are an example of an exaggerated immune response to a drug to which an individual is sensitised. The reaction is IgE mediated, resulting in degranulation of mast cells and basophils which lead to the release of histamine, serotonin and other vasoactive substances. There is usually a history of prior exposure to the drug.

Anaphylactoid reactions

Anaphylactoid reactions are clinically indistinguishable from anaphylactic reactions. The difference between them however, is that it is not IgE mediated.

Incidence

There are approximately 319 cases per year in the United Kingdom, 55 of which are directly related to anaesthetic agents.

Clinical presentation

The clinical features of an anaphylactic/anaphylactoid reaction usually occur immediately following induction but can occur at any time during anaesthesia. The most common presentation is of cardiovascular collapse with bronchospasm. Table 10 shows the common features at presentation of such a reaction.

Management

The Association of Anaesthetists of Great Britain and Ireland has produced an anaphylaxis drill. Every physician should be competent at managing anaphylaxis. The severity of the reaction may vary but early use of oxygen and epinephrine are advocated. Figure 7 details such a drill.

MANAGEMENT OF A PATIENT WITH SUSPECTED ANAPHYLAXIS DURING ANAESTHESIA:
MODEL OPERATING PROCEDURE/GUIDELINE

1. Stop administration of all agents likely to have caused the anaphylaxis.

2. Call for help

3   Maintain airway, give 100% oxygen and lie patient flat with legs elevated.

4. Give epinephrine (adrenaline). This may be given intramuscularly in a dose of 0.5 mg to 1 mg (0.5 to 1 ml of 1:1,000) and may be repeated every 10 minutes according to the arterial pressure and pulse until improvement occurs.

    Alternatively, 50 to 100 micrograms intravenously (0.5 to 1 ml of 1:10,000) over 1 minute has been recommended for hypotension with titration of further doses as required.

    Never give undiluted epinephrine 1:1000 intravenously

    In a patient with cardiovascular collapse, 0.5 to 1 mg (5 to 10 ml of 1:10,000) may be required intravenously in divided doses by titration. This should be given at a rate of 0.1 mg/minute stopping when a response has been obtained.

    Paediatric doses of epinephrine depend on the age of the child. Intramuscular epinephrine 1:1000 should be administered as follows

>12 years	500 micrograms IM (0.5ml)
6-12 years	250 micrograms IM (0.25ml)
>6 months-6 years	120 micrograms IM (0.12ml)
<6 months	50 micrograms IM (0.05ml)

    Start rapid intravenous infusion with colloids or crystalloids. Adult patients may require 2 to 4 litres of crystalloid.

Secondary Therapy

1. Give antihistamines (chlorpheniramine 10-20 mg by slow intravenous infusion)

2. Give corticosteroids (100 to 500 mg hydrocortisone slowly iv).

3. Bronchodilators may be required for persistent bronchospasm.

Statement

This guideline is not a standard of medical care. The ultimate judgement with regard to a particular clinical procedure or treatment plan must be made by the clinician in light of the clinical data presented and the diagnostic and treatment options available. The guideline will be reviewed in the light of new knowledge and will be reissued in 2008.

Fig. 7.   Management of a patient with suspected anaphylaxis during anaesthesia.[13]

Table 10.   Clinical Features at Presentation of Anaphylaxis

Feature	Percentage
No pulse	25.9
Difficult to inflate lungs	23.7
Flush	18.1
Desaturation	10.6
Cough	6.7
Rash	4.2
ECG abnormality	2.2
Urticaria	1.8
Subjective	1.5
Swelling	1.18
No bleeding	0.3
Other	3.2

The investigation of a patient following such a reaction should take place immediately. Three samples should be taken for mast cell tryptase, the timing of which should be immediately following treatment, 1 hour and between 6 and 24 hours after the reaction. Tryptase is an enzyme found within mast cells. Following degranulation tryptase is released into the circulation. This occurs in both anaphylactic and anaphylactoid reactions. A negative result however does not exclude anaphylaxis. The anaesthetist is responsible for referral to the anaphylaxis services within their hospital. The patient should be fully investigated, informed and counselled.

Latex Allergy

Latex is derived from the lactiferous cells of the rubber tree, *Hevea brasiliensis*. Latex contains a vast number of polypeptides which all vary in the potential to produce an allergic response. The incidence of latex allergy is increasing. Those at greatest risk are:

- atopic individuals,
- patients with spina bifida,
- congenital urological abnormalities,

- frequent urological surgery, and
- health care workers.

The incidence in the US is less than 5% of the general population but between 10–30% in health care workers. Latex allergy is increased in populations with chronic exposure to latex.

Latex is found in abundance in the hospital environment. Gloves, tourniquets, blood pressure cuffs, ECG electrodes, stethoscopes, catheters, IV tube ports, syringes, goggles, wound drains, dressings, multidose vials, tires, handgrips, balloons, condoms and many other pieces of equipment to name but a few.[14]

Two types of clinical syndromes are seen:

Type IV Delayed Hypersensitivity — This develops within 1–2 days of exposure of cutaneous or mucus membranes to latex. The chemicals are processed within Langerhans cells of the skin and mucus membranes. The antigens are then presented to cutaneous T-cells leading to the formation of dermatitis.

Type I Hypersensitivity Reactions — The clinical features of these have been discussed earlier under anaphylaxis. The clinical scenario occurs approximately 30 minutes following induction of anaesthesia, usually when the patient has had a body cavity opened, for example, at laparotomy. A full-blown type I hypersensitivity reaction will develop.

Treatment

The aims of treatment should be prevention and thus commenced preoperatively. Admission to hospital should be on the morning of surgery, thereby limiting exposure to environmental latex. The patient should be first on the operating list for the same reason. Latex free equipment should be utilised. Pre-medication with histamine 1 and 2 receptor type blockers can be utilised although these are not proven to be effective. Treatment of any reaction is as described above under the management of anaphylaxis.

Malignant Hyperpyrexia

Malignant hyperpyrexia is an inherited disorder of skeletal muscle that can be triggered by anaesthetic drugs (all inhalational agents and suxamethonium). It is very rare (around 1 in 50,000 anaesthetics) but potentially fatal. Clinical features arise as a consequence of loss of skeletal muscle homeostasis leading to a raised intracellular calcium concentration. This causes muscle rigidity, hypermetabolism and muscle breakdown. Clinically these lead to oxygen desaturation, excessive production of CO_2 leading to acidosis, excessive heat production, raised serum potassium levels leading to arrhythmias, acute renal failure and disseminated intravascular coagulation. Morbidity and mortality are reduced by prompt intervention. Treatment is supportive. All triggering agents should be discontinued and 100% oxygen administered. Active cooling measures should be commenced. The only drug that is effective in limiting the accumulation of intracellular calcium is dantrolene. Up to 10 mg/kg may be required. At the same time acidosis and hyperkalaemia should be treated with hyperventilation, bicarbonate and insulin/dextrose.

Hepatitis

Hepatic injury is a rare complication of repeat anaesthesia. It may be precipitated by all the commonly used volatile agents, although halothane is the most common cause. Two forms of hepatic injury have been described: a more common mild form and a rare fulminant form with massive hepatic necrosis. Obese patients and being female increases the risk. Medication that increases cytochrome P450, such as isoniazid, phenobarbitone or dexamethasone, all increase the risk of hepatic injury. Treatment is essentially symptomatic. It is best to avoid all agents in patients who sustain hepatic injury after the use of one of the volatile agents. A total intravenous technique is suitable for such cases.

Massive Blood Transfusion

Major haemorrhage is a rare complication of surgery and trauma. There are no fixed definitions of a major haemorrhage but many would include:

- the use of "O" negative blood,
- the use of more than 10 units of blood in 24 hours, and
- the immediate use of 4 units.

The problems associated with massive blood transfusion can be considered as early or late complications.

Early complications

These can be either rate- or volume-related. Rate-related complications are shown in Table 11 and volume-related complications in Table 12.

   Blood should be administered through a blood warmer to prevent the effects of hypothermia. Calcium and magnesium may require to be supplemented and hyperkalaemia treated. In addition, transfused haemoglobin will not carry oxygen as efficiently, the oxygen dissociation curve having shifted to the left due to depletion of 2,3-diphosphoglycerate and hypothermia and acidosis.

Late complications

- Adult respiratory distress syndrome (ARDS)
- Allergy: haemolytic and non-haemolytic transfusion reactions
- Depression of immune function
- Disease transmission: vCJD, HIV, CMV, hepatitis, parasites and syphilis[15]

Table 11.   Rate-Related Complications

Complications	Triggering Rate
Hypocalcaemia	1 ml/kg/min
Hyperkalaemia	0.3 ml/kg/min
Hypothermia	1 unit decreases core temperature by 0.4°C
Acidosis	1 ml/kg/min
Hypomagnesaemia	Undefined

Table 12.   Volume-Related Complications

Complications	Triggering Volume
Procoagulant dilution (fibrinogen < 1.0 g/dl)	> 1.4 blood volumes
Thrombocytopaenia (platelets < 50,000)	> 2.3 blood volumes

The volumes relate to patients where euvolaemia was maintained.

COMPLICATIONS OF LOCAL AND REGIONAL ANAESTHESIA

Local anaesthetic agents block conductance along all types of nerves. Motor, sensory and autonomic nerves are all affected to a varying degree. It is advocated for high-risk patients as neuraxial blockade reduces postoperative mortality and other serious complications. However, it must be recognised that regional anaesthesia itself carries risks of its own. In all cases there is a risk of introducing infection, a potential for greater than expected spread, and intravascular or intraneural injection. The incidence of cardiac arrest is 6 per 10,000 following a spinal anaesthetic. Transient neurological sequelae have a similar incidence. Damage to surrounding structures (e.g. pleura) also needs to be considered. In addition, it is time consuming and most blocks have a failure rate, at best, of 5%. Clearly the operator needs to understand the regional anatomy and be able to deal with any complication that may arise. Proper training and supervision to acquire the necessary experience and competence is essential. Rarely serious and permanent damage may occur. One of the most significant risk factors is multiple attempts at performing a block. Three unsuccessful attempts warrant a call for help, a different approach or abandonment.

When a regional block is used to supplement general anaesthesia it should be placed before induction. Exceptions to this include poorly co-operative patients, children and an inability to correctly position the patient, for example, due to pain from fractures. The potential for undetected nerve damage is much greater when the patient is unconscious as postoperative neurological dysfunction is strongly associated with paraesthesia on needle placement or pain on injection.

Spinal Anaesthesia

A spinal anaesthetic leads to motor, sensory and autonomic nerve block-ade. Autonomic nerve dysfunction may require bladder catheterisation. More importantly, the systolic blood pressure may fall and require support with intra-venous fluids and vasoconstrictor agents. If the spread of the local anaesthetic is too high, respiratory failure may result.

A complication of spinal anaesthesia is post-dural puncture headache. This risk is reduced by the use of pencil point needles. However, in turn, these increase the risk of spinal cord injury, as they have to be inserted further into the intrathecal space. Other complications include meningitis and arachnoiditis.

Epidural Anaesthesia

The most commonly sited epidurals are in the lumber region, especially for the relief of pain during labour and delivery. However, epidurals may also be sited in the thoracic and cervical regions. In the latter case, the incidence of side effects is high and include hypotension, bradycardia, respiratory failure and dural puncture. An epidural infection is very rare (1 in 150,000). An abscess requires urgent evacuation and aggressive antibiotic therapy.

The use of catheters prolongs the duration of the block. However, these catheters may penetrate blood vessels or pass through the dura into the CSF. This may lead to a "total" spinal as described below. The insertion or removal of these catheters increases the risk of an epidural haematoma. This is very rare (1 in 200,000) but may cause paraplegia and requires urgent evacuation. It may also occur after a straightforward epidural or spinal anaesthetic. The increasing use of prophylactic anti-thrombotic agents has lead to an increased incidence, especially when low molecular weight heparins were introduced.

Strict guidelines are required to permit the safe use of regional anaesthesia in patients who are receiving medication for DVT prophylaxis. Aspirin has an antiplatelet effect that persists for 7 days while platelet function returns to normal within 3 days of stopping NSAIDs. It is safe to proceed with central blockade in patients taking these drugs. COX-2 inhibitors do not affect platelet function. Clopidogrel is a potent anti-platelet agent. There are reports of fatal bleeding complications associated with it. It should be stopped 7 days before surgery or central neural blockade is performed. Guidelines regarding low molecular weight heparins recommend waiting 12 hours after administration before a central block is undertaken or a catheter removed. Warfarin should be stopped and surgery or central blockade only performed once the INR is 1.5 or less.

Upper Limb Blocks

The brachial plexus can be blocked at a variety of levels. In general, the higher the level the more complete is the block. However there are major variations in the anatomy that may lead to failure or significant side effects.

The interscalene approach tends to fail to achieve an adequate block on the ulnar side of the arm. It may also lead to a Horner's syndrome and phrenic nerve palsy. The latter may lead to respiratory compromise. In addition, rarely the injection may be made into the subarachnoid/epidural space or the vertebral artery. Spread to the recurrent laryngeal nerve may lead to hoarseness and the possibility of aspiration.

The supraclavicular approach provides a more reliable block of the arm. However, it has the highest incidence of pneumothorax and phrenic nerve palsy is also possible. The subclavian artery may also be punctured.

The infraclavicular approach carries a much less risk of pneumothorax while the axillary approach, though having few side-effects, is only useful for surgery to the hand, wrist and lower forearm. In the latter case the artery may be punctured and lead to a haematoma.

In addition, the peripheral nerves can all be blocked distally at the anticubital fossa and wrist. The most important complication is when performing a block of the ulnar nerve at the elbow where it runs behind the medial epicondyle. The risks of intraneural injection or ischaemia are higher because of the limited space available.

Cervical plexus

Regional anaesthesia can be used for operations in the neck, including carotid artery surgery. Potential complications include intravascular injection, producing immediate unconsciousness and seizures, subarachnoid injection producing a total spinal and phrenic nerve palsy. Other potential complications can be predicated from a knowledge of the local anatomy and include hoarseness, dysphagia, stellate ganglion block and a Horner's syndrome.

Lower Limb

In many respects, lower limb blocks are safer than upper limb blocks because surrounding structures are less important.

Intravenous regional anaesthesia (Bier's block) — This can be very useful in certain situations. However, it is of limited duration and there is the potential of leakage of the local anaesthetic with significant systemic toxicity. When using a double tourniquet care must be taken that the wrong cuff is not deflated.

Local Anaesthetic Toxicity

The toxicity of local anaesthetics is manifested when they are injected inadvertently into the circulation. The main effects are on the central nervous and cardiovascular systems. Symptoms include visual disturbances, dizziness, circumoral tingling and tinnitus. Signs include agitation or sedation, tremor and epileptic fits. Eventually apnoea and coma ensue. From a cardiovascular viewpoint there may be collapse, with hypotension, tachyarrhythmias, ventricular fibillation and later cardiac arrest. Therapy is again non-specific and supportive. The most important aspect of management, however, is prevention through awareness of the blood vessels in the vicinity of the injection.

Total Spinal

A "total" spinal results from the inadvertent injection into the CSF of a large volume of local anaesthetic when performing epidural, paravertebral or psoas compartment blocks. It may also rarely occur when performing cervical or interscalene brachial plexus blocks. There is typically motor blockade with a high sensor block. If it reaches the cervical spine, respiratory failure due to block of the phrenic nerves may result. Spread to the cerebral CSF will lead to unconsciousness, respiratory arrest and severe hypotension leading to cardiac arrest. Treatment is supportive.

THEATRE ENVIRONMENT AND EQUIPMENT

All equipment needs to be maintained on a regular basis by appropriately trained personnel. For example, heated humidifiers are thermostatically controlled. If the temperature is incorrectly set too low there is a risk of infection, while if set too high there is a risk of airway burns. Condensation may also accumulate in the inspiratory limb, potentially leading to obstruction.

Electricity

There are potential dangers associated with the direct application of electrical equipment to the human body, whether a patient or a member of staff. Electricity can cause morbidity or mortality by one of three processes: electrocution, burns or ignition of flammable materials. Damage depends upon the density, type and duration of current.

The effects of electrocution occur when a connection is made between a live wire and earth. There are two potential sources: faulty equipment, where a live wire may be touching the casing, or leakage currents, which arise because equipment is at a higher potential than earth. In the UK, all medical equipment should meet the requirements of the *British Standard 5724: Safety of Medical Equipment* which is identical to the corresponding international standard (International Electro-technical Committee standard in IEC 601). The degree of protection is defined by the type designation. Type CF provide the highest degree of protection and have a maximum leakage current of $< 10\,\mu A$.

The current density (amount of current flowing per unit area) has different effects, varying from a tingling sensation (1 mA, 50 Hz AC) to ventricular fibrillation (75 mA). If the current flows directly or in close proximity to the heart, the current density will be very much greater and a substantially smaller amount ($50\,\mu A$) can cause ventricular fibrillation. This is known as microshock. Equipment which may allow this include central venous catheters (which should be filled with dextrose rather than saline), intracardiac pacemakers with an external lead and even an oesophageal temperature probe.

When an electrical current is passed through a resistance, heat is produced. Electrical burns are most marked on or near the skin. Surgical diathermy equipment uses the heating effects of high frequency electrical current but accidents may result in burns, fires or by effecting pacemakers. Unipolar diathermy can inhibit or damage pacemakers and thus if essential, bipolar diathermy should be used but if so should be applied distant from the pacemaker. The defibrillation and anti-tachycardia functions of implantable cardioverter defibrillators should be deactivated if diathermy is to be used to avoid the misinterpretation of electrocautery as ventricular fibrillation with a resultant counter-shock.

Sparks can ignite inflammable vapours such as old anaesthetic gases (no longer in use), skin cleaning solutions and bowel gas.

Infusion Devices

Infusion devices are used extensively throughout the hospital but have a high incidence of critical incidents, mainly attributable to human error. The standard luer lock connection system allows misconnections between epidural, intrathecal, intravenous and enteral infusions. Proper documentation, with accurate and clear prescribing, is essential. There should be a regular written record of the progress of an infusion. The use of pre-filled syringes and infusion bags reduces the risk of dosage miscalculations. The setting up of an infusion device requires training as there are several potential pitfalls.

Syringe drivers should never be placed above the level of the patient. Anti-siphon valves are used to reduce the risk of inadvertent free flow. This can occur if the syringe barrel or plunger is not fully engaged or if the pump is placed more than 100 cm above the patient. Siphoning can also occur if there is a crack in the system allowing air entry. An anti-reflux valve should also be inserted to prevent back flow up another infusion line connected to the syringe driver line.

The infusion rate should not be too low (at least > 10 ml/hr) to prevent a delay in the onset of treatment. With respect to volumetric pumps, it is essential that a check is made that there is no flow with the clamp fully open when the pump is not running *before* it is attached to the patient. A further problem with these devices is the risk of entrainment of air and subsequent embolism. Most devices should be fitted with in-line air detectors. These can detect single bubbles of 0.1 ml.

Occlusion of an infusion device may lead to harm, not only from failure of treatment but also because of the delivery of a sudden bolus when the occlusion is subsequently relieved. Extravasation only causes a slight increase in infusion pressure which is usually insufficient to trip the occlusion alarm. Hence, regular direct visualisation of the infusion site is necessary.

Finally, locking systems should be in place to ensure accidental or malicious tampering is avoided while regular maintenance should help to minimise device faults.

REFERENCES

1. Mallory S, *et al.* (2003) The individual, the system, and medical error. *BJA CEPD Rev* **6**: 179–182.
2. Rollin A, *et al.* (1998) *Risk Management* (The Association of Anaesthetists of Great Britain and Ireland, UK), pp. 1–36.
3. Dodds C, *et al.* (2001) *Anaesthesia and Perioperative Care of the Elderly* (The Association of Anaesthetists of Great Britain and Ireland, UK), pp. 1–8.

4. Scott WE, *et al.* (2001) *Pre-operative Assessment: The Role of the Anaesthetist* (The Association of Anaesthetists of Great Britain and Ireland, UK), pp. 1–17.
5. Carter JA, Birks RJS. (2004) *Checking Anaesthetic Equipment*, 3rd edn (The Association of Anaesthetists of Great Britain and Ireland, UK), pp. 1–17.
6. Mills GH. (2001) Respiratory physiology and anaesthesia. *BJA CEPD Rev* **1**: 35–39.
7. Aitkenhead AR, Smith G. (1996) *Textbook of Anaesthesia*, 3rd edn (Churchill Livingston, London), pp. 377–406.
8. Vaughan RS. (2001) Predicting difficult airways. *BJA CEPD Rev* **2**: 44–48.
9. Marik PE. (2001) *Handbook of Evidence-Based Critical Care* (Springer-Verlag, New York), pp. 67–74.
10. Calvey TN, Williams NE. (1997) *Principles and Practice of Pharmacology for Anaesthetists*, 3rd edn (Blackwell Science, London), pp. 209–283.
11. Nolan J, Baskett P, Gabbott D, *et al.* (2005) *Advanced Life Support Course Provider Manual*, 5th edn (European Resuscitation Council, London), pp. 34, 112, 113.
12. Reinecke H, Breithardt G. (2003) Cardiological aspects in preoperative anaesthesiological evaluation: old heroes, new shadows. *Eur J Anaesthesiol* **8**: 595–599.
13. Bodog D, *et al.* (2003) *Suspected Anaphylactic Reactions Associated with Anaesthesia*, 3rd edn (The Association of Anaesthetists of Great Britain and Ireland, UK), pp. 1–20.
14. Behrman AJ. (2001) *Latex Allergy* (www.emedicine.com).
15. Thomas D, *et al.* (2001) *Blood Transfusion and the Anaesthetist: Red Cell Transfusion* (The Association of Anaesthetists of Great Britain and Ireland, UK), pp. 1–17.

FURTHER READING

1. Boumphrey S, Langton JA. (2003) Electrical safety in the operating theatre. *BJA CEPD Rev* **3**(1): 10–14.
2. Keay S, Callander C. (2004) The safe use of infusion devices. Continuing education in anaesthesia. *Crit Care Pain* **4**(3): 81–85.
3. Scottish Audit of Surgical Mortality Annual Report (2002).
4. Cullinane M, *et al.* (2003) Who operates when? In: *National Confidential Enquiry Into Perioperative Death* (Royal College of Surgeons, England).

Chapter 3

CARDIOPULMONARY COMPLICATIONS

Carlos M. H. Gómez

I   INTRODUCTION

Cardiopulmonary complications following surgery are common; their incidence is directly proportional to the magnitude of the surgical procedure. An estimated suffer significant cardiopulmonary complications. Conversely, of all the complications that follow a surgery, approximately are principally cardiovascular and respiratory.

The impact of these complications on the length of stay in hospital, and the cost, mortality rate and unplanned admissions to intensive care is considerable.

Their incidence is highest in patients with pre-existing heart or lung disease or with risk factors for these, such as hypercholesterolaemia, arterial hypertension, obesity, sedentary lifestyle and smoking.

The necessity for investigation and optimisation of chronic heart and lung conditions cannot be overemphasised, especially in those undergoing elective high risk non-cardiac surgery.

II   GENERAL PRINCIPLES

1.   Diagnosis

It is critical that complications are detected early, to establish a probable cause, proper diagnosis and to exclude other similar conditions.

It is important to determine the history of events leading to the particular complication and detect the factors commonly associated with cardiopulmonary deterioration. This includes pain and its many variations, laboured breathing, blood loss, changes in body temperature and signs and symptoms of hypovolaemia. These must be integrated with pre-existing risk factors, such as coronary artery disease (CAD) and its causes, arterial hypertension and its causes and systemic consequences, obstructive airway disease, chronic renal impairment, and excessive alcohol and tobacco consumption.

Physical examination must not be overlooked and should be tailored to the clinical scenario, depending on the urgency and gravity of the illness. It is possible to obtain considerable information from careful examination of the heart rate and rhythm, heart sounds, mucous membranes and peripheral perfusion and jugular venous pressure. Some clinicians find the bedside estimation of pulse volume and vascular resistance along with cardiac output reliable, reproducible and useful.

Similarly, a careful examination of the respiratory system can yield valuable information on the respiratory rate and pattern, pain or discomfort, air entry and presence and quality of added sounds.

The importance of mentation to gauge cerebral perfusion, and consequently cardiovascular and respiratory performance cannot be overemphasised. While there are multiple causes of cerebral dysfunction, especially in the critically ill, lethargy, confusion, agitation and other symptoms of dysfunction are reported, cardiovascular insufficiency or respiratory failure as the primary or principal cause must be considered.

Laboratory investigations, in particular blood count and serum chemistry, can indicate the cause of the complication.

Non-invasive tests such as an electrocardiogram (ECG) and chest X-ray should be performed as soon as possible. They often confirm or exclude other significant complications such as myocardial infarction, pneumothorax, pneumonia, atelectasis etc.

Echocardiography is a minimally invasive test which offers a useful assessment of the cardiac structure and function, flows and pressures by

Doppler interrogation as well as visualisation of chambers, their surroundings, and the great vessels. It is especially useful in detecting pericardial effusion, valve lesions, cardiac trauma and acute myocardial infarction. Transthoracic echocardiography is non-invasive and ideal for examining the anterior structures of the heart (right-sided chambers and their valves) and the aorta in long axis. In contrast, trans-oesophageal echocardiogram is more invasive (without upper gut morbidity) but is ideally suited for examination of the posterior structures (left sided chambers, mitral valve and thoracic aorta). It occupies an important role as a perioperative tool, especially in high-risk cardiac and vascular surgery.

2. Management

The general principle in the treatment of complications is to support organ function while awaiting recovery. The real challenge is in identifying patients who can wait for recovery and those who cannot. The principal determinants of outcome are magnitude of injury, cardiopulmonary reserve, adequacy of antibiotics and timely drainage or control of the source of infection and prevention of cross-infection.

For the patient, critical care involves a delicate trade-off between achievable and acceptable physiology. This precarious balance not only varies with each individual patient but changes over the course of the illness.

Some specific trade-offs are worth considering, such as the optimum intravascular volume which carries a certain price in terms of potentially excessive pulmonary, peripheral and cerebral oedema. Similarly, a certain perfusion pressure can only be achieved at the expense of increased cardiac work and peripheral vasoconstriction. Acceptable acid-base chemistry requires an increase in intrathoracic pressure (ventilation), cardiac work and tissue oedema.

There are of course intrinsic dangers within the specific treatments employed in every day intensive care. These are associated with sedation, mechanical ventilation, over treatment of chronic conditions and over- or under treatment of acute conditions.

a) Initial management

This is geared towards stabilising the critical functions of the airway, breathing and circulation followed by the transfer to a suitable ward. Initial interventions therefore, must be practical, swift, realistic and tailored for use of available resources and equipment. There is always a difficult balance between too much stabilisation and too early a transfer.

The state of the airway normally dictates the course of action. An assessment of the factors contributing to a patent airway is pertinent; these are mentation and general central nervous system function, pharyngeal and laryngeal neuromuscular function and respiratory capacity. When one of these is deficient, controlling the airway becomes the single most important intervention. Many simple manoeuvres such as jaw positioning and introduction of oropharyngeal or nasopharyngeal tubes can be useful as short term interventions.

Definitive airway control is achieved by tracheal intubation. Theoretically, intubation indicators fall into three inter-related categories. First, cerebral dysfunction which can be primary (epilepsy, infection, space occupying lesion or vascular insufficiency) or secondary (cardiopulmonary insufficiency, chemical or acid-base imbalances, sepsis, etc.). Second, inadequate gas exchange; hypoxaemia and hypercapnia may impact cerebral function adversely, perpetuating a vicious cycle leading to worsening airway and cardiopulmonary function. Third, when mechanical ventilation is likely to be prolonged, it necessitates tracheal intubation.

Once the airway is controlled, due attention is paid to ventilation, to facilitate gas exchange in the lungs without damaging them. There is a fundamental trade-off here, between improving blood gas chemistry by ventilation with greater airway pressures and lung volumes and contributing to injuring already weakened lungs. This is perhaps one of the most extensively discussed topics in critical care and is reviewed in more detail later in this chapter.[1,2]

It is important to pay attention to the circulation. Circulatory collapse is often a combination of decreased stroke volume and/or heart rate, abnormal rhythm and functional hypovolaemia, the latter often associated with sepsis. It is important to try and rectify it during the initial management of a complication. However, it is prudent to consider that an increasing proportion of hospital in-patients have longstanding heart disease and heart failure, and their deterioration may be due to postoperative decompensation. The dilemma therefore between too much and too little fluid is a very real one.

In the end, successful management relies on understanding the cause of a particular complication. This can be challenging and is normally achieved by a combination of pattern recognition and diagnostic tests. In each individual, the balance between treating supposed causes and excessive and time consuming investigations that detract from therapeutic interventions is difficult and variable. Blind interventions carry a cost but so do diagnostic tests.

b)   Medium term management

The goal is to minimise damage and unnecessary intervention while allowing physiological recovery. This is done by constantly reassessing patients who are not progressing or responding as expected. This may occur because of a more serious manifestation of the underlying condition, a wrong diagnosis, a new complication or a recurrence of an old one. In particular, haemodynamic and respiratory interventions deserve special attention.

Haemodynamic management

i   *Oxygen transport*

The main objective of circulation management is to maximise oxygen transport to all tissues and its consumption while avoiding an increase in potentially damaging and unnecessary excess work on the heart. The amount of cardiac work that constitutes too much is not known until signs of myocardial ischaemia develop; this amount varies greatly among individuals, depending upon the critical balance between coronary artery blood supply and heart muscle oxygen consumption.

Factors affecting the coronary artery blood flow are:

i) Coronary perfusion pressure gradient which is determined by the mean arterial — left ventricular diastolic pressure gradient for the left ventricle, and mean arterial — right ventricular diastolic pressure gradient for the right ventricle
ii) Coronary filling time which is the diastolic duration for the left ventricle, essentially the duration of the entire cardiac cycle for the right ventricle

Factors affecting myocardial oxygen consumption are:

i)   High afterload, determined by the systemic vascular resistance, left ventricular outflow tract obstruction, aortic stenosis or aortic coarctation
ii) Left ventricular hypertrophy
iii) Tachycardia
iv) Basal metabolic rate

Therefore, the conditions commonly associated with good myocardial oxygenation are:

i) Good, but not high, systemic blood pressure with adequate, but not high, left and right ventricular filling pressures to maintain a favourable coronary perfusion gradient

ii) Slow heart rate because as the heart rate falls there is a proportionately greater increase in duration of diastole and therefore coronary filling

iiii) Sufficient vascular resistance to maintain adequate, but not excessive, systemic blood pressure. In an aortic or left ventricular outflow obstruction there is a clear need for greater vasoconstriction in view of the pressure drop across the obstruction

iv) Conditions in which oxygen consumption is reduced, such as hypothermia, and balanced general anaesthesia

The following are commonly associated with poor myocardial oxygenation:

• Low systemic blood pressure combined with high ventricular filling pressure leading to an unfavourable coronary perfusion gradient
• High ventricular filling pressures, due either to fluid overload or reduced ventricular compliance
• High ventricular wall tension as occurs in a dilated ventricle
• Tachycardia where there is a relative shortening of diastole and therefore of coronary filling time
• Pain
• Respiratory distress because increased breathing can increase oxygen consumption dramatically
• Conditions in which oxygen consumption is increased such as fever, convulsions and shivering

It is therefore important to recognise that the postoperative patient suffering from pain, anxiety, respiratory distress, hypoxaemia and relative hypovolaemia is at high risk of myocardial ischaemia.

Another important factor is oxygen consumption by different vascular beds and transport to them. The governing principles of perfusion pressure gradient, work, metabolism and consumption are the same as for the myocardium.

However, it is less easy to measure the adequacy of oxygenation, and the clinician often has to rely on indirect signs of dysoxia, such as the presence of anaerobic metabolism highlighted by a lactic acidaemia.

ii   Circulation

The question of the patient's intravascular volume often arises. In principle the correct filling status is determined by the balance between the amount of fluid required to generate an adequate cardiac output, but not so much that it contributes to pulmonary, cerebral or peripheral tissue oedema, and systemic perfusion. Clearly this balance varies among individuals and clinical situations. Often, the most vulnerable organ determines which aspect of this balance is most critical, as seen in the following examples.

- Left ventricular dysfunction normally requires judicious fluid restriction, at the expense of peripheral tissues and kidneys
- Right ventricular dysfunction usually benefits from cautious fluid administration, especially in acute right ventricular infarction. However, chronic right ventricular failure leads to fluid overload which responds to fluid restriction and diuresis
- Acute renal failure normally requires fluid administration at some risk to the cardiorespiratory systems
- Sepsis and acute inflammatory states are characterised by gross functional hypovolaemia, often responding to treatment with several litres of intravenous fluids. Furthermore, severe sepsis is almost always accompanied by capillary leak and is associated with pulmonary and general tissue oedema.
- In the postoperative stages, the renin-aldosterone axis drives water retention, which can lead to oliguria and renal hypoperfusion

In the presence of symptoms consistent with impaired contractility, echocardiography is necessary to check for regional wall motion abnormalities suggestive of coronary artery disease.

Blood pressure — determined by the product of cardiac output and systemic vascular resistance — should be high enough to drive tissue perfusion in all vascular beds but low enough so as not to increase the afterload on the heart (see above). It is important to state the nonlinear relationship between blood pressure and flow. In particular the phenomenon of autoregulation needs to be considered, i.e. all pressure beds have pre-capillary arterioles capable of vasodilating or constricting with change in pressure, to maintain a relatively constant flow. Diseased vascular beds have greatly reduced autoregulation, often due to arteriosclerosis, and therefore are much more sensitive to changes in pressure.

Vasoactive drugs or inotropes are often used to optimise circulatory status. They can be used to facilitate the achievement of the primary goal or to offset expected or observed side-effects of other treatments aimed at achieving a primary goal. The decision of which and how much inotrope to use is determined by the cause and state of circulatory derangement and the side effects of the inotrope. Table 1 outlines some aspects of commonly used inotropes.

Table 1.   Commonly Used Vasoactive Agents

Agent	Pharmacology	Effects	Indications	Disadvantages
Adrenaline	Equipotent α/β	Tachycardia Increased cardiac output Raised blood pressure	Resuscitation shock	Arrhythmias Acidaemia Hyperglycaemia
Noradrenaline	$\alpha_1 > \beta_1$	Raised blood pressure Reflex bradycardia	SIRS/sepsis	Vasoconstriction
Dobutamine	β_1, β_1	Tachycardia Increased cardiac output vasodilatation	Cardiac failure sepsis	Arrhythmias Myocardial Ischaemia
Dopamine	$DA_1, DA_2, \beta_1, \alpha_1$	Renal vasodilatation Tachycardia Raised blood pressure	Circulatory support	Arrhythmias Vasoconstriction
Dopexamine	$\beta_2 > DA_1 > \beta_1$	Vasodilatation Renal vasodilatation Tachycardia	Circulatory support Cardiac failure Gut perfusion	Arrhythmias
Milrinone	PDE III inhibitor Increased cAMP	Cardiac contractility Vasodilatation	Cardiac failure	Vasodilatation

Ventilatory management

i   General aspects

Mechanical (positive pressure) ventilation (MV or PPV) can be thought of as a predominantly inspiratory support along with some form of expiratory support. The objective of the former is to inflate the lungs to allow gas exchange without causing airway or lung trauma. The latter is aimed at reducing end-expiratory airway closure without causing impaired exhalation and air-trapping. Expiration, both in spontaneous and in PPV, is passive and depends on elastic lung recoil and airway resistance. The first is difficult to manipulate while the second can be altered pharmacologically.

Therefore, MV can be useful in treating conditions associated with inspiratory abnormalities. In contrast, with a predominantly expiratory disease MV may not be as useful, because it cannot alter elastic recoil. Theoretically, the greater the intrathoracic pressure the greater the adverse effect on right heart filling and emptying.

ii   Definitions

Airway resistance is the pressure gradient required to generate a certain flow; it is increased in asthma.

Compliance is the ratio of change in volume to change in pressure (dV/dP); it is decreased in parenchymal or interstitial diseases such as infection, oedema, collapse or fibrosis, and is increased in airway diseases such as emphysema and bronchitis.

Shunt occurs when poorly ventilated alveoli are adequately perfused; if causes hypoxaemia, the treatment for which necessitates recruitment of underventilated areas. Typical in pneumonia and lung collapse.

Deadspace occurs when adequately ventilated alveoli are insufficiently perfused; causes effective fall in alveolar ventilation with consequent hypoxaemia and hypercapnia.

Positive end expiratory pressure (PEEP) is applied to maintain alveoli open at the end of every breath. It increases intrathoracic pressure and can adversely reduce venous return and cardiac output.

Continuous positive airway pressure (CPAP) is the equivalent term when applied to spontaneous ventilation.

Pressure support refers to ventilator applied inspiratory pressure bursts triggered by a spontaneous effort. The actual tidal volume delivered depends on lung compliance.

Pressure control is the equivalent term when applied to mandatory or controlled ventilation. The tidal volume also depends on compliance.

Equivalent considerations apply to **volume support and control**, but here the tidal volume is fixed and the pressure is a function of compliance.

Modern ventilators enable the clinician to combine inspiratory and expiratory manoeuvres and synchronise these with spontaneous breathing efforts.

c)   Long term management

Here the objectives are to minimise chronic organ failure, reduce the impact of existing irreversible organ failure and understand the interdependence of organ failures.

3.   Monitoring

a)   Clinical

This is unquestionably the most important type of monitoring. Considerations like the nature of the ward, nurse to patient ratio, presence of junior doctors, adequate consultant guidance and supervision and general familiarity and experience with the patient's condition are crucial to success. The most important monitoring is that provided by trained, caring and vigilant health professionals. The issue of clinical examination has been mentioned earlier but it must be emphasised that substantial and valuable information about cardiorespiratory well-being can be extracted from close observation of the functioning of all the end-organs. Subtle changes in end-organ function are often the first tell tale signs of cardiorespiratory complications.

b)   Less invasive

The importance of echocardiography has been discussed above (see Diagnosis).

In the last decade transoesophageal Doppler has gained wide acceptance.[3] By measuring the descending aortic flow it calculates a number of useful parameters, such as stroke volume, peak aortic blood velocity and ejection time, all of which are related to cardiac filling and performance. Its information is near-continuous but it cannot enable visualisation of cardiac structures. Complications are low and learning is rapid.

Newer technologies loosely based on the principle of thermodilution but necessitating only arterial and central venous access have also emerged. They are centred on the lithium dilution cardiac output technique which relies on an in-line lithium electrode.[4] Other variants rely on mathematical analysis of the arterial waveform. All of these can provide a continuous calculation of stroke volume and haemodynamic indices, such as systemic vascular resistance.

c) Invasive

Pulmonary artery catheters (PAC) have long been used at the patient's bedside[5] and have always attracted interest and controversy.[6]

PAC measures pulmonary artery pressures, including pulmonary artery wedge pressure (PAWP), and haemodynamic indices such as cardiac output. They can also be used to calculate haemodynamic indices such as vascular resistances and oxygen transport values. PAWP often reflects left atrial pressure which in turn is proportional to left ventricular end-diastolic pressure and filling. Pulmonary artery pressure is a determinant of right ventricular afterload and left ventricular preload and therefore, its measurement provides an unrivalled assessment of the relationship between both ventricles. However, it is important to recognise that in mitral valve pathology or left heart disease PAWP may not reflect true left ventricular preload.

Despite their frequent use there is no compelling evidence supporting the notion that therapy guided by PAC offers a survival advantage in heterogeneous critically ill patients.[7,8] Their use is, therefore, determined by the characteristics of the patient and local preference, experience and training.

Notwithstanding all the available monitoring options, the response to therapy is the best indicator of patient condition.

III SPECIFIC COMPLICATIONS

1. Systemic Inflammatory Response

This is a hyperdynamic state characterised by varying degrees of vasodilatation and consequent functional intravascular fluid depletion, increased cardiac output, heart rate and stroke volume, elevated temperature and metabolic rate. There is a mobilisation of fatty stores and fluid retention.

A mild form of the condition is very common post-surgery, especially after a major surgery. Moderate to severe forms have a reported incidence of between and depend on many variables, including magnitude of surgery, blood loss and probably genetic predisposition.

Post-surgery inflammation is the protective response of vascularised living tissue to destroy injurious substances and facilitate repair of damaged local structures.[9] This is done via delivery of neutrophils and monocyte-macrophages to the site of tissue trauma. Just how much inflammation is necessary and when is it excessive and damaging depends on the nature and magnitude of the insult as well as on the host's physiological reserve. There are finely tuned in-built systems to modulate the inflammatory response. Nevertheless, some individuals produce insufficient response and are overwhelmed by the injurious process, while others mount an excessive inflammatory reaction, which leads to widespread tissue destruction and dysfunction.[10]

An excessive host response with multi-system involvement characterised by varying degrees of circulatory instability and end-organ insufficiency is referred to as systemic inflammatory response syndrome (SIRS).[11] In the USA, the incidence of SIRS from all causes has been estimated at 400,000 cases annually with a mortality rate as high as 40%.[12]

Clinically, SIRS is said to be present when certain criteria exist. These include central temperature greater than 38°C or lower than 36°C; heart rate greater than 90 beats per minute; respiratory rate greater than 20 per minute; or requirement of mechanical ventilation, elevated (greater than 12×10^9/L) or severely reduced (less than 4×10^9/L) white cell count, along with hypotension or a requirement of inotropes and evidence of impaired end-organ perfusion such as metabolic acidaemia (pH $\leq$ 7.3), hypoxaemia, coagulopathy or acute deterioration of mental state.[13]

SIRS constitutes a spectrum of conditions mediated primarily by the immune system and involving activation of the host defences,[14] including the cytokine network,[15] endothelium,[16] the complement and coagulation cascades[17] and the neutrophil-monocyte system.[18] These result in the release of arachidonic acid metabolites,[19] oxygen radicals, leukotrienes, proteases and nitric oxide (NO),[20] endothelial dysfunction, altered microvascular flow and

Table 2.   Conditions Associated with the Systemic
Inflammatory Response Syndrome (SIRS)

Major Surgery
Trauma
Infection
Cardiopulmonary bypass
Pancreatitis
Burns
Acute poisoning
Chemical injury

---

aggregation of platelets.[21] The final common result is vasodilatation;[22] tissue dysoxia;[23] and mitochondrial dysfunction.[24]

SIRS need not be caused by infection although in intensive care it most often is, and in this context it is termed sepsis. Many conditions have been associated with the onset of SIRS. They are listed in Table 2.

Management of the condition is mainly supportive and geared towards maintaining adequate circulation.

2.   Acute Lung Injury/Acute Respiratory Distress Syndrome

Acute respiratory distress syndrome (ARDS) and acute lung injury (ALI) encompass a clinical spectrum of elevated pulmonary alveolocapillary permeability characterised by refractory hypoxaemia, widespread alveolar infiltrate on the chest X-ray, and respiratory distress which is not caused by but may co-exist with raised left atrial or pulmonary capillary pressure.[25] ARDS has an incidence of 2–75 cases per 100,000 individuals each year, depending on the patient population and diagnostic criteria.[26] Although the mortality of ARDS has remained constant, at around 50–60%, the cause of death has changed from respiratory failure to multiple organ dysfunction related to the underlying illness.[27]

The initial insult to the lungs results in an inflammatory response which causes the alveolar deposition of fibrin and collagen, pulmonary microthrombi, and acute destruction of the alveolocapillary membrane leading to increased permeability and widespread inflammatory alveolar exudate.[28] There may follow a fibrotic response characterised by repair and proliferation of fibroblasts and Type II pneumocytes.[29]

The consequences of such changes are alveolar oedema and collapse, reduced lung compliance, increased venous admixture, and hypoxaemia. Pulmonary vasoconstriction also occurs, which increases the alveolar deadspace, exacerbates the ventilation-perfusion mismatch and may lead to pulmonary hypertension and increased right ventricular work.

Currently, there is no treatment to reverse the raised capillary permeability or the hyperinflammatory reaction. The management of ALI is essentially supportive, directed towards minimising the accumulation of alveolar exudates, inducing pulmonary vasodilatation to reduce the severity of pulmonary hypertension, minimising potential damage to lungs and circulation associated with ventilation, treatment of infection and use of supportive measures while awaiting lung recovery.

Much attention has been directed to establishing the best modes of ventilation for patients with ARDS. A gentle ventilation with lower tidal volumes (around 6 ml/kg) and plateau or peak pressures (not higher than 30 cm water)[2,30] is now considered beneficial. The general consensus is that there is little to gain with PEEP greater than 13–14 cm water, and it is also potentially damaging.[1] Avoiding ventilator induced lung injury[31] seems more important than pursuit of ideal gas exchange.

Correct fluid balance is also very important but difficult to achieve. Excessive fluid reduction may worsen cardiovascular performance and compromise organ perfusion.[32] However, because alveolar flooding is one of the main structural manifestations of ARDS, therapy leading to resolution of alveolar fluid should improve gas exchange.

Imaging by computed tomography (CT) scans[33] can play an important role in diagnosis and response to treatment, and in determining whether the pattern of alveolar infiltrate is gravitational and therefore likely to benefit from turning the patient prone.[34]

Inhaled NO was received with great enthusiasm[35,36] but has not proven to be effective in larger trials.[37,38] It has nevertheless improved our understanding of pulmonary endothelial dysfunction in ARDS/ALI.[39]

3. Pneumonia and Ventilator Associated Pneumonia (VAP)

VAP has an incidence of 9–28% of all intubated patients and accounts for 25% of all ICU infections. The risk of developing VAP is the highest during the first five days of ventilation (3%). Various studies have observed mortality indices in the range of 24–76%, with a 2- to 10-fold increased risk of death.[40] Others have calculated an incremental risk of pneumonia, at about 1% per day of ventilation.[41]

The incidence, severity and organisms vary greatly between units, mostly as a function of patient characteristics, type of surgery and antibiotic policy. However, extensive studies suggest that the organisms commonly associated with VAP are *Pseudomonas aeruginosa* (24%); *Staphylococcus aureus* (at least 55% resistant to methicillin–MRSA-); the *Entrobacteriaceae* species (*E. coli*, *Proteus* spp, *Enterobacter* spp, *Klebsiella* spp, *Serratia* spp), *Haemophilus* spp (10%), *Streptococcus* spp (8%) and *Acinetobacter* spp (8%), and various fungi (1%).

Many organisms are multidrug resistant (MDR) and this is becoming an increasingly grave problem with tremendous implications for duration of stay, outcome, staffing and cost. Their resistance is of many types; some organisms, such as the *Pseudomonas* spp, have high intrinsic resistance often mediated by a variety of membrane channels and pumps susceptible to upregulation by mutation.[42] Another mechanism of resistance is by acquisition of enzymes, such as extended spectrum ß-lactamases (ESBL, *Klebsiella*), other inducible ß-lactamases (*E. coli*), Carbapenemases (*Acinetobacter* and *S. maltophila*), often mediated or transmitted by plasmids.

There are many factors contributing to VAP. Tracheal intubation, despite an adequately functioning cuff, provides a port of entry for organisms from both the environment and aero-digestive tract. Respiratory cilia motility and macrophage function are reduced with tracheal intubation and ventilation. Prolonged ventilation is also associated with muscle weakness and fatigue and in general, critical illness is associated with impaired immune response.

The diagnosis is clinical and microbiological. Clinical signs of pneumonia include progressive respiratory distress, gas exchange and ventilator requirements with an increase in tracheal secretions and auscultation signs of consolidation (bronchial breathing) along with a change in radiological appearances, usually because of alveolar infiltrate. Microbiological diagnosis is by identification of an organism from suitable specimens of respiratory secretions, often from a bronchoalveoalr lavage because it is less likely to contain contaminant organisms. Finally, as in any infection, there may be signs of systemic inflammation or infection, most importantly temperature, leukocytosis, cardiovascular instability, increase in fluid and inotrope requirements and impaired mentation.

The treatment of VAP is by continued ventilation, often with increased assistance, general supportive measures and antibiotics. It is crucial to distinguish between colonising organisms which do not normally produce systemic signs of infection, and truly pathogenic or infective ones which do.

If VAP is suspected, a decision must be made with respect to genuine infection; institution of empirical antibiotics depending on the characteristics displayed by the patient and the illness as well as local prevalence; and commencement of antibiotics upon confirmation of organism and antimicrobial sensitivities. There is a delicate balance between premature and inadequate antibiotics leading to a consequent increase in dangerous drug resistance, versus a delayed and insufficient treatment after the systemic infection has set in. Another very important decision is to know when to discontinue antimicrobial therapy, and this is associated with development of resistance to strains and toxic or unwanted drug side effects. In general, and especially in relapsed cases of VAP, short courses of single agent treatment guided by antibiogrammes in all but the most severe cases of overwhelming systemic infections are recommended.[43]

Finally in all infections in intensive care, it is particularly important to avoid cross-contamination of patients by healthcare personnel or equipment.

4.   Acute Coronary Syndrome/Myocardial Infarction

The incidence of postoperative myocardial ischaemia varies greatly with type and magnitude of surgery and patient cardiac risk factors. Repeated studies reveal that the predictors associated with an increased risk of postoperative cardiac (but not necessarily ischaemic) events include recent myocardial infarction — especially in the preceding three months — congestive heart failure and major vascular surgery. Among patients with or at risk of coronary artery disease having non-cardiac surgery, myocardial ischaemia is detected in about 40% while about 3% suffer ischaemic events (death, myocardial infarction or unstable angina).[44] It follows therefore that there is a strong indication to estimate and check for cardiac risk in the preoperative stage, and to optimise cardiac management in patients with established coronary artery disease.

The wide spectrum of clinical scenarios caused by coronary artery disease, ranging from myocardial ischaemia through unstable angina to acute myocardial infarction, is loosely encompassed by the term acute coronary syndrome.[45] Clearly, a given patient's condition can fluctuate between the two extremes of this spectrum.

Outside the intensive care unit and perioperative period, the definition of myocardial infarction is often clear, more so since the definition and nomenclature of myocardial infarction have been revisited recently.[46,47] The presence of two of the following three features constitutes myocardial infarction: symptoms of cardiac ischaemia such as pain; characteristic electrocardiographic changes such as Q waves or specific T wave changes; and elevation of biochemical markers of myocardial necrosis such as creatinine kinase isoenzyme MB (CKMB) or cardiac troponin T. In addition, echocardiographic or angiographic signs of regional wall motion abnormalities are highly suggestive of the diagnosis.

However, in many postoperative or critically ill patients the diagnosis is difficult and relies heavily on the clinical course and exclusion of confounding conditions. An asymptomatic patient with elevated serum troponin concentrations must be handled with care because the condition is known to cause non-cardiac conditions such as renal failure, sepsis, pulmonary embolism, acute cerebrovascular accidents, subarachnoid bleeding, hypertension and drug toxicity.[48] In addition, cardiac surgery or manipulation is associated with elevated troponin concentrations but without demonstrable ischaemia.

Cardiac troponin measurement has also enabled easier recognition of critically ill patients with minor cardiac damage. This is relevant because raised serum cardiac troponin appears to be associated with an independent increase in mortality. However, risk stratification using cardiac troponins, is not widely accepted. Additional treatment for troponin-positive critically ill patients has not been established.[49]

Myocardial infarction is usually caused by coronary artery occlusion in patients with a sufficiently small coronary artery reserve leading to myocardial ischaemia and consequent necrosis. This can lead to regional wall motion abnormalities and reduced cardiac output.

The treatment, like the diagnosis, is standardised for primary acute myocardial infarction, but not so much in the postoperative period or during critical illness. Nevertheless, it is determined by the general condition of the patient, surgical considerations such as haemostasis, drains, anastomosis, etc. and, above all, the magnitude of the impact on cardiovascular haemodynaics.

The general principles of management of an AMI in the postoperative period are:

i) Relief of coronary ischaemia by manipulation of myocardial oxygen supply and demand. This involves reduction of heart rate, alleviation of pain and anxiety, preferential coronary vasodilators (nitrate compounds), increase in systemic perfusion pressure, and optimisation of fluid status. Although preoperative ß blockers are advocated,[44] the benefits of these drugs in a complicated postoperative setting needs to be considered carefully in each patient, in view of the importance of maintaining cardiac output.
ii) Anticoagulation, inhibition of platelet aggregation and thrombolysis.
iii) Coronary revascularisation, either percutaneous coronary intervention or coronary artery bypass grafts.

The wide variation in clinical circumstances surrounding the AMI will determine the therapy to be applied. However, the preferred option is a judicious combination of coronary and general haemodynamic manoeuvres along with partial heparinisation and anti-platelet therapy. Coronary imaging and revascularisation are used when the patient has recovered from surgery and acute conditions. However, in a small minority of patients angiography and percutaneous coronary intervention is the only successful strategy to improve cardiac output sufficiently to wean from organ support.

5. Dysrrhythmias

The incidence of dysrrhythmias in general intensive care is unclear but varies significantly depending on admission diagnosis, type of surgery and pre-existing risk factors. In critically ill patients with arrhythmias, the two most common irregularities are atrial fibrillation and ventricular tachycardia although the relative incidences vary among studies.[50,51] Atrial flutter, supraventricular tachycardia, ventricular fibrillation and cardiac arrest are less common. From another perspective, a significant number of deaths due to cardiovascular disease are attributed to sudden acute ventricular tachyarrhythmias.[52]

a)   Atrial fibrillation (AF)

The predisposing factors for atrial fibrillation are ischaemic, valvular or hypertensive heart disease, diabetes, certain types of surgery, in particular heart and lung surgery, increased inflammatory response[53] and drugs such as dopamine.[54] There is also a rare familial type.[55]

The principal pathophysiological disturbance in AF is loss of atrioventricular synchrony with rapid and irregular ventricular contraction leading to a reduction in stroke volume.[56] In addition, atrial stasis along with hypercoagulability is predisposed to thrombus formation, especially in the left atrial appendage.[57]

Treatment is aimed at cardioversion in the first instance as it improves symptoms. Electrical cardioversion with direct current shocks is particularly indicated if there is haemodynamic compromise. The pro-thrombotic risk is low if the patient has been in AF for less than 48 hours. In AF of longer duration the risk is higher so anticoagulation is normally commenced, and the decision to cardiovert depends on the clinical circumstances and should be preceded by transoesophageal echocardiography to exclude thrombi, especially in the left atrial appendage.

Pharmacological cardioversion is normally attempted when there is little or no haemodynamic compromise. However, it is unlikely to be effective if AF has persisted longer than 48 hours.[58] In the critically ill, amiodarone is used most commonly. However, occasional acute severe pulmonary toxicity is well described.[59] Flecainide and propafenone have been more efficacious than amiodarone in conversion to sinus rhythm, in a wider population.[60]

The maintenance of sinus rhythm after cardioversion is conventionally achieved with a β blocker, sodium channel blockers like flecainide or with amiodarone.

When cardioversion is unsuccessful, the focus is on rate control, normally with digoxin, calcium channel or ß-blockers, along with anticoagulation with heparin, warfarin or aspirin.[58,61]

The following is a suggested strategy for new-onset AF in the postoperative period:

- Identify patients at risk
- Assess haemodynamic impact
- Ensure adequate serum potassium concentration
- Ensure adequate position of indwelling right atrial pressure "central" lines, intercostal chest drains and tracheal tube as these can trigger AF mechanically
- Consider magnesium supplementation (intravenously)
- Intravenous amiodarone infusion
- Synchronised electrical defibrillation under general anaesthesia
- Look for signs of acute coronary syndrome as atrial fibrillation can be the presenting feature of coronary artery disease
- Low threshold for performing echocardiogram to assess heart size and function
- Consider anticoagulation if cardioversion is unsuccessful

Irrespective of the perceived wisdom of cardiovert to sinus rhythm, recent evidence from two major studies indicates no significant benefit from rhythm control when compared with rate control in terms of death or cardiovascular complications.[62,63]

b)   Ventricular tachyarrhythmias

Predisposing factors are coronary artery disease, dilated and hypertrophied cardiomyopathies and, less commonly, valvular heart disease. Another important trigger that is not very common is the Wolff-Parkinson-White syndrome (re-entry type atrial fibrillation potentially leading to malignant ventricular tachyarrhythmias). Congenital and infiltrative abnormalities are rare, as is the acquired long-QT syndrome.[64] Genetically determined ion-channel abnormalities exist but are very rare.[65]

In critically ill patients ventricular ectopics are not unusual and often associated with electrolyte abnormalities or rapid fluctuations. Ventricular tachycardia and fibrillation are more unusual but serious and often reflect underlying coronary ischaemia or low cardiac output.

Its management depends greatly on haemodynamic impact of arrhythmis. In principle, it rests on the removal of cause and triggers, observation — which may not be possible if sudden pulseless VT or ventricular fibrillation (VF) occur — minerals and drugs: amiodarone, adenosine is useful in slowing ventricular rhythm (profound AV block) to distinguish atrial flutter from VF, ß blockers (metoprolol, sotalol), disoppyramide and bretyllium. Immediate defibrillation is required in VF or sustained VT. Survivors should be investigated for placement of internal cardiac defibrillators.[66]

Refractory atrial[67] and ventricular tachyarrhythmias can also be treated by various forms of electrophysiological mapping and radiofrequency ablation of aberrant pathways performed using conventional percutaneous approaches. Surgery is also a well established option for atrial fibrillation.[68]

6.   Atelectasis

Alveolar collapse can be radiological and/or clinical. There is an ill defined and variable relationship between the two.

Normally there is a satisfactory balance between the tendency of alveoli to collapse due to their elastic recoil and chest wall tug to anchor them and keep them open. This is the concept of functional residual capacity (FRC) at end expiration. Hypoventilation, which in the postoperative period is normally associated with CNS depression, pain, sputum retention, opioids, muscle weakness, shifts this balance unfavourably towards collapse. It is a vicious cycle where impaired cough causes sputum plugging, which in turn causes segmental collapse that further worsens the cough by reducing vital capacity. The consequence is further hypoventilation with increased work of breathing, hypercapnia and exhaustion.

It is important to remember the law of Laplace which dictates the relationship between intraluminal pressure (P), wall tension (T) and radius (R):

$$P = 2T/R.$$

Careful inspection of this formula reveals that as the radius becomes smaller there comes a point at which the wall tension pushing in outweighs the intraluminal pressure keeping the alveolus open and airway collapse ensues.

Management of atelectasis is geared towards removing the cause. The cornerstone therefore is adequate analgesia and oxygen. Maintenance of a relatively high end expiratory pressure, by continuous positive airway pressure (CPAP), is often useful in reversing the cycle and generating lung expansion and alveolar recruitment. Severe forms require inspiratory support which can be delivered by noninvasive ventilation (face mask bilevel positive airway pressure — BIPAP) or tracheal intubation and mechanical ventilation.

Physiotherapy can be very useful but is short lived and required regularly and frequently. The treatment of infection, especially if nosocomial, is by using broad-spectrum antibiotics, guided by microbiological results whenever possible.

7. Deep Vein Thrombosis (DVT)

This is the formation of a clot in a large vein, usually the popliteal, femoral or iliac veins of the lower limb. It is due to a combination of i) hypercoagulability associated with dehydration, malignancy, platelet aggregation, atrial fibrillation, inherited or acquired abnormalities in coagulation and certain types of surgery such as orthopaedic, urological and vascular ii) venous stasis associated with immobility and venous insufficiency.

There is a well described but incompletely understood relationship between the inflammatory and coagulation cascades such that activation of one results in activation of the other. Furthermore, within the coagulation cascade the balance between excessive bleeding and clotting is so delicate that one often generates correction mechanisms which almost invariably lead to the other.

Thrombosis *per se* cannot only cause circulatory instability characterised by venous engorgement and limb ischaemia but also a self-perpetuating cycle of further thrombosis. However, the real impact of thrombosis is that proximal — downstream-migration can give rise to embolism which can be life-threatening.

The diagnosis involves a combination of history and clinical assessment, ultrasonography (particularly compression ultrasonography) and ultimately venography. There are numerous coagulation parameters which become activated in DVT and fibrinogen degradation products and d-dimers have been used in early diagnostic tests. However, in the post-operative period and in critical illness these are difficult to interpret due to the simultaneous activation of the coagulation cascade by the inflammatory process.[69]

Its management is by prevention, aggressive diagnosis, anticoagulation and thrombolysis. Prevention includes identification of patients at risk, good hydration, early mobilisation, mechanical compression to assist venous return (compression devices or stockings), aspirin and various forms and doses of heparin. The standard treatment is complete anticoagulation in confirmed cases and thrombolysis in high (proximal) venous thrombosis.

8. Pulmonary Embolism

This is the migration of a clot through the right heart into a pulmonary arterial vessel. The larger the clot, the more proximal (upstream) its seating and therefore the more pronounced its haemodynamic impact.

The incidence is unknown but probably higher than reported. When untreated or presenting haemodynamic compromise, mortality is in the region of 20–30%.[70] It commonly arises from previously undetected DVT.

Table 3 lists the various risk factors associated with venous thromboembolism.

Pulmonary embolism creates an obstruction across the pulmonary arterial vasculature. This causes an increased pulmonary vascular resistance which creates increased work for the right heart, strain and, ultimately, right heart failure. In addition, there is an increase in areas which are ventilated but

Table 3.   Risk Factors for Venous Thromboembolism[71]

- Age greater than 40 years
- Prior history of venous thromboembolism
- Prolonged immobilisation
- Cerebrovascular accident
- Congestive heart failure
- Cancer
- Fracture of pelvis, femur or tibia
- Obesity
- Pregnancy or recent delivery
- Oestrogen treatment
- Inflammatory bowel disease
- Genetic or acquired thrombophilia
    - Antithrombin III deficiency
    - Protein C deficiency
    - Protein S deficiency
    - Factor V Leiden
    - Anticardiolipin antibody
    - Lupus anticoagulant

underperfused; this constitutes alveolar deadspace leading to hypoxaemia. The compensatory tachypnoea is normally insufficient to correct hypoxaemia but does cause a relative or absolute reduction in arterial carbon dioxide (hypocarbia). This therefore gives rise to the hallmark hypoxaemia/hypocarbia which is not always seen but should raise suspicion when observed.

The diagnosis can be notoriously difficult as many of the classical features are highly ubiquitous.[71] It is based on a combination of clinical suspicion, electrocardiographic signs of right ventricular strain[72] impaired gas exchange with a relatively normal chest X-ray, echocardiographic visualisation of an embolus and/or impairment of right ventricular systolic function, presence of deep venous thrombosis, suggestive CT pulmonary angiogram and, ultimately, ventilation/perfusion scan.

The management is complicated, and often close collaboration between several specialists is required. The principles of managements are: i) removal of reversible risk factors; ii) anticoagulation with heparin initially before switching to warfarin. In an emergency, systemic or localised thrombolysis (tissue plasminogen activator) should be contemplated,[73] with careful consideration given to potentially catastrophic haemorrhage;[74] iii) treatment of right heart failure and pulmonary hypertension,[75] and of consequent reduced cardiac output and cardiovascular failure; iv) pulmonary thromboendarterectomy is performed only in highly specialised centres and can yield favourable results in some cases.[76]

9. Pleural Effusion

This is fluid, serosanguineous, lymphatic or exudative, in the pleural space, and can be bilateral or unilateral. The incidence is difficult to specify as definitions vary and only a few studies are available. A large number of patients in intensive care have pleural effusion, which is either clinically silent or not considered significant enough to drain.

Bilateral pleural effusions are often associated with capillary leak, cardiogenic pulmonary oedema (heart failure), fluid overload and reduced oncotic pressure or a combination of these. Other causes include hypothyroidism and pericarditis. Unilateral effusions imply local pathology such as pneumonia, cancer and pulmonary infarction. Effusion fluid low in protein (below 30 g/L) is known as transudate while an exudate is high in protein (above 30 g/L).

The management in intensive care is dictated by cause, physiological impact on clinical condition and timing of weaning. In the end, the decision to drain depends on whether the benefits in terms of diagnosis and reduction of work of breathing outweigh the risks of infection and haemopneumothorax. There are many techniques for drainage and three are discussed. First, a one-shot needle aspiration mostly indicated for diagnosis and short-term relief. Second, a pigtail type small bore catheter usually inserted using the Seldinger technique or a variant. Third, a large bore surgical type intercostal chest drain. There is a good case for ultrasound marking of the point of safest entry.

10.   Weaning Difficulties

There are many weaning strategies but few are superior or confer survival advantage. Crucial to weaning is an attempt to understand the pathophysiology of respiratory failure (RF), of which there are essentially three forms.

- Postoperative RF is characterised by a combination of pain, basal atelectasis, altered intravascular and extracellular volume, hypothermia, drowsiness and most importantly, capillary leak leading to pulmonary and peripheral oedema. Correction of these abnormalities and/or physiological support until recovery or compensation is the cornerstone of management.
- Obstructive RF (ObRF) is commonly seen in chronic obstructive airway disease (COAD) and asthma. These are predominantly diseases of the airways characterised by abnormal expiration caused by airway narrowing and/or excessive secretions. When significant, expiratory disease leads also to inspiratory weakness. The role of MV in obstructive RF is limited to provision of inspiratory assistance to reduce work of breathing while the expiratory pathology is reversed and the general condition, muscle weakness and nutrition improve. In principle, ventilation parameters for ObRF are low inspiratory pressure because compliance and inspiration are not normally affected, and low expiratory pressure, sufficient to prevent airway collapse and trigger inspiratory effort but not too high so as to cause air-trapping. Because MV does not treat the principle abnormality in obstructive RF, weaning is often slow and difficult.
- Restrictive RF (ReRF) is the physiological hallmark in diseases of the chest wall and neuromuscular disorders marked by predominantly inspiratory difficulties. Parenchymal Infection (pneumonia) is a form of restrictive lung

disease in that lung consolidation leads to reduced compliance and airway collapse, difficulty in drawing in air and fatigue. Therefore, in ReRF mechanical ventilation plays an important role, particularly in the setting of pneumonia. The ventilation parameters for ReRF due to pneumonia are a high mean or plateau airway pressure (but low enough to prevent trauma) and a high expiratory pressure to prevent airway collapse and facilitate gas exchange. Current research favours cautious ventilation and acceptance of certain physiological derangement (permissive hypercapnia) in an attempt to avoid excessively high pressure and volume with consequent iatrogenic lung damage.

In reality there is a spectrum of conditions with varying degrees of inspiratory and expiratory abnormalities. For example, patients with asthma or COAD can develop serious pneumonia, and those with kyphoscoiosis can also have asthma or undergo surgery.

The acute respiratory distress syndrome (ARDS) poses particular challenges for ventilation and weaning. Capillary leak leads to lifethreatening non-cardiogenic pulmonary oedema with increased lung water. This leads to decreased compliance and altered alveolar-capillary membrane, both of which can cause reduced alveolar ventilation and consequent ventilation/perfusion match leading to shunt and hypoxaemia. The ventilation strategy is as for ReRF/pneumonia.

Tracheostomies

Tracheostomies are now being performed early in patients likely to require ventilation for several days.[77] Recent evidence supports the general belief that the benefits of reduced sedation, improved mouth and secretion care and reduced deadspace outweigh the risks (early bleeding and pneumothorax and potential late development of tracheal infection and stenosis).[78]

Similarly, the advantages of percutaneous tracheostomies at the bedside, such as logistics and a perceived reduction in tracheal infections, must be weighed against the advantages of the traditional surgical technique, which are safety and access, especially in unfavourable neck and airway anatomy.[79] The technique, experience of the operator, the institution as well as timing are the most important factors in preventing complications, which can be catastrophic.

11. Slow Progress

Following complications, it is not uncommon for patients to develop multiple organ failure from which recovery is prolonged. This is characterised by a combination of severe sepsis and SIRS, multi-resistant ventilator associated pneumonia, ileus, inotrope dependence, wasting and malnutrition, renal failure and global central nervous dysfunction. Survival is often possible but requires a well orchestrated and enthusiastic multidisciplinary approach with an emphasis on organ support until physiological recovery ensues. Often, the central determinant of resolution of illness is freedom from infection.

REFERENCES

1. National Heart L, and Blood Institute ARDS Clinical Trials Network. (2004) Higher versus Lower Positive End-Expiratory Pressures in patients with the acute respiratory distress syndrome. *N Engl J Med* **351**: 327–336.
2. Network ARDS. (2000) Ventilation with lower tidal volumes as compared with traditional tidal volumes for acute lung injury and the acute respiratory distress syndrome. *New Engl J Med* **342**: 1301–1308.
3. Singer M, Bennett ED. (1991) Noninvasive optimization of left ventricular filling using esophageal Doppler. *Crit Care Med* **19**: 1132–1137.
4. García Rodriguez C, Pittman J, Cassell C, *et al.* (2002) *Crit Care Med* **30**: 2199–2204.
5. Bradley RD. (1964) Diagnostic right heart catheterisation with miniature catheters in severely ill patients. *The Lancet* **2**: 941–942.
6. Gómez C, Palazzo M. (1998) Pulmonary artery catheterisation in anaesthesia and intensive care. *Br J Anaesth* **81**: 945–956.
7. Harvey S, Harrison D, Singer M, *et al.* (2005) Assessment of the clinical effectiveness of pulmonary artery catheters in management of patients in intensive care (PAC-Man): a randomised controlled trial. *The Lancet* **366**: 472–477.
8. Sandham J, Douglas Hull R, Brant R, *et al.* (2003) A randomized, controlled trial of the use of pulmonary-artery catheters in high-risk surgical patients. *New Engl J Med* **348**: 5–14.
9. Robbins S, Cotran R, Kumar V. (1984) *Pathologic Basis of Disease*, 3rd edn. (W B Saunders Company, Philadelphia).
10. Manthous CA, Hall JB, Samsel RW. (1993) Endotoxin in human disease. Part 1: biochemistry, assay, and possible role in diverse disease states. *Chest* **104**: 1572–1581.

11. Bone RC, Balk RA, Cerra FB, *et al.* (1992) Definitions for sepsis and organ failure and guidelines for the use of innovative therapies in sepsis. *Chest* **101**: 1644–1655.

12. Blackwell TS, Christman JW. (1996) Sepsis and cytokines: current status. *Br J Anaesth* 77: 110–117.

13. Rangel-Frausto MS, Pittet D, Costigan M, *et al.* (1995) The natural history of the systemic inflammatory response syndrome. *JAMA* **273**: 117–123.

14. Galley HF, Webster NR. (1996) The immuno-inflammatory cascade. *Br J Anaesth* 77: 11–16.

15. Wheeler AP, Bernard GR (1999) Current concepts: treating patients with severe sepsis. *N Engl J Med* **340**: 207–214.

16. Hack CE, Zeerleder S. (2001) The endothelium in sepsis: source of and a target for inflammation. *Crit Care Med* **29**: S21–S27.

17. Esmon C, Taylor FJ, Snow T. (1991) Inflammation and coagulation: linked processes potentially regulated through a common pathway mediated by protein. *J Thromb Haemost* **66**: 160–165.

18. Parrillo JE. (1993) Pathogenic mechanisms of septic shock. *N Engl J Med* **328**: 1471–1477.

19. Bone RC. (1992) Phospholipids and their inhibitors: a critical evaluation of their role in the treatment of sepsis. *Crit Care Med* **20**: 884–889.

20. Titheradge MA. (1999) Nitric oxide in septic shock. *Biochim Biophys Acta* **1411**: 437–455.

21. van der Poll T, Butler HR, ten Cate HT. (1990) Activation of coagulation after administration of TNF to normal subjects. *N Engl J Med* **322**: 1622–1627.

22. Landry DW, Oliver JA. (2001) The patogenesis of vasodilatory shock. *N Engl J Med* **345**: 588–595.

23. Sair M, Etherington PJ, Peter WC, Evans TW. (2001) Tissue oxygenation and perfusion in patients with systemic sepsis. *Crit Care Med* **29**: 1343–1349.

24. Fink MP. (2001) Cytopathic hypoxia. Mitochondrial dysfunction as mechanism contributing to organ dysfunction in sepsis. *Crit Care Clin* **17**: 219–237.

25. Bernard GR, Artigas A, Brigham KL, *et al.* (1994) The American-European Consensus Conference on ARDS. Definitions, mechanisms, relevant outcomes, and clinical trial coordination. *Am J Respir Crit Care Med* **149**: 818–824.

26. Beale R, Grover ER, Smithies M, Bihari D. (1993) Acute respiratory distress syndrome ("ARDS"): no more than a severe acute lung injury? *Br Med J* **307**: 1335–1339.

27. Kollef MH, Schuster DP. (1995) The acute respiratory distress syndrome. *N Engl J Med* **332**: 27–37.

28. Bigatello LM, Zapol WM. (1996) New approaches to acute lung injury. *Br J Anaesth* 77: 99–109.

29. Schuster DP. (1995) What is acute lung injury? What is ARDS? *Chest* **107**: 1721–1726.

30. Amato MBP, Barbas C, Medeiros D, *et al.* (1998) Effect of a protective ventilation strategy on mortality in the acute respiratory distress syndrome. *N Engl J Med* **338**: 347–354.

31. Pinhu L, Whitehead T, Evans TW, Griffiths M. (2003) Ventilator associated lung injury. *The Lancet* **366**: 249–260.

32. Schuster DP. (1995) Fluid management in ARDS: "keep them dry" or does it matter? *Intensive Care Med* **21**: 101–103.

33. Goodman L, Fumagalli R, Tagliaube P, *et al.* (1999) Adult respiratory distress syndrome due to pulmonary and extrapulmonary causes: CT, clinical and functional correlations. *Radiology* **213**: 545–552.

34. Gattinoni L, Tognoni G, Pesenti A, *et al.* (2001) Effect of prone positioning on the survival of patients with acute respiratory failure. *N Engl J Med* **345**: 568–573.

35. Bigatello LM, Hurford WE, Kacmarek RM, *et al.* (1994) Prolonged inhalation of low concentrations of nitric oxide in patients with severe adult respiratory distress syndrome. Effects on pulmonary hemodynamics and oxygenation. *Anesthesiology* **80**: 761–770.

36. Puybasset L, Stewart T, Rouby JJ, *et al.* (1994) Inhaled nitric oxide reverses the increase in pulmonary vascular resistance induced by permissive hypercapnia in patients with acute respiratory distress syndrome. *Anesthesiology* **80**: 1254–1267.

37. Dellinger RP, Zimmerman JL, Taylor RW, *et al.* (1998) Effects of inhaled nitric oxide in patients with acute respiratory distress syndrome: results of a randomized phase II trial. *Crit Care Med* **26**: 15–23.

38. Payen D, Vallet B, Group G. (1999) Results of the French prospective multicentric randomized double-blind placebo-controlled trial on inhaled nitric oxide in ARDS. *Intensive Care Med* **25**(Suppl): S166.

39. Brett SJ, Evans TW. (1995) Inhaled vasodilator therapy in acute lung injury: first, do NO harm? *Thorax* **50**: 821–823.

40. Chastre J, Fagon J. (2002) Ventilator associated pneumonia. *Am J Respir Crit Care Med* **165**: 867–903.

41. Fagon J, Chastre J, Domart Y, *et al.* (1989) Nosocomial pneumonia in patients receiving continuous mechanical ventilation. Prospective analysis of 52 episodes with use of a protected specimen brush and quantitative culture techniques. *Am Rev Respir Dis* **139**: 877–884.

42. Livermore D. (2002) Multiple mechanisms of antimicrobial resistance in *Pseudomona Aeruginosa*: our worst nightmare? *Clin Infect Dis* **34**: 634–640.

43. Chastre J, Wolff M, Fagon J, *et al.* (2003) Comparison of 8 vs 15 days of antibiotic therapy for ventilator associated pneumonia in adults. A randomized trial. *JAMA* **290**: 2588–2598.

44. Mangano D, Browner W, Hollenberg M, *et al.* (1990) Association of perioperative myocardial ischaemia with cardiac morbidity and mortality in men undergoing noncardiac surgery. *N Engl J Med* **323**: 1781–1788.

45. Hamm C, Bertrand M, Braunwald E. (2001) Acute coronary syndrome without ST elevation: implementation of new guidelines. *The Lancet* **358**: 1533–1538.

46. Bertrand M, Simoons M, Fox K, *et al.* (2000) Management of acute coronary syndromes: acute coronary syndromes without persistent ST segment elevation; recommendations of the Task Force of the European Society of Cardiology. *Eur Heart J* **21**: 1406–1432.

47. Braunwald E, Antman E, Beasley J, *et al.* (2000) ACC/AHA guidelines for the management of patients with unstable angina and non-ST segment elevation myocardial infarction. A report of the American College of Cardiology/American Heart Association Task Force on Practice Guidelines (Committee on the Management of Patients with Unstable Angina). *J Am Coll Cardiol* **2000**: 970–1062.

48. Collinson PO, Stubbs PJ. (2003) Are troponins confusing? *Heart* **89**: 1285–1287.

49. Klein J, van der Hoeven J. (2004) Cardiac troponin elevations among critically ill patients. *Curr Opin Crit Care* **10**: 342–346.

50. Baine W, Yu M, Weis K. (1998) *J Am Geratr Soc* **49**: 763–770.

51. Reinet P, Karth G, Geppert A. (2001) Incidence and type of cardiac arrhythmias in critically ill patients: a single center experience in a medical-cardiological ICU. *Intensive Care Med* **27**: 1466–1473.

52. Huikuri H, Castellanos A, Myeburg J. (2001) Sudden death due to cardiac arrhythmias. *N Engl J Med* **345**: 1473–1482.

53. Yared J, Starr N, Torres F, *et al.* (2000) Effects of single dose, postinduction dexamethasone on recovery after cardiac surgery. 2000. *Ann Thorac Surg* **69**: 1420–1424.

54. Argalious MMM, Pablo MD, Khandwala, *et al.* (2005) "Renal dose" dopamine is associated with the risk of new-onset atrial fibrillation after cardiac surgery. *Crit Care Med* **33**: 1327–1332.

55. Brugada R, Brugada J, Roberts R. (1999) Genetics of cardiovascular disease with emphasis on atrial fibrillation. *J Interv Card Electrophysiol* **3**: 7–13.

56. Daoud E, Weiss R, Bahu M, *et al.* (1996) Effect of an irregular ventricular rhythm on cardiac output. *Am J Cardiol* **15**: 1433–1436.

57. Li-Saw-Hee F, Blann A, Lip G. (2000) Effects of fixed low-dose warfarin, aspirin-warfarin combination therapy, and dose-adjusted warfarin on thrombogenesis in chronic atrial fibrillation. *Stroke* **31**: 828–833.

58. Peters N, Schilling R, Kanagaratam P, Markides V. (2002) Atrial fibrillation: strategies to control, combat, and cure. *The Lancet* **359**: 593–603.

59. Trappe H, Brandts B, Weismueller P. (2003) Arrhythmias in the intensive care patient. *Curr Opin Crit Care* **9**: 345–355.

60. Martinez Marcos F, García Garmendia J, Ortega Carpio A, *et al.* (2000) Comparison of intravenous flecainide, propafenone, and amiodarone for conversion of acute atrial fibrillation to sinus rhythm. *Am J Cardiol* **86**: 950–953.

61. Hart R. (2003) Atrial fibrillation and stroke prevention. *New Engl J Med* **349**: 1015–1016.

62. Investigators AFF-uIoRMA. (2002) A comparison of rate control and rhythm control in patients with atrial fibrillation. *N Engl J Med* **347**: 1825–1833.

63. van Gelder I, Hagens V, Bosker H, *et al.* (2002) A comparison of rate control and rhythm control in patients with recurrent persistent atrial fibrillation.

64. Zipes D, Wellens H. (1998) Sudden cardiac death. *Circulation* **98**: 2334–2351.

65. Chen Q, Kirschott G, Zhang D, *et al.* (1998) Genetic basis and molecular mechanism for idiopathic ventricular fibrillation. *Nature* **392**: 293–296.

66. Investigators A. (1997) The antiarrhythmics versus implantable defibrillators (AVID) investigators: a comparison of antiarrhythmic drug therapy with implantable defibrillators in patients resuscitated from near fatal ventricular arrhythmias. *N Engl J Med* **337**: 1576–1583.

67. Lau C, Tse H, Ayers G. (1999) Defibrillation-guided radiofrequency ablation of atrial fibrillation secondary to an atrial focus. *J Am Coll Cardiol* **33**: 1217–1226.

68. Cox J, Boineau J, Schuessler R, *et al.* (1993) Five-year experience with the maze procedure for atrial fibrillation. *Ann Thorac Surg* **56**: 814–823.

69. Kelly J, Rudd A, Lewis R, Hunt BJ. (2002) Plasma d-dimers in the diagnosis of venous thromboembolism. *Arch Intern Med* **162**: 747–756.

70. Carson J, Kelley M, Duff A, *et al.* (1992) The clinical course of pulmonary embolism. *N Engl J Med* **326**: 1240–1245.

71. Fedullo P, Tapson V. (2003) The evaluation of suspected pulmonary embolism. *N Engl J Med* **349**: 1247–1256.

72. Zimetbaum P. (2003) Use of the electrocardiogram in acute myocardial infarction. *N Engl J Med* **348**: 933–940.

73. Konstantinides S, Geibel A, Heusel G, *et al.* (2002) Heparin plus alteplase compared with heparin alone in patients with submassive pulmonary embolism. *N Engl J Med* **347**: 1143–1150.

74. Goldhaber S. (2002) Thrombolysis for pulmonary embolism. *N Engl J Med* **347**: 1131–1132.

75. Vieillard-Baron A, Jardin F. (2003) Why protect the right ventricle in patients with acute respiratory distress syndrome. *Curr Opin Crit Care* **9**: 15–21.

76. Luckraz H, Dunning J. (2001) Pulmonary thromboendarterectomy. *Ann R Coll Surg Engl* **83**: 427–430.

77. Frutos VF, Esteban MA, Apezteguía C, *et al.* (2005) Outcome of mechanically ventilated patients who require a tracheostomy*. *Crit Care Med* **33**: 290–298.

78. Griffiths J, Barber V, Morgan L, Young J. (2005) Systematic review and meta-analysis of studies of the timing of tracheostomy in adult patients undergoing artificial ventilation. *Br Med J* **330**: 1243–1247.

79. Freeman B, Isabella K, Cobb J, *et al.* (2001) A prospective, randomized study comparing percutaneous with surgical tracheostomy in critically ill patients. *Crit Care Med* **29**: 926–930.

Chapter 4

SURGICAL INFECTIONS

Nazar A. Mustafa, Vasillios E. Papalois and Nadey S. Hakim

INTRODUCTION

In the old days, surgery was associated with high mortality caused by infection, because the concept of asepsis was not appreciated. Joseph Lister (1827–1912) demonstrated that using carbolic acid as an antiseptic before surgery reduces the chances of infection. In the 1880s and 90s, sterilisation of surgical instruments became another milestone towards aseptic surgery.[1]

William Stewart Halsted (1852–1912) and his student, Joseph Bloodgood were the first surgeons to introduce gloves for the operating theatre staff to protect them from the corrosive sublimate used for sterilisation. They demonstrated that this further reduced postoperative infection.[2]

Penicillin, discovered by Alexander Fleming in 1928 and used by Howard Florey in 1940, was a giant step in controlling infection and subsequently reducing mortality from surgery.[3]

Continuous improvement of anaesthetics since its use by Long (1842) and Molin (1846), increased the scope of surgery and helped combat infection by allowing surgeons more time to handle tissues gently and adopt measures that reduce the risk of infection.

More recently, the last few decades witnessed great advances in modern surgical practice, refined anaesthetics and potent antimicrobial therapy, but surgical infections continue to occur especially among immuno-compromised patients.

By definition, surgical infection is infection caused by surgery or requiring surgical treatment. This does not eliminate other modalities of treatment and it is possible for surgical infection to be treated solely by antimicrobial or conservative therapy. Among surgical patients, surgical site infections are the most common (38%) nosocomial infections. Each year, an estimated 2–5% of the patients undergoing surgical procedures develop infection.[4]

Surgical infections are associated with substantial morbidity and mortality with rates varying widely, depending upon the characteristics of patient population, size of the hospital and the surgeon's experience. Non-teaching hospitals generally have a lower rate of infection when compared with small (<500 beds) or large (>500 beds) teaching hospitals (4.6% versus 6.4% and 8.2% respectively).[5] Several studies have noted an increased risk of surgical infection in patients with cancer especially those undergoing surgical procedures.[6]

Surgical infections prolong hospital stay and increase the chances of patients contracting other nosocomial infections, such as respiratory and urinary infections. In one study of postoperative wound infection following orthopaedic procedures in a community and a tertiary care teaching hospital, the occurrence of surgical site infection accounted for a median 14-day increase in total hospitalisation.[7]

This confirms that surgical infections increase the overall cost of patient care as documented in several studies.[8]

PATHOPHYSIOLOGY OF SURGICAL INFECTION

Definition

Surgical infection is infection that requires operative treatment or results from operative treatment.

Defence Mechanisms

The human body is continuously in a state of defence against pathogens; in general, human defences can keep pathogens away and destroy them if they gain entry to the body. However, large numbers of pathogens live within the human body, under complete control of human defence mechanisms, and some of them even help in the defence mechanisms.

Infection occurs when human defence mechanisms are impaired or if powerful pathogens attack the human body. There are many factors that can tip this balance either way.

The host defence mechanisms are mechanical barriers, commensal microbial flora, cellular elements and humoral elements.

Skin, mucous membranes and the epithelial lining of hollow organs act as physical barriers preventing microbial entry into tissues either from outside the body or from within the lumen of organs containing a heavy microbial load. This is the first line of defence that is usually breached by the surgeons giving access to microbial invasion of the human body.

The human body harbours large quantities of microbial flora especially at either end of the gastrointestinal tract and the skin. An intact normal flora prevents possible pathogenic bacteria from multiplying by utilising available resources for growth themselves. However, beneficial bacteria that leave their natural environment and gain access to other organs or tissues can also cause infections. For example, normally harmless *Escherichia coli* present in the intestinal flora may cause urinary tract infection.

Cell-mediated immunity is an immune response that involves the activation of macrophages and natural killer (NK) cells, the production of antigen-specific cytotoxic lymphocytes, and the release of various cytokines in response to an antigen. Cellular immunity protects the body by:

- Activating antigen-specific cytotoxic T-lymphocytes that can lyse body cells
- Displaying foreign antigen, such as virus infected cells, cells with intracellular bacteria, and cancer cells with tumour antigens, on their surface
- Activating macrophages and natural killer cells, enabling them to destroy intracellular pathogens
- Stimulating cells to secrete a variety of cytokines that influence the function of other cells involved in adaptive and innate immune responses

Cell-mediated immunity is directed primarily at microbes that survive in phagocytes and those that infect non-phagocytic cells. It is most effective in removing virus-infected cells, and also participates in defending against fungi, protozoa, tumour cells and intracellular bacteria. It also plays a major role in transplant rejection.

Humoral immunity consists of antibodies, mainly immunoglobulins, a complement system with a cascade of reactions that lead to opsonization of pathogens and cytokines released by different cells of the immune system. It is a complex system but the basic principle is that phagocytic cells ingest a foreign antigen, process it and present it to the T helper cells, which stimulate B cells to produce antibodies against that specific antigen.

The pathogen must be extremely potent to overcome all these barriers in a healthy person. However, in patients debilitated by disease or major surgery and in immuno-suppressed patients, these barriers can be easily overcome and infection ensues.

Even in the presence of competent defence mechanisms infection can occur by less virulent pathogens and with less microbial load.

The factors that favour surgical infection are:

- Presence of devitalised tissues after trauma or surgery
- Fluid collection like haematoma or lymphocele
- Foreign bodies introduced by trauma or by the surgeon
- Oedema
- Impaired circulation due to ischemia or shock

It is obvious that surgical technique plays an important role in preventing or facilitating infection. Gentle tissue handling, good haemostasis, excision of devitalised tissues, appropriate use and removal of drains and non-tension in anastomotic lines will reduce the chances of postoperative infection.

SURGICAL MICROBIOLOGY

Most surgical site infections begin at the time of surgery and usually, the patient himself is the source of infection.

In clean wounds, the most common cause of infection is *Staphylococcus aureus* and coagulase negative *Staphylococci* from the skin flora of the patient. When surgery involves opening a viscus, bacteria present here is the usual suspect, leading to polymicrobial infection.

With the widespread use of prophylactic antibiotics, there is increasing incidence of infections caused by antibiotic resistant pathogens. Typical examples are methicillin-resistant *Staphylococcus aureus* (MRSA), methicillin-resistant *Staphylococcus epidermidis* (MRSE) and vancomycin-resistant *Enterococci* (VRE).[9,10] In addition, fungi, particularly *Candida albicans*, have been isolated from an increasing percentage of surgical site infections.[11]

Wound infection can also be caused by an exogenous source of pathogens from the operating room environment or personnel. An outbreak of wound infection with the same organisms can frequently be traced back to an infected theatre staff and rarely to contaminated dressing, antiseptic solution or drapes.

The common pathogens that cause surgical infection are *Staphylococcus aureus*, *Pseudomonas aeruginosa*, *Escherichia coli*, *Staphylococcus epidermidis* and *Enterococcus faecalis*.[12]

CLINICAL MANIFESTATION OF INFECTION

Stimulation of the immune system by microbial invasion of the human body leads to release of inflammatory mediators and consequent local or systemic inflammatory reaction. Classic symptoms of surgical infection are fever and pain at the site of infection. An examination of superficial infection may reveal a tender, red area, which is hot to touch and with or without discharge from the wound. Blood investigations may indicate a high level of inflammatory markers. The severity of infection depends on its intensity, the site of the infection and the competence of the immune system.

In immuno-compromised patients, infection can progress remarkably before any of these signs appear and the patient may collapse suddenly of overwhelming infection.

The immune reaction of the body can progress uncontrollably, as in systemic inflammatory response syndrome, due to severe sepsis and the patient might end up with septic shock and multi-organ failure.

Postoperative fever can be the first sign of infection and must be investigated thoroughly. Its common causes are:

Postoperative days 0 to 2

Mild fever (temperature less than 38°C) (Common)

- Tissue damage and necrosis at operation site
- Haematoma

Persistent fever (temperature more than 38°C)

- Atelectasis
  This is an extremely common postoperative complication, caused by partial pulmonary collapse that occurs after almost every abdominal or transthoracic procedure. Retained mucus in the bronchial tree blocks the finer bronchi and the alveolar air is absorbed resulting in collapse of the lung segments, usually the basal lobes. The collapsed lung may further face secondary infection from inhaled organisms.
- Specific infections related to the surgery

  - Biliary infection post-liver surgery
  - UTI post-kidney stones surgery

- Blood transfusion/Drug reaction

Postoperative days 3–5

- Bronchopneumonia
- Sepsis

  - Wound infection
  - Canula site infection/phlebitis
  - Abscess formation (e.g. subphrenic or pelvic, depending on type of surgery)

Postoperative days 5–7

- Deep venous thrombosis
- Specific complications related to surgery (bowel anastomosis breakdown, fistula formation)

Following the first postoperative week (less likely to be related to the specific operation)

- Wound infection
- Distant sites of sepsis
- Deep venous thrombosis

TYPES OF SURGICAL INFECTION

A. Surgical Site Infection
B. Soft Tissue Infection
C. Body Cavity Infection
D. Prosthetic Device related Infection
E. Miscellaneous

A. Surgical Site Infection

Postoperative wound infection is usually localized to the incision site but it can extend into adjacent deeper structures. Therefore, the term surgical wound infection has now been replaced with the more suitable name, surgical site infection. It is defined as an infection related to the operative procedure that occurs at or near the surgical incision within 30 days of an operative procedure or within one year if an implant is left in place.[13]

Types of Surgical Wounds

Clean wounds are uninfected surgical wounds without any evidence of inflammation and where the surgical wound was closed. Surgery here does not involve opening a viscus, such as the bowel, bladder or vagina. A good example is the hernia repair operation.

Clean contaminated wounds are wounds where a viscus is opened but without gross contamination, e.g. bowel surgery.

Contaminated wounds include open, fresh, accidental wounds, operations with major breaks in sterile technique or gross spillage from a viscus. Wounds in which acute, purulent inflammation was encountered are also included in this category.

Dirty wounds are defined as old traumatic wounds with retained devitalised tissue, foreign bodies, or faecal contamination or wounds that involve existing clinical infection or perforated viscus.

surgical site infections are either incisional or organ/space. Incisional infections are further divided into superficial (those involving only the skin or subcutaneous tissue) and those involving deep soft tissues of an incision. An organ/space infection may involve any part of the anatomy other than the incision that was opened or manipulated during the operative procedure.

The criteria of diagnosis of surgical site infection are:

— Purulent discharge from the wound or drain
— Positive culture of exudates from the wound
— Wound dehisces spontaneously or is opened deliberately by the surgeon to drain collection unless culture is negative
— Radiological evidence of collection with temperature over 38°C unless culture is negative
— Surgeon diagnoses infection on clinical suspicion

A surgical site infection is usually diagnosed by examination of the wound and a thorough assessment of the patient's charts. Imaging may be needed in some cases. Ultrasound has proved to be very efficient as first line investigation because it is non-invasive, can be done in the ward and is not expensive. However, in obese patients with deep-seated infection a computed tomography (CT) scan may be required.

The infected wound should be laid open to release pus and exudates. This is done by removing the stitches partially or totally in minor wound sepsis with no obvious collection. In other cases, it should be done in the operating room, with the patient anaesthetised, and the wound adequately opened, explored, irrigated, debrided, properly dressed, and the need for antibiotic therapy assessed.

Irrigation is usually done with saline because it is isotonic and does not interfere with wound healing. However, sterile water can also be used.[14] Irrigation should be under pressure to remove pus, loose clots, and dead tissue, using a syringe.

Debridement is the mechanical removal of devitalised tissue and foreign bodies by excision using scissors, scalpel or forceps. The tissue will not heal properly and infection will not be eradicated in the presence of dead tissue. Debridement can be done repeatedly and should stop only when healthy granulation tissue is in view.

The dressing of an infected surgical wound must be done carefully, repeatedly and by an experienced nurse or doctor who can differentiate between types of dressing and decide its frequency. Wet-to-dry gauze dressings are often used for continuing debridement of necrotic tissue from the wound bed. The gauze is moistened with normal saline or tap water, placed inside the wound and covered with dry layers of gauze.[15] As the moistened gauze dries out, it adheres to surface tissues, which are then removed when the dressing is changed. This process is repeated two to three times daily until the wound surface is covered with granulation tissue. However, wet-to-dry debridement can also remove developing granulation tissue, resulting in re-injury.

Exudate of wounds may contain factors that promote healing, and keeping wounds moist may hasten the healing process. Common categories of modern dressings that retain moisture include transparent films, hydrocolloids, foams, absorptive wound fillers, hydrogels, and collagens. While there is no clear recommendation for use of one over another, the ideal dressing should absorb exudate without leakage, be impermeable to water and bacteria, lack particulate contaminants that could be left in the wound upon removal, and not be traumatic to granulation tissue.

Antibiotics are usually not required in a superficial wound infection with no systemic signs of infection; simple local measures are sufficient for a good outcome. If there are signs of the infection spreading to adjacent tissues or in case of symptomatic infection, antibiotics are required.

A broad-spectrum antibiotic with coverage of the expected flora at the site of surgery should be started. Definitive antimicrobial treatment is guided by the clinical response of the patient and, when available, culture and sensitivity results. However, wound swab cultures often reveal polymicrobial growth, making it difficult to distinguish colonisation from true infection. There is no evidence that local antibiotics are beneficial in surgical site infection and their use should be restricted.

Following an infection, the wound can either be left to heal by secondary intention or closed if it looks healthy.

Novel Therapies

Negative pressure wound vacuum therapy is a procedure for evacuating wound fluid to expedite the healing of complex wounds, including those in previously irradiated tissue. There are no data from randomised trials evaluating the efficacy of this approach, but small observational series have been promising.[16,17]

Prevention of Surgical Site Infection

The incidence of infection varies from surgeon to surgeon, hospital to hospital, one surgical procedure to another, and most importantly patient to patient.

Although difficult to quantify, the critical factors in the prevention of surgical site infections are sound judgment and proper technique from the surgeon and the team, the type and severity of the primary illness, existing co-morbidities such as coincident remote site infections or colonisation, diabetes, cigarette smoking, systemic steroid use, obesity (20% over the ideal body weight), extremes of age, poor nutritional status, and perioperative transfusion of certain blood products.[18–20]

In clean surgical procedures, for which the infection rate should be less than 3%, infections may be solely due to airborne exogenous microorganisms.

Prevention of infection should be maximally tried at three levels:

Preoperative measures to reduce the risk of surgical site infection:

Treatment of pre-existing infections that may act as possible sources of infection.

Improving the general nutritional status of the patient, believed by some surgeons as a means to reduce the risk of infection,[21] although studies failed to confirm this despite a period of Total Parentral Nutrition.[22,23]

In diabetic patients, a good control of the condition should be achieved at least 48 h before surgery.[24]

Longer hospital stay is associated with a higher risk of postoperative infection. However, the length of the preoperative stay is likely to be a surrogate for severity of illness and co-morbid conditions requiring inpatient work-up and/or therapy before the operation.

Patients on steroids are at a higher risk of surgical site infection.[25] A short break off or a reduction in dosage if clinically feasible will reduce the risk of postoperative wound infection.

Smokers should be advised to stop smoking before surgery as some studies showed an increased risk of wound infection in tobacco smokers.[26]

Staphylococcus aureus is a frequent cause of postoperative surgical site infection. This pathogen is carried in the nares of 20%–30% of healthy humans. A recent study demonstrated that such a means of transport was the most powerful independent risk factor for infection following cardiothoracic operations.[27] A recent report suggested that risk of infection was reduced in patients who had undergone cardiothoracic operations when mupirocin (a topical ointment which is effective in eradicating *Staphylococcus aureus* from the nares of colonised patients or healthcare workers) was applied pre-operatively to their nares, regardless of carrier status.[28]

Pre-operative shower with antiseptic soap the night before surgery is advisable.

Hair removal should be avoided before surgery unless it interferes with the surgery. If so, it should be removed immediately before surgery and preferably using an electrical clipper.

The use of antibiotic prophylaxis before surgery has evolved greatly in the last 20 years.[29] Improvement in the timing of initial administration, the appropriate choice of antibiotic agents, and shorter durations of administration have defined the value of this technique in reducing postoperative wound infections more clearly. The choice of parentral prophylactic antibiotic agents and the timing and route of administration have become standardised on the basis of well-planned prospective clinical studies. In elective clean surgical procedures using a foreign body and in clean-contaminated procedures, a single dose of a cephalosporin, such as cefazolin, is recommended for intravenous administration by the anaesthetist just before incision. Additional doses are generally recommended only when the operation lasts longer than two or three hours.[30]

Intraoperative measures that reduce the risk of surgical site infection:

It is routine practice for surgeons to wash their hands with an antiseptic soap like povidone-iodine or chlorohexidine, before surgery (surgical scrubbing) ideally for 10 minutes. Scrubbing removes dirt and desquamated skin and reduces bacteria on the skin. Although there are no trials to prove the benefits of scrubbing in infection protection, it is considered as acceptable practise.[31] A recent trial in France showed that hand rubbing with 75% alcohol aqueous solution is superior to antiseptic soap scrubbing in the prevention of postoperative infection.[32]

The skin should be free of gross contamination by substances such as dirt, soil, or any other debris. The patient's skin is prepared by applying an antiseptic solution in concentric circles, beginning in the area of the proposed incision. The prepared area should be large enough to extend the incision or create new incisions or drain sites, if necessary. Various antiseptic solutions such as the iodophors (e.g. povidone-iodine), alcohol-containing products and chlorohexidine gluconate, are used. However, there have been no studies so far to prove the superiority of one over the other.

Surgical instruments are not a source of infection if sterilized properly. Strict control and check measures should be applied to ensure this is done.

Gloves play the dual role of protecting patients from a massive amount of hand pathogens[33] and protecting the surgeon as well. Surgical gloves provide a mechanical barrier against communicable diseases. Pooled data indicate the average probability of transmission after needle stick exposure as 0.2%–0.5% for HIV-1; 30% for hepatitis B, and between 5%–10% for hepatitis C.[34] An estimated 14% of the surgical gloves will have punctures after surgery[35] and double gloves are recommended, especially in an emergency, when bleeding is anticipated, in a long surgery and on patients with a high risk of HIV or hepatitis. Gloves should fit snugly and end over the cuff of the surgical gown.

Sterile surgical drapes are used to prevent contamination of the surgical site by migration of pathogens from outside the surgical field. Two types of drapes are usually used, disposable drapes with a plastic lining and cloth drapes. Cloth drapes should have tight weaves and must be dry to prevent bacterial migration. There is no evidence indicating the superiority of one type over the other and usage depends on hospital preferences and costs.

Gowns, masks and caps are traditionally used by surgeons to prevent shedding of microbes, desquamated skin and nasal droplets into the surgical wound although there are no studies to prove their benefit. There have been a few studies that indicate no difference in the incidence of postoperative infection if surgeons operate without wearing masks.[36]

Filters to provide ultra clean air in the operating room, laminar flow to move particle-free air over the aseptic operating field at a uniform velocity (vertically or horizontally) and positive pressure in the operating room to prevent entry of air from the theatre corridors are some of the advanced measures to prevent infection in orthopaedic theatres. In ordinary operating theatres, these may not be cost-effective.

Oxygen supplementation during surgery was proved to improve wound healing and reduce postoperative infection by increasing subcutaneous oxygen tension.[37]

Surgical technique: Surgery is a kind of physical trauma and the human body reacts to it in the same way as it reacts to other types of trauma. Surgery should be performed such that the goals of surgery are fulfilled with the minimum possible damage to tissues. The surgeon should be gentle in dealing with tissues, must understand the physiology of healing and remember that fluid collections and devitalised tissues are an open invitation to infection. Drains should be used appropriately and removed as soon as their work is done. There is no doubt that good surgical technique is the key to uneventful recovery from surgery.

Postoperative measures to reduce risk of wound infection:

Strict adherence to hand hygiene protocols should be followed while dealing with postoperative patients. Ideally, such patients should be nursed in a separate ward and discharged as soon as possible. Routine use of postoperative antibiotics should be discouraged unless indicated.

B. Soft Tissue Infection

Cellulitis is a superficially spreading skin infection, usually caused by streptococci. It starts as a minor insignificant wound infection, and can be accompanied by systemic symptoms of fever, chills, rigor and local pain at the site of infection. On examination, the area is warm with erythema that fades gradually into the adjacent healthy skin. Cellulitis responds to penicillin and its derivatives and if left untreated can progress to an abscess. Failure to respond to antibiotics may indicate an underlying abscess.

Necrotizing Infections

These are a spectrum of infectious diseases that result in necrosis of the skin and soft tissues. They include clostridial infections, which are rare, and necrotizing soft tissue infections of various types, which are more common. The broad categories within the latter group include necrotizing fasciitis, bacterial synergistic gangrene, and streptococcal gangrene. This entire spectrum is designated as infectious gangrenes or necrotizing soft tissue infections.

Necrotizing infections are uncommon and difficult to diagnose. They cause rapidly progressive morbidity until the infectious process is diagnosed and treated medically and surgically. A delay in diagnosis is associated with a grave prognosis and increased mortality.

For the clinician, the challenge in evaluating a necrotizing skin infection is the lack of diagnostic external signs or symptoms suggestive of the infection in the initial stages. The most important clinical approach to treating a skin and soft tissue infection is suspicion of a possible necrotizing soft tissue infection. Patients with malignancies, with chronic liver disease and immunocompromised patients are especially prone to necrotizing infections.

The majority of infections resulting in necrotizing fasciitis are due to a combination of [beta]-haemolytic *Streptococci* (90%), anaerobic Gram-positive *Cocci*, aerobic Gram-negative *Bacilli*, and the *Bacteroides* spp. A single organism, with the unusual exception of Group A [beta]-haemolytic *Streptococci*, rarely causes an infection resulting in necrotizing fasciitis.

Here, the patient appears ill and has a rapid pulse and significant temperature elevation. Some patients with necrotizing fasciitis may present with localized pain of the involved site, and the overlying skin is erythematous, hot, and oedematous. Severe pain and systemic symptoms that not proportional to the local infection characterise clostridial infections. An occasional symptom is numbness of the involved area, probably due to infarction of the cutaneous nerves that are located in the necrotic subcutaneous fascia and soft tissue. As the clostridial infection progresses, the skin may develop a bronze colour, followed by haemorrhagic bullae, dermal gangrene, and finally crepitus. The clinical sign of crepitus is found in 50% of the patients. Bullae, skin necrosis, sero-purulent exudates, and foul odour are common in the late presentation of skin and soft tissue necrotizing infections.

Several reliable diagnostic tests for necrotizing infection are available, such as CT and magnetic resonance imaging (MRI) scans, tissue biopsy, and needle aspiration. Biopsy can identify fungus in the tissue and fungal invasion with thrombosis of blood vessels. Tissue biopsy with Gram's stain of the exudate may also reveal the characteristic finding of clostridia organisms, which appear as Gram-positive rods with blunt ends resembling boxcars. Fine-needle or large-bore needle aspiration is another method by which to establish the diagnosis and direct antimicrobial therapy. CT scans provide an accurate picture of the presence and extent of abnormal soft tissue gas dissecting along fascial planes, which is almost always diagnostic of necrotizing fasciitis. MRI is most useful in stable, conscious, cooperative, and not seriously septic patients.

Once the diagnosis of necrotizing skin and soft tissue infection is made or highly suspected, fluid resuscitation and cardiovascular stabilisation of the patient is necessary before surgery. Frequently, this requires placement of a central line or a Swan-Ganz catheter and preoperative fluid resuscitation in an intensive care unit (ICU) if the patient is unstable. Appropriate IV antibiotics are always administered prior to surgery, and a triple regimen of IV antibiotic coverage is appropriate to cover the diverse and varied causative bacteria.

Penicillin or ampicillin for *Clostridia*, *Streptococci*, and *Peptostreptococcus*
Clindamycin or metronidazole for anaerobes, *Bacteroides fragilis, Fusobacterium* and *Peptostreptococcus*.
Gentamicin or another aminoglycoside for *Enterobacteriaceae* (i.e. Gram-negative organisms). Gentamicin has a synergistic effect with penicillin against *Streptococci*.

Imipenem and meropenem by virtue of their high [beta]-lactamase resistance, wide-spectrum efficacy, and inhibition of endotoxin release from aerobic (i.e. Gram-negative) *bacilli*, may be the initial agents of choice for treatment. Amputation of an extremity should be considered early in the treatment of clostridial gangrenous infections, because it may be lifesaving. High-dose intravenous penicillin should be administered; clindamycin or metronidazole is substituted for patients with penicillin allergy.

The management of any infectious gangrene requires an urgent surgical procedure. As soon as the patient's condition permits administration of a general anaesthetic, complete surgical debridement of the area is performed in the operating room. Occasionally, a patient may remain in septic shock after resuscitation and intravenous antibiotics are initiated. Surgical debridement should not be delayed, because correction of the septic state may not occur until the infectious gangrenous process is completely excised.

The surgeon must always follow three surgical principles, which are complete excision of all necrotic tissue; establishment of wide surgical drainage; and meticulous attention to haemostasis. A critical element in the successful treatment of patients with soft tissue necrotizing infections is time. Early recognition and aggressive medical and surgical therapy are the primary determinants of a successful outcome in the treatment of all patients with skin and soft tissue necrotizing infections. A delay between admission and the first complete surgical debridement would significantly increase morbidity and mortality.

Hyperbaric oxygenation should be administered post-surgery to a patient with clostridial gangrene, because it is bacteriostatic to the clostridial organism and seems to hinder the production of [alpha] toxin. However, residual necrotic tissue left after debridement of clostridial gangrene reduces or neutralizes the beneficial effect of hyperbaric oxygenation. In non-clostridial soft tissue infection, hyperbaric oxygenation shortens the time taken for closure of the wound after surgical debridement. Therefore, it is important to emphasise that primary treatment in all patients with infectious gangrene is meticulous, with complete surgical debridement at the initial surgical procedure.[38]

Abscess is a collection of pus in tissue, organ or confined space and is usually caused by bacteria. It often presents as painful swelling or lump that develops over a period, from a few hours to a few days. If it is superficial, signs of inflammation will be obvious in surrounding tissues but if it is deep, systemic signs of infection like fever and anorexia may be present initially.

Abscess is usually caused by disruption of a normal tissue barrier through penetrating trauma, haematogenous spread or by migration of normal flora to other sterile areas of the body. Leukocytes form a wall around infectious agents in tissue, organs or body space to localise pus in an attempt to prevent further spread of infection. This may resolve the inflammation and the exudates may be reabsorbed. In a more severe infection, more leukocytes will be drawn into the area. Dead bacteria, leukocytes and tissue will liquefy to form pus. Bacteraemia occurs if an abscess develops deep in the body and ruptures allowing infectious agents to enter the blood stream. If the pathogen continues to multiply in the blood and release toxins, the result is septicaemia.

The causative organisms are varied and may reflect the area where the abscess is located. Cutaneous and soft tissue abscess are commonly associated with *Staphylococcus aureus*, while those of the abdomen may be due to a combination of both anaerobic and aerobic Gram-negative *bacilli* such as *Klebsiella* and *Escherichia coli*, and anaerobes such as *Bacteroides fragilis*. Oral and perineal abscesses may be produced by anaerobic bacteria and contain a brown foul smelling pus.

Surgical treatment is mandatory if an abscess is diagnosed. The abscess should be incised and drained and the necrotic wall must be curettaged. Antibiotics are not effective in treatment because they do not penetrate the abscess wall. Antimicrobial therapy is needed only if there are signs and symptoms of systemic infection.

C. Body Cavity Infection

Peritonitis is the inflammation of the peritoneal lining of the abdominal cavity. The different types of peritonitis are:

Spontaneous or primary peritonitis affects children and patients with ascites with intact body wall and internal organs. It is usually caused by a single type of bacteria that probably migrated haematogenously or via the lymphatic circulation to the peritoneal cavity. This type of peritonitis usually responds to antibiotic therapy.

Secondary peritonitis is usually polymicrobial due to inflammation or rupture of an internal organ. It can also be due to penetrating injuries of the abdominal wall or surgery.

Peritonitis associated with dialysis is usually caused by skin flora, mainly *Staphylococcus*, with an average incidence of one episode per patient every 19.2 months in Scotland.[39] The Renal Association standard is one episode per patient every 18 months or more. It may respond to antibiotic therapy; however, removal of the peritoneal dialysis catheter may be required.

Sclerosing peritonitis is a rare but serious complication of peritoneal dialysis. Small-bowel obstruction due to encapsulation, dense adhesions, or mural fibrous are characteristics often associated with peritonitis. In plain abdominal film, diffuse calcification of the peritoneum and small-bowel dilatation are indicative of sclerosing peritonitis. A CT scan of the abdomen showed both peritoneal and mesenteric thickening with dilated bowel.

The treatment of peritonitis involves treatment of the original cause along with fluid resuscitation and antibiotic therapy.

D. Prosthetic Device Related Infection

Infections related to prosthesis, such as artificial valves and joints as well as simple peritoneal and haemodialysis catheters or vascular grafts are difficult to treat and often the device (foreign body) has to be removed. Foreign bodies reduce the inoculums of *Staphylococcus aureus* required to induce infection to as little as 100 colony-forming units.[40] In addition, the interaction of neutrophils with the foreign body can induce a neutrophil defect that may enhance the susceptibility to infection.[41]

Bacteria attach themselves to the surface of the foreign body, and as they multiply, they produce exopolysaccharides, which are also known as glyocalyx. Microcolonies of bacteria encased in glycocalyx coalesce to form a structure known as a biofilm.[42,43] The biofilm isolates the multiplying bacteria from host defences and antibiotics. Diffusion of antimicrobial agents through a biofilm is often slow or limited.

In some cases, treatment may involve washing out of the prosthesis combined with antibiotic therapy. However, recurrence of the infection is common and the only effective treatment is removal of the foreign body.

E. Hospital Acquired Infection

Nosocomial infections can be defined as those occurring within 48 h of hospital admission, three days of discharge or 30 days following an operation. They affect 10% of patients admitted to hospitals. In the United Kingdom, this results in 5,000 deaths annually with a cost of one billion pounds per year to the National Health Service. On average, a patient with hospital acquired infection spent 2.5-times longer in hospital, incurring additional costs of £3,000 more than an uninfected patient.[44] The study, carried out by the Public Health Laboratory Service and London School of Hygiene and Tropical Medicine on behalf of the Department of Health in the United Kingdom, found that infected patients incurred higher personal costs and returned to normal daily activities and/or paid employment much later than uninfected patients.

The highest prevalence of hospital-acquired infections is seen in the ICU. The European Prevalence of Infection in Intensive Care Study (EPIC), involving over 4,500 patients, demonstrated that nosocomial infection prevalence rate in the ICU was 20.6%.[45] ICU patients are particularly at risk because of mechanical ventilation, use of invasive procedures and their own immuno-compromised status.[46]

The cause of nosocomial infection is the high prevalence of pathogens in the hospital environment in the presence of compromised hosts and effective mechanisms of transmission from patient to patient.

Nosocomial infections are primarily caused by opportunistic organisms, particularly the *Enterococcus* and *Pseudomonas* spp., *Escherichia coli*, and *Staphylococcus aureus*. These pathogens also tend to become incorporated into the normal flora of hospital workers, which makes it available for transmission to patients. Once infection has set in, it is not easy to treat.

The common sites of nosocomial infections, in order of frequency, are the urinary tract, surgical wounds, the respiratory tract, skin, blood (bacteraemia), the gastrointestinal tract and the central nervous system. Immuno-compromised patients and those with broken skin or mucous membranes are at higher risk of infection.

The chain of transmission of pathogens from patients to patients and from patients to hospital staff and back to patients should be broken and every hospital should have a set of procedures and guidelines on how to break it.

The methods of prevention of nosocomial infections and breaking the chain of transmission include:

- Observance of aseptic technique
- Frequent hand washing especially between patient examinations
- Careful handling, cleaning, and disinfection of fomites
- Use of single-use disposable items where possible
- Patient isolation
- Avoidance of medical procedures that can increase the probability of nosocomial infections, where possible
- Various institutional methods, such as air filtration within the hospital
- General awareness that prevention of nosocomial infections requires constant personal surveillance
- Active oversight within the hospital

Examples of Hospital Acquired Infection

Urinary Tract Infection

Urinary tract infection (UTI) is the most common hospital acquired infection. The clinical spectrum of UTI is broad, ranging from asymptomatic bacteriuria to symptomatic UTI, pyelonephritis, renal abscess, and sepsis.

Bacteriuria is an inevitable consequence of urethral catheters that are commonly inserted in very ill patients and postoperatively after a major surgery. The risk of bacteriuria with a single insertion of urethral catheter is 5%, increasing by an additional 5% for each day of catheterisation. Bacteriuria will eventually become symptomatic and progress to frank UTI.

Although less than 5% of catheter-associated UTIs result in bacteraemia, 15% of all nosocomial bacteraemia are attributable to nosocomial UTI as the initial source. Catheter-associated UTIs have a major impact on healthcare. They are a source of antibiotic-resistant organisms in the hospital and, as a result, a major economic burden on hospital costs.

Some factors that increase the risk catheter-related infection significantly are duration of catheterisation; lack of systemic antibiotics during short catheter courses; lack of a closed system urinemeter drainage; sex (females are at higher risk); diabetes mellitus; microbial colonisation of the drainage bag; serum creatinine levels (greater than 2 mg/dl at the time of catheterisation); and the reason for catheterisation.[47]

The pathogens associated with UTIs have changed over the past decade with a shift to more fungal and Gram-positive infections and fewer Gram-negative rods. *Escherichia coli* is responsible for 17.5% of UTIs; *Candida albicans* for nearly 16%; the *Enterococcus* spp. for nearly 14%; *Pseudomonas aeruginosa* for 11%; and the *Enterobacter* spp. for 5%.[48] The other pathogens, including coagulase-negative *Staphylococci* and *Staphylococcus aureus*, account for approximately 30%.[49] Nonetheless, most complications of urinary catheterisation remain a direct result of the patient's own bacteria, which colonise in the external and internal surfaces of indwelling catheters.

The use of systemic antibiotics is shown to postpone the development of UTIs and, consequently bacteraemia in catheterised patients. However, the preventive use of antibiotics is generally effective only for the first few days and subsequently, resistant organisms begin to arise. The rapid emergence of resistance and the cost of antibiotic prophylaxis have resulted in many authorities recommending against this practice, except in transplant patients and those who are granulocytopenic.[50]

Lower Respiratory Tract Infections

Pneumonia is the second most common nosocomial infection in general and the third in surgical patients, after UTI and surgical site infection. It is associated with considerable morbidity and mortality.

Some conditions associated with higher risk of nosocomial pneumonia are:

- Extremes of age
- Severe underlying disease
- Immuno-suppression
- Diminished consciousness
- Cardiopulmonary disease
- Thoracoabdominal surgery
- Pulmonary oedema
- Nasogastric tube insertion

Although those receiving mechanically assisted ventilation do not represent a major proportion of patients with nosocomial pneumonia, they are at the highest risk for acquiring the infection.

Most bacterial nosocomial pneumonias occur because of aspiration of bacteria colonising the oropharynx or upper gastrointestinal tract of the patient, in the presence of a diminished cough reflex due to anaesthesia and sedation. Intubation and mechanical ventilation increase the risk for nosocomial bacterial pneumonia greatly.

The most common bacteria in hospital-acquired pneumonia are *Staphylococcus aureus*, *Pseudomonas aeruginosa*, *Escherichia coli*, and the *Klebsiella* and *Enterobacter* spp. More than one-half of cultured *Enterobacteriaceae*, *Pseudomonas*, and *Staphylococcus aureus* were obtained in patients diagnosed with pneumonia before the fifth postoperative day.

Nosocomial bacterial pneumonia has been difficult to diagnose.[51] The criteria for diagnosis are fever, cough, and development of purulent sputum, in conjunction with radiological evidence of a new or progressive pulmonary infiltrate. A suggestive Gram's stain and positive cultures of sputum, tracheal aspirate, pleural fluid or blood help in establishing the diagnosis.[52,53] Cultures of blood or pleural fluid have very low sensitivity.[54]

The traditional preventive measures for nosocomial pneumonia include decreasing aspiration by the patient, preventing cross-contamination or colonisation via the hands of healthcare workers, appropriate disinfection or sterilisation of respiratory-therapy devices, use of available vaccines to protect against particular infections, and education of hospital staff and patients. New measures being investigated involve reducing oropharyngeal and gastric colonisation by pathogenic microorganisms.[55]

Intravascular Line Infection

Vascular catheters and central venous lines are increasingly being used in modern surgical and medical practice for monitoring ill patients, dialysis, parentral nutrition, chemotherapy and fluid therapy. This has led to an increase in the incidence of line infections. The skin flora (*Staphylococcus aureus* and *Staphylococcus epidermis*) are the most common cause of infection. However, Candida and other organisms like *Klebsiella*, *Pseudomonas*, *Serratia*, *Acinetobacter*, *Stenotrophomonas maltophilia* and other *Enterobacteria* can also infect vascular catheters. Once the infection is established and the biofilm has formed it will be difficult to eradicate it; the vascular line will have to be removed.

Systemic antibiotic and antibiotic lock therapy may sometimes help in treating intravascular line infection. Antibiotic lock therapy involves the use of antibiotics after an anticoagulant solution is flushed through the catheter. This "locks" a high concentration of the antibiotics in the lumen of the catheter at least once daily day.[56]

A careful insertion of these lines by an experienced practitioner, under strict aseptic conditions is the only way to reduce the risk of such an infection. An antibiotic cover should be considered for immuno-compromised and severely ill patients.

CONCLUSION

Surgical infections can range from mild cellulitis to overwhelming sepsis with variable degrees of morbidity and even mortality. They draw on a considerable portion of the healthcare budget. The key is to try all the necessary pre-, intra- and postoperative measures to prevent their incidence. However, even with all the preventive measures on board, surgical infections are sometimes inevitable. When they do occur, it is vital to diagnose early and to treat the infections promptly before they escalate and have a considerable effect on patients.

REFERENCES

1. Lister J. (1867) On a new method of treating compound fractures, abscesses, etc. *The Lancet* **1**: 326–329.
2. Koehler BM, Roderer NK, Ruggere C. (2004) A short history of the William H. Welch Medical Library. *Neurosurgery* **54**(2): 465–479.
3. Chain E, Florey HW, Gardner AD, *et al.* (2005) The classic: penicillin as a chemotherapeutic agent. *Clin Orthop Rel Res* **439**: 23–26.
4. Consensus paper on the surveillance of surgical wound infections. (1992) The Society for Hospital Epidemiology of America; The Association for Practitioners in Infection Control; The Centers for Disease Control; The Surgical Infection Society. *Infect Control Hosp Epidemiol* **13**: 599.
5. Whitehouse JD, Friedman ND, Kirkland KB, *et al.* (2002). The impact of surgical-site infections following orthopedic surgery at a community hospital and a university hospital: adverse quality of life, excess length of stay, and extra cost. *Infect Control Hosp Epidemiol* **23**: 183.

5. Perencevich EN, Sands KE, Cosgrove SE, *et al.* (2003) Health and economic impact of surgical site infections diagnosed after hospital discharge. *Emerg Infect Dis* **9**: 196.

6. Whitehouse JD, Friedman ND, Kirkland KB, *et al.* (2002) The impact of surgical-site infections following orthopedic surgery at a community hospital and a university hospital: adverse quality of life, excess length of stay, and extra cost. *Infect Control Hosp Epidemiol* **23**: 183.

7. Vegas AA, Jodra VM, Garcia ML. (1993) Nosocomial infection in surgery wards: a controlled study of increased duration of hospital stays and direct cost of hospitalisation. *Eur J Epidemiol* **9**: 504.

8. Poulsen KB, Bremmelgaard A, Sorensen AI, *et al.* (1994) Estimated costs of post-operative wound infections. A case-control study of marginal hospital and social security costs. *Epidemiol Infect* **113**: 283.

9. Cruse PJ, Foord R. (1980) The epidemiology of wound infection. A 10-year prospective study of 62,939 wounds. *Surg Clin North Am* **60**: 27.

10. Culver DH, Horan TC, Gaynes RP, *et al.* (1991) Surgical wound infection rates by wound class, operative procedure, and patient risk index. National Nosocomial Infections Surveillance System. *Am J Med* **91**: 152S.

11. Jarvis WR. (1995) Epidemiology of nosocomial fungal infections, with emphasis on Candida species. *Clin Infect Dis* **20**: 1526.

12. Giacometti A, Cirioni O, Schimizzi AM, *et al.* (2000) Epidemiology and microbiology of surgical wound infections. *J Clin Microbiol* **38**(2): 918–922.

13. Horan TC, Gaynes RP, Martone WJ, *et al.* (1992) CDC definitions of nosocomial surgical site infections, 1992: a modification of CDC definitions of surgical wound infections. *Am J Infect Control* **20**: 271.

14. Fernandez R, Griffiths R, Ussia C. (2002) Water for wound cleansing. *Cochrane Database Syst Rev* CD003861.

15. Ovington LG. (2001) Hanging wet-to-dry dressings out to dry. *Home Healthc Nurse* **19**: 477.

16. Schimp VL, Worley C, Brunello S, *et al.* (2004) Vacuum-assisted closure in the treatment of gynecologic oncology wound failures. *Gynecol Oncol* **92**: 586.

17. Lambert KV, Hayes P, McCarthy M. (2005) Vacuum assisted closure: a review of development and current applications. *Eur J Vasc Endovasc Surg* **29**: 219.

18. Nichols RL. (1982) Postoperative wound infection. *N Engl J Med* **307**: 1701–1702.

19. Nichols RL. (1991). Surgical wound infection. *Am J Med* **91**(Suppl 3B): 54S–64S.

20. Nichols RL. (1982) Techniques known to prevent postoperative wound infection. *Infect Control* **3**: 34–37.

21. Moore EE, Jones TN. (1986) Benefits of immediate jejunostomy feeding after major abdominal trauma. A prospective, randomized study. *J Trauma* **26**: 874.

22. Brennan MF, Pisters PW, Posner M, *et al.* (1994) A prospective randomized trial of total parenteral nutrition after major pancreatic resection for malignancy. *Ann Surg* **220**: 436.

23. The Veterans Affairs Total Parenteral Nutrition Cooperative Study Group. (1991) Perioperative total parenteral nutrition in surgical patients. *N Engl J Med* **325**: 525.

24. Zerr KJ, Furnary AP, Grunkemeier GL, *et al.* (1997) Glucose control lowers the risk of wound infection in diabetics after open heart operations. *Ann Thorac Surg* **63**: 356.

25. Post S, Betzler M, vonDitfurth B, *et al.* (1991) Risks of intestinal anastomoses in Crohn's disease. *Ann Surg* **213**: 37.

26. Nagachinta T, Stephens M, Reitz B, Polk BF. (1987) Risk factors for surgical-wound infection following cardiac surgery. *J Infect Dis* **156**: 967.

27. Perl TM, Golub JE. (1998) New approaches to reduce Staphylococcus aureus nosocomial infection rates: treating *S. aureus* nasal carriage. *Ann Pharmacother* **32**: S7.

28. Kluytmans JA, Mouton JW, Ijzerman EP, *et al.* (1995) Nasal carriage of *Staphylococcus aureus* as a major risk factor for wound infections after cardiac surgery. *J Infect Dis* **171**: 216.

29. Nichols RL, Condon RE. (1971) Preoperative preparation of the colon. *Surg Gynecol Obstet* **132**: 323–337.

30. Nichols RL. (1996) Surgical infections: prevention and treatment — 1965 to 1995. *Am J Surg* **172**: 68–74.

31. Boyce JM, Pittet D. (2002) Guideline for hand hgiene in healthcare settings: recommendations of the Healthcare Infection Control Practices Advisory Committee and the HICPAC/SHEA/APIC/IDSA Hand Hygiene Task Force. *Infect Control Hosp Epidemiol* **23**: S3.

32. Parienti JJ, Thibon P, Heller R, *et al.* (2002) Hand-rubbing with an aqueous alcoholic solution vs traditional surgical hand-scrubbing and 30-day surgical site infection rates: a randomized equivalence study. *JAMA* **288**: 722.

33. Thomas S, Agarwal M, Mehta G. (2001) Intraoperative glove perforation-single versus double gloving in protection against skin contamination. *Postgrad Med J* **77**: 458–460.

34. Dalgleish AG, Malkovsky M. (1988) Surgical gloves as a mechanical barrier against human immunodeficiency viruses. *Br J Surg* **75**: 171–172.

35. Alrawi S, Houshan L, Satheesan R, *et al.* (2001) Glove reinforcement: an alternative to double gloving. *Infect Control Hosp Epidemiol* **22**: 526.

36. Edmiston CE Jr., Seabrook GR, Cambria RA, *et al.* (2005) Molecular epidemiology of microbial contamination in the operating room environment: is there a risk for infection? *Surgery* 138(4): 573–582.

37. Hopf HW, Hunt TK, West JM, *et al.* (1997) Wound tissue oxygen tension predicts the risk of wound infection in surgical patients. *Arch Surg* 132: 997.

38. Majeski JA, John JF Jr. (2003) Necrotizing soft tissue infections: a guide to early diagnosis and initial therapy. *South Med J* 96(9): 900–905.

39. Kavanagh D, Prescott GJ, Mactier RA, on behalf of the Scottish Renal Registry. (2004) Peritoneal dialysis-associated peritonitis in Scotland (1999–2002). *Nephrol Dial Transpl* 19(10): 2584–2591; doi:10.1093/ndt/gfh386.

40. Zimmerli W, Waldvogel FA, Vaudaux P, Nydegger UE. (1982) Pathogenesis of foreign body infection: description and characteristics of an animal model. *J Infect Dis* 146: 487.

41. Zimmerli W, Lew PD, Waldvogel FA. (1984) Pathogenesis of foreign body infection. Evidence for a local granulocyte defect. *J Clin Invest* 73: 1191.

42. Costerton JW, Stewart PS, Greenberg EP. (1999) Bacterial biofilms: a common cause of persistent infections. *Science* 284: 1318.

43. Donlan RM. (2001) Biofilm formation: a clinically relevant microbiological process. *Clin Infect Dis* 33(8): 1387 (Epub 2001 Sep 20).

44. Plowman R, Graves N, Griffin M, *et al.* (2000) The socio-economic burden of hospital acquired infection. London: PHLS. (Executive summary: http://www.doh.gov.uk/haicosts.htm).

45. Louis V, Bihari MB, Suter P, *et al.* (1995) The prevalence of nosocomial infections in intensive care units in Europe. European Prevalence of infection in intensive care (EPIC) study. *JAMA* 274: 639–644.

46. Kollef MH (2004) Prevention of hospital-associated pneumonia and ventilator-associated pneumonia. *Crit Care Med* 32(6): 1396–1405.

47. Platt R, Polk BF, Mudock B, Rosner B. (1986) Risk factors for nosocomial urinary tract infection. *Am J Epidemiol* 124(6): 977–985.

48. NNIS System. (1999) National nosocomial infections surveillance (NNIS) system report, data summary from January 1990–May 1999, issued June 1999. *Am J Infect Control* 27: 520–532.

49. Tambyah PA, Maki DG. (2000) Catheter-associated urinary tract infection is rarely symptomatic. *Arch Intern Med* 160: 678–682.

50. Warren JW. (1997) Catheter-associated urinary tract infections. *Infect Dis Clin North Am* 11: 609–622

51. Chastre J, Fagon JY, Soler P, *et al.* (1988) Diagnosis of nosocomial bacterial pneumonia in intubated patients undergoing ventilation: comparison of the usefulness

of bronchoalveolar lavage and the protected specimen brush. *Am J Med* **85**: 499–506.

52. Schaberg DR, Culver DH, Gaynes RP. (1991) Major trends in the microbial etiology of nosocomial infection. *Am J Med* **91**(suppl 3B): 72S–75S.

53. Bartlett JG, O'Keefe P, Tally FP, *et al.* (1986) Bacteriology of hospital-acquired pneumonia. *Arch Intern Med* **146**: 868–871.

54. Higuchi JH, Coalson JJ, Johanson WG Jr. (1982) Bacteriologic diagnosis of nosocomial pneumonia in primates: usefulness of the protected specimen brush. *Am Rev Respir Dis* **125**: 53–57.

55. Montravers P, Veber B, Auboyer C, *et al.* (2002) Diagnostic and therapeutic management of nosocomial pneumonia in surgical patients: results of the Eole study. *Crit Care Med* **30**: 368.

56. Krzywda EA, Andris DA, Edmiston CE, Quebbeman EJ. (1995) Treatment of Hickman catheter sepsis using antibiotic lock technique. *Infect Control Hosp Epidemiol* **16**: 596–598.

Chapter 5

SURGICAL WOUND COMPLICATIONS

Umraz Khan

THE VASCULAR SUPPLY OF SKIN

Interest in the arterial input to the skin and sub-cutaneous fat has been investigated by surgical scientists for over a century. However, it appears to have been ignored as an important piece of surgical knowledge. The works of Manchot[1] and Salmon[2] were amongst the first published accounts of the vascular tree inherent in the skin. Since one of the many functions of the skin is to maintain body temperature, the skin must be enabled with a mechanism for changes in its blood flow of a hundred fold. Skin is capable of these great changes in the flow of blood because of the presence of a number of plexi within the subcutaneous fat, the dermis and the dermo-epidermal junction (Fig. 1). As can be seen from the cartoon figure and the clinical photograph, there are at least three sources of blood which feed into a section of skin and fat. These are the direct perforating vessels (sometimes referred to as septo-cutaneous vessels) which end with the skin; the in-direct perforating vessels (sometimes referred to as musculo-cutaneous perforating vessels); and the random feeding vessels.

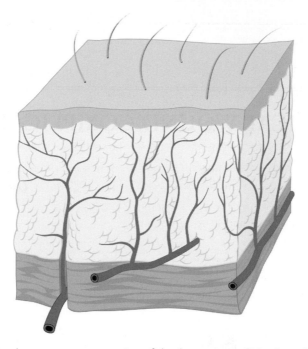

Fig. 1. Shown is a cartoon representation of the three sources of blood supply to the skin. The three arteries are the septocutaeous perforators (in the lower left corner of the block of skin). These vessels are given off from the axial vessel which itself is travelling between adjacent muscle groups. These septocutaneous perforators travel to the skin in a septum to end in the skin. The second group of vessels are the musculo-cutaneous perforators (shown in the middle of the cartoon). These vessels reach the skin after travelling through the muscle which they also supply). The last source of arterial input to the skin is shown in the cartoon towards the right. These are the random vessels which lie in the surrounding tissue but provide branches into the index block of skin.

The control of the blood flow is regulated by pre-capillary sphincters which in turn are responsive to both local and systemic factors. Among the local factors which exert an important influence is the accumulation of lactic acid and CO_2. The sphincters are innervated by the sympathetic nervous system and thus respond to demands declared by that system. When one makes a surgical incision into the skin one must be aware of this basic physiology of the skin circulation, the importance of the underlying musculature and where the "mother" vessels lie.

WOUND HEALING

Following either intentional (i.e. surgical) or unintentional (i.e. traumatic) wounding, the tissues of the body respond in a predictable manner. Thus one refers to phases of wound healing which orchestrate the closure of the open wound. Prior to giving consideration to the phases of wound healing it is important to respect the function of skin. The skin separates "inner" space from "outer" space. The basic structure of the skin is shown in Fig. 1. The skin has a number of important functions, including:

- acting as a physical barrier to infection
- thermo-regulation
- keeping the internal organs in place
- vitamin D metabolism
- the suppleness affords underlying joint motion

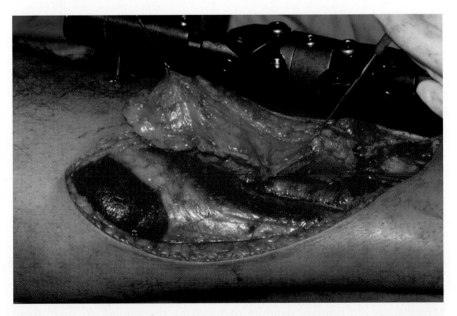

Fig. 2.   This is a clinical illustration showing the two most important sources of blood supply to the skin. In the centre is a septocutaneous perforating blood vessel. This septocutaneous blood vessel has emerged between two adjacent muscle groups to end in the skin. To the left one can see a musculo-cutaneous perforator travelling through the gastrocnemius muscle to end in the fat of the skin. The random input has been cut by the surgical incision.

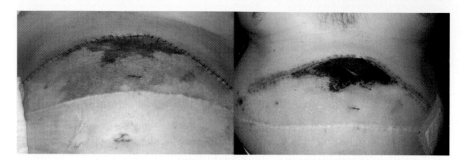

Fig. 3. This case illustrates the point of appreciating the vascular supply to the skin. This patient has undergone oesophageal surgery for malignancy. The access incision was via a "roof-top" approach. He had previously undergone a lower mid-line incision for prostate surgery. Whilst the lower incision would have resulted in severance of the deep inferior epigastric vessels, the "roof-top" incision would have further de-vascularised the skin edge by severance of the superior epigastric vessels. This resulted in full-thickness necrosis and more importantly, necrosis of the rectus abdominis muscles.

The first and third are important functions to consider when making elective surgical incisions. The first and last functions become important when dealing with tissue loss following trauma. An important fact about the skin is that the epidermal thickness remains constant while the dermis thickness varies throughout the body.

The Phases of Wound Healing are:

- Haemostasis
- Inflammation
- Fibrosis
- Reepithelialisation
- Remodelling of the extracellular matrix

Haemostasis

Haemostasis is a primary requisite to surviving the wound. As such, there are powerful intrinsic and extrinsic mechanisms to arrest haemorrhage. More importantly, trapped platelets complement components and the prostaglandin system act as signals which recruit cells into the inflammatory phase of wound healing.

The cells that are important for the inflammatory phase of wound healing are:

- Neutrophils
- Macrophages

Neutrophils appear in the first wave of cell activity at the wound site.[3] Their function is to contain invading bacteria and to set the scene for the removal of damaged extracellular matrix (ECM). Neutrophils are bone marrow derived, and once activated, leave the circulation by a process termed diapedesis. Once at the wound site, neutrophils undertake phagocytosis of debris; they contain enzymes within their cytoplasm, these enzymes being contained in lysosomes. The enzymes termed lysozymes can degrade structural molecules and can thus degrade any bacteria as well as begin the process of ECM degradation. Neutrophils also have a number of important "respiratory" enzymes; a collection called superoxide dysmutase when activated can generate oxygen free radicals which are cytotoxic. Activated neutrophils produce signals for other circulating neutrophils to enter the wounded area and thus recruitment occurs to replenish nascent cells.

Macrophages are also bone marrow derived. Although some appear in the circulation as monocytes, they are confined to specific sites. Macrophages have a longer half-life than neutrophils and so in chronic wounds the exudates contain a majority of macrophages. As well as the phagocytosis of debris and organisms, macrophages can set the milieu of the healing wound such that the process of fibrosis proceeds. The macrophage is a pivotal cell requisite for optimum wound healing.[4]

Fibroblasts

Fibrosis. Beginning on day 2–3 after wounding, mesenchymal cells found in the pervascular space divide and begin to populate the wound edges. Cell migration occurs with the help of a glycoprotein called fibronectin. Fibronectin is thought to facilitate cell adhesion and is believed by some to be a substrate upon which fibroblasts migrate and deposit collagen.[5] Both neo-collagen and glycosaminoglycan production form the basis for the important role played by these cells in this phase of wound healing. During this phase of wound healing, there is a progressive increase in the tensile strength of the wound. This increase in tensile strength can be attributed to the accumulation of collagen. There are over 17 types of collagen (at the last count). Types 1 and 3 predominate in healing wounds and initially there is more type 3. The collagen production continues over a 3-week period. Wound contraction occurs via the coordinated efforts of a specialised type of fibroblast called a myofibroblast.[6] These cells have, in addition to normal fibroblast attributes, cytoplasmic microfilaments similar to those of smooth muscle cells. Myofibroblasts are present throughout the entire surface of a granulating wound and the entire surface is thought to progressively contract.[7]

Kertinocytes

Epithelialisation itself occurs in a predictable sequence of cellular responses as follows: mobilisation, migration, mitosis and cellular differentiation. Mobilisation of keratinocytes occurs from the skin immediately adjacent to the wound edge by loss of contact inhibition. Mitosis occurs away from the wound in the basal layer of the epidermis. Once the initial layer of epidermal covering has formed subsequent cellular recruitment provides differentiation from basal to surface layers.

Skin Wounds

Generally speaking skin wounds can be categorised as follows:

- Acute
- Chronic
- Surgical
- Special wounds

In any case consider the following:

- Location of wound
- Structures involved
- Is the wound killing the patient?
- Is the patient killing the wound?
- Can the "KISS" principle be applied?

Acute

Acute wounds are produced as a result of trauma or by surgical election. Some "special" wounds can also be placed in this category.

Traumatic wounds can affect any part of the anatomy, and thus a working knowledge of surface anatomy of certain vital or important structures is of paramount importance. When the underlying organ is a vital one (for example, calvarial injuries or chest trauma) the care and attention to the overlying wound may ultimately determine the final outcome. It is less obvious (but equally important) when the underlying structure(s) are not vital to survival. In this instance, if neglected, loss of the overlying integument will impact tremendously upon the patient's lifestyle. This can be seen in the victims of road traffic accidents who sustain open fractures of long bones in the upper and lower limbs (Fig. 4). Thus, traction on nerves and tendons as well as the potential for infection to prevent bone repair may result in a useless limb. Neglect in patients with multiple injuries may result in compartment syndrome within the limbs which will further compromise the ultimate outcome.

Surgical wounds are produced in lines of election (Fig. 5). These enable easy surgical access to the pathology but must also result in minimal damage to the integument. Thus, care when entering the anatomical site as well as when

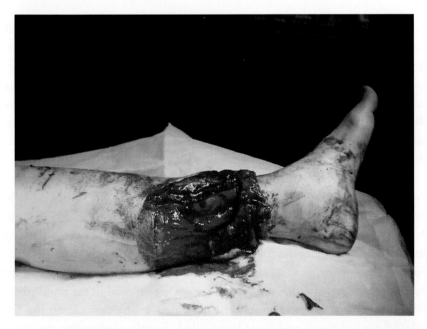

Fig. 4.   This is a case of high energy trauma to the lower limb. The traumatic wound has resulted in a fractured long bone (tibia) but importantly has resulted in loss of skin and crushing of the muscle/tendons and nerves. Attention to these "soft tissues" will ultimately determine whether the limb can be saved.

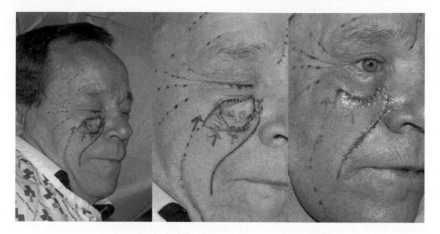

Fig. 5.   This series of pictures is of a gentleman who has a skin malignancy arising in the right cheek area. The dotted lines indicate the natural lines of election for excision and tension-free closure. However, the simple closure of this wound would have resulted in ectropion of the lower eyelid. To prevent this a local flap advancement was undertaken. Correct planning of this flap ensured that the final scars were in the lines of election and that there was no ectropion.

leaving the site will ensure that the overlying integument has been minimally handled. This in turn will result in sound primary healing. This statement may sound banal but consider the consequences when rough handling of a median sternotomy during coronary artery by-pass surgery (CABG) results in sternal dehiscence and subsequent mediastinitis (carrying a mortality of over 80%; see Fig. 6). The incidence of this tragic complication is higher in those patients who are diabetic and where the internal mammary vessels have been used to revascularise the myocardium.

Besides the careful handling of tissue another often under-recognised reason for poor wound healing is excessive tension at the suture line. This holds true for any viable structure which is being sutured (bowel, viscera, muscle, skin). Another variable which the surgeon has some control over is the care, during the procedure of the tissues, which may not be receiving surgical attention. Neglect of these tissues will lead to tissue desiccation. Under the warm theatre lights, tissue (which normally does not get exposed to the atmosphere) will dry out as its inherent moisture evaporates. Tissue desiccation is a true killer of normal tissue and must be avoided. Simply placing the tissue in a moist pack may not be sufficient and regular irrigation with a balanced salt solution will be needed.

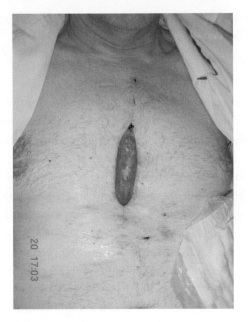

Fig. 6. This is a case of sternal wound dehiscence following coronary artery bypass grafting (CABG). Note that the lower part of the surgical wound has dehisced. This is because this is the part of the wound where most tension is exerted during wound closure. If one source of blood supply has been removed by the surgeon (internal mammary vessel used for the CABG) and the second source compromised by a tight closure then one can predict dehiscence.

Another factor that is often not accounted for is the fact that traumatised tissue continues to swell after the traumatic event (this may be a surgical incision). Thus, if the closure was tight during the operation then one can see that it will be even more so during the first 24 hours after surgery. An allowance for this must be made.

Of the complicated "special" wounds known, those produced by necrotising skin infections are amongst the worst. Not only are they a true, life-threatening emergency which requires urgent surgical attention, they may also be difficult to diagnose in the early stages. These wounds may be localised or generalised and may be monomicrobial or polymicrobial. The commonest organisms are β-haemolytic streptococci; however, there may be synergism between bacteria to induce the rapid onset of frank tissue necrosis. Terms such as Meleneys gangrene and Fourniers gangrene should not be used as they only add to the confusion of this spectrum of disease. Simply view these as either localised or generalised and mono- or polymicrobial. Urgent excision of all devitalised tissue is required.

Chronic

Wounds remain unhealed and thus become chronic for a number of defined reasons which may all interplay in the same patient. The wounds are "stuck" in the first two phases of healing. Chronic inflammation results in oedematous, hostile, friable tissue. When investigated the cells within the open wound appeared to respond to growth factors normally produced in the inflammatory phase of wound healing but there was surprisingly a high output of enzymes called metalloproteinases (MMP).[8] Thus chronic wounds perpetuate their own existence if left unchecked. A chronic open wound impacts a patient's lifestyle (malodourous, painful wounds requiring regular dressing); and may render the patient in a state of catabolism. When faced with a wound which remains unhealed, there are a number of basic questions which need to be asked and answered. Ask yourself: Is this a benign wound or is it malignant? If unsure, a biopsy (punch) will be required to establish this. Once it has been established that the wound is "benign" the quality of the underlying and surrounding tissue needs to be taken into account. Hence, an area which has received radiation therapy cannot afford prompt primary healing, nor can it withstand standard plastic surgical attention (for example, skin grafts). Also consider the factors outlined in the next section.

FACTORS WHICH LEAD TO POOR WOUND HEALING

The factors which compromise the pathways requisite for sound primary healing may be divided into general and local factors. General factors that need to be taken into account include:

- Nutrition
- Anaemia
- Cardiorespiratory compromise
- The presence of malignancy
- Sepsis
- Immunosuppression
- Age

The recognised local factors which contribute to poor tissue healing are:

- Poor vascularity
- Poor quality tissues
- Oedema
- Haematoma
- Local radiation therapy
- Underlying infection
- Tension at the wound site

As a rule of thumb if an elective surgical wound has not completely healed after two weeks then consideration must be given to factors which have acted to delay healing.

Considering each of these factors in turn will illuminate the pitfalls which are to be avoided. Poor vascularity needs little qualification since without adequate vascular nourishment tissue necrosis occurs with a resultant dehiscence of the wound. One can influence the vascularity of the wound edges by paying attention to the tension to which the wound edges are subject. A tension-free repair is the ideal provided that no further incisions are made to achieve this end. Poor attention to tissue handling such as crushing, tearing and poor retraction all contribute to a poor substrate (tissue). Poor quality tissue whether present prior to the operation or after the operation will fail to heal. Oedema occurs in all viable tissue subjected to trauma. It is an obligate response to tissue disruption at a basic level; the capillaries become incompetent and fluid leaks out into the tissue. This extravascular water either weeps out onto the wound surface or remains within the interstices of the tissue, which effectively produces tissue swelling. Even when the tissue handling is exemplary, there is a degree of tissue oedema. The extent of this oedema is dependent upon, amongst other things, the tissue itself. Thus little, if any, oedema occurs in injured bone, but muscle undergoes extensive oedema for a given amount of tissue disruption. Another important variable in terms of inducing tissue oedema is the type of injury that is imparted upon the tissue. Tissue subject to a burn will become significantly more swollen than tissue which has been sharply incised (Fig. 7).

Every time one uses a diathermy one is causing a focus of burnt tissue. When this occurs over a large surface area, a burn is essentially created over a

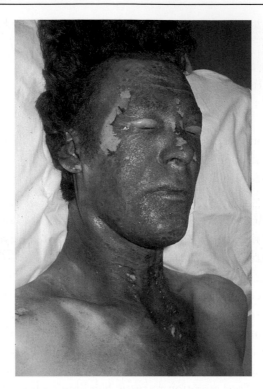

Fig. 7.   A victim of a flash burn. Note the periorbital oedema.

large surface area. Thus one must take this into account when considering the best method of repairing tissue.

Haematomas deserve special mention here. Haematomas can be of two basic types: **expanding** haematomas or **established** haematomas. The former must be controlled urgently as they are the result of a reactionary (usually) arterial bleed. As the name would suggest, an expanding haematoma may collect in a "dead-space" until it is filled with blood, after which pressure is exerted on the walls of the confined space. If the walls are composed of compliant tissue, then the pressure building up will expand the walls. This will produce problems for a number of reasons. Firstly, if as a result of this expansion natural conduits are obstructed by the expanding haematoma, applying external pressure will be required so as to impede flow. Secondly, the application of pressure itself will result in tissue tension which may impede vascularity and thus directly lead to tissue necrosis.[8] Haematomas can cause tissue damage by means other

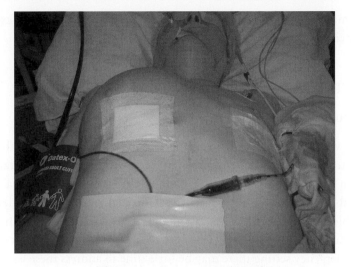

Fig. 8.   Shown here is a case of expanding haematoma following elective breast surgery. Note the obvious difference in size between the breasts and that despite the surgeon inserting a drain the haematoma was not prevented. This graphically demonstrates the fallacy of the myth that drains prevent haematoma formation.

than their physical presence. A haematoma which is unrelieved will lead to the production of oxygen free radicals. This occurs because the Fe^{2+} readily loses an electron to give rise to Fe^{3+}. The electron that is lost attaches to O_2 molecules. This will produce superoxides which damage cell membranes and thus can lead to cellular and thus tissue loss.[9,10]

Haematomas are to be avoided or anticipated. Simply placing a drain in a "dead space" will not guard against the formation of haematoma. A meticulous surgical technique will reduce haematoma rates. Clearly if patients have a bleeding tendency (on anticoagulants or is thrombocytopenic), then attention must be paid to correcting these deficiencies prior to embarking on surgery as the bleeding may become difficult to control.

Local radiation therapy causes a pericapillary fibrosis.[11] This places post-radiotherapy tissue at a disadvantage to normal tissue in terms of its healing potential. Tissue which has had external beam radiation is less compliant than normal tissue, which will make the achievement of a tension-free repair of such tissue difficult. As natural planes of dissection are not easily established in post-radiotherapy tissue, this dissection of the tissue becomes very demanding, and often tissue is inadvertently injured. The undesirable result is a larger zone of oedematous tissue. For these reasons and others, one must take extra care when incising into tissue which has had radiotherapy.

ELECTIVE VERSUS EMERGENCY SURGERY

The Situation

Patients who undergo elective surgery are usually optimised for the surgical event. Thus even if there is a malignant stricture in the alimentary canal nutrition is corrected by enteral or parenteral means. Any anaemia or electrolyte abnormalities are also bought to a normal level for the patient. Any co-morbidity is also attended to. All phases of the surgical journey from pre-incision to pre-op to post-op recovery are controlled to favour a swift recovery. In the emergency setting there may be little time to address these issues. Thus the "work-up" of a patient may be far from ideal. The old cliché "fail to prepare … prepare to fail" is most aptly applied in these situations. Extensive emergency surgery in elderly patients carries significant risk.

The Reconstructive Ladder

Traditionally reconstructive plastic surgeons approach tissue reconstruction by paying due attention to the reconstructive ladder. This was viewed as a ladder with each successive rung representing an increasingly complex mode of treatment (see Fig. 9). This concept was principally introduced as an aid to obtaining wound closure. Thus the simplest method represented on the ladder is by primary closure and the most sophisticated is by way of free tissue transfer. It was envisaged that one "climbed" this "ladder" when attempting to close wounds. Thus only after the simplest technique has failed should one try the next level of complexity. Free tissue transfer is in essence an autotransplantation of blocks of tissue. An increased level of anatomical knowledge and surgical skill are required when undertaking free tissue transfer. Whilst undoubtedly the reconstructive ladder principle was of help, modern reconstructive plastic surgeons suggest that one gets to the most appropriate rung of the ladder at the beginning. This represents a shift in the attitudes in modern reconstructive plastic surgery and some have re-named the ladder as a "toolbox" or "elevator". We should do the right operation for the patient at the outset rather than the simplest. Clearly these may be inclusive.

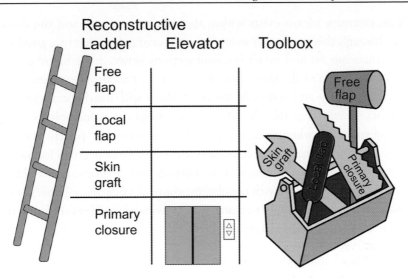

Fig. 9.   The reconstructive ladder/elevator/toolbox concept.

Pressure Ulcers

Pressure sores, decubitus ulcers and bed sores are some of the different terms referring to the consequences of unrelenting pressure on vulnerable skin points (Fig. 10). The commonest areas where they occur are the sacrum, heels and ischial tuberosities, and the greater trochanteric areas. The normal capillary pressure which has to be overcome to result in tissue ischaemia is 32 mmHg.[12] This capillary pressure is easy to overcome over boney prominences. If one recalls the vascularity of the skin and subcutaneous fat (Fig. 1) it can be seen

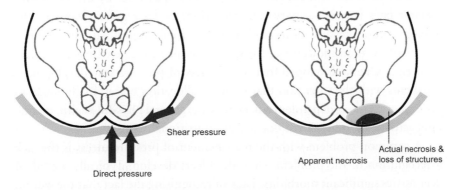

Fig. 10.   The basic mechanism for the development of a pressure ulcer.

that an extensive plexus exists within the subcutaneous fat and the dermis. Thus although this pressure is overcome in everyday life, due to a good layer of subcutaneous fat and intact interconnections between the blood capillaries, true ischaemia of the tissue does not occur. In the conscious patient with normal sensibility and mobility, however, there will also be conscious and subconscious efforts at relieving the pressure from the vulnerable points. In contra-distinction, when there is poor nutrition, when the patient is unconscious, and when there is poor sensibility/mobility, tissue necrosis followed by local sepsis will results. Ultimately there will be loss of integument as well as loss of any underlying muscle with possible exposure of underlying bone/joints. A grading system exists to help in management plans for patients suffering from pressure ulcers. It is graded 1–4 as follows[13]:

(1) Non-blanchable erythema of the intact skin. This is a red or violaceous area that does not blanch upon pressure with the finger, indicating blood has escaped form the capillaries into the interstitial tissue.
(2) Partial-thickness skin loss.
(3) Full-thickness skin loss and extension into the subcutaneous fat.
(4) Extension into the muscle and bone.

Prevention is far better than any attempts to cure these ulcers. It is incumbent on the attending surgeon to ensure appropriate nursing care such that pressure is relieved from the commonest points and the patient is turned regularly. The patient must be placed on an appropriate pressure relieving mattress. Malnourishment needs to be alleviated. If there is loss of continence of bowel or bladder then the effluent needs to be controlled either by diversion into reservoir bags (stoma, urinary catheterisation) or by regular cleaning. The development of pressure ulcers in otherwise normal surgical patients has been used by some as an indicator of the quality of medical care delivery.[14] There has been a schema developed to assess the risk of pressure sore development in patients with the intention that resource allocation be rationally made to those most at risk. Independent risk factors are: general physical health, mental state, activity, mobility, incontinence and nutritional status.

A common problem with the management of pressure ulcers is the lack of recognition of the problem when the ulcers develop. Typically a grade 4 ulcer carries significant morbidity. Lack of recognising the fact that the wound surface will have many deep fissures/sinuses means that they are inadequately treated and therefore recur rapidly. The apparent wound surface will only be a small portion of the true wound surface. This is explained by the fact that during their natural history, the skin and subcutaneous fat are destroyed, but the fat is destroyed to a greater extent than the skin and thus there will be some amount of undermining. Colonised or frankly infected ulcers will lead to further fat necrosis to differing depths surrounding the ulcer.

Surgical management of pressure ulcers must be undertaken if the patient is acutely septic from an infected pressure ulcer and/or when the patient has been optimised for surgery. Again the principle of "tumour" excision of the wound has to be applied. Various aids have been developed to ensure complete wound excision. In essence all the aids to a comprehensive excision relate to revealing the true extent of the wound surface. The so-called bursa of the wound needs to be excised. Thus sewing a gauze swab soaked in either betadine or hydrogen peroxide and India ink will delineate the bursa. Tumour excision can then be effectively undertaken by excising around this construct and ensuring that no pigmented tissue is seen. After a comprehensive excision one must remember that primary and reactionary haemorrhage is common and these must be anticipated during and after the surgery. In paraplegic patients, there is profound hypotension during anaesthesia and thus during wound excision cut blood vessels may be concealed and a reactionary bleed will occur post-op.

When considering the reconstruction of pressure ulcers one must apply the KISS principle. A defensive approach will ensure that should the ulcer recur, options have not been exhausted. The usual reconstructive ladder/elevator/ toolbox can be applied in these cases. An algorithm is shown and the important aspect is to diagnose the condition accurately.

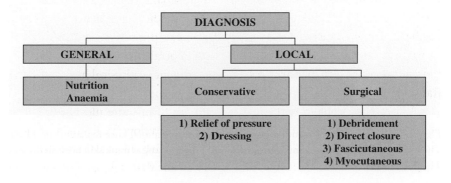

POST-SURGICAL COMPLICATIONS — SPECIFIC SITUATIONS

Orthopaedics

Wound complications in orthopaedics can relate to either the elective cases or the trauma cases. Those which affect elective cases often relate to infection of the underlying metalwork (arthroplasty prosthesis/plate and screw fixation devices). Infection can either arise from within, i.e. as a result of the introduction of pathogenic microbes by the operating surgeon or via the blood-stream (haematogenous). These infections manifest either as a sinus or multiple sinuses where frank pus discharges to the surface, or as an indolent infection which leads to loosening of the indwelling prosthesis (see Fig. 11). The picture is of a patient who had undergone a knee replacement. There is obvious skin necrosis with multiple sinuses. An algorithm has been proposed for managing these cases and like most implant related problems, the greater the extent of infection/tissue necrosis, the greater the threat to the implant.[15]

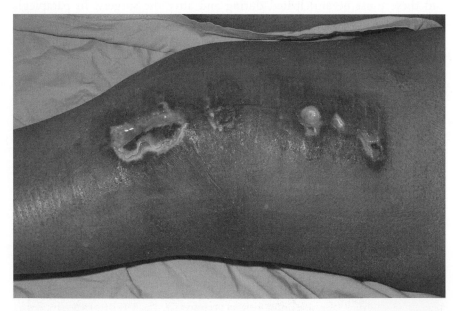

Fig. 11. Shown is a case of wound edge necrosis overlying a total knee replacement (TKR). There are a number of sinuses both proximally and distally as well as frank skin necrosis distally. The knee is swollen.

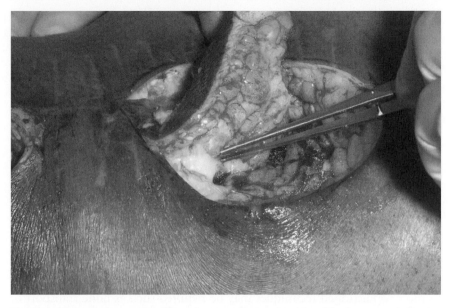

Fig. 12.   Shown is the process of "pseudotumour" wound excision. The forceps are indicating a pocket of pus in an area of liquifactive fat necrosis.

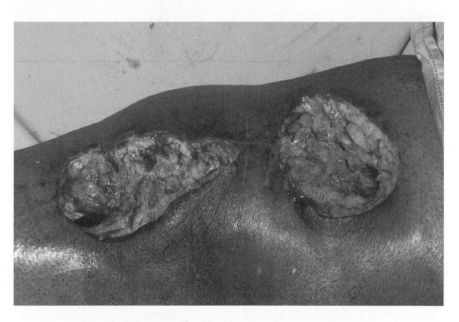

Fig. 13.   The result after "pseudotumour" type wound excision.

Each wound was excised as shown in Fig. 12, until the wound was found to be healthy (Fig. 13). The lower wound required coverage with a gastrocnemius flap and skin grafts as shown in an effort to rescue the underlying implant.

The main organisms responsible for these complications are *Staphylococcal* bacteria (*Aureus/Epidermidis*). Inevitably the metalwork will need to be removed and the sinuses excised. All colonised surfaces will have to be excised. This approach is described as a pseudotumour **excision** of the wound. The word "debridement" should be dropped in favour of excisional surgery. The reconstruction of the resultant defects may be complicated. Not only will the underlying skeleton be managed but the soft-tissue defect also reconstructed.

Infected non-union. In this situation the same principle applies as that for elective orthopaedics. Thus the pseudoarthrosis (the non-union) needs to be resected and then a decision made about the feasibility of obtaining infection-free bony union. This may be a simple matter of cancellous bone grafting or more sophisticated techniques may be required such as bone transport or vascularised bone grafting (such as a free fibula transfer). Figure 15 shows a leg

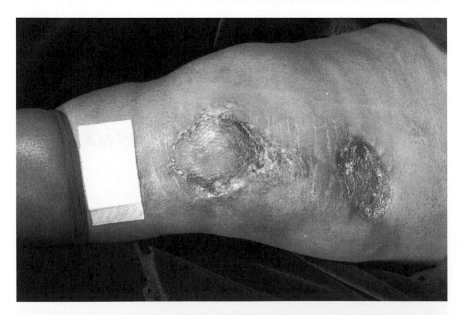

Fig. 14. The result after reconstruction. The distal wound was reconstructed using a local muscle flap with a split-thickness skin graft, whereas the proximal wound was suitable for a split-thickness graft only. The underlying TKR was thus salvaged.

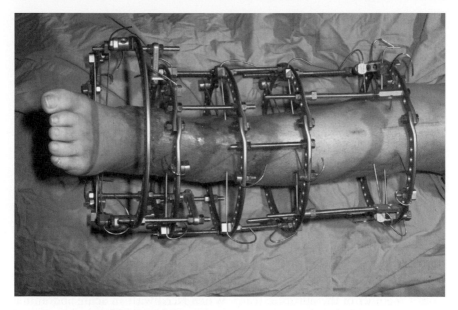

Fig. 15.   Using complex "Ortho-Plastic" techniques one can salvage badly traumatised limbs which would have otherwise been amputated. This is an illustration of such a case. The traumatised limb has been fixed with a circular frame and the "soft-tissue" loss has been reconstructed by way of a free-tissue transfer. The circular frame allows stretching the fractured bone even after the bone has been acutely shortened.

which was salvaged after a high energy collision. The tibia was acutely shortened by 5 cm, and the soft-tissue was reconstructed with a chimeric muscle transfer (two muscle flaps supported by a common vascular pedicle) and skin grafts.

The shortened limb is finally lengthened using the circular frame method.

GENERAL SURGERY

Open operations on the abdominal viscera usually involve a breach of the anatomy of the anterior abdominal wall. When we review this anatomy there is an intricate relationship between the three anatomical layers that make up the musculoaponeurotic system. A fine balance exists between the actions of the groups of muscles. This balance is upset when access through the muscles into the peritoneal cavity is sought. This imbalance often results in lower abdominal weakness with the potential for herniation and it may occasionally lead to low back pain. The commonest incision is for a midline laparotomy. Although this can be the least destructive method (in as much as no muscle is incised), it nevertheless weakens the most vulnerable part of the anterior abdominal envelope. The problems arising from this weakening are either manifested as acute or chronic. Acutely, there can be a dehiscence of the entire wound with the dramatic results of exposure of the viscera. In the acute setting, what is required is an urgent return to the theatre with particular attention being to the presence of infection and the state of the wound edges. What must also be asked is a reason for the acute dehiscence. Quite often it is due to a combination of factors which are not conducive to pristine wound healing (see above). Poor tissue handling along with too tight a closure and poor patient nutrition are the usual culprits. Pre-op malnutrition may not be easy to reverse particularly if there is an underlying malignant condition; however, postoperative nutrition is a variable which may be addressed with the input from a member of the nutrition team. When faced with an acute abdominal dehiscence the wound edges can be freshened and the wound re-sutured only if the surgeon is confident of obtaining a tension-free repair of healthy, well-vascularised tissue. What is required in this unfortunate situation is to try and correct the factors which lead to the breaking down of the suture line. What must be avoided is a large fistula forming between the epithelial lining of the peritoneal cavity and the epithelial lining of the skin. This is best achieved by serial visits to the theatre where the wound is critically assessed. The peritoneal cavity must be sutured; this is usually achieved by approximating the linea alba with sutures that can take the majority of the tension across the wound site. For this purpose the author recommends using a looped mattress suturing technique (see Fig. 16). This technique spreads the load of one strand of suture over three strands per stitch. The remaining layers of tissue (Scarpa's fascia, fat and skin) can remain open and when ready will need a split-thickness skin graft to obtain healing.

A chronic problem related to poor wound healing in the abdominal wall is ventral herniation (Fig. 17). This latter problem can either be a minor nuisance or a major problem.

In the latter case a detailed working knowledge of the vascular anatomy of the abdominal wall is required (see Fig. 18).

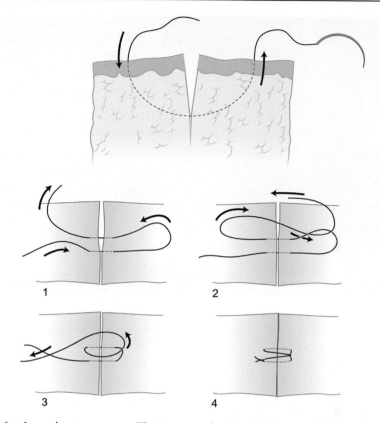

Fig. 16. Looped mattress suture. The sets are outlined in this diagram of creating this useful suture. Note that at the end there should be 4 strands of suture material crossing the wound.

It can be seen from this diagram (Fig. 18) that the neurovascular bundles run transversely between the external oblique and the transverses abdominus. To obtain a sound reconstruction, what is recommended is the technique described by Ramirez *et al.*,[16] referred to as the "separation of components". This technique allows the midline to be advanced up to 10 cm on each side, thus affording the safe closure of massive defects.

Ent, Head and Neck Surgery

Specific wound healing problems in head and neck surgery relate to the care of the complex oncoplastic patient. These patients are affected by a primary

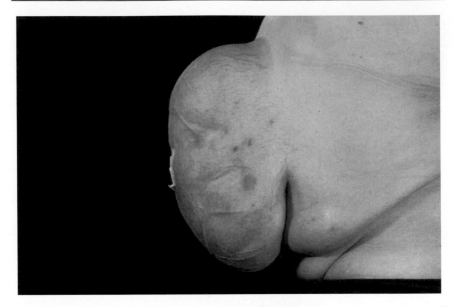

Fig. 17. Shown is a gross case of ventral herniation following a laparotomy. Almost half the abdominal contents are in the hernial sac. Addressing this problem requires a detailed understanding of the anatomy of the anterior abdominal wall musculature.

carcinoma in the aerodigestive tract which will necessitate a wide resection, followed by a form of neck dissection, then followed by reconstruction. When they have recovered from the destructive and reconstructive surgery, they may need a course of radiotherapy. Wound problems can arise at any stage of the treatment. Thus acutely after the combined oncoplastic surgery, there may be a wound infection in the access incisions in the neck. A reason must be sought for the poor wound healing. Quite often one must look for abnormal fluid leaks such as chyle and saliva. This cause can be excluded by a chemical analysis of the effluent (a high triglyceride in the former and a high amylase in the latter). A chyle leak should be treated expectantly with nutritional adjustments but a salivary leak is more worrisome as the risk of a fatal secondary haemorrhage in the neck (effectively a "blow-out" of the carotid artery) is high. The fistula should be controlled by opening the neck wound. If the volume of the fluid remains high and the neck skin remains inflamed, then formal closure of the fistula by excision and closure with a "waterproofing" layer (usually with a pectoralis major flap transfer) is needed.

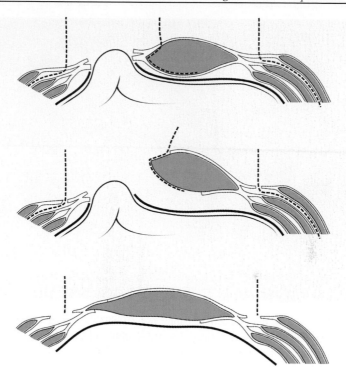

Fig. 18. These cartoons illustrate sequentially the technique of "component separation" of the anterior abdominal musculature. The dotted lines indicate where the components should be separated.

Breast Surgery

Problems arising from wound complications relating to breast surgery can essentially be split into cases of surgery undertaken for size (breast augmentation/breast reduction) and those undertaken for breast malignancy.

Breast Reduction Surgery

Early

- Haematoma collection of blood within the substance of the breast. Of the early ones, the risk of haematoma will necessitate an urgent return to the theatre for the removal of the blood and a search for the bleeding points.

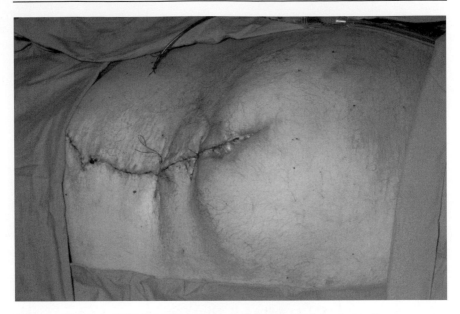

Fig. 19. This is the end result of herniorrhaphy and anterior abdominal wall reconstruction using the Ramirez technique. Note the looped mattress sutures which help disperse the tension at the wound edge.

- Infection. This can occur in any aspect of the surgical field either in the skin wound or the breast (deep) wound. If extensive, this may require further surgical intervention as well as intravenous treatment.
- Nipple loss. Should the nipple be found to be compromised, then there is a risk of partial or total loss of the nipple. Should this happen, the wound should be allowed to heal either with skin grafts of by itself.
- Loss of nipple sensation is to be expected as there is a circumareolar incision iatrogenic injury to the cutaneous nerves supplying the nipple.
- Delayed wound healing. Although there can be a delay in the healing in any aspect of the wounds due to infection, delayed wound healing is commonest at the junction of the vertical and horizontal wound, as this area experiences the greatest tension. These usually heal with regular dressing but sometimes may need skin grafts.
- Chest wall pain. This occurs as a result of trapment of the nerves within the chest wall and may be severe enough to warrant surgical exploration at a later date.

Late

- Asymmetry of the nipple height and gland. This is usually due to the lack of predictability of the response of the breast to the surgery on each side. The process of fat necrosis is usually responsible (slow loss of the fat of the breast after surgery) but infection (if present) may also play a role. If marked, a re-operation will have to be planned in order to address this.
- Inability to breastfeed. Although some ladies have reported being able to breastfeed after breast reduction surgery, this should be considered a bonus. If breastfeeding is possible, one must wait between 6–12 months after the surgery.

Breast Augmentation

Augmentation is achieved by placing a silicone gel filled implant into a surgically created pocket (either subglandular or subpectoral).

Infection of the implant will necessitate either removal of or rescue with an irrigating system.

Implant rupture is a recognised complication which can affect any gel-filled implant. Current medical literature reports that silicone implants are safe[18] and thus the presence of gel is not deleterious to health; however, due to the loss of volume, the implant will have to be replaced. A much more vexing problem with breast implants is the presence of "capsule" formation. The capsule is essentially a scar that forms internally and on the surface of the implant. The thickness of the scar can vary from a flimsy thin layer to a thick, calcified coating. A thick capsule will lead to loss of beast consistency. The capsule can also undergo a process called capsular contracture where the implant shape is distorted by the capsule undergoing progressive contraction (Fig. 20). In any of these cases, the capsules will have to be comprehensively excised and the implants replaced.

Breast Cancer

The incidence of breast cancer is high in the UK.[19] The majority of these patients will need some form of surgical treatment. Some controversy exists over how much tissue should be removed during the excision of the tumour as well as the role of adjuvant treatments. The role of sentinel node biopsy is

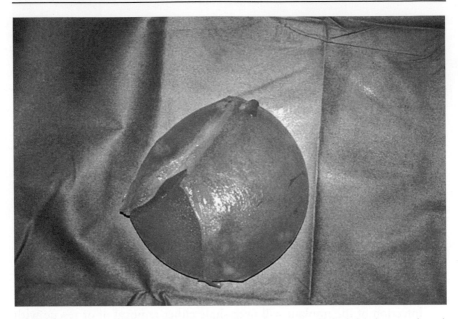

Fig. 20. This is a picture of a silicone gel filled breast implant which has been explanted. The breast implant is covered in a membrane called a capsule. Also note that the capsule has contracted to distort the implant. All foreign materials (joint replacements, heart valves) in the body will induce the formation of such a membrane.

also being evaluated. Regardless of the treatment chosen, the patient is often left with a distorted breast, the skin of which may be further disfigured due to the late effects of external radiotherapy (Fig. 21).

These postoperative and post-radiation consequences must be communicated to the patient. Partial breast defects are much more difficult to correct than complete mastectomy defects.

Breast reconstruction: Wound complications in cases of breast reconstruction can largely be a mixture of those arising from reduction and augmentation. When tissue transfer is employed, morbidity relating to the donor sites becomes an issue. The common transfers are the pedicled latissimus dorsi muscle and the free flap transfer of the lower abdominal skin and fat (TRAM flap). The morbidity in the former relates to the seroma collection at the flank and back as well as the loss of this muscle which will be missed when undertaking the front stroke in swimming or reaching for the top compartments in a cupboard. The TRAM flap donor morbidity relates to the potential loss of

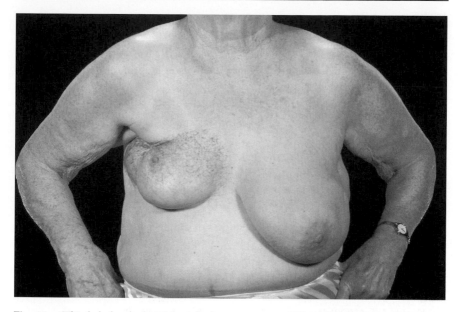

Fig. 21. This lady has had excision of a breast tumour of the right side. This was followed by chest wall irradiation. The combined result of tumour excision and irradiation is a retracted breast and telangiectasia of the skin. The texture and suppleness of the skin has changed from soft and compliant to hard and non-compliant.

the rectus muscle and the imbalance this may cause in the equilibrium of the muscle tone around the abdominal girth.

REFERENCES

1. Manchot C. (1889) *Die Hautarterien des Menschlichen Korpers* (Leipzig, FCW Vogel).
2. Salmon M. (1936a) *Arteres de la Peau* (Masson et Cie, Paris).
3. Simpson DM, Ross R. (1972) The neutrophilic leukocyte in wound repair. A study with anti-neutrophil serum. *J Clin Invest* **51**: 2009.
4. Clarke RA, *et al.* (1976) Role of macrophages in wound healing. *Surg Forum* **27**: 16.
5. Kurkinen M, Vaheri A, Roberts PJ, Stenman S. (1980) Sequential appearance of fibronectin and collagen in experimental granulation tissue. *Lab Invest* **43**: 47.
6. Gabbiani G, Ryan GB, Majno G. (1970) Presence of modified fibroblasts in granulation tissue, and possible role in wound contraction. *Experimentia* **27**: 549.

7. McGrath MH, Hundahl SA. (1982) The spatial and temporal quantification of myofibroblasts. *Plast Reconstr Surg* **69**: 975.

8. Tengore NJ, Stacey MC, MacAuley S, *et al.* (1999). Analysis of the acute and chronic wound environments: the role of proteases and their inhibition. *Wound Repair Regen* **7**: 442–452.

9. Hillelson RL, Glowacki J, Healey NA, Mulliken JB. (1980) A microangiographic study of haematoma-associated flap necrosis and salvage with isoxsuprine. *Plast Reconstr Surg* **66**: 528–533.

10. Angel MF, Narayanan MD, Swartz WM, *et al.* (1986). The etiologic role of free radicals in haematoma-induced flap necrosis. *Plast Reconstr Surg* **77**: 795–801.

11. Miller SH, Rudolph R. (1990) Healing in the irradiated wound. *Clin Plast Surg* **17**: 503.

12. Landis EM. (1930) Microinjection studies of capillary blood pressure in human skin. *Heart* **15**: 209.

13. National Pressure Ulcer Advisory Panel. (1989) Pressure ulcers prevelance, cost and risk assessment: consensus development conference statement. *Decubitus* **2**: 24.

14. Kenkle JM. (1999) Pressure sores. *Sel Read Plast Surg* **8**: 39.

15. Norton D, McLaren R, Exton-Smith AN. (1962) *An Investigation of Geriatric Nursing Problems in Hospital* (London Churchill Livingstone, 1962), pp. 194–236.

16. Laing JH, Hancock K, Harrison DH. (1992) The exposed total knee replacement prosthesis: a new classification and treatment algorithm. *Br J Plast Surg* **45**: 66–69.

17. Ramirez OM, Ruas E, Dellon AL. (1990) Component separation method for closure of abdominal wall defects: an anatomic and clinical study. *Plast Reconstr Surg* **86**: 519–526.

18. Janrowsky EC, Kupper LL, Hulka BS. (2000) Meta-analyses of the relation between silicone breast implants and the risk of connective tissue diseases. *N Engl J Med* **342**: 781–790.

19. Botha JL, Bray F, Sankila R, Parkin DM. (2003) Breast cancer incidence and mortality trends in 16 European countries. *Eur J Cancer* **39**: 1718–1729.

Chapter 6

COMPLICATIONS IN BREAST SURGERY

Lisa A. Newman and Vernon K. Sondak

BACKGROUND

The breast is a relatively clean organ, comprising skin, fatty tissue and mammary glandular elements that do not have a direct connection with any major body cavity or visceral structures. In the absence of concomitant major reconstruction, breast surgery is usually not accompanied by large-scale fluid shifts, infectious complications, or haemorrhage. Thus, the breast is largely perceived as being associated with a relatively low risk of surgical morbidity. However, it is the site of the most common cancer afflicting American women, and a myriad of complications can occur with the procedures performed to detect and treat the malignancy. Some of these complications are related to the breast itself, and others are associated with axillary staging procedures. This chapter addresses some general non-specific complications (wound infections, seroma formation, haematoma), followed by a discussion of the complications that are specific to breast-related procedures (lumpectomy, including both diagnostic open biopsy and breast conservation therapy for cancer, mastectomy; axillary lymph node dissection (ALND), lymphatic mapping/sentinel lymph node biopsy, and reconstruction). A few conditions, such as immediate breast reconstruction and neoadjuvant chemotherapy, that require special surgical considerations will also be presented.

GENERAL WOUND COMPLICATIONS RELATED TO BREAST AND AXILLARY SURGERY

As a peripheral, soft tissue organ, many wound complications related to breast procedures are relatively minor and frequently managed on an outpatient basis. Therefore it is difficult to establish the accurate incidence rates for these events. However, as discussed below, studies have reported that surgical morbidity from breast and/or axillary wound infections, seromas, and haematomas occur in up to 30% of the cases. Fewer than half of these will require an extension in hospital stay or readmission for inpatient care. Besides the ones mentioned above, a fourth complication, chronic incisional pain, is also possible in conjunction with various surgical breast procedures.

A few rare complications that occur along with various breast procedures are mentioned here, but will not be discussed in depth. Pneumothorax can be related to either inadvertent pleural puncture during wire localization, or inadvertent deep dissection within an intercostal space. Patients can also develop brachial plexopathy related to stretch injury of a malpositioned arm in the operating room.[1] The American Society of Anesthesiology recommends upper extremity positioning such that maximal abduction at the shoulder with neutral forearm position is 90°, and the use of padded armboards.[2]

Mondor's disease, or thrombosis of the thoracoepigastric vein, can occur spontaneously, or following a breast procedure such as lumpectomy or even percutaneous needle biopsy.[3–7] While the disease is not an established breast cancer risk factor, there are reports of patients presenting with this condition at the time of diagnosis.[4] It typically presents as a palpable, sometimes tender cord running vertically from the mid-lower hemisphere of the breast toward the abdominal wall. Mondor's disease is usually a self-limited condition and resolution can be expedited by soft-tissue massage.

Wound Infections: The rate of postoperative infections in breast and axillary incisions range from less than 1% to nearly 20% of the cases, as shown in Table 1.[8–21] A meta-analysis by Platt *et al.* (1993) analysed data from 2,587 surgical breast procedures to arrive at an overall wound infection rate of 3.8%.[22] Staphylococcal organisms, introduced via skin flora, are usually implicated in these infections.[8,17] Obesity, age, and diabetes mellitus are some of the most consistently identified risk factors for breast wound sepsis. Several researchers[11,14,21] have found that patients undergoing definitive surgery for cancer had a lower risk of wound infection if their diagnosis was established by prior needle biopsy as opposed to an open surgical biopsy; however, one researcher observed the opposite effect.[20] Nicotine and other components of cigarettes have an adverse effect on the small vessels of the skin, with an almost four-fold increase in the risk of wound infection following breast surgery.[19] As demonstrated by the various studies summarised in Table 1, there is no consistent correlation between the risk of wound infection and mastectomy versus lumpectomy as definitive breast cancer surgery.

The use of preoperative antibiotics to minimise the rate of infection has been evaluated in multiple retrospective as well as prospective, randomised controlled trials. These studies have yielded disparate results; many have shown that a single dose of a preoperative antibiotic (usually a cephalosporin, administered approximately 30 min before surgery) will effectively reduce the infection rate by 40% or more,[8,13,21,22] while the Platt *et al.*[22] meta-analysis revealed that antibiotic prophylaxis (with antibiotics used in high risk cases) reduced the infection rate by 38%. Furthermore, the lowest reported rate of breast wound infections occurred in a Phase III study[16] of a long-acting versus short-acting cephalosporin, revealing the greatest risk reduction with the former (0.45% vs 0.91%). In contrast, Wagman *et al.*[10] found no effect with perioperative cephalosporin in a placebo-controlled Phase III trial involving 118 breast cancer patients (5% vs 8%), however, the onset of infection was delayed (17.7 days vs 9.6 days). Gupta *et al.*[17] reported similar wound infection rates in a Phase III study of prophylactic amoxicillin/clavulinic acid (17.7%) versus placebo (18.8%); and concluded that perioperative antibiotics are unnecessary in elective breast surgery. Because of these disparate results, and in an attempt to minimise cost, many clinicians have adopted the practice of limiting antibiotic prophylaxis to high-risk patients, and in cases involving foreign bodies, such as wire localisation biopsies. Despite this common practice, it should be noted that wire localisation procedures have not been specifically identified as a risk factor for wound infection.[21]

Table 1.   Selected Studies Evaluating Wound Infection Rates Following Breast Surgery

Study	#Cases	Type of Procedures Analysed	Type of Study	Wound Infection Rate	Study Findings/Risk Factors for Infection
Platt et al.[8]	606	Lumpectomy Mastectomy ALND Reduction mammoplasty	Phase 3 study of preoperative antibiotics	9.4%	Preoperative antibiotic coverage reduced wound infection rate (6.6% vs 12.2%)
Hoefer et al.[9]	101	Mastectomy	Retrospective review	8.9%	Risk Factor: Cautery
Wagman et al.[10]	118	Mastectomy	Phase 3 study of preoperative antibiotics	6.8%	Preoperative antibiotics had no effect on wound infection rates (5% vs 8%)
Chen et al.[11]		Mastectomy Lumpectomy	Retrospective review	2.6–11.1%	Risk Factors: Old age Surgery performed in 1970s vs 1980s Prior open diagnostic biopsy vs single-stage surgery
Vinton et al.[12]	560	Mastectomy Lumpectomy ALND	Retrospective review	15% (mastectomy) 13% (lumpectomy)	Risk Factors: Old age Mastectomy vs lumpectomy Tobacco smoking Obesity

Table 1. (*Continued*)

Study	#Cases	Type of Procedures Analysed	Type of Study	Wound Infection Rate	Study Findings/Risk Factors for Infection
Platt et al.[13]	1,981	Mastectomy Lumpectomy ALND Reduction mammoplasty	Retrospective review	3.4%	Preoperative antibiotic coverage reduced wound infection rate (odds ratio 0.59; 95% confidence interval 0.35–0.99)
Lipshy et al.[14]	289	Mastectomy	Retrospective review	5.3%	*Risk Factor:* Prior open diagnostic biopsy vs diagnostic needle biopsy (6.9% vs 1.6%)
Bertin et al.[15]	18 cases 37 controls	Mastectomy Lumpectomy	Case-Control	NA	Preoperative antibiotic coverage reduced wound infection rate *Risk Factors:* Obesity Old age
Thomas et al.[16]	1,766	Mastectomy Lumpectomy ALND	Phase 3 study of preoperative antibiotics	0.6%	Short-acting vs long-acting preoperative cephalosporin (0.91% vs 0.45%)
Gupta et al.[17]	334	Mastectomy Lumpectomy ALND	Phase 3 study of preoperative antibiotics	18.3%	Preoperative antibiotics had no effect on wound infection rates (17.7% vs 18.8%)

Table 1. (*Continued*)

Study	#Cases	Type of Procedures Analysed	Type of Study	Wound Infection Rate	Study Findings/Risk Factors for Infection
Nieto et al.[18]	107	Mastectomy Lumpectomy ALND	Prospective observational study	7% (mastectomy) 17% (lumpectomy)	*Risk Factors:* Lumpectomy vs mastectomy Old age Obesity
Sorenson et al.[19]	425	Mastectomy Lumpectomy ALND	Retrospective review	10.5%	*Risk Factors:* Tobacco smoking Diabetes mellitus Obesity Heavy ethanol consumption
Witt et al.[20]	326	Mastectomy Lumpectomy ALND	Prospective observational study	15.3%	*Risk Factors:* Old age Obesity Diabetes mellitus Prior diagnostic core needle biopsy vs open diagnostic biopsy
Tran et al.[21]	320	Mastectomy Lumpectomy	Retrospective review	6.1%	Preoperative antibiotic coverage reduced wound infection rate *Risk Factors:* Prior open diagnostic biopsy vs diagnostic needle biopsy (11.1% vs 9.7%)

ALND = Axillary lymph node dissection; NA = not applicable.

Mild incisional cellulitis can be treated with oral antibiotics, but non-responding or extensive soft tissue infection will require intravenous therapy. A small percentage of breast wound infections will progress into a fully-developed abscess. The pointing, fluctuant, and exquisitely tender mass of a breast abscess will usually become apparent one- to two-weeks postoperatively, and occur at the site of lumpectomy, mastectomy, or axillary incision. When there is an uncertainty regarding the diagnosis (as with deep-seated abscesses following lumpectomy), ultrasound imaging may be helpful, but the complex mass that will be visualised can appear as identical to a consolidating seroma or haematoma. Aspiration may also confirm the diagnosis, but the possibility of sampling error can mislead clinicians. The definitive management of an abscess will usually require drainage. Occasionally, curative aspiration of purulent material is successful especially if accomplished with ultrasound-guided insertion of a percutaneous drainage catheter, and many clinicians will opt for this as the initial treatment. Patients with an abscess require close follow-up because if it reaccumulates, it may warrant a more aggressive intervention. When necessary, incision and drainage can be accomplished by reopening the original surgical wound, and the resulting cavity must be left open to heal by secondary intention. If recurrent cancer is a concern, a biopsy of the cavity wall of the abscess is recommended.

Chronic recurrent periareolar abscess formation, or Zuska's disease, does not necessarily develop as a consequence of primary breast surgical procedures, but is significant for its high risk of complications following surgical treatment attempts. This condition has been associated with cigarette smoking, and afflicted patients should also be checked for tuberculosis as a factor in recurrent superficial soft tissue infections. A resection of the involved subareolar ductal system(s) is frequently offered to break the cycle of repeated abscesses, but these procedures are often complicated by wound infections, and chronically draining sinus tracts. In the most refractory cases, a complete resection of the entire nipple-areolar complex is performed, but this strategy should certainly be reserved as a last-ditch attempt.

Seroma: The rich lymphatic drainage of the breast from intramammary lymphatics to the axillary, supraclavicular, and internal mammary nodal basins establishes the tendency for seroma formation within any closed space that results from breast surgery. It has been proposed that the low fibrinogen levels and net fibrinolytic activity within lymphatic fluid collections account for seroma formation.[23,24] The closed spaces of the lumpectomy cavities, axillary wounds, and the anterior chest wall cavity under the mastectomy skin flaps will harbour seroma. Following a lumpectomy, this seroma is advantageous to the patient, as it usually preserves the normal breast contour even after a large-volume resection; it is eventually replaced by scar formation as the cavity consolidates. Occasionally the lumpectomy seroma is overly exuberant, and if the patient experiences discomfort from a bulging fluid collection, simple aspiration of the excess can be performed.

Seroma formation under the skin flaps of axillary or mastectomy wounds impairs the healing process, and drains are usually left in place to evacuate postoperative fluid collection. Most breast cancer surgery is performed in an outpatient setting, and patients must be instructed on proper drainage catheter care. After one to three weeks, the skin flaps will heal and adhere to the chest wall, as evidenced by diminished drain output. Once the drain is removed, the seroma collections that develop, can be managed by percutaneous aspiration. Usually, the mastectomy and axillary incisions tend to be insensate; these procedures can be repeated as frequently as necessary to ensure that the skin flaps adher densely to the chest wall. On an average, seroma aspiration is required in 10% of ALND and mastectomy cases, although this can go up to as high as 80%. Pogson *et al.* have reviewed studies on this subject.[23] Axillary surgery limited to the sentinel lymph node biopsy appears to confer a lower risk of seroma formation, but this is usually performed without drain insertion, and therefore patients may require subsequent seroma aspiration.[25]

Several researchers have studied strategies that may minimise seroma formation to decrease the duration for which drainage catheters are needed, or to obviate them completely. Talbot *et al.*[26] subjected 90 consecutive breast cancer patients undergoing ALND to conventional, prolonged closed suction drainage (Group 1) two-day short-term drainage (Group 2) and no drainage (Group 3). There was no difference in the rate of infectious wound complication among the three groups; at a follow-up one year later, there was no difference in the risk of lymphedema. In Group 1, the drain was removed at a median of nearly 10 days, with 73% of the cases requiring subsequent seroma aspiration. As expected, the short-term and no-drain groups required more frequent seroma aspirations (86% and 97%, respectively). The mean duration of suction drainage and/or aspiration drainages was similar for all three groups (25–27 days). In all the groups, fluid accumulation was mostly resolved in four weeks, but each group had a few patients (approximately 16%) requiring prolonged drainage (an additional two- to three weeks). Similar findings have been reported in previous studies.[27,28] The number of drains utilised and low- versus high-vacuum suction do not appear to affect the results achieved with drainage catheters.

Shoulder immobilisation with slings or special wraps to decrease seroma formation have also been proposed, but these carry the risk of possible long- term motion limitations and may even increase the risk of lymphedema.[29] A reasonable alternative approach endorsed by most breast surgeons is that patients limit motion at the shoulder to no greater than 90°, and delay active upper extremity physiotherapy until the drainage catheters are removed. This strategy appears to decrease seroma formation compared to early phys- iotherapy programs, and does not adversely affect the long-term motion development.[30,31]

The effects of electrocautery on tissues are an acknowledged risk factor for seroma formation.[23] Two prospective clinical trials[32,33] were conducted where randomised breast cancer patients underwent surgery with electrocautery and scalpel respectively; they confirmed a lower incidence of seroma formation with the latter technique. However, few surgeons are willing to relinquish the convenience and improved haemostasis associated with electrocautery dissection.

Classe *et al.*[34] reported the successful use of axillary padding in lieu of catheter drains in 207 breast cancer patients undergoing ALND, with seroma formation in 22.2%. In contrast, the Memorial Sloan Kettering Cancer Cen- ter conducted a clinical trial where 135 randomised ALND patients received a compression dressing for four days instead of the standard wound cover- age (all patients had conventional catheter drainage as well), and found no benefit.[35] Both arms of this study had similar total drainage volumes and drainage catheter durations. Furthermore, the compression arm had increased seroma aspiration requirements (mean number of aspirations 2.9 in the com- pression arm compared to 1.8 in the standard dressing arm; $p < 0.01$).

Chemical manoeuvers to decrease seroma formation have also been investigated. The application of tetracycline as a sclerosing agent has been ineffective,[36] as has bovine thrombin.[37] The use of fibrin glues, patches, and/or sealants have appeared promising, but clinical studies in man have yielded inconsistent results.[23,38–40] Therefore, it is unclear whether the added expense and potential infectious risks of these agents justify their routine use.

Haematoma: The widespread utilisation of electrocautery has dramatically reduced the incidence of haematoma formation in breast surgery, but this complication continues to occur in 2–10% of cases. Some low-volume haematoma cases carry low morbidity, leaving the patient with a more extensive ecchymosis because the adjacent soft tissue absorbs the haematoma. At the other end of the spectrum, large haematomas can be quite painful because of their rapid expansion through the closed wound space; they should be surgically evacuated, with aggressive wound irrigation and re-closure to optimise cosmesis.

An ongoing debate in breast surgery revolves around defining the optimal technique for lumpectomy cavity closure. The conventional wound closure strategy is to leave the cavity open to fill with seroma and close the overlying skin with deep dermal sutures and a final subcuticular layer. This method allows for prompt restoration of the breast contour through rapid filling of the lumpectomy cavity by seroma. However, it requires meticulous attention to ensure that haemostasis takes place along the lumpectomy cavity walls prior to skin closure. Therefore, many advocate the use of absorbable sutures to reapproximate the deeper lumpectomy tissues, and this manoeuvre is reported to decrease the risk of haematoma complications.[41] The disadvantage of employing the deep cavity sutures is the potential for compromising the final cosmetic result by altering the underlying breast architecture and causing focal areas of retraction. Hence, closure of the lumpectomy cavity is not usually recommended.

The use of a support brassiere in the postoperative period will bolster efforts to sustain haemostasis, and also relieve tension on the skin closure imposed by the weight of the breast. It can be especially important with large, pendulous breasts, where blood vessels running alongside the cavity can be avulsed mechanically if allowed to suspend unsupported. The patient should be encouraged to wear the support brassiere day and night for several days.

The use of specific medication in the perioperative period has also been implicated as a risk for bleeding complications. Aspirin-containing products and non-steroidal anti-inflammatory drugs (NSAID), such as ibuprofin have well-known antiplatelet activity, and should be avoided for one- to two-weeks prior to surgery (the lifespan of the affected platelets). Another such agent, ketorolac, which is a popular intravenous substitute for opiate analgesics during the postoperative period, should be used cautiously to minimise the risk of haematoma.[42] In addition, several over-the-counter medication and products that are widely used as "herbal supplements" have recently been recognised as contributors to bleeding diathesis; these include ginseng, ginkgo biloba, and garlic.[43,44]

Chronic Pain: A small percentage of breast cancer patients will experience postoperative chronic incisional pain, lasting from several months to years, that can be quite debilitating and refractory to standard analgesics. The exact aetiology of this syndrome remains obscure, although it is commonly assumed to be neuropathic. It is frequently described as a "burning", "constricting", or "lancing" pain, reported among mastectomy and lumpectomy patients, and is often accompanied by ipsilateral upper extremity symptoms. The incidence of this chronic pain syndrome is uncertain, but it has been reported to afflict 20–30% of patients who were specifically queried.[45–49] Surprisingly, it has also been reported more commonly following lumpectomy.[45,49] The risk factors identified with this syndrome include older age, larger tumours, radiation therapy, chemotherapy, depression and poor coping mechanisms.[46,49,50] The occasionally intractactable quality of this syndrome causes substantial frustration for both patients and surgeons. Recently, successful management has been reported with the use of serotonin uptake inhibitors, such as the antidepressants, amitryptalline and venlafaxine.[51]

COMPLICATIONS SPECIFIC TO MASTECTOMY PROCEDURES

Incisional dog-ears: Heavyset patients with thick axillary fat pads are especially prone to being left with triangular or cone-shaped flaps of redundant skin and fatty tissue along the lateral aspect of their mastectomy incisions, commonly known as "dog-ears". The incisional dog-ear is often not readily apparent while the patient is lying supine on the operating room table, but when she sits or stands upright postoperatively, these unsightly protrusions become obvious. They also create significant discomfort for the patient because they are irritating to the ipsilateral upper extremity. In many patients these redundant skin flaps were actually present preoperatively as excess subaxillary fat pads, however, the breast pulls this tissue forward, making them less noticeable; following mastectomy, they become "unmasked" and are apparent. As with the inframammary fold prior to mastectomy, dog-ears can be the site for recurrent candidal/yeast infections.

Numerous surgical approaches have been recommended to either prevent or eliminate the dog-ear problem. One option is to bring the redundant axillary tissue forward and create a "T" or "Y" configuration at the lateral aspect of the transverse mastectomy incision.[52] Alternatively, the redundant axillary skin and fatty tissue can be resected either by elongating the standard elliptical mastectomy wound, or by utilising a broad "tear-drop" incision, with the point of the tear-drop oriented medially.[53,54]

COMPLICATIONS SPECIFIC TO LUMPECTOMY PROCEDURES

Breast fibrosis, breast lymphedema, and chronic/recurrent breast cellulitis: The satisfaction with the final cosmetic result achieved by breast conservation therapy is difficult to define, and there may be dramatic differences in the perception of the surgeon and the patient. Ultimately, the acceptability must be in accord with the aesthetic standards of the patient, and the role of the surgeon is to advise the patient regarding the probable long-term appearance. Several features influence the final result, including the extent of breast volume resected, radiation-related fibrosis, infectious and/or hemorrhagic complications, and the ratio of the primary breast tumour size versus breast size.

The presence of long-term adverse sequelae related to breast conservation therapy for cancer is increasingly being acknowledged and reported.[55,56] These complications are secondary to the combined tissue effects of surgery and radiation therapy. The European Organisation for Research and Treatment of cancer and the Radiation Therapy Oncology Group have proposed that the late effects of breast conservation therapy (including breast oedema, fibrosis, and atrophy/retraction) be graded according to the Late Effects of Normal Tissue-Subjective, Objective, Management, and Analytic (LENT-SOMA) scales.[57] The LENT-SOMA system stratifies breast symptoms on the basis of pain magnitude as reported by the patient, measurable differences in breast appearance, intervention requirement for control of pain and/or lymphedema, and the presence of image-documented breast sequelae (e.g. photos, mammography, CT/MRI, etc.).

Using the LENT-SOMA four-point grading system, Fehlauer *et al.*[56] reported grades 3–4 toxicity in 4–18% of the breast cancer patients treated between 1983–84 (XRT fractionation schedule 2.5 Gy 4x/week to 60 Gy, with median follow-up after 171 months), and ≤2% for patients treated between 1994–95 (XRT fractionation schedule 2.0 Gy 5x/week to 55 Gy, with median follow-up 75 months). This suggests that the extent of side effects is a function of both follow-up duration and radiation delivery technique. Similarly, Meric *et al.*[55] reported chronic breast symptoms that lasted for at least one year post-treatment in 9.9% of breast cancer patients treated by lumpectomy and radiation from 1990–92.

Recurrent episodes of breast cellulitis occurring several months-to-years after lumpectomy and/or breast radiation therapy are reported to afflict fewer than 5% of the patients, but this unusual and delayed complication causes significant concern because of the need to rule out inflammatory breast cancer recurrence.[58–62] This condition can present in a myriad of scenarios, such as acutely inflamed seroma formation, localised mastitis, or diffused breast pain and swelling. Repeated breast imaging is required to check for parenchymal features, such as an underlying spiculated mass, calcifications, etc. that suggest recurrence; if any of these are present, an image-guided biopsy should be pursued. The cases that appear benign but are refractory to a standard course of antibiotics should undergo punch biopsy for further evaluation. Occasionally patients do request a mastectomy because of the intractable pain and inflammation.

The cause of delayed breast oedema and cellulitis is incompletely understood, but presumed related to lymphatic obstruction affecting intramammary drainage. The risk factors for this condition include a history of early postoperative complications such as haematoma and seroma, upper extremity lymphedema, and large-volume lumpectomies.[59] In most of the cases there has been a resection of upper outer quadrant tumours. Rarely, the causative agent is identified as a bacterial pathogen, but conventional management covers this by including antibiotics for skin flora. The development of this complication does not appear to carry any cancer-related prognostic significance.

Lumpectomy and brachytherapy-related complications: Several breast programs are currently exploring strategies of partial breast irradiation that allow for shortening of the conventional 5–6 week external beam program. One such strategy involves the insertion of a balloon-type catheter (the MammoSite applicator) into the lumpectomy cavity for delivery of brachytherapy. This device is typically inserted in the operating room at the time of lumpectomy to achieve margin control; if this is not done during lumpectomy, additional surgery and a second implantation is required. Computed tomography (CT) imaging is subsequently performed to ensure adequate balloon placement, as defined by a minimum applicator-skin distance of 5 mm and appropriate conformance, with uniform contact between the balloon and lumpectomy walls. The optimal positioning can be challenging, but is essential for delivery of the therapy with a minimal risk of local complications.

While investigations of the long-term efficacy of the accelerated breast irradiation programs are being conducted, the experience related to catheter-related risk is accumulating. The results from a prospective, multicenter study of the MammoSite device[63] revealed that of the 70 patients who enrolled, 21 (30%) could not complete the study because of lumpectomy-related issues (cavity size, skin spacing, or conformance). Of the 54 patients with an inserted balloon, 57% experienced overlying skin erythema and two developed wound infections, including one abscess.

Breast conservation therapy-related angiosarcoma: Reviewed in detail by Monroe *et al.*,[64] angiosarcomas of the breast following lumpectomy and XRT for breast cancer were very rare, but are now being reported with increasing frequency. These secondary angiosarcomas must be distinguished from primary breast angiosarcomas, which occur in relatively younger women and do not have well-defined risk factors. Secondary angiosarcomas occur 4–10 years after the primary breast cancer treatment.[64–66] Lymphedema-related extremity angiosarcoma (Stewart-Treves syndrome, discussed below) has a longer latency period from the time of breast cancer treatment. Furthermore, the occurrence of breast angiosarcomas in the irradiated field coupled with the implications for genetic predisposition to radiation-induced tumorigenesis (e.g. ataxia-telangiectasia) have prompted speculation that these lesions have an aetiology different from the Stewart-Treves syndrome. However, the median survival is equally poor in both, at 1–3 years.[64]

COMPLICATIONS SPECIFIC TO DIAGNOSTIC OPEN BIOPSY PROCEDURES

Sampling error: The primary potential risk specifically associated with a diagnostic open biopsy is related to misdiagnosis, by missing a cancerous lesion and resecting adjacent fibrocystic tissue. This complication exists with palpable masses as well as screen-detected non-palpable lesions.

The risk of misdiagnosis with palpable breast masses can be minimised by complete preoperative breast imaging, including mammography and ultrasonography. In palpable lesions with a suspicious imaging correlate, diagnosis should be confirmed with an initial attempt at percutaneous core needle biopsy. If malignancy is confirmed, cancer-directed management options can be addressed promptly. Neoadjuvant chemotherapy is an option for patients with measurable disease in the breast, because the potential benefits of tumour downstaging to improve the success rate of breast conservation therapy as well as to monitor chemosensitivity, remain available to them.[67] If the percutaneous biopsy was performed freehand and returned non-diagnostic, an image-guided (either by ultrasound or stereotactic/mammographic) needle biopsy may be attempted. Alternatively, and if resources are available, a percutaneous biopsy may be performed with image guidance as the initial manoeuvre to improve the diagnostic accuracy.

If the palpable lesion does not have an imaging correlate, or if needle biopsy strategies are unavailable, a diagnostic open biopsy must be performed. Sampling errors with these procedures are uncommon, but in patients with extensive fibrocystic changes, especially where the lesion was a self-detected mass that is less dominant on clinical examination, it can be challenging. In these cases, the breast should be assessed and marked just prior to surgery by the surgeon and patient together, but intraoperative surgical judgement remains critical and any suspicious masses identified within the open breast wound should be biopsied and oriented appropriately.

The risk of sampling error with non-palpable breast lesions is greater. Establishing a diagnosis for clinically occult lesions that are identified by the mammogram or ultrasound depends on image guidance. As mentioned earlier, an image-guided percutaneous needle biopsy as the initial diagnostic strategy has certain advantages; patients whose diagnosis has been made via needle biopsy are more likely to have successful breast conservation therapy and require fewer re-excisions for margin control compared to patients that undergo an initial open biopsy.[68] A core needle biopsy is preferable to a fine needle aspiration biopsy because of a larger tissue yield, which can distinguish *in situ* from invasive architecture, and the sampling error is only 5–10% here as opposed to 30% with a fine needle aspiration biopsy. If the targeted lesion is small and can be completely resected within the core specimens, a radioopaque clip should be left in place to facilitate subsequent localisation in the event of surgery.

When high-risk lesions, such as atypical hyperplasia, radial scar, or lobular carcinoma *in situ* are identified on core needle biopsy, a follow-up open surgical biopsy should be performed. The sampling error rates associated with these findings are substantial, and 10–40% will be upstaged to invasive cancer or ductal carcinoma *in situ* on subsequent open biopsy.[69]

The open surgical biopsies of non-palpable, image-detected breast lesions require image-guided wire localisation. The localising wire can be inserted under ultrasound or mammographic guidance, depending on which modality images the abnormal lesion best. Magnetic resonance imaging (MRI)-guided wire localisation technology is available in some centres. In the past, strategies for localisation have included external skin markings and preoperative injection of a dye in the vicinity of the lesion, but these have been largely abandoned because of higher sampling error rates. The insertion of a hooked wire, with a two-view confirmatory mammography of the wire position in relation to the abnormal lesion, followed by mammographic (and/or ultrasonographic) imaging of the biopsy specimen to document the inclusion of the suspicious target, is the most common routine employed in contemporary breast programs. With this algorithm, the failure to sample the target should occur in fewer than 5% of the cases. Despite these precautions, the risk factors for a sampling error complication include suboptimal wire localisation, localising wire migration between the time of insertion and surgical resection, and migration of a previously-inserted clip intended to mark the site of a prior core needle biopsy. When a sampling error is recognised intraoperatively, based on specimen imaging, it is quite difficult to reorient the breast anatomy without the localising wire. In such circumstances it is prudent to resist multiple attempts at "blind" biopsies, as the likelihood of success is low and the additional tissue resections will compromise cosmesis. The patient should be informed of the failed procedure, and imaging should be repeated 2–4 weeks postoperatively, and a further wire localisation planned accordingly.

COMPLICATIONS RELATED TO AXILLARY STAGING PROCEDURES

The axillary nodal status remains the most powerful prognostic feature in staging patients with invasive breast cancer. Surgical staging of the axilla is necessary for a majority of newly-diagnosed patients, because the available imaging modalities can easily miss small nodal metastases. The conventional Level I/II ALND is the gold standard means of evaluating the axilla, but sentinel lymph node biopsy has recently emerged as a viable alternative strategy for accurately determining the nodal status. Each of these staging procedures is associated with risks for various complications, and will be discussed separately.

Complications associated with ALND: The level I/II ALND is the conventionally-accepted staging procedure. Random axillary sampling procedures or ALND limited to Level I can miss metastases in 20–25% of the cases where nodal disease is present. On the other hand, a Level III dissection is generally considered unnecessary (unless there is grossly apparent disease present in the axillary apex) because "skip" metastases to Level III occur only in 2–3% of node-positive cases. The presence of an "axillary arch" has been proposed as an anatomic variant that can increase the risk of sampling error when a standard level I and II ALND is performed.[70] The axillary arch is formed by an aberrant segment of the latissimus dorsi muscle that extends toward the pectoralis. If the axillary dissection does not encompass the lymphatic tissue lateral to these fibres, significant nodal tissue can be missed; the failure to appreciate this anatomic variant has been implicated as a cause for subsequent axillary recurrence.[71]

Of the complications following ALND, upper extremity lymphedema has generated the most concern because it is a lifelong risk and can be quite refractory to treatment. Lymphedema has been reported to develop in 13–27% of breast cancer patients,[25,72–75] but detection rates will vary based on how closely patients are monitored and the duration of follow-up. The risk of lymphedema increases after a higher-level axillary dissection compared with a less extensive surgery, but is reported to occur even after axillary surgery limited to the sentinel lymph nodes.[25] Other risk factors include obesity and regional radiation therapy. Patients can minimise the risk of lymphedema by participating in an aggressive and regulated physical therapy program, but the onset of this problem can be initiated by upper extremity trauma or infection.

One of the most feared long-term sequelae of chronic lymphedema is the development of upper extremity angiosarcoma.[76,77] This condition is also known as Stewart-Treves syndrome,[78] named for the researchers who first reported a series of cases demonstrating the association between postmastectomy lymphedema and the onset of this malignancy. It typically appears as bluish-reddish macular lesions or nodules on the skin of the ipsilateral upper extremity, and develops approximately 10 years after the breast cancer treatment. Usually (but not always) it is seen in patients where the risk of lymphedema is amplified by regional irradiation in addition to ALND. Various treatment strategies, including wide local excision, amputation, chemotherapy, and/or radiation, have met with disappointing results. Most patients succumb to haematogenously-disseminated metastases to lung and visceral organs, with a median survival of approximately two years.

The axillary dissection surgical bed exposes the thoracodorsal, long thoracic ("nerve of Bell"), and intercostal-brachial nerves, the axillary vein as well as the neurovascular bundle to the pectoralis musculature. The intercostobrachial nerves are routinely sacrificed during a conventional ALND as they course directly through the nodal tissue *en route* to the skin of the axilla and upper inner arm, leaving patients with sensory deficits in this distribution. Attempts to preserve these nerves can result in damage that leaves the patient with chronic neuropathic pain of the involved skin. The axillary vein is at risk for haemorrhagic complications as a consequence of direct injury, or thrombosis secondary to traction and/or compression. The axillary artery and brachial plexus are relatively protected from intraoperative damage because of their deeper and more superior location. The thoracodorsal neurovascular bundle, which courses along the inner aspect of the latissimus dorsi muscle, should be completely exposed and preserved intact unless there is gross encasement by nodal metastases. Sacrificing these structures will denervate the latissimus (leaving the patient with weakness of internal rotation and shoulder abduction), and eliminate the availability of the thoracodorsal vessels for possible future use in free flap reconstructions (with microvascular anastomoses). Disruption of the long thoracic nerve results in the loss of serratus anterior function and a "winged scapula" deformity, with an unsightly posterior shoulder bony protrusion. When both the medial and lateral pectoral nerves are transected, denervation atrophy of the pectoral muscles will eventually become apparent and may compromise the patient's cosmetic result substantially. This risk can be minimised by preserving the neurovascular bundle that curves medial to the pectoralis.

Axillary webs are bands of scar tissue that develop after ALND in fewer than 10% of cases. They are readily apparent as cordlike structures coursing from the surgical bed toward the forearm, and occasionally reaching the thumb.[79] These webs cause significant tightness and limitation of motion but often resolve within a few months. Physical therapy and massage are frequently helpful in alleviating symptoms.

One final, and rather rare, complication of the ALND is chyle leak,[80] reputed to be secondary to thoracic duct injury. Recently, octreotide has been recommended to control extensive lymphorrhea.[81]

Complications associated with lymphatic mapping and sentinel lymph node biopsy: Krag *et al.* (1993) and Giuliano (1994) reported lymphatic mapping and sentinel lymph node biopsy for breast cancer patients using radiolabelled isotope,[82] and blue dye[83] respectively. This technology was recognised as a promising strategy to identify node-negative patients and spare them the morbidity of a conventional ALND. Since these pioneering studies were published, dozens of other researchers have reported their experiences with lymphatic mapping and sentinel lymph node biopsy in conjunction with a completion ALND to define the accuracy and optimal technique for performing the procedure. A meta-analysis of these studies[84] presented at the American Society of Clinical Oncology 2002 annual symposium revealed an overall identification rate of 96% and an overall false negative rate of 8.4%; this analysis included data from 69 studies involving 10,454 patients. Surgeons with limited experience with the procedure and/or early in the learning curve with lymphatic mapping technology, and the use of a single mapping agent (blue dye or isotope versus use of both) were identified as risk factors for complications from either a failed mapping procedure or a false negative sentinel lymph node result.

Table 2 summarises the results of studies that have evaluated specific causes for the inability to identify the sentinel lymph node, and features that predict a greater risk of a falsely negative result. As with the meta-analysis findings, inexperience with lymphatic mapping and use of a single mapping agent rather than two agents are repeatedly implicated with unsuccessful sentinel lymph node biopsies. The steep learning curve, and the benefits of dual versus single mapping agents, are explored and presented in detail by Cox *et al.*[85] and Derossis *et al.*,[86] respectively.

Table 2.   Selected Studies Reporting Risk Factors for Failed Lymphatic Mapping and/or False Negative Sentinel Lymph Node Biopsy

Study	Total # Cases	SLN Id Rate (%)	SLN FN Rate (%)	Factors Associated with SLN Non-identification						Factors Associated with SLN FN Risk					
				Learning Curve	Tumour Location (Medial Worse)	Older Age Pt	Prior Excisional Biopsy	Single vs Dual Mapping Agent	Larger Size Tumour	Learning Curve	Tumour Location (UOQ Worse)	Older Age Pt	Prior Excisional Biopsy	Single vs Dual Mapping Agent	Larger Size Tumour
Canavese[119]	212*	97.1%	6.5%	No	NR	NR	NR	Yes	No	No	NR	NR	NR	No	Yes
Albertini[120]	62	92%	0%	NR	NR	NR	NA*	Yes	NR	No	No	No	No	No	No
McMasters[121]	806	88%	7.2%	No	No	Yes	No	Yes	No	No	Yes	No	No	Yes	No
Veronesi[91]	163	98%	4.7%	No	No	No	No	NA (Tc only used)	Yes	No	Yes	No	No	NA	Yes
Veronesi[92]	376	98.7%	6.7%	No	No	NR	NR	No	No	No	No	No	NR	No	No
Cox[122]	465	94.4%	UK	Yes	NR	NR	No	Yes	NR	Yes	NR	NR	NR	NR	NR
Giuliano[83]	174	65.5%	8.1%	Yes	NR	NR	NR	NA (dye only used)	NR	Yes	NR	NR	NR	NR	NR
Bedrosian[93]	104*	99%	3.3%	NR	NR	NR	NR	NR	No	NR	No	NR	NR	NR	No
Haigh[87]	284**	81.0%	3.2%	NR	No	NR	No	NR	No	Yes	No	NR	No	NR	No
Wong[88]	2206	92.5%	8.0%	NR	No	NR	No	NR	Yes	NR	No	NR	No	NR	No
Krag[123]	443	93%	12.8%	NR	Yes	Yes	Yes	NA (isotope-only used)	No	NR	Yes	No	No	NA (isotope-only used)	No
O'Hea[124]	59	93%	15%	NR	No	NR	No	Yes	No	Yes	No	NR	No	No	Yes
Guenther[125]	260	81.9%	NR***	Yes	Yes	NR	No	NA (dye only used)	NR	***	***	***	***	***	***

*Patients with prior excisional biopsy excluded from study.

*All T2 and T3 tumours.

**Including 181 lymphatic mapping cases with prior excisional biopsy.

***Analyses limited to 47 patients with unsuccessful mapping procedures.

The original studies of sentinel lymph node biopsy involved intra-parenchymal, peritumoral injections of the mapping agent(s), since the goal was to replicate the pathway traversed by tumour cells along intramammary lymphatic channels *en route* to the sentinel node. If the mapping procedure was being performed after a prior excisional biopsy, there was a risk of inadvertent injection into the biopsy cavity in which case the mapping agent will not reach the nodal basin. As experience with lymphatic mapping grew, these techni-cal failures declined and researchers have specifically documented the ability to reliably identify the sentinel lymph node in the setting of prior excisional biopsy.[87,88] Injections of skin overlying the tumour sites will further improve sentinel node identification rates, because of exuberant uptake by dermal lymphatics.[89] With age, lymph nodes can become fatty-replaced and difficult to recognise, also contributing to a failed identification. For tumours located in the upper, outer quadrant of the breast, extensive background radioactivity (shine-through) impairs the ability to discriminate focal uptake by the sentinel node; and the likelihood of missing the true sentinel node and obtaining a false-negative result is increased. In contrast, medially-located tumours have been associated with the risk of mapping failure, because of the increased like-lihood of primary lymphatic drainage to non-axillary sites. Other reports[90] have found no relationship between tumour location and sentinel node accu-racy. An additional factor implicated in mapping inaccuracy is the size of the primary tumour; with large lesions there is risk of tumour embolisation caus-ing obstructed lymphatic vessels, thereby altering the pathway that a mapping agent would follow. While early studies[91] did suggest a correlation between breast tumour size and the risk of a false negative sentinel lymph node biopsy, recent studies have indicated none.[92–94] Grube *et al.*[95] have also confirmed the accuracy of sentinel lymph node biopsy for invasive lobular carcinoma.

Most of the potential pitfalls in lymphatic mapping procedures have been obviated by the development of newer mapping techniques, such as subare-olar injections of the mapping agent.[96–98] The basis for this strategy is the embryologic development of the breast and its lymphatic drainage system, which begins as the centrally-located nipple bud, followed by radial exten-sion peripherally. The concept is that each breast has a primary drainage to a discrete cluster of sentinel lymph nodes, as opposed to separate drainage pathways for different areas of the breast. The model further opens the door for improving lymphatic mapping in multicentric breast cancer, which was previously considered as a contraindication to sentinel node biopsy.

Recent studies on lymphatic mapping in patients with multifocal and/or multicentric disease have demonstrated that sentinel lymph node biopsy is accurate in this setting.[99–103] It also appears that the sentinel node can be identified by the subareolar technique or an injection targeting the different breast tumours.

Other complications that have been reported following a sentinel lymph node biopsy are identical to those associated with ALND, including seroma, lymphedema, axillary web formation and neurosensory disturbances, but the magnitude of risk is lower. Data on long-term follow-up of patients who have undergone sentinel lymph node biopsy alone now reveal adverse sequelae occurring in fewer than 5% of cases.[25,74,104]

The risk of allergic reactions to the blue dye for mapping procedures must be considered. Table 3 demonstrates the reported series, involving both isosulfan blue and patent blue dye. Within a few minutes-to-an-hour following blue dye injection, up to 2% of patients may experience sudden haemodynamic instability and other sequelae of intraoperative anaphylaxis. Despite the dramatic presentation, these episodes are usually responsive to

Table 3. Selected Studies of Allergic Reactions to Blue Dye in Breast Cancer Cases

Study	Blue Dye Type	# Cases (Type)	Incidence	# 2nd Reactions
Lyew[126]	Isosulfan blue	1 (anaphylactic)	NR	No
Mullon[127]	Patent blue			
Cimmino[108]	Isosulfan blue	5 (3 anaphylactic*; 2 blue urticaria)	2%	No
Albo[128]	Isosulfan blue	7 (all anaphylactic)	1.1%	2/7 (%)
Montgomery[129]	Isosulfan blue	39 (27 blue hives; 12 anaphylactic)	1.6%	NR
Efron[106]	Isosulfan blue	1 (anaphylactic)	NR	No
Laurie[105]	Isosulfan blue	2 (anaphylactic)	NR	No
Stefanutto[130]	Isosulfan blue	1 (anaphylactic)	NR	No
Crivellaro[131]	Patent blue	1 (anaphylactic)	NR	No
Sprung[132]	Isosulfan blue	1 (anaphylactic)	NR	Possibly; protracted hypotension noted

*Series includes two cases of lymphatic mapping performed for breast cancer.

supportive care, which includes discontinuation of the gaseous anaesthetics, 100% oxygen, aggressive fluid resuscitation and pressor support as well as histamine blocking agents and even corticosteroids. In most cases the anaesthesia and surgical procedure have been resumed and completed uneventfully after the patient had stabilised. However, some surgeons have elected to abort the surgical procedure[105] and reschedule the mapping without blue dye, and in one reported case[106] a planned lumpectomy was converted to a mastectomy so that the allergen focus would be completely resected. Many patients have undergone successful lumpectomies despite a blue dye allergic reaction, but they should be monitored closely for 24 h because continued uptake of the blue dye from skin and soft tissue can result in protracted or delayed secondary (biphasic) reactions.

Blue urticaria, a less severe form of blue dye allergy characterised by blue-tinged hives, is another pattern that has been reported.[107,108] There is no correlation with past allergy history, and preoperative skin testing is unreliable in identifying highest-risk patients. One hypothesis is that many individuals have prior sensitisation from exposure to industrial dyes in cosmetics, textiles, detergents, etc. Routine premedication of all mapping cases with steroids, antihistamines, and/or histamine receptor blockade has been proposed, but the added expense and risk for a low-incidence allergic reaction has not been justified; as noted by Raut *et al.* this prophylactic strategy may increase wound infection rates.[109] Known allergy to triphenylmethane is a contraindication to blue dye use. So far, methylene blue appears to be less allergenic,[110] but caution must be exercised to avoid skin necrosis from dermal injections of this agent.

Blue dyes can also cause a spurious decline in pulse oximetry measurements, related to intravascular uptake and interference with spectroscopy; arterial blood gases in these circumstances will reveal normal oxygenation. In addition, blue dyes are considered relatively contraindicated during pregnancy, because the risk of teratogenicity is unknown and because an anaphylactic reaction during pregnancy could have catastrophic consequences for the fetus.

COMPLICATIONS SPECIFIC TO IMMEDIATE BREAST RECONSTRUCTION (IBR)

A detailed discussion of breast reconstruction options and risk of complications is beyond the scope of this chapter, but a few issues warrant mention. Smoking, obesity, and chest wall irradiation increase the risk of wound complications associated with any type of reconstruction.

Skin-sparing mastectomy: The skin-sparing mastectomy technique has become increasingly popular to improve the cosmetic results achieved by IBR, but the surgeon should pay attention while raising the elongated skin flaps so that risk of retained breast tissue and increased local recurrence rates is minimised. When the oncologic principles of the mastectomy are upheld, breast cancer outcome is equivalent for patients undergoing skin-sparing and conventional mastectomy with IBR.[111–113] Localised wound problems such as minor infections, focal epidermolysis, and fat necrosis are usually managed successfully without the need for additional surgery. A needle or excisional biopsy may be necessary when fat necrosis associated with a mass is equivocal for local recurrence.

IBR and chest wall irradiation: Chest wall irradiation can compromise reconstruction outcome regardless of whether the mastectomy and IBR are performed before or after the radiation exposure. Mastectomy and IBR performed on a previously irradiated chest wall (as in the setting of patients undergoing surgery for local recurrence after prior BCT, or in breast cancer patients with a history of therapeutic chest wall irradiation for Hodgkin's disease) is more challenging because of the stiffer, less compliant chest wall skin. Autogenous tissue reconstructions are usually preferred in this setting, because of the difficulty in expanding the chest wall to accommodate an implant.

Mastectomy and IBR are performed prior to irradiation in cases requiring postmastectomy irradiation (extensive nodal disease, locally advanced breast cancer, or cases mastectomy flaps with inadequate margin control). In this setting, irradiation of the reconstructed breast increases the risk of fat necrosis and wound infection. Implant reconstructions are particularly sensitive to this effect, and up to one half will require ultimate explantation because of contractures and/or recurrent infections.[114] Some researchers have reported that TRAM flap reconstructions will tolerate irradiation with acceptable early results,[115] but recent studies have indicated that on long-term follow-up there is increased morbidity, including high rates of fibrosis/shrinkage and progressive deformity.[116] Therefore, if there is a likelihood of postmastectomy irradiation, patients should be informed of the risks associated with IBR and delayed reconstruction should be encouraged. An alternative is the insertion of a tissue expander during mastectomy for the sole purpose of skin expansion, and with a plan for final surgery upon completion of chest wall irradiation, by either autogenous tissue reconstruction or exchange to the final implant. While this strategy seems reasonable in concept, the long-term results and rates of attendant infectious morbidity remain undefined.

OTHER ISSUES RELATED TO BREAST SURGERY COMPLICATION RATES

Neoadjuvant chemotherapy: The benefits of increased breast preservation rates (because of primary tumour downstaging) and monitoring for chemosensitivity have led to broadened applications for induction chemotherapy regimens. Numerous studies have demonstrated the oncologic and medical safety of this approach. However, patients should time their surgery following the last chemotherapy cycle so that adequate bone marrow recovery has occurred (usually 3–4 weeks post-treatment), as evidenced by a platelet count greater than 75,000 and an absolute neutrophil count greater than 1,500. Broadwater *et al.*[117] reported wound complication rates in a retrospective study of nearly 200 patients from the M.D. Anderson Cancer Center receiving treatment for locally advanced breast cancer; approximately half of these patients underwent primary mastectomy followed by postoperative chemotherapy, while the remainder received treatment in the reverse sequence. The wound infection rates were similar for both groups while the seroma rates were actually lower for the neoadjuvant chemotherapy patients.

Patients with unifocal breast cancers and no mammographically-suspicious calcifications who are receiving induction chemotherapy to improve their eligibility for breast preservation should have radio-opaque clips inserted into the tumour bed prior to the first or second course of chemotherapy (while the tumour site is still radiographically apparent). If no markers are inserted and the patient shows a complete clinical response, she may require a mastectomy because of the inability to localise the tumour bed at the time of lumpectomy. Alternatively, at the time of diagnosis, patients with diffuse suspicious microcalcifications associated with their cancer, or with multicentric disease, should be informed that mastectomy will be required regardless of the magnitude of response to induction chemotherapy, because of the limited ability to accurately monitor the response in these clinical scenarios.[118]

Table 4. Selected Studies of Lymphatic Mapping and Sentinel Lymph Node Biopsy Performed After Neoadjuvant Chemotherapy

Study	T Status	Sample Size	Sentinel Node Identification Rate	False Negative Rate	Metastases Limited to Sentinel Node(s)
Breslin[133]	2,3	51	85% (42/51)	12% (3/25)	40% (10/25)
Nason[134]	2,3	15	87% (13/15)	33% (3/9)	11%*(1/9)
Haid[135]	1–3	33	88% (29/33)	0% (0/22)	50% (11/22)
Fernandez[136]	1–4	40	90% (36/40)	20% (4/20)	20% (4/20)
Tafra[137]	1,2	29	93% (27/29)	0% (0/15)	NR
Stearns[138]	3,4	T4d (inflammatory) 8	75% (6/8)	40% (2/5)	24% (5/21)
		Non-inflammatory 26	88% (23/26)	6% (1/16)	
Julian[139]	1–3	34	91% (31/34)	0% (0/12)	42% (5/12)
Miller[140]	1–3	35	86% (30/35)	0% (0/9)	44% (4/9)
Brady[141]	1–3	14	93% (13/14)	0% (0/10)	60% (6/10)
Piato[142]	1,2	42	98% (41/42)	17% (3/18)	0% (0/18)
Balch[143]	2–4	32	97% (31/32)	5% (1/19)	56% (10/18)
Schwartz[144]	1–3	21	100% (21/21)	9% (1/11)	64% (7/11)
Reitsamer[145]	2,3	30	87% (26/30)	7% (1/15)	53% (8/15)
Mamounas[146] (abstract)	1–3	428	85% (363/428)	11% (15/140)	50% (70/140)

The optimal strategy for integrating lymphatic mapping technology into neoadjuvant chemotherapy protocols remains to be defined. As shown in Table 4, numerous researchers have documented the accuracy of sentinel lymph node biopsies performed after the delivery of neoadjuvant chemotherapy, but the success rates have varied. While the identification rates range from 70–100%, the false negative rates range between 0–33%, with averages approximating 90% and 9%, respectively. Nonetheless, many of these series reveal axillary metastases limited to the sentinel node at rates which are comparable to primary surgery cases, and support the validity of the technology from a biologic perspective. An alternative is to perform the axillary staging via sentinel lymph node biopsy prior to the delivery of the neoadjuvant chemotherapy. Unfortunately, this sequence commits many patients to an "unnecessary" completion axillary dissection, as the sentinel node(s) is often the isolated site of metastases, and chemotherapy sterilizes the axillary metastases in approximately one-quarter of cases. This issue remains to be further evaluated in prospective clinical trials.

REFERENCES

1. Grunwald Z, Moore JH, Schwartz GF. (2003) Bilateral brachial plexus palsy after a right-side modified radical mastectomy with immediate TRAM flap reconstruction. *Breast J* **9**(1): 41–43.
2. Warner M, *et al.* (2000) Practice advisory for the prevention of perioperative peripheral neuropathies. A report by the American Society of Anesthesiologists' Task Force on the prevention of perioperative peripheral neuropathies. *Anesthiology* **92**: 1168–1182.
3. Bejanga BI. (1992) Mondor's disease: analysis of 30 cases. *J R Coll Surg Edinb*, **37**(5): 322–324.
4. Catania S, *et al.* (2003) Mondor's disease and breast cancer. *Cancer* **69**(9): 2267–2270.
5. Harris AT. (2003) Mondor's disease of the breast can also occur after a sonography-guided core biopsy. *Am J Roentgenol* **180**(1): 284–285.
6. Hou MF, *et al.* (1999) Mondor's disease in the breast. *Kaohsiung J Med Sci* **15**(11): 632–639.
7. Jaberi M, Willey SC, Brem RF. (2002) Stereotactic vacuum-assisted breast biopsy: an unusual cause of Mondor's disease. *Am J Roentgenol* **179**(1): 185–186.

8. Platt R, *et al.* (1990) Perioperative antibiotic prophylaxis for herniorrhaphy and breast surgery. *N Engl J Med* **322**(3): 153–160.

9. Hoefer R, *et al.* (1990) Wound complications following modified radical mastectomy: an analysis of perioperative factors. *J Am Osteopath Assoc* **90**: 47–53.

10. Wagman LD, *et al.* (1990) A prospective, randomized double-blind study of the use of antibiotics at the time of mastectomy. *Surg Gynecol Obstet* **170**(1): 12–16.

11. Chen J, Gutkin Z, Bawnik J. (1991) Postoperative infections in breast surgery. *J Hosp Infect* **17**: 61–65.

12. Vinton AL, Traverso LW, Jolly PC. (1991) Wound complications after modified radical mastectomy compared with tylectomy with axillary lymph node dissection. *Am J Surg* **161**(5): 584–588.

13. Platt R, *et al.* (1992) Prophylaxis against wound infection following herniorrhaphy or breast surgery. *J Infect Dis* **166**(3): 556–560.

14. Lipshy KA, *et al.* (1996) Complications of mastectomy and their relationship to biopsy technique. *Ann Surg Oncol* **3**(3): 290–294.

15. Bertin M, Crowe J, Gordon S. (1998) Determinants of surgical site infection after breast surgery. *Am J Infect Control* **26**: 61–65.

16. Thomas R, *et al.* (1999) Long-acting versus short-acting cephalosporins for pre-operative prophylaxis in breast surgery: a randomized double-blind trial involving 1,766 patients. *Chemotherapy* **45**(3): 217–223.

17. Gupta R, *et al.* (2000) Antibiotic prophylaxis for post-operative wound infection in clean elective breast surgery. *Eur J Surg Oncol* **26**(4): 363–366.

18. Nieto A, *et al.* (2002) Determinants of wound infections after surgery for breast cancer. *Zentralbl Gynakol* **124**(8–9): 429–433.

19. Sorensen LT, *et al.* (2002) Smoking as a risk factor for wound healing and infection in breast cancer surgery. *Eur J Surg Oncol* **28**(8): 815–820.

20. Witt A, *et al.* (2003) Preoperative core needle biopsy as an independent risk factor for wound infection after breast surgery. *Obstet Gynecol* **101**(4): 745–750.

21. Tran CL, *et al.* (2003) Does reoperation predispose to postoperative wound infection in women undergoing operation for breast cancer? *Am Surg* **69**(10): 852–856.

22. Platt R, *et al.* (1993) Perioperative antibiotic prophylaxis and wound infection following breast surgery. *J Antimicrob Chemother* **31**(Suppl B): 43–48.

23. Pogson CJ, Adwani A, Ebbs SR. (2003) Seroma following breast cancer surgery. *Eur J Surg Oncol* **29**(9): 711–717.

24. Bonnema J, *et al.* (1999) The composition of serous fluid after axillary dissection. *Eur J Surg* **165**: 9–13.

25. Giuliano AE, *et al.* (2000) Prospective observational study of sentinel lymphadenectomy without further axillary dissection in patients with sentinel node-negative breast cancer. *J Clin Oncol* **18**(13): 2553–2559.

26. Talbot ML, Magarey CJ. (2002) Reduced use of drains following axillary lymphadenectomy for breast cancer. *ANZ J Surg* **72**(7): 488–490.

27. Cameron AE, *et al.* (1988) Suction drainage of the axilla: a prospective randomized trial. *Br J Surg* **75**(12): 1211.

28. Somers R, Jablon L, Kaplan M. (1992) The use of closed suction drainage after lumpectomy and axillary dissection for breast cancer: a prospective randomized trial. *Ann Surg* **215**: 146–149.

29. Flew J. (1979) The effect of restriction of shoulder movement. *Br J Surg* **66**: 302–305.

30. Lotze M, *et al.* (1981) Early versus delayed shoulder motion following axillary dissection. *Ann Surg* **193**: 288–295.

31. Schultz I, Barrholm M, Grondal S. (1997) Delayed shoulder exercises in reducing seroma frequency after modified radical mastectomy: a prospective randomized study. *Ann Surg Oncol* **4**: 293–297.

32. Porter KA, *et al.* (1998) Electrocautery as a factor in seroma formation following mastectomy. *Am J Surg* **176**(1): 8–11.

33. Keogh G, *et al.* (1998) Seroma formation related to electrocautery in breast surgery — A prospective, randomized trial. *Breast* **7**: 39–41.

34. Classe J, *et al.* (2002) Axillary padding as an alternative to closed suction drain for ambulatory axillary lymphadenectomy. *Arch Surg* **137**: 169–173.

35. O'Hea BJ, Ho MN, Petrek JA. (1999) External compression dressing versus standard dressing after axillary lymphadenectomy. *Am J Surg* **177**(6): 450–453.

36. Rice DC, *et al.* (2000) Intraoperative topical tetracycline sclerotherapy following mastectomy: a prospective, randomized trial. *J Surg Oncol* **73**(4): 224–227.

37. Burak WE Jr., Goodman P, Young D. (1997) Seroma formation following axillary dissection for breast cancer: risk factors and lack of influence of bovine thrombin. *J Surg Oncol* **64**: 27–31.

38. Langer S, Guenther JM, DiFronzo LA. (2003) Does fibrin sealant reduce drain output and allow earlier removal of drainage catheters in women undergoing operation for breast cancer? *Am Surg* **69**(1): 77–81.

39. Berger A, *et al.* (2001) Sealing of postoperative axillary leakage after axillary lymphadenectomy using a fibrin glue coated collagen patch: a prospective randomised study. *Breast Cancer Res Treat* **67**(1): 9–14.

40. Moore M, *et al.* (2001) Fibrin sealant reduces the duration and amount of fluid drainage after axillary dissection: a randomized prospective clinical trial. *J Am Coll Surg* **192**(5): 591–599.

41. Paterson ML, Nathanson SD, Havstad S. (1994) Hematomas following excisional breast biopsies for invasive breast carcinoma: the influence of deep suture approximation of breast parenchyma. *Am Surg* **60**(11): 845–848.

42. Sharma S, *et al.* (2001) Incidence of hematoma associated with ketorolac after TRAM flap breast reconstruction. *Plast Reconstr Surg* **107**(2): 352–355.

43. Hodges P, Kam P. (2002) The perioperative implications of herbal medicines. *Anaesthesia* **57**(9): 889–899.

44. Ang-Lee M, Moss J, Yuan C. (2001) Herbal medicines and perioperative care. *JAMA* **286**(2): 208–216.

45. Tasmuth T, von Smitten K, Kalso E. (1996) Pain and other symptoms during the first year after radical and conservative surgery for breast cancer. *Br J Cancer* **74**(12): 2024–2031.

46. Tasmuth T, Blomqvist C, Kalso E (1999) Chronic post-treatment symptoms in patients with breast cancer operated in different surgical units. *Eur J Surg Oncol* **25**: 38–43.

47. Stevens P, Dibble S, Miastowski C. (1995) Prevalence, characteristics, and impact of postmastectomy pain syndrome: an investigation of women's experiences. *Pain* **61**: 61–68.

48. Carpenter J, *et al.* (1998) Postmastectomy/postlumpectomy pain in breast cancer survivors. *J Clin Epidemiol* **51**: 1285–1292.

49. Tasmuth T, *et al.* (1995) Pain and other symptoms after different treatment modalities of breast cancer. *Ann Oncol* **6**: 453–459.

50. Bishop SR, Warr D. (2003) Coping, catastrophizing and chronic pain in breast cancer. *J Behav Med* **26**(3): 265–281.

51. Tasmuth T, Hartel B, Kalso E. (2002) Venlafaxine in neuropathic pain following treatment of breast cancer. *Eur J Pain* **6**(1): 17–24.

52. Farrar WB, Fanning WJ. (1988) Eliminating the dog-ear in modified radical mastectomy. *Am J Surg* **156**(5): 401–402.

53. Chretien-Marquet B, Bennaceur S. (1997) Dog ear: true and false. A simple surgical management. *Dermatol Surg* **23**(7): 547–551.

54. Mirza M, Sinha KS, Fortes-Mayer K. (2003) Tear-drop incision for mastectomy to avoid dog-ear deformity. *Ann R Coll Surg Engl* **85**(2): 131.

55. Meric F, *et al.* (2002) Long-term complications associated with breast-conservation surgery and radiotherapy. *Ann Surg Oncol* **9**(6): 543–549.

56. Fehlauer F, *et al.* (2003) Long-term radiation sequelae after breast-conserving therapy in women with early-stage breast cancer: an observational study using the LENT-SOMA scoring system. *Int J Radiat Oncol Biol Phys* **55**(3): 651–658.

57. No authors listed. (1995) LENT-SOMA scales for all anatomic sites. *Int J Radiat Oncol Biol Phys* **31**: 1049–1091.

58. Zippel D, *et al.* (2003) Delayed breast cellulitis following breast conserving operation. *Eur J Surg Oncol* **29**(4): 327–330.
59. Brewer VH, *et al.* (2000) Risk factor analysis for breast cellulitis complicating breast conservation therapy. *Clin Infect Dis* **31**(3): 654–659.
60. Staren ED, *et al.* (1996) The dilemma of delayed cellulitis after breast conservation therapy. *Arch Surg* **131**(6): 651–654.
61. Rescigno J, *et al.* (1994) Breast cellulitis after conservative surgery and radiotherapy. *Int J Radiat Oncol Biol Phys* **29**(1): 163–168.
62. Miller SR, *et al.* (1998) Delayed cellulitis associated with conservative therapy for breast cancer. *J Surg Oncol* **67**(4): 242–245.
63. Keisch M, *et al.* (2003) Initial clinical experience with the MammoSite breast brachytherapy applicator in women with early-stage breast cancer treated with breast-conserving therapy. *Int J Radiat Oncol Biol Phys* **55**(2): 289–293.
64. Monroe AT, Feigenberg SJ, Mendenhall NP. (2003) Angiosarcoma after breast-conserving therapy. *Cancer* **97**(8): 1832–1840.
65. Edeiken S, *et al.* (1992) Angiosarcoma after tylectomy and radiation therapy for carcinoma of the breast. *Cancer* **70**(3): 644–647.
66. Feigenberg SJ, *et al.* (2002) Angiosarcoma after breast-conserving therapy: experience with hyperfractionated radiotherapy. *Int J Radiat Oncol Biol Phys* **52**(3): 620–626.
67. Fisher B, *et al.* (1997) Effect of preoperative chemotherapy on local-regional disease in women with operable breast cancer: findings from National Surgical Adjuvant Breast and Bowel Project B-18. *J Clin Oncol* **15**(7): 2483–2493.
68. Liberman L, Goodstone S, Dershaw D. (2002) One operation after percutaneous diagnosis of nonpalpable breast cancer: frequency and associated factors. *Am J Roentgenol* **178**: 673–679.
69. Newman L. (2004) Surgical management of high-risk breast lesions. In *Problems in General Surgery, Benign Breast Disease*. Lippincott, Williams, Inc., Philadelphia, 2003, Vol. 20, No. 4, pp. 99–112.
70. Petrasek AJ, Semple JL, McCready DR. (1997) The surgical and oncologic significance of the axillary arch during axillary lymphadenectomy. *Can J Surg* **40**(1): 44–47.
71. Wright FC, *et al.* (2003) Outcomes after localized axillary node recurrence in breast cancer. *Ann Surg Oncol* **10**(9): 1054–1058.
72. Erickson VS, *et al.* (2001) Arm edema in breast cancer patients. *J Natl Cancer Inst* **93**(2): 96–111.
73. Beaulac SM, *et al.* (2002) Lymphedema and quality of life in survivors of early-stage breast cancer. *Arch Surg* **137**(11): 1253–1257.

74. Sener SF, *et al.* (2001) Lymphedema after sentinel lymphadenectomy for breast carcinoma. *Cancer* **92**(4): 748–752.

75. Roses DF, *et al.* (1999) Complications of level I and II axillary dissection in the treatment of carcinoma of the breast. *Ann Surg* **230**(2): 194–201.

76. Grobmyer SR, *et al.* (2000) Role of surgery in the management of postmastectomy extremity angiosarcoma (Stewart-Treves syndrome). *J Surg Oncol* **73**(3): 182–188.

77. Janse AJ, *et al.* (1995) Lymphedema-induced lymphangiosarcoma. *Eur J Surg Oncol* **21**(2): 155–158.

78. Stewart FW, Treves N. (1981) Classics in oncology: lymphangiosarcoma in post-mastectomy lymphedema: a report of six cases in elephantiasis chirurgica. *CA Cancer J Clin* **31**(5): 284–299.

79. Moskovitz AH, *et al.* (2001) Axillary web syndrome after axillary dissection. *Am J Surg* **181**(5): 434–439.

80. Caluwe GL, Christiaens MR. (2003) Chylous leak: a rare complication after axillary lymph node dissection. *Acta Chir Belg* **103**(2): 217–218.

81. Carcoforo P, *et al.* (2003) Octreotide in the treatment of lymphorrhea after axillary node dissection: a prospective randomized controlled trial. *J Am Coll Surg* **196**(3): 365–369.

82. Krag DN, *et al.* (1993) Surgical resection and radiolocalization of the sentinel lymph node in breast cancer using a gamma probe. *Surg Oncol* **2**(6): 335–340.

83. Giuliano AE, *et al.* (1994) Lymphatic mapping and sentinel lymphadenectomy for breast cancer. *Ann Surg* **220**(3): 391–401.

84. Kim T, Agboola O, Lyman G. (2002) Lymphatic mapping and sentinel lymph node sampling in breast cancer. In: *Proceedings of the American Society of Clinical Oncology 2002 Annual Symposium*. American Society of Clinical Oncology, Orlando, Florida.

85. Cox CE, *et al.* (1999) Implementation of new surgical technology: outcome measures for lymphatic mapping of breast carcinoma. *Ann Surg Oncol* **6**(6): 553–561.

86. Derossis AM, *et al.* (2001) A trend analysis of the relative value of blue dye and isotope localization in 2,000 consecutive cases of sentinel node biopsy for breast cancer. *J Am Coll Surg* **193**(5): 473–478.

87. Haigh PI, *et al.* (2000) Biopsy method and excision volume do not affect success rate of subsequent sentinel lymph node dissection in breast cancer. *Ann Surg Oncol* **7**(1): 21–27.

88. Wong SL, *et al.* (2002) The effect of prior breast biopsy method and concurrent definitive breast procedure on success and accuracy of sentinel lymph node biopsy. *Ann Surg Oncol* **9**(3): 272–277.

89. Linehan DC, *et al.* (1999) Intradermal radiocolloid and intraparenchymal blue dye injection optimize sentinel node identification in breast cancer patients. *Ann Surg Oncol* **6**(5): 450–454.

90. Chao C, *et al.* (2001) Reliable lymphatic drainage to axillary sentinel lymph nodes regardless of tumor location within the breast. *Am J Surg* **182**(4): 307–311.

91. Veronesi U, *et al.* (1997) Sentinel-node biopsy to avoid axillary dissection in breast cancer with clinically negative lymph-nodes. *Lancet* **349**(9069): 1864–1867.

92. Veronesi U, *et al.* (1999) Sentinel lymph node biopsy and axillary dissection in breast cancer: results in a large series. *J Natl Cancer Inst* **91**(4): 368–373.

93. Bedrosian I, *et al.* (2000) Accuracy of sentinel lymph node biopsy in patients with large primary tumors. *Cancer* **88**: 2540–2545.

94. Chung MH, Ye W, Giuliano AE. (2001) Role for sentinel lymph node dissection in the management of large (> or = 5 cm) invasive breast cancer. *Ann Surg Oncol* **8**(9): 688–692.

95. Grube BJ, Hansen NM, Ye X, Giuliano AE. (2002) Tumor characteristics predictive of sentinel node metastases in 105 consecutive patients with invasive lobular carcinoma. *Am J Surg* **184**(4): 372–376.

96. Klimberg VS, *et al.* (1999) Subareolar versus peritumoral injection for location of the sentinel lymph node. *Ann Surg* **229**(6): 860–865.

97. Bauer TW, *et al.* (2002) Subareolar and peritumoral injection identify similar sentinel nodes for breast cancer. *Ann Surg Oncol* **9**(2): 169–176.

98. Kern KA. (2001) Breast lymphatic mapping using subareolar injections of blue dye and radiocolloid: illustrated technique. *J Am Coll Surg* **192**(4): 545–550.

99. Jin Kim H, *et al.* (2002) Sentinel lymph node drainage in multicentric breast cancers. *Breast J* **8**(6): 356–361.

100. Kumar R, *et al.* (2003) Retrospective analysis of sentinel node localization in multifocal, multicentric, palpable, or nonpalpable breast cancer. *J Nucl Med* **44**: 7–10.

101. Tousimis E, *et al.* (2003) The accuracy of sentinel lymph node biopsy in multicentric and multifocal invasive breast cancers. *J Am Coll Surg* **197**: 529–535.

102. Zavagno G, *et al.* (2002) Subareolar injection for sentinel lymph node location in breast cancer. *Eur J Surg Oncol* **28**: 701–704.

103. Schrenk P, Wayand W. (2001) Sentinel node biopsy in axillary lymph node staging for patients with multicentric breast cancer. *Lancet* **357**: 122.

104. Leidenius M, *et al.* (2003) Motion restriction and axillary web syndrome after sentinel node biopsy and axillary clearance in breast cancer. *Am J Surg* **185**(2): 127–130.

105. Laurie SA, *et al.* (2002) Anaphylaxis to isosulfan blue. *Ann Allergy Asthma Immunol* **88**(1): 64–66.

106. Efron P, *et al.* (2002) Anaphylactic reaction to isosulfan blue used for sentinel node biopsy: case report and literature review. *Breast J* **8**(6): 396–399.

107. Sadiq TS, *et al.* (2001) Blue urticaria: a previously unreported adverse event associated with isosulfan blue. *Arch Surg* **136**(12): 1433–1435.

108. Cimmino VM, *et al.* (2001) Allergic reactions to isosulfan blue during sentinel node biopsy — A common event. *Surgery* **130**(3): 439–442.

109. Raut CP, *et al.* (2004) Anaphylactoid reactions to isosulfan blue dye during breast cancer lymphatic mapping in patients given preoperative prophylaxis. *J Clin Oncol* **22**(3): 567–568.

110. Mostafa A, Carpenter R. (2001) Anaphylaxis to patent blue dye during sentinel lymph node biopsy for breast cancer. *Eur J Surg Oncol* **27**: 610.

111. Newman LA, *et al.* (1998) Presentation, treatment, and outcome of local recurrence afterskin-sparing mastectomy and immediate breast reconstruction. *Ann Surg Oncol* **5**(7): 620–626.

112. Medina-Franco H, *et al.* (2002) Factors associated with local recurrence after skin-sparing mastectomy and immediate breast reconstruction for invasive breast cancer. *Ann Surg* **235**(6): 814–819.

113. Rivadeneira DE, *et al.* (2000) Skin-sparing mastectomy with immediate breast reconstruction: a critical analysis of local recurrence. *Cancer J* **6**(5): 331–335.

114. Newman LA, *et al.* (1999) Feasibility of immediate breast reconstruction for locally advanced breast cancer. *Ann Surg Oncol* **6**(7): 671–675.

115. Hunt KK, *et al.* (1997) Feasibility of postmastectomy radiation therapy after TRAM flap breast reconstruction. *Ann Surg Oncol* **4**(5): 377–384.

116. Tran NV, *et al.* (2000) Postoperative adjuvant irradiation: effects on tranverse rectus abdominis muscle flap breast reconstruction. *Plast Reconstr Surg* **106**(2): 313–320.

117. Broadwater JR, *et al.* (1991) Mastectomy following preoperative chemotherapy. Strict operative criteria control morbidity. *Ann Surg* **213**(2): 126–129.

118. Newman LA, *et al.* (2002) A prospective trial of preoperative chemotherapy in resectable breast cancer: predictors of breast-conservation therapy feasibility. *Ann Surg Oncol* **9**(3): 228–234.

119. Canavese G, Gipponi M, Catturich A, Di Somma C, Vecchio C, Rosato F, Percivale P, Moresco L, Nicolo G, Spina B, Villa G, Bianchi P, Badellino F. (2000) Sentinel lymph node mapping in early-stage breast cancer: technical issues and results with vital blue dye mapping and radioguided surgery. *J Surg Oncol* **74**(1): 61–68.

120. Albertini JJ, *et al.* (1996) Lymphatic mapping and sentinel node biopsy in the patient with breast cancer. *JAMA* **276**(22): 1818–1822.
121. McMasters KM, *et al.* (2000) Sentinel lymph node biopsy for breast cancer: a suitable alternative to routine axillary dissection in multi-institutional practice when optimal technique is used. *J Clin Oncol* **18**(13): 2560–2566.
122. Cox CE, *et al.* (1998) Guidelines for sentinel node biopsy and lymphatic mapping of patients with breast cancer. *Ann Surg* **227**(5): 645–653.
123. Krag D, *et al.* (1998) The sentinel node in breast cancer — A multicenter validation study. *N Engl J Med* **339**(14): 941–946.
124. O'Hea BJ, *et al.* (1998) Sentinel lymph node biopsy in breast cancer: initial experience at Memorial Sloan-Kettering Cancer Center. *J Am Coll Surg* **186**(4): 423–427.
125. Guenther JM. (1999) Axillary dissection after unsuccessful sentinel lymphadenectomy for breast cancer. *Am Surg* **65**(10): 991–994.
126. Lyew MA, Gamblin TC, Ayoub M. (2000) Systemic anaphylaxis associated with intramammary isosulfan blue injection used for sentinel node detection under general anesthesia. *Anesthesiology* **93**(4): 1145–1146.
127. Mullon. (2001) Anaphylaxis to patent blue dye during sentinel lymph node biopsy for breast cancer. *Eur J Surg Oncol* **27**: 218–219.
128. Albo D, *et al.* (2001) Anaphylactic reactions to isosulfan blue dye during sentinel lymph node biopsy for breast cancer. *Am J Surg* **182**(4): 393–398.
129. Montgomery LL, *et al.* (2002) Isosulfan blue dye reactions during sentinel lymph node mapping for breast cancer. *Anesth Analg* **95**(2): 385–388.
130. Stefanutto TB, Shapiro WA, Wright PM. (2002) Anaphylactic reaction to isosulphan blue. *Br J Anaesth* **89**(3): 527–528.
131. Crivellaro M, *et al.* (2003) Anaphylaxis due to patent blue dye during lymphography, with negative skin prick test. *J Investig Allergol Clin Immunol* **13**(1): 71–72.
132. Sprung J, Tully MJ, Ziser A. (2003) Anaphylactic reactions to isosulfan blue dye during sentinel node lymphadenectomy for breast cancer. *Anesth Analg* **96**(4): 1051–1053.
133. Breslin TM, *et al.* (2000) Sentinel lymph node biopsy is accurate after neoadjuvant chemotherapy for breast cancer. *J Clin Oncol* **18**(20): 3480–3486.
134. Nason KS, *et al.* (2000) Increased false negative sentinel node biopsy rates after preoperative chemotherapy for invasive breast carcinoma. *Cancer* **89**(11): 2187–2194.
135. Haid A, *et al.* (2001) Is sentinel lymph node biopsy reliable and indicated after preoperative chemotherapy in patients with breast carcinoma? *Cancer* **92**(5): 1080–1084.

136. Fernandez A, *et al.* (2001) Gamma probe sentinel node localization and biopsy in breast cancer patients treated with a neoadjuvant chemotherapy scheme. *Nucl Med Commun* **22**(4): 361–366.

137. Tafra L, Verbanac KM, Lannin DR. (2001) Preoperative chemotherapy and sentinel lymphadenectomy for breast cancer. *Am J Surg* **182**(4): 312–315.

138. Stearns V, *et al.* (2002) Sentinel lymphadenectomy after neoadjuvant chemotherapy for breast cancer may reliably represent the axilla except for inflammatory breast cancer. *Ann Surg Oncol* **9**(3): 235–242.

139. Julian TB, Dusi D, Wolmark N. (2002) Sentinel node biopsy after neoadjuvant chemotherapy for breast cancer. *Am J Surg* **184**(4): 315–317.

140. Miller AR, *et al.* (2002) Analysis of sentinel lymph node mapping with immediate pathologic review in patients receiving preoperative chemotherapy for breast carcinoma. *Ann Surg Oncol* **9**(3): 243–247.

141. Brady EW. (2002) Sentinel lymph node mapping following neoadjuvant chemotherapy for breast cancer. *Breast J* **8**(2): 97–100.

142. Piato JR, *et al.* (2003) Sentinel lymph node biopsy in breast cancer after neoadjuvant chemotherapy. A pilot study. *Eur J Surg Oncol* **29**(2): 118–120.

143. Balch GC, *et al.* (2003) Lymphatic mapping and sentinel lymphadenectomy after preoperative therapy for stage II and III breast cancer. *Ann Surg Oncol* **10**(6): 616–621.

144. Schwartz GF, Meltzer AJ. (2003) Accuracy of axillary sentinel lymph node biopsy following neoadjuvant (induction) chemotherapy for carcinoma of the breast. *Breast J* **9**(5): 374–379.

145. Reitsamer R, *et al.* (2003) Sentinel lymph node biopsy in breast cancer patients after neoadjuvant chemotherapy. *J Surg Oncol* **84**(2): 63–67.

146. Mamounas E, *et al.* (2002) Accuracy of sentinel lymph node biopsy after neoadjuvant chemotherapy in breast cancer: updated results from NSABP B-27 (abstract #140). in American Society of Clinical Oncology 38th annual meeting, Orlando FL.

Chapter 7

COMPLICATIONS OF HEAD AND NECK SURGERY

Patrick J. Bradley and Antony A. Narula

INTRODUCTION

Head and neck surgery involves the investigation, diagnosis, and surgical treatment of congenital, inflammatory, infective and neoplastic conditions and processes that affect the anatomical area between the clavicle and the cranium. In this chapter surgery specific to the ear and the nose/paranasal sinuses has been excluded.

COMPLICATIONS AND SEQUELAE

The spectrum of surgery in the head and neck, especially for neoplasms, ranges from simple excision with secondary healing to complex resections combined with equally complex reconstructive techniques. As a result of these surgical interventions complications and sequelae will occur; however, they do not always imply negligence.

Sequelae are defined as a logical consequence of a particular procedure, whereas a complication constitutes an unexpected untoward event. The complication is the bane of good surgery while sequelae are the result of it. We can strive to eliminate complications, and sequelae can be reduced or improved by modifying the therapy, using new and less destructive surgical approaches or even non-surgical substitutes. In today's medico-legal climate, surgical patients must be informed of possible complications and sequelae.[1] Many factors, such as poor nutritional health, prior irradiation, extensive ablation and complex reconstruction may predispose to a higher incidence of surgical complications even in the hands of the most experienced surgeon. It also stands to reason that the incidence of complications will be less in a more experienced surgeon's hands.

Avoiding complications is largely dependent on a thorough knowledge of the physiology and patho-physiology of health and disease, surgical anatomy, the common complications, and a humble appraisal of one's ability to help a patient in a particular circumstance.

CLASSIFICATION OF HEAD AND NECK SURGERY

A classification of head and neck surgery is useful in discussing the likelihood of complications with colleagues and patients.

Type I "Simple" excision	a) External (skin or deeper structures) with primary or secondary healing
	b) Internal excision (mucosal) with primary or secondary healing
Type II "Intermediate" Excision	a) Excision of skin with the need for a local flap of skin to close defect
	b) Excision with the need to replace mucosal defect with a local flap
Type III "Complex"	a) Excision of a "tumour" or "viscus" employing a through approach
	b) Excision of the skin through mucus membrane, with primary closure of both defects

Type IV "Complex Major"   a) Excision of a "tumour" or "viscus" with
loss of covering surfaces that requires
additional tissue, from elsewhere to
be brought in to close the surgical defect

USE OF FLAPS

The use of regional, myocutaneous flaps and free tissue transfers has been one of the most significant advances in the last three decades, in the rehabilitation of extensive wounds in head and neck surgery.[2,3] It permits the immediate resurfacing of extensive skin and mucous membrane defects, protects the carotid artery system, facilitates the restoration of physiology, and provides the foundation for future reconstructive techniques. The introduction of flap surgery allowed for immediate single stage ablation and reconstruction to be performed. Because of the time and expertise required, it has developed as a specialisation within the discipline of head and neck surgery.

INDICATION FOR ANTIBIOTICS

The use of antibiotics prophylactically is routine in cases where the likelihood and degree of wound contamination can be assessed. Wounds can be classified as clean, clean contaminated, contaminated and dirty, according to the risk and degree of contamination at the time of operation. Clean wounds are usually elective and are type I and II procedures. They do not show contamination from the lumen of the respiratory or alimentary tracts, inflammation or a break in the aseptic technique. These wounds can be closed primarily and drained within the closed system. Clean wounds have an infection rate of 1–5%. Clean contaminated wounds are operations where the oropharyngeal, respiratory and alimentary tracts are entered under controlled conditions, type III and IV procedures. The infection rate documented is 8–11%, but may go up 25–80% in complex procedures requiring extensive reconstruction.[4]

   Dirty wounds are those in which the organisms causing the postoperative infection are present prior to the operation. They carry an infection rate of more than 25%. Host and local wound factors play an important role in determining the risk of infection in addition to the degree of contamination.

Perioperative chemoprophylaxis is used when there is a definite risk of infection. However, their use in clean head and neck wounds is not supported. In dirty or traumatic wounds, antibiotics are considered therapeutic rather than prophylactic.[5]

It has been shown that the use of perioperative prophylactic antibiotics is essential during major head and neck surgery when the wound is contaminated by saliva. The duration of the prophylaxis is not important, and a short course (24 hrs) is as effective as prolonged prophylaxis (two to seven days). The preferred antibiotic has not been identified, but should be based on the type of pathogens; the pathogens cultured from wound infections represent those found in the oral cavity and oropharynx. Infection can result from perioperative contamination via the mucosal incision and, more significantly from a persistent postoperative leakage of saliva. The majority of infections are polymicrobial in nature, consisting primarily of anaerobes and some aerobic Gram-positive cocci. Gram-negative organisms appear to colonise the infected wounds but are usually not the causative organisms.[6]

Potential risk factors for postoperative wound infections are related to tumour size and stage of disease, closure using flaps, nutritional status and alcohol consumption, duration of surgical procedure, intraoperative risk such as poor surgical technique, classification of the procedure and antibiotic use. The incidence of postoperative infections is not statistically significant among patients receiving preoperative radiation therapy despite the severity of the infections.[7]

SPECIFIC PROCEDURES

1) Complications of Endoscopy

Technique

A meticulous, gentle technique is the key to avoiding complications during endoscopy, beginning with proper patient preparation. Because most of the instruments used are rigid metallic objects, pressure trauma is a potential problem. Eyelids must be taped closed, with lubrication applied to prevent corneal abrasions.

Dental injury is a common complication.[8] All patients must have their dentition examined carefully and a written documentation of loose, carious or capped teeth must be recorded prior to consenting to the procedure. A tooth guard must be used if dentition is present. In children or edentulous adults, a gauze sponge can be used, and the teeth should never be used as a fulcrum. This is the most common problem with the central incisors. At the end of the procedure, if a tooth is missing, an extensive search must be made to find it, including an X-ray of the chest and neck. It should never be assumed that the tooth was swallowed.

The endoscopist needs to exercise gentle care during patient positioning. A rapid, forceful extension of the cervical spine in elderly patients or those with degenerative disease may result in atlanto-axial instability resulting in neurological deficits. Children with Down's syndrome are at special risk of atlanto-axial subluxation. A radiologic evaluation and clinical consultation prior to the operation may minimise the patient's postoperative discomfort.

2) Transoral Examination and Biopsy

The examination of the oral cavity and oropharynx is most commonly undertaken in the clinic without the need for anaesthetic. Most patients are tolerant of the process and allow biopsy procedures to be performed using local anaesthetic. When other conditions are present, such as leucoplakia, asymmetrical tonsils, ulceration of unknown origin, symptoms such as pain whose cause cannot be determined, an examination under general anaesthetic may be required. The key to successful transoral surgery requiring resection is adequate exposure, usually necessitating the use of mouth gags, cheek retractors and tongue depressors. An excision may be accomplished using a scalpel, electrocautery, or laser. Following resection the defect may be allowed to heal by secondary intention, be closed primarily, or be skin grafted.

Complications may occur from the exposure, resection or repair.

1) Exposure

Exposure of the anterior oral cavity is usually accomplished easily, but there can be a problem in accessing the posterior oral cavity and oropharynx. Although a variety of gags are available, the most commonly used is the Jennings gag, which enable the mouth to be stented open while the tongue is depressed by the Crowe-Davis gag giving better access to the roof, the palate and the lateral oropharyngeal areas, or allows for the use of a traction tongue stitch and cheek retractors to facilitate surgery on the tongue and floor of mouth. The most common complication is contusion or possible laceration of the posterior pharyngeal wall due to rough or blind insertion of the gag without adequately visualising the tip of the tongue blade, or slippage of the gag from the teeth resulting in chipping or even broken teeth. This can be minimised or avoided by having the patient adequately anaesthetised, selecting the correct and appropriate length of blade and inserting the blade under direct vision with ample lighting. Another complication from the gag is prolonged pressure on the tongue during a long procedure. This may affect the lingual nerve, resulting in aberration in taste and tongue sensation, which may persist for weeks or even months after the procedure.[9]

2) Resection

Haemorrhage occurs to some degree with any resection but is usually easily manageable. Although haemorrhage is associated with intraoral resection, the posterior tongue is more at risk because of the extensive vasculature. Excessive uncontrolled haemorrhage may present either at the time of surgery, in the immediate postoperative period, or after 7–10 days (secondary haemorrhage). If significant bleeding is encountered intraoperatively, cautery and/or ligation of the offending vessel is usually possible. However, if the bleeding site cannot be identified because of retraction of the vessel, "blind" clamping or cautery should be avoided, and instead, a deep judiciously placed suture ligature should be used. A similar approach works for postoperative or secondary haemorrhage. If the bleeding cannot be controlled, angiography with embolization or open exploration of the neck and ligation of the relevant external carotid artery branches may be necessary.

Damage to the lingual or hypoglossal nerves may occur if "blind" surgery is performed. Inadvertent damage to the submandibular ducts may result in stenosis with resultant submandibular sialadenitis. This can be avoided by dissecting the submandibular ducts, marsupialisating the openings and relocating the ducts to the wound edges. An alternative is to use a CO_2 laser while transecting the ducts, resulting in a low incidence of duct stenosis.

Alteration to the oropharyngeal function from defects of the soft palate, will result in velopharyngeal incompetence with hypernasal speech and possible reflux of food and liquids through the nose. The corrective mechanism may include the use of an obturator or local or regional flaps.

3) Repair

Most small defects that develop can be allowed to heal by secondary intention with no sequelae or complications. However, if the underlying musculature is damaged, the resultant scarring can cause distortion of the anatomy and may affect its function (e.g. velopharyngeal incompetence, secondary Eustachian tube dysfunction, dysphagia and dysarthria). Rarely, nasopharyngeal stenosis may result if a circumferential dissection has been performed. To overcome some of these problems, a skin graft may be placed and stabilised by a bolster or "quilted" into place.

4) Direct Laryngoscopy

Direct laryngoscopy may be performed for diagnostic or therapeutic purposes. There are many different types of rigid laryngoscopes. The endoscopist should use a laryngoscope that gives the largest field of vision, but is small enough to pass through the oral cavity. If the scope is too large or inappropriate, it may cause oral or pharyngeal oedema and dental trauma.

The larynx is extremely sensitive to stimulation. Cardiac arrhythmias are a well-known risk, especially in hypoxic patients. Two techniques can reduce this complication — spraying the larynx with lignocaine prior to instrumentation, and avoiding hypoxia during the procedure. Surgical procedures on the vocal cords should usually be performed using a microscope, because magnification reduces the likelihood of injury to normal tissue. Certain anatomical areas, such as the anterior and posterior commissure should not be violated during biopsy; disruption of the anterior commissure will result in web formation and alteration of voice.

5) Oesophagoscopy

The proper technique for rigid oesophogoscopy begins with the positioning of the patient. Most commonly, a shoulder roll is used to extend the neck, thereby placing the oesophagus in a slightly direct line. Over manipulation of the cervical spine must be avoided. The use of a flexible oesophagoscopy may be considered an alternate procedure in such circumstances. The risk of perforation is less than 1% for both flexible and rigid oesophogoscopy.

There are two procedures that deserve special attention, oesophogeal dilatation and foreign body removal. Dilatation should not be performed without viewing the structured area endoscopically, as radiographs alone are insufficient. A useful rule for passing the bougies is to end the dilatation after three consecutive sizes have been passed or when blood is first seen on the bougie.

The endoscopic removal of pointed foreign bodies is especially associated with an increased risk of complication.[10] The use of the point sheath technique is advocated, where the pointed foreign body is brought into the lumen of the scope and withdrawn together. After the oesophageal foreign bodies are removed, an immediate evaluation of the area is "not recommended, especially if the foreign bodies were present for some time." This is because the granulation tissue may be hiding a severely damaged portion of the wall leading to a higher risk of perforation.

The risk of oesophageal perforation is primarily related to the extent of the lesion for which the oesophogoscopy is indicated. This is especially true for sharp foreign bodies, oesophageal malignancy and severe caustic ingestion. Other predisposing factors include cervical spinal disease, craniofacial anomalies that can affect the mandible, and being unaware of the presence of a pharyngeal pouch.

Cervical oesophageal perforations usually occur in the posterior wall or through the piriform fossae. Contamination begins in the retropharyngeal or pretracheal space and can spread to the mediastinum. Thoracic oesophageal perforations spread directly into the pleural space and/or the mediastinum.

The clinical manifestations of oesophageal perforations vary with the site and the size of the tear.[11] Patients with cervical perforations complain of neck pain and swelling, usually associated with surgical crepitus. Fever and an elevated WBC follow within hours; thoracic perforations cause severe chest pain, dysphagia and dyspnoea, and physical and radiographic signs of pneumothorax may be present. Morbidity and mortality due to mediastinitis remains high despite aggressive medical and surgical therapy. The physical signs of mediastinal involvement include asymmetrical chest movement during respiration and an audible rub due to pericardial effusion. Hypotension develops early and responds poorly to intravenous fluid hydration.

The plain radiographs of the chest and neck will show free air in the peri-oesophageal soft tissue. The site and extent of the perforation can be demonstrated with a contrast oesophagram using a water-soluble dye such as gastrograffin.

With the possible exception of a small cervical perforation, all patients should undergo surgical exploration with repair and drainage of the injury. Cervical injuries warrant a lateral cervical approach to the retropharyngeal space. The tear should be repaired in two layers and the site must be drained. Thoracic perforations are usually approached through a left thoracotomy. Severe thoracic lesions require a diverting pharyngostomy and a feeding gastrostomy. Postoperatively, all patients require intravenous fluids and antibiotics. Oral feeding can commence once the contrast oesophagram has documented the closure of the perforation without leakage.

6) Bronchoscopy

An inspection of the tracheobronchial passages may be indicated for diagnostic or therapeutic reasons, and rigid or flexible bronchoscopies are available for the procedure. Flexible bronchoscopy is most commonly used in adults, usually as an outpatient procedure, and is associated with a major complication rate of 0.08%. In contrast, rigid bronchoscopy under a general anaesthetic is mostly indicated for removal of foreign bodies, paediatric endoscopy and intraoperative evaluation.

Before passing a bronchoscope, the larynx should be sprayed with lignocaine to minimise the chance of laryngospasm. The bronchoscope can be safely positioned into the trachea by using a Negus laryngoscope or a Mackintosh for a child. Gentle manipulation is most important because this is both the anatomic and temporal point in rigid bronchoscopy where most of the tissue oedema is created. Biopsies are frequently performed during bronchoscopy. Bleeding usually ceases within a few minutes, although occasionally tamponade may be necessary, which is easier when a rigid scope is used. Pneumothorax is also a risk after transbronchial lung biopsy, and a post-biopsy chest X-ray is indicated.

Following fiberoptic bronchoscopy, fever occurs in 10–25% of the patients, sometimes due to bacteraemia, or involving the transfer of toxins to the intravenous space. While bacteraemia is more common after bronchoalveolar lavage, cardiac arrhythmias have been reported in 40% of the patients undergoing bronchoscopy. The use of topical lignocaine during flexible bronchoscopy appears to have a protective effect.

Poor technique can contribute to postoperative oedema, and is a major risk in the glottic/subglottic area in children. It can be minimised by using the correct bronchoscope. Modern bronchoscopes with optical forceps are mandatory for removal of foreign bodies these days.

Foreign body removal during bronchoscopy presents the greatest risk of any airway procedure creating an uncontrolled airway. Suction or the use of long forceps is recommended to grasp objects lodged in the bronchus. The preferred anaesthetic during foreign body removal is general anaesthesia. Should the foreign body move into the trachea, it is wise to push it back into one of the bronchi rather than risk losing control of the airway. A finite amount of time should be allocated to the removal of a foreign body from a tracheobronchial tree. Considerable oedema can result from extensive instrumentation, and it is often wiser to return to the endoscopy after a course of steroids and antibiotics.

Complications of Laser Surgery

As laser technology advances, its use in surgery of the head and neck continues to expand. Many lasers have been described, including the argon, carbon dioxide, neodymium: yttrium-aluminium-garnet (Nd:YAG), potassium titanyl phosphate (KTP), dye (argon and flash lamp-pumped) and holmium-Yag (Ho:YAG), to treat lesions in the oral cavity, pharynx, larynx, oesophagus tracheobronchial tree, and skull base. The potential clinical application of each of these surgical lasers are determined by their wavelength, the output pulse length, and the specific tissue absorption characteristics.

Lasers are precise but potentially dangerous surgical instruments that must be used with extreme caution. There is no question that certain, distinct advantages are associated with their use in the management of selected benign and malignant diseases of the head and neck. However, these advantages must be balanced against the possible risks of complications. The surgeon must first decide whether the use of laser offers any advantage over conventional surgical techniques. Laser education and training is a prerequisite to use this technology, not only for the surgeon, but the anaesthetist and other theatre staff. The correct choice of anaesthetic techniques, protection of the endotracheal tube during surgery, and the selection of the proper instruments are critical for successful laser therapy.

The eyes and facial skin require protection and a double layer of saline-moistened eye pads and surgical sponges and towels are recommended to protect all the exposed skin and mucus membranes of the patient outside the surgical field. All laser cases should be equipped with two separate suction set-ups, one for smoke and steam evacuation from the operative field, and another connected to the surgical suction tip for the aspiration of blood and mucus from the operative wound. Constant suction is required to remove laser-induced smoke from the operating field when performing surgery with a closed anaesthetic system. However, when working with an open anaesthetic or with a jet ventilation system, suction should be limited to an intermittent basis to maintain the forced inspiratory oxygen (FiO_2) at a safe level. Risk factors include airborne particulate debris from CO_2 ablation of lesions and possible dispersal of the human papillomavirus DNA onto adjacent normal local tissue or to the operator. Anaesthetic risks include the possibility of fire, the inspired concentration of oxygen, a potent oxidising gas, as well as the risk of ignition to the endotracheal tube.

Inadvertent CO_2 laser beam irradiated on the tissue of the perioperative field can lead to excessive local scarring; on the anterior commissure it can result in an acquired glottic web.

Complications of Tracheostomy

Tracheostomy represents the surgical introduction of an artificial airway into the trachea to direct the path of airflow from the upper airway structures. Complications from tracheostomy frequently result from improper execution of the procedure or inadequate postoperative care.[12] Most retrospective studies have addressed the incidence of overall complications, ranging from 5–40%, the most common being haemorrhage, tube obstruction or tube displacement. Pneumothorax, atelectasis, aspiration, tracheal stenosis and tracheooesophageal fistula occur with less than 1% frequency each. Death occurs in 0.5–1.6% of cases and is often caused by haemorrhage or inadvertent tube displacement. An emergency tracheostomy carries an additional two- to five-fold increase in the incidence of complications over an elective procedure. The seriousness and frequency of tracheostomy-associated morbidity and mortality compare with those of major abdominal procedures, and in this respect tracheostomy must be considered a major operation.

Surgical Technique

Adequate preparation and meticulous attention to detail are imperative for safe and successful tracheostomy. In an emergency a cricothyrotomy may be performed. The surgeon must have adequate lighting and suction equipment. In addition to preoperatively securing an airway and ensuring ventilation, endotracheal intubation provides a recognisable target for the surgeon and helps protect the posterior tracheal wall and oesophagus from inadvertent injury. The patient must be supine with the shoulders on a roll, the neck extended and the occiput supported. This position brings the cricoid cartilage antero-superiorly, aiding in its identification while drawing the trachea out of the mediastinum. Neck extension may be compromised in the trauma patient when a cervical spin injury is suspected and not excluded radiologically.

When the situation demands it, a midline vertical skin incision is recommended, beginning at the lower border of the cricoid cartilage, and extended approximately 2–3 cm inferiorly. This avoids the transection of many vertical orientated subcutaneous vessels and more importantly, allows for the tracheostomy tube to glide unimpeded in the vertical plane as it ascends and descends during swallowing. Straying off the midline can lead to transection of vessels, the oesophagus, or recurrent laryngeal nerves. A tracheostomy placed too high, through the first tracheal ring or even the cricoid cartilage, can lead to injury to the cricoid or other cartilage structures, causing late stenosis. If placed too low, the tracheostomy may cause right main stem bronchial intubation, laceration, or later erosion of the innominate artery or entry into the apical pleura.

The thyroid isthmus, located at the second and third tracheal rings, is mobilised by bluntly inserting a haemostat from above and lifting it off the anterior tracheal wall; it is then clamped on each side, divided, and its edges suture-ligated. A failure to divide the thyroid isthmus invites its erosion, bleeding, or tube displacement when the patient is taken out of the neck extension. The pre-tracheal fascia is lifted and divided, exposing the anterior tracheal wall. Any dissection required below the isthmus should be done bluntly or with a scalpel blade pointed superiorly to minimise injury to the vascular structures of the mediastinum.

The use of a hook to elevate the cricoid and deliver a low-lying trachea aids tracheotomy, and ensures the safe placement of the tracheal tube into the trachea. In adults, a small circular window of cartilage is removed from the second and third tracheal rings using a scalpel or heavy scissors while the segment to be removed is grasped firmly with a clamp. Sometimes, in the presence of calcified cartilage rings, a vertical midline incision is made from the lower edge of the window and the fourth and sixth tracheal rings are split. This procedure allows for an atraumatic entry of the tracheal tube into the trachea without excessive pressure, reduces the risk of in-fracture of the cartilage window or the lower tracheal rings, formation of tracheal granulations, and prevents or delays subsequent decannulation.

When the tracheostomy tube has been placed, the incision must be left open lest expired air becomes trapped and forced into the exposed fascial planes, causing expanding subcutaneous or mediastinal emphysema. A post-tracheostomy chest X-ray may help, when there is anxiety about the patients breathing following surgery, as it may reveal the possibility of undetected subcutaneous emphysema, pneumomediastinum, or pneumothorax.

Early Complications

Minor bleeding or oozing is not uncommon and is usually venous involving the anterior jugular vein or thyroid isthmus, and occurs near the stoma. Reducing the venous pressure by raising the patient into the semirecumbant position and applying haemostatic gauze is usually adequate management. Major haemorrhage is more unusual, and often involves thyroid arteries, especially if the surgeon has not maintained a midline surgical approach. In this case, immediate surgical re-exploration and ligation of the injured vessel is warranted. This exploration is made easier if the patient can be intubated orotracheally and the tracheostomy tube can be removed.

Late Complications

Occasionally, a massive haemorrhage may indicate bleeding from the innominate artery. This may be caused by erosion of the vessel at the distal end of the tracheostomy tube through the anterior tracheal wall (usually 7–10 days), mediastinal infection, intraoperative disruption when the artery is high lying, or if the normal anatomy is distorted or obscured by tumour, previous operation, radiation. In this situation, the airway should first be secured by the insertion of a longer, usually endotracheal tube. Digital pressure is applied against the artery, and the patient is returned to the theatre for ligation of the offending vessel by using a median sternotomy approach.

Death due to tube displacement is reported in 2–5% of the patients. While it can occur any time, it is most common in the immediate postoperative period (especially between the third and fifth day) before a stable tract has matured between the skin and the tracheal lumen. The tube should be secured with sutures for at least 48 hrs to minimise tube displacement.

Tube displacement is frequently caused by the failure to secure the tube adequately to the patient or by excessive traction applied to the tube from dependent ventilatory apparatus. These events are usually signalled by high airway resistance, decreasing oxygen saturation, inability to pass a suction catheter, air trapping, or in the awake-patient, signs of respiratory distress. These signs should prompt an immediate search for a misdirected tube, which should then be replaced under direct vision. Blind reinstatement invites the creation of a false passage in the pretracheal tissue that can further distort the anatomy and lead to subcutaneous emphysema, enormously amplifying the difficulty in re-establishing the airway. Since the diameter of the tracheostomy tube often approximates the size of the opening in the trachea, it may be difficult to insert the tube under direct vision. A tube with a smaller calibre, such as a "red rubber" catheter or even a No. 5 endotracheal tube can be inserted more easily and used as a guide; the tracheostomy tube is then be passed over the guide into the tracheal lumen.

Cardiopulmonary dysfunction or arrest can occur during or soon after tracheostomy. Even a transitory period of oxygen desaturation in a haemo-dynamically unstable patient has the potential to trigger the collapse of vital functions. Increased myocardial irritability, arrhythmia and even cardiac arrest can occur because of a delay in obtaining an adequate airway by an improperly placed or dislodged tube, resulting in hypoxia and acidosis. Pneumothorax or pneumomediastinum can impede cardiac functioning to a critical threshold with the same result. In certain situations, relieving the airway obstruction itself may cause fatal respiratory depression. In a patient suffering from chronic upper respiratory obstruction, tracheostomy can cause a sudden loss of the hypoxic stimulation to which chemoreceptors have acclimated, leading to a loss of the ventilatory drive. Ventilatory assistance may be required temporarily until the chemoreceptors are reset to a lower level of PCO_2. The sudden relief of upper airway obstruction may cause pulmonary oedema. The mechanism is incompletely understood but is thought to involve a rapid change of capillary-alveolar transmural pressure gradients and a catechol-mediated shift in pulmonary blood volume leading to a rapid egress of fluid out of the pulmonary capillary bed. The patient should be maintained on continuous positive airway pressure ventilation and weaned over 24–36 hrs gradually, depending on the arterial blood gas measurements.

Complications of Neck Surgery

Neck surgery is the most common procedure conducted by the head and neck surgeon. Thus, complications from neck surgery occur in every surgeon's practice.[13] The types and severity vary with the procedure involved, patient factors and the clinical judgment and technical expertise of the surgeon. Because radical neck dissection and its modifications encompass the contents of the neck, the complications associated with these procedures will be emphasised here. They are related to a multitude of predisposing factors but proper surgical technique and patient selection are the foremost determinants of a satisfactory outcome. One of the most profound predictors is whether the surgery involves entry into the oral cavity, larynx, or pharynx. Although prophylactic antibiotics have had a dramatic effect on diminishing the incidence of infection, it is unlikely that postoperative infections and wound problems will ever be eliminated. Patient factors, such as smoking and alcohol intake also play a major role in the tolerance of surgical interventions and wound healing. The majority of patients with head and neck neoplasms, especially cancer are chronic smokers and with excessive alcohol intake. These patients also have several co-morbidities such as pulmonary, cardiac, liver and vascular diseases. Many are malnourished because of their lifestyles and because the tumour that has affected their swallowing and mastication abilities. Any history of bleeding disorders must be established because familial bleeding disorders, liver dysfunction, and anticoagulant medication may set the stage for haemorrhage and haematoma. Previous treatment by radiotherapy is associated with higher rates of wound infection, breakdown, haematoma, and fistula formation.

The standard surgical principles cannot be violated without an attendant increase in morbidity and possible mortality. These include use of the natural tissue planes for dissection, gentle tissue manipulation, maintenance of tissue moistness, proper haemostasis, relaxed tissue closure, proper antibiotic prophylaxis, irrigation of contaminated wounds, and appropriate drainage techniques. A careful management of the patient's fluid and nutritional status in the perioperative period is also crucial for a successful surgical outcome. In general, the risk of complications in an isolated neck dissection is low. The incidence of complications increases significantly if the dissection is performed with resection of a primary tumour in the upper aerodigestive tract due to the bacterial contamination and increases further, if this is in a post-radiated patient.

Planning the Neck Surgery

The type of incision to be used in a given procedure should not be arbitrary; the surgeon must be cognisant of the different incisions so that the most advantageous cervical flap can be used. A poorly planned incision may lead to flap ischaemia and possible infection, most notably in the diabetic or irradiated patient, and possible wound dehiscence and carotid artery exposure. The skin incision should be selected such that it provides adequate exposure for the excision and protect the carotid artery. Flaps elevated in the subplatysmal plane enhance skin viability. While cosmesis should be a concern, it is secondary to the issues of oncologic principles, exposure and wound healing. The incisions for a lesser procedure, such as a cervical node biopsy should be given the same degree of careful consideration regarding exposure, appearance, and possible incorporation into a future neck dissection. A more limited exposure with such incisions increases the likelihood of inadvertent nerve and vessel injury.

Where feasible, incisions should be made in skin creases or in the relaxed skin tension lines for both cosmesis and grater wound strength. If separate limbs are needed, they must meet at right angles to avoid ischaemia at the corners and the trifurcation point placed away from the carotid artery, to avoid possible exposure. Vertical limbs should be made in a gentle curve to avoid scar contracture. The use of prophylactic antibiotics has been shown to decrease the incidence of infection dramatically in patients whose oral cavity or pharynx has been entered.

A watertight closure of the oral cavity or pharynx is necessary; in the case of cervical flaps only healthy tissue should be closed without any tension. If the viability of the peripheral skin flap is an issue, a small portion of the edge can be excised. The closure includes the platysma, either incorporated into the dermal closure or as a separate layer. The type and size of suture material used during the procedure are less important than the technique. Because all suture material act as a foreign body to some degree, the fewest number of sutures required should be used. In addition, tissue should be brought only into apposition, not strangulated, because it leads to ischaemia and necrosis, with an increase in the risk of infection and fistula formation.

The appropriate placement and care of suction drains is critical in the care of patients. When used, their intent is to keep the skin flaps coapted with the underlying tissue, eliminating dead space, and reducing the incidence of haematoma and seroma formation. Drains should be inserted via a separate stab incision and placed in dependent portions of the wound to facilitate drainage. Sometimes, an absorbable suture may be used to anchor the drain so that it is not in contact with major vessels or areas of vascular or viscus anastemosis. Suction drainage should never be placed over the line of closure. While there have been no reports on unnecessary suffering from over drainage, patients may suffer serious complications due to the lack of drains or hasty removal of them. Numerous methods of affixing the drains to the patient have been devised, and in choosing the right one, the criteria are the drain must be fixed to the patient such that accidental removal is unlikely, the method of attachment should not damage the skin, there should be no air leakage at the drain site, and the drain should be easily removable when it is no longer needed.

Drain failure is usually due to inadequate care of the drain but also occurs when a haematoma blocks it. A poorly functioning drain may be remedied by aspiration with a syringe using a sterile technique, or by injecting a small amount of sterile saline to clear it. If this cannot be accomplished, the drain should be cut off beyond the skin exit wound and converted into a passive drain, and a compression dressing applied (if the flaps are not at significant risk of ischaemia, or contraindicated by an underlying vascular pedicle flap). The postoperative care of closed suction drains is simple but if ignored, can lead to major wound infection. The drainage must be measured and recorded accurately so that decisions regarding the removal of the drains can be made. A suction drain should be removed when it is no longer needed; the duration can vary from removing it when it drains 10–40 cc per 24 hrs or a minimum of four days regardless of output, as some surgeons insist. The most important thing is not to remove the drain too early.

COMPLICATIONS

Haematoma/Seroma

Haematoma formation occurs in approximately 1% of radical neck dissections and about 4% of all head and neck surgical cases. It is critical to recognise haematoma formation early by careful inspection of the neck, and observing the character and amount of drainage. The pressure from a haematoma may cause necrosis of a flap, disrupt a suture line, and obstruct the airway. The rate of infection also increases in the presence of a haematoma secondary to tissue ischaemia.

Numerous factors, including medication may influence the likelihood of haematoma formation. Salicylates exert their antiplatelet effect for two weeks, and surgery should be delayed for this period. Patients should also be warned about non-steroidal anti-inflammatory products. Hypertension at the conclusion of the surgery or in the postoperative period may contribute to excessive bleeding and result in a haematoma. If cervical swelling, flap eleva-tion, discolouration or significant bloody drainage are observed, postoperative haematoma should not be ruled out. Suction drains may become occluded due to clot, causing further accumulation of blood. Bleeding around the drain site may also signal problems. Following evacuation of the clot, major bleeding may not be seen but a diffuse generalised oozing is fairly common.

The key to avoiding haematoma formation lies in identifying any coag-ulation disorder prior to surgery and ensuring meticulous haemostasis at the close of the surgery. The wound should be irrigated repeatedly, and each aspect inspected for bleeding, taking extra care to visualise the under-surface and base of all cervical flaps. The placement of suction drains in dependant areas is important but does not substitute for good haemostasis.

Chyle Leak

Chyle leaks have been reported to occur following neck dissections in 1–2.5% of cases, with 25% occurring on the right.[14] Chyle is a mixture of lymph from interstitial fluid and emulsified fat from interstitial lacteals. It is mildly alkaline and on standing forms three layers, a cream top layer, milky middle layer, and a lower layer of cellular sediment. The fat content is 1–3%, largely triglycerides, which are responsible for the milky appearance and greasy feel. The daily drainage may reach two to four litres.

Anatomy

The thoracic duct begins at the cisterna chyli and continues upwards into the thorax posterior to the aorta through the aortic hiatus of the diaphram. It runs in the posterior mediastinum along the right anterior aspect of the vertebral bodies between the aorta and the azygous vein. The thoracic duct crosses the midline at the fifth or sixth thoracic vertebra and continues to extend superiorly along the left posterior border of the oesophagus. It exits the thorax posterior to the left common carotid artery between this vessel and the left subclavian artery. As it enters the neck, it arches superior, anterior and lateral to form a loop that terminates into the venous system. This loop is anterior to the vertebral artery and the thyrocervical trunk. It courses between the internal jugular vein and the anterior scalene muscle superficial to the deep cervical fascia overlying the phrenic nerve. The loop is always found within 2 cm of the internal jugular-subclavian vein junction, and its maximal height is usually 3–5 cm above the clavicle.

The right jugular, subclavian, and the tracheobronchial trunks form the right lymphatic ducts. These usually terminate separately in the region of the right internal jugular — subclavian vein junction. A single duct on the right is thought to be rare.

Presentation

A chyle leak may present in the neck, chest or abdomen. If left untreated, it may result in a metabolic, nutritional and immunologic complication. Patients will eventually become weak, dehydrated, oedematous, and emaciated. Chylotho-rax can result from injury in the chest or neck. It may progress from the neck by tracking along fascial planes to the mediastinum, where it causes tissue maceration and inflammation, resulting in rupture of the pleura. The dangers of a chylothorax include cardiopulmonary compromise because of compression of the lungs, leading to a mediastinal shift with distortion of the great vessels.

The diagnosis of a chyle leak can be intra or postoperative. During dissection of the lower left portion of the neck, chyle may macroscopically be recognised as a milky substance, or the thoracic duct itself may be seen with a tear in it. If a leak is suspected it can be confirmed by asking the anaesthetist to apply a continuous positive airway pressure and place the patient in the Trendelenburg position. Postoperatively, chyle may present in the drainage bottle, but if it is a low volume leak, it can be missed initially because it is mixed with blood. Even chemical analysis of the fluid may not be conclusive. However, >100 ng/dL triglycerides or $>4\%$ chylomicrons indicate possible chylous leakage.

Management

It is universally accepted that the optimum management of a chylous fistula is by prevention. If the leak is identified during surgery, every effort should be made to arrest it immediately. Ligation with 3-0 or 4-0 non-absorbable suture without going through the duct wall should be performed. It has been suggested that inclusion of the medial edge of the anterior scalene muscle will help prevent duct laceration during ligation. Leakage may continue to occur postoperatively, even when the procedure is apparently successful because of unidentified injuries to the duct or additional terminations.

Medical management involves an elemental diet supplemented with medium chain triglycerides (MCT). These are absorbed directly into the portal circulation, bypassing the lymphatic system. Total parentral nutrition (TPN) is an alternative, but is not recommended by all. In theory, interruption of entral alimentation should reduce intestinal peristalsis and lymph flow. However, the disadvantages are the need for central venous access, associated morbidity, and cost. The application of pressure dressings to encourage closure and the formation of chyle collection are usually futile, as the anatomy is not contoured for such an efficient dressing to be applied continuously. Instead, the use of continuous suction drainage is recommended to prevent chyloma formation and avoid the associated intense inflammatory reaction.

The indications and timing for surgical intervention, when a chyle leak is diagnosed in the postoperative phase, remain controversial. Surgery is appropriate if the leak is in excess of 500 ml per day for four or more consecutive days, or if a chyloma formation could not be controlled with pressure dressings or serial aspirations. Surgery is also recommended when chyle drainage is in excess of 500 ml per day after one week of medical management, in case of persistent low-output drainage for a prolonged period, or if complications develop. In these situations, a thorascopic approach to the thoracic duct, on the right side of the chest is considered the definitive management option, with minimal morbidity.

Carotid Artery "Blow Out"

Carotid rupture or blow out is one of the most feared complications (approximately 5% of the cases) of neck surgery.[15] Most ruptures occur when the neck dissection is accompanied by resection of oral, pharyngeal, or laryngeal structure. Mortality rates with spontaneous rupture can reach 50%; the time of rupture is often in the early postoperative period with a median time of 16 days. However, rupture has been reported as late as 200 days post-surgery.

The most common aetiological factors contributing to rupture are *en-bloc* resection of the tumour coupled with preoperative radiotherapy to the overlying tissues and the artery. Wound breakdown and necrosis of overlying tissue and flaps are other major contributors, followed by infection, fistula formation and wound dehiscence. An overzealous manipulation of the carotid artery can damage the aventitia and compromise the vascular wall. Some patients will present a "sentinel bleed," which is the classic warning sign of impending rupture. This will not be as dramatic as an actual "blow-out" and may even appear as a minor bleed. However, if the wound has breaks, the surgeon should initiate steps to minimise or prevent a "blow out" from occurring.

Carotid rupture is a surgical emergency. If a "sentinel bleed" is encountered, surgical exploration is indicated. If a rupture occurs spontaneously, pressure should be applied immediately to slow the bleeding, a large-bore intravenous line established, and support for haemodynamic stability initiated. Transfusion with blood type O should be used if it cannot be cross-matched. Any attempt to clamp or ligate the arterial bleeding without visualising the source is condemned. One of the keys to avoiding cerebrovascular complications is to maintain the patient haemodynamically before formal exploration.

The suggested surgical interventions include ligation and excision of the ruptured area to prevent subsequent bleeds. If rupture is imminent, an elective ligation of the carotid is recommended. Postoperative morbidity and mortality is lower for elective surgery. Emergency ligation should be considered if the eroded area is suspected to be infected, ischemic or involved with tumour. Suturing or repair of the involved arterial segment is usually fruitless and probably dangerous. In case with an early "sentinel bleed" phase the carotid artery can be resected and bypassed. However, the association of a pharyngeal fistula would contraindicate such a procedure.

The prevention of carotid rupture in patients at risk is beneficial and the frequency of its occurrence has been reduced. At its bifurcation, the carotid artery is covered by a dermal graft, or by the rotation of the laevator scapulae muscle at the end of the neck dissection.

Air Embolism

In a surgical setting, where the patient's head is above his or her heart and venous structures are in the operative field, the risk of air embolism is increased.[16]

Air embolism has an unknown incidence because there are many unreported events. The reverse Trendelenburg position is common for head and neck surgical procedures because it decreases the amount of bleeding secondary to decreased orthostatic pressure. If the head is slightly elevated, the pressure within the venous structures of the head and neck is greater than that in the right heart. In most neck dissections the internal jugular vein is exposed, manipulated, and/or sacrificed (requiring ligature and division). With higher pressures within the vein and a point of entry for air into the venous system, air embolization is likely to occur. The pressure gradient which develops is directly proportional to the height of the opening in relation to the heart and inversely proportional to the central venous pressure. Therefore, most of the air that is introduced enters during inspiration.

Once air enters the vein, it travels via the anatomic pathway to reach the heart where it has three major pathways available. The first — is to continue through the heart, pass through the pulmonary artery and reach the lungs. If the amount of air is small, it may diffuse into the alveoli and be expired, or cause platelet aggregation in the small capillaries. If this occurs, microemboli form and inflammatory mediators are released leading to vasoconstriction, increased pulmonary resistance, and decreased compliance. If a large amount of air enters the system and proceeds to the lung, an intense pulmonary artery vasoconstriction with resulting cor pulmonale and oedema are likely. Air embolus and cor pulmonale may also initiate cardiac dysrrhythmias and obstruct the right ventricular outflow tract.

The second alternative is for the air to remain in the heart. Air which passes into the heart may initially be lodged within the right atrium resulting in dilatation of the atrium with associated dysarrhythmias. If the air enters the right ventricle an airlock phenomenon appears that prevents proper venous return and reduces cardiac output. Subsequently, haemodynamic instability ensues leading to cardiovascular failure.

The third pathway requires a patent foramen ovale, estimated to be present in 20% of the normal population. When the right atrial pressure exceeds the left the embolized air can pass through this foramen and enter the arterial circulation. Once here, embolization can occur. This is also known as paradoxical embolization because the air has originated on the right side of the heart. Embolization to the cerebral and other vital arterial circulation routes may have significant sequelae. Air emboli, of as little as 100 ml of air has proven lethal in humans.

It may be difficult to recognise air embolism in anaesthetised patient. If a major vein is torn or if a ligature becomes dislodged and a sucking noise is heard, embolism should be suspected. Auscultation may elicit a millwheel cardiac murmur indicative of air mixing with blood in the heart. Sudden cardio-respiratory collapse in this setting can indicate embolization. A sudden rise in central venous pressure and/or a decrease in end-tidal carbon dioxide should also draw the attention of the anaesthetist. Tachycardia, arrhythmias, cyanosis, and hypotension are associated classic signs and symptoms.

The treatment begins by placing the patient in the left decubitus position and Trendelenburg. This reduces the risk of paradoxical embolus through a patent foramen ovale and has the ability to shift the embolus out of the right ventricular outflow tract into the apex of the right ventricle and allow antegrade blood flow. An occlusion of the torn vein, either by direct pressure or repair will prevent further air entry. If nitrous oxide (NO) is being used as anaesthesia, it should be discontinued immediately and replaced with 100% oxygen, because NO can increase and sustain the air bubbles. Closed-chest cardiac massage has been suggested as an alternative treatment of choice, because speed is crucial. As a last resort trans cardiac aspiration of air may be attempted by placing a needle into the right ventricle to aspirate the air. Central nervous system sequelae may respond to hyperbaric oxygen therapy.

The prevention of embolus is best achieved by careful dissection of the jugular vein, by identifying the hidden tributaries and following the proper plane of dissection. Preoperative placement of pulmonary artery catheters is helpful in the recognition and treatment of air embolus but is not advocated for routine use in neck surgery.

CRANIAL NERVE INJURY

Vagus Nerve

The vagus nerve exits the skull through the jugular foramen and runs in the carotid sheath along with the major vessels in the neck. In the neck, it lies between the common carotid and the internal jugular vein. The first branch of the vagus is the superior laryngeal nerve, which in turn has two branches, the internal branch of a special visceral afferent from the supraglottic larynx, and the external branch that innervates the cricothyroid muscle. In the lower part of the neck, the vagus has smaller superior and inferior cardiac branches, which pass behind the subclavian artery and join the cardiac plexus. The recurrent laryngeal arises at the base of the neck, loops behind the subclavian artery (from anterior to posterior) and runs medially and superiorly in the tracheooesophageal groove to reach the larynx. The left recurrent laryngeal nerve runs below and behind the arch of the aorta and then follows a similar path to the larynx. The recurrent laryngeal nerves innervate all the intrinsic muscles of the larynx, except the cricothyroid muscle, which is innervated by the extrinsic branch of the superior laryngeal nerve. They also innervate the pharyngeal constrictors. Finally, the recurrent nerves supply special visceral afferent sensation to the glottis and subglottic larynx.

An inadvertent injury to the vagus nerve may occur while ligating the internal jugular vein, resulting in ipsilateral laryngeal and pharyngeal paralysis and loss of sensation in the larynx at the level of the true cord and below. This is characterised by a breathy voice, inefficient cough, and a subjective sense of dyspnoea result. Dysphagia may also occur due to inefficient pharyngeal paralysis together with a tendency for laryngeal penetration during swallowing, especially thin liquid. The loss of more distal vagal innervation has little clinical effect.

The immediate neurorrhaphy of the transected vagus nerve is not often considered to be useful. The intraoperative medialisation of the vocal cord to preserve voice quality is a more critical issue. Gelfoam or Bioplastic injection or some other procedure may be considered electively in the postoperative period after the situation has been explained to the patient.

Spinal Accessory Nerve

Pain and weakness of the shoulder are among the most common postoperative complications following neck dissection.[17] Unfortunately similar complications may result from excision biopsy of cutaneous or lymph nodes in the posterior triangle of the neck. The damage to or sacrifice of the spinal accessory nerve (cranial nerve XI) is a major factor for complaints related to the shoulder.

Anatomy

The accessory nerve exits the skull through the jugular foramen with the IX and X nerves, and the jugular vein, running lateral or medial to the internal jugular vein. It then moves posterior and downward to enter the deep surface of the sternomastoid muscle (SCM), usually running through or deep to the SCM. After supplying the SCM, the nerve runs turns inferiorly and laterally, running through the posterior triangle and deep to the trapezius, which it innervates. The spinal accessory nerve may receive branches from the cervical plexus, which help in supplying the SCM and the trapezius muscle. Most of the cervical plexus derives from the C-2, C2-3, or C-3. Usually the branches join the accessory nerves deep to the SCM and not in the posterior triangle; it is not clear these branches also carry motor or sensory fibres into the accessory nerve.

In the posterior triangle, the nerve can be located best by three landmarks, the distance between the clavicle and the point where the nerve passes under or pierces the trapezius is generally 2–4 cm, the greater auricular nerve is easily located during neck surgery and is found emerging on the posterior border of the SCM and curving forward across the muscle the accessory nerve is found approximately 2 cm above the exit point of the greater auricular nerve, and lastly, the nerve can nearly always be found along the top half of the posterior border of the SCM.

Patients who suffer from damage to the accessory nerve are often afflicted with the classic "shoulder syndrome," consisting of pain in the shoulder, limited abduction of the shoulder, a full passive range of motion, anatomic deformity (including scapular flaring, droop and protraction) and an abnormal electromyogram of the trapezius.

The treatment of patients with transection of the accessory nerve is twofold. The immediate options consist of preservation of the cervical plexus to preserve any existing alternatives muscular innervations as long as this appears to be oncologically feasible. Primary reanastamosis of the severed nerve endings or cable grafting have also been recommended. Aggressive physical therapy following surgery is shown to be useful in strengthening supportive musculature (serratus anterior, deltoid, levator scapulae, and rhomboids) and maintaining the trapezius function in modified and grafting techniques.

Sympathetic Nerve Injury

The sympathetic trunk lies deep in the neck posterior and medial to the carotid artery, between the prevertebral fascia and the carotid sheath. It runs upwards superficial to the longus coli and longus capitis muscles behind the common carotid artery. In some instances, the superior sympathetic ganglion lies deep to the prevertebral fascia. Care must be taken not to transect or remove the superior cervical ganglion inadvertently because it can resemble a lymph node at the level of C-1 and C-3.

Postoperatively, this injury is recognised by several signs and symptoms related to the classic Horner's syndrome. The physical findings resulting from loss of sympathetic innervation include meiosis (papillary constriction), ptosis (eyelid drooping secondary to paralysis of Muller's muscle), transient blushing, anhydrosis, and nasal congestion. If the lesion is below the stellate ganglion, Horner's syndrome will not occur.

The treatment of Horner's syndrome is supportive care.

Phrenic Nerve Injury

The phrenic nerve originates from the cervical roots C3–5. It descends on the anterior surface of the anterior scalene muscle beneath the fascia. As the nerve roots leave the foramina they may join to form the phrenic nerve or remain separated on the anterior scalene for some distance. Therefore, it may appear that two phrenic nerves are running beneath the fascia. In this instance, the lower of the two branches is usually referred to as an accessory nerve. The incidence of accessory phrenic nerves is between 5–50%.

Injury to the phrenic nerve may occur during neck dissection or surgery in this region. The phrenic nerve carries motor innervation to the diaphram a well as somatic afferent fibres (pain fibres) from the pericardium, the mediastinum, the diaphragmatic portions of the parietal pleura, and the parietal peritoneum on the inferior surface of the diaphram. The signs and symptoms of phrenic nerve injury are cough, dyspnoea, chest pain, cyanosis, palpitations, tachycardia, dyspepsia, abdominal discomfort, nausea, vomiting, excessive belching, paralysis, and/or elevation of the ipsilateral diaphram and mediastinal shift. The four classical signs described are elevated hemidiaphram, absent or paradoxical diaphram movement, mediastinal shift, and positive Hitzenberger sign (paradoxical movement of the diaphram when sniffing).

Although the patient rarely notes the symptoms, the surgeon should be aware of the increased incidence of atelectasis on the involved side and take precautions to prevent postoperative pneumonia. If the nerve has been sectioned, immediate neurorrhaphy or cable grafting is indicated.

Pharyngocutaneous Fistula

All major oral, pharyngeal, hypopharyngeal and laryngeal ablative surgery can lead to pharyngocutaneous fistulae.[18] The breakdown of the mucosal closure, resulting in saliva and secretion leakage into surrounding soft tissue, ultimately causes communication of the salivary tract with the skin, resulting in a pharyngocutaneous fistula. It is the most frequent complication after total laryngectomy but can occur after all oncologic oropharyngeal or hypopharyngeal surgery. Non-oncologic surgery with mucosal entry, such as open techniques for the treatment of Zenker Diverticulum can also result in fistula formation.

The causes of the pharyngocutaneous fistula are multifactorial. Comorbid patient factors can predispose patients to fistula occurrence, as can local factors that affect wound healing. The identification of high-risk patients is imperative to anticipate difficulties in wound healing and attempt to prevent or minimise them. High-risk patients can be identified by the presence of obvious comorbidity factors. A preoperative haemoglobin level lower than 12.5 g/dL has been reported to carry an additional nine-fold increase in the risk of fistula development. Increased frequency of pharyngocutaneous fistula has also been reported in patients who have received radiotherapy. It has been reported that the rate of fistula formation may be related to the radiation dosage but the fractionation protocols are poorly analysed and reported.

The presence of a fistula will usually become clinically apparent 5–11 days after surgery. The diagnosis of pharyngocutaneous fistula may be confirmed by barium swallow, or rarely with a CT scan. In some cases the patient has not yet resumed oral intake, whereas with late fistulae, the patient has. The first clinical signs are wound erythema in combination with neck and facial oedema and soft tissue swelling. Although tenderness of the skin incision is the classic hallmark of soft tissue infection, the intensity of pain and tenderness is lesser because of the resultant neck paraesthesia. Often patients may present with fever, particularly if there is significant purulence associated with the fistula; fever during the first 48 hrs postoperatively has been shown to correlate with the development of pharyngocutaneous fistula and wound infection. With further fistula progression, surgical wound contamination by oropharyngeal contents leads to wound dehiscence, skin flap necrosis, and soft tissue necrosis. A barium swallow performed 1–2 weeks after laryngectomy, when an impending fistula is suspected, is reported to be an excellent predictor of a clinical fistula. A sinus tract longer than 2 cm is predictive of fistula formation.

Prevention

Preoperative recognition of a patient at risk may reduce the incidence of fistula. The standard care for laryngectomy patients is prophylactic antibiotics treatment, which reduces the incidence of severe wound infections by 50%. Gastro-oesophageal reflux prophylaxis (ranitidine and metoclopramide hydrochloride parentral for seven days) has been shown to reduce fistula formation dramatically. The commencement of oral feeding remains contentious, in the non-irradiated patient it may commence within 48 hrs, but in the preoperative irradiated patient, it is usually withheld for 10 days. One of the most important factors in repairing the surgical mucosal area is surgical technique, with meticulous haemostasis, atraumatic handling of the mucosa, the closure type (T vs. linear), the two-layer technique, minimal tension, adequate use of drains to eliminate dead space, and a watertight suture line.

MANAGEMENT

Conservative Management

Early recognition of a fistula can prevent secondary wound complications and reduce the incidence of catastrophic complications. The areas suspected with fluid collection should be aspirated, exteriorised immediately by opening the suture line if purulent or salivary contamination is detected. Early drainage and aggressive wound care with debridement are important; drainage will divert the fistula from critical structures such as the carotid artery and the posterior tracheal wall. The lateralisation of the fistula tract to the neck side with its better soft tissue cover will maintain the integrity of the posterior tracheal wall and reduce the risk of aspiration and pneumonia. The placement of a cuffed tracheostomy tube may help reduce aspiration in situations where the fistula is close to the tracheostomy. Sometimes the use of a Montgomery salivary bypass tube inserted into the pharynx may prevent leakage of the secretions. Antibiotics should be reinstated and nutritional support with nasogastric tube feeding or gastrostomy feeding will optimise the host response and improve healing. Wound packing, with proflavine or such antiseptic product, is imperative and should be performed twice a day, and in exceptional circumstances increased to four times a day. Most small fistulae in non-irradiated tissues will heal by secondary intention with aggressive wound care.

Surgical Repair

The primary closure of a fistula is rarely possible but may be considered in small fistulae in which there is minimal surrounding loss of soft tissue and the mucosa seems healthy. However, even a small fistula will turn out to be bigger than it appears at first inspection. Fistulae are often associated with extensive overlying skin loss and mucosal dehiscence. Residual or recurrent disease must be considered a possibility when a large fistula fails to close by secondary intention. A complete debridement of the devascularised and necrotic tissue and closure of the mucosal and skin sites can result in significant soft tissue loss, resulting in the need for local, regional or microvascular flap reconstruction. Unless a critical structure is exposed, flap reconstruction should not be undertaken until the process of secondary healing and healthy granulation tissue has occurred. The flap type or combination of flaps will depend on the surgeon's preference and previous experience.

Late Effects after Pharyngocutaneous Fistula

Pharyngocutaneous fistulae result in minimal functional late effects on swallowing or speech. Pharyngeal stenosis is uncommon after pharyngocutaneous fistula although scarring of the pharyngo-oesophageal complex occurs. The degree and extent of stenosis may necessitate surgical intervention if there is obstructive dysphagia or limitation in voice rehabilitation after tracheooesophageal speech. Dilatation of the pharyngo-oesophageal stenosis or even reconstruction of the pharyngeal segment with free tissue transfer may be necessary in a small number of patients. Jejunal interposition free flap, tubed gastro-omental free flap, or tubed anterolateral thigh flap are possible options for reconstructive surgery.

Complications of Flap Surgery

The defects created by oncologic surgery in the head and neck often require repair by local or distant tissue to maintain or restore function. Myocutaneous pedicled flaps using the pectoralis major, deltoid, latissimus, trapezius, and platysma muscles are used to repair many defects but are associated with complications. The local and pedicled flaps are tethered and therefore the distal portion of the flap is often inset with some tension. The flaps also have a limited ability to reconstruct the pre-existing anatomy, possess inappropriate tissue bulk, and lack vascularised bone for replacement. Because the distal portion of a local and pedicle flap is located one angiosome distal to the vascular territory of the pedicle, complications arise from partial muscle or cutaneous necrosis at the distal aspect of the flap. Distal necrosis results in dehiscence that is often followed by fistula formation.

The use of free tissue flaps overcomes many of these problems by being centred over the vascular pedicle, and therefore the entire transferred tissue is well vascularised. Free tissue also offers several distinct advantages in head and neck reconstruction, such as tissue dimensions and thickness can be tailored to the size of the defect, vascularised bone can be used to reconstruct composite defects, free tissue can be rotated and contoured to fit the defect, and the free flap is typically centred on the pedicle, allowing superior blood supply and limiting incidence of partial necrosis.

Donor Site Complications

In free tissue flaps, the donor site has fewer associated complications, compared to pedicled flaps, because it is usually not involved in the diseased process being treated, undergoes one procedure instead of two (resections and reconstruction at the recipient site, each with their own imperatives) and is free from the challenges of respiration, mastication, swallowing, and salivation posed by the upper aerodigestive tract.

Ultimately the reconstructive technique should be driven by functional results and subsequent impact on quality of life.

Complications of Major Salivary Gland Surgery

The prevention of complications from salivary gland surgery begins with a thorough understanding of the complex regional anatomy of the parotid and submandibular areas, and in some instances, the infratemporal fossa, temperomandibular joint, and external ear.[19] A thorough familiarity with pathophysiology, including malignant and benign tumours, primary and secondary tumours, and infectious and inflammatory processes, will guide in the appropriate selection of patients as well as preoperative evaluation and postoperative management.

NERVE INJURY

Parotid Surgery: Facial Nerve

Regardless of the indication for the surgery, the key to the prevention of facial paralysis is formal identification and preservation of the branches of the facial nerve. It is easier when there is no inflammation, no prior surgery or prior irradiation, if the process is limited to the superficial lobe and the tumour is

small. Many surgeons find it useful to have available a disposable nerve stimulator to assist in the identification of branches. This is especially useful in
the event of prior surgery, or in cases of sialadenitis. The facial nerve exits the
temporal bone through the stylomastoid foramen, which lies just posterior to
the styloid process and just anterior to the digastric ridge. The attachment of
the posterior belly of the digastric muscle to the inferior end of the tympanomastoid suture is 6–8 mm lateral to the stylomastoid foramen. After first
identifying the tragal pointer, this is the most common location for identifying the facial nerve trunk. The tragal pointer is the anteroinferior portion of
the cartilage of the external auditory canal. The facial nerve is located about
1 cm deep and slightly inferior to it. The tympanomastoid suture is palpated,
as is the styloid process. Once the nerve is identified, it is followed anteriorly to the pes, where it branches. Because there are considerable variations
of the nerve, it is important to follow each branch as far as necessary towards
the periphery to facilitate the removal of the tumour with-a-cuff of normal
gland around it. Tumours arising from or extending deep to the plane of the
branches of the facial nerve are said to be "deep lobe." Retracting branches superiorly and inferiorly may be necessary to dissect such tumours. The division of
the stylomastoid ligament affords additional exposure to the parapharyngeal
space.

If a major branch or trunk of the facial nerve is transected intraoperatively,
it should be repaired at the end of the procedure; a simple microsurgical neurorrhaphy between the two ends should be done without tension. The next best
choice is a cable graft, usually using the greater auricular nerve. The management of facial paralysis depends in part on the branches involved (whether it is
partial or complete) and for how long it is expected to persist. Paralysis of the
marginal mandibular branch and the branches to the orbiculus oculi are most
likely to be symptomatic, with paralytic ectropian, conjunctivitis, exposure
keratosis, and epiphora. The initial management is aimed at the prevention of
corneal ulcers by keeping the conjunctiva moist. Artificial tears administered
frequently during the day and lubricating ointment during the night are often
effective. If recovery is expected to be delayed (or permanent) an upper lid
gold weight may be placed at or soon after surgery. Other surgical oculoplastic
procedures may be required to correct the facial cosmetic deformity, which
will become unsightly with time.

Parotid Surgery: The Greater Auricular Nerve

During parotidectomy the greater auricular nerve is usually scarified, and the numbness of the ear lobe is permanent. It has been recommended that the posterior branch of the greater auricular nerve should be preserved if possible because it significantly minimises the resultant morbidity.

Often, months or even years following surgery, a small 0.5–1.5 cm mass, often painful, may be palpated over the sternomastoid muscle at the amputated greater auricular nerve. The initial presentation of this neuroma may be pain radiating from a trigger point in the area. Because the differential diagnosis includes recurrent tumour, excision of the lesion cures the pain and reassures the patient.

SUBMANDIBULAR GLAND

Facial Nerve, Lingual Nerve, and Hypoglossal Nerve

The three cranial nerves located in close proximity to the submandibular gland are to be preserved if they are not affected by tumour while excising the submandibular gland.

The marginal mandibular branch of the facial nerve courses superficial to the fascia overlying the gland and should be specifically sought and preserved by raising the submandibular gland fascia with the platysma, which includes the nerve, towards the inferior border of the mandible. Even if the nerve is not traumatised the corner of the lower lip may not depress normally, due to inadequate functioning of the transacted playtsma muscle or temporary neuropraxia of the nerve from trauma or devascularisation.

The hypoglossal nerve is found between the hyoglossus and the mylohyoid muscle. It is in close proximity to the external facial artery as one ligates it. Inferior retraction of the anterior belly of the digastric muscle and tendon should expose the nerve. Ipsilateral loss of the hypoglossal nerve is usually well tolerated in the absence of other neuromuscular deficit associated with speech or swallowing.

While retracting the submandibular inferiorly, the anterior retraction of the mylohyoid muscle exposes the lingual nerve, the submandibular ganglion and the submandibular duct. While ligating the ganglion, care must be taken to avoid clamping the lingual nerve. A ligature is preferred to cautery to handle the venous bleeding, as heat transmitted to the nerve may result in its damage. Injury to the nerve results in hypaesthesia of the anterior two thirds of the tongue. As a result, the patient may occasionally bite their tongue, leading to trophic ulcers.

Haematoma

Adequate intraoperative haemostasis using bipolar cautery and ligatures prevents most postoperative bleeding. If the posterior facial vein has to be ligated to resect a deep-sited tumour, there may be increased venous pressure, making complete haemostasis more difficult to achieve. A haematoma should be suspected in case of facial swelling over the surgical field, accompanied by pain. In this case, blood may have clotted and the suction tubes fail to drain it adequately. Often, a haematoma will require re-exploration and evacuation.

Salivary Leak or Sialocoele

A salivary leak may manifest as clear drainage from the incision or drain site or as a sialocoele beneath a healed flap. Both are likely to respond within a week or two to treatment with pressure dressings. Aspiration of the sialocoele may either be helpful or serve as a means to distinguish it from possible seroma. A persistent salivary fistula can be a nuisance but may respond to pressure dressings. The use of Botox is reported to be useful if the flow does not abate after several weeks. If re-exploration and completion total parotidectomy are required, the risk of injury to the facial nerve increases.

Gustatory Sweating (Frey's Syndrome)

Gustatory sweating or Frey's syndrome involves post-parotidectomy facial sweating and skin flushing while eating.[21] It may be present along the distribution of the greater auricular nerve or branches of the cervical plexus. The symptoms usually occur several months or even years after parotid surgery.

Minor's starch/iodine test can be used to measure the extent of the gustatory sweating. The likely pathophysiology is aberrant regeneration of postganglionic secretomotor parasympathetic nerve fibres (originating from the otic ganglion) misdirected through severed axonal sheaths of post-ganglionic sympathetic fibres feeding the sweat glands. For Frey's syndrome, these sympathetic fibres are to the sweat glands of the skin in the dissected field.

The current treatment involves the use of Botox injections administered to the area after the Minor's Starch Test has delineated it. Repeat treatments may be required. The use of a thicker skin flap or the interposition of a sternomastoid rotation muscle flap is associated with a lesser incidence of symptomatic Frey's' syndrome. Many patients will not volunteer the symptoms or seek an opinion, but if the problem is explained, they are reassured, especially since it does not require further treatment.

Thyroid and Parathyroid Surgery

The risk of complications from the surgery of the thyroid and parathyroid glands varies depending on the extent of the operation (i.e. lobectomy vs. subtotal or total thyroidectomy). However, complications from this type of surgery are rare, but when they occur can be life threatening or cause severe functional impairment;[20] the risk is greater when a re-operation is required. Currently, most complications from thyroid and parathyroid surgery are related to metabolic derangements or injury to the recurrent laryngeal nerves. Others include superior laryngeal nerve injury, infection, airway compromise, and bleeding. Although the principal goal of surgery is not the prevention of these complications, prompt recognition and intervention will minimise morbidity and provide the patient with the best chance of a satisfactory outcome.

Intraoperative Bleeding

Haemorrhage is a concern during any surgical procedure, and any bleeding is not desirable during thyroid and especially parathyroid surgery. The presence of blood in the operative field increases the possibility of injuring the nerves. In addition, the resulting tissue staining makes it more difficult to identify the parathyroid glands.

Adequate exposure and careful ligation of the individual vessels is paramount to avoid bleeding in this area. It may be necessary to divide the sternothyroid muscles near their superior insertion to improve exposure. Some of the small vessels, especially when locating and operating around the parathyroid glands, should be isolated and ligated by passing a ligature around the vessel before division. The thyroid lobe has to be mobilised medially, and before it can be removed, profuse bleeding can occur from small branches of the inferior thyroid artery, which courses medial to the recurrent nerve, in the suspensory ligament of Berry. The proximity of the nerve usually precludes the use of electrocautery and clamping may be cumbersome because the thyroid may adhere to the trachea. Clamping and ligation of the branches of the inferior thyroid artery can be facilitated by dividing the thyroid isthmus, and dissecting the lobe off the trachea from medial to lateral.

Postoperative Bleeding

Postoperative bleeding occurs in less than 2% of all thyroidectomy cases. Small or moderate size collections of blood in the wound are usually inconsequential; however, large haematomas can be life threatening due to airway compromise. It is assumed that the resulting increase in venous pressure produces laryngeal oedema thus causing the airway obstruction.

Postoperative bleeding may result from faulty intraoperative haemostasis or from increased venous pressure caused by coughing or gagging prior to or after extubation.

The insertion of drains or bulky dressings may not prevent the formation of haematoma when bleeding commences. Furthermore, dressings may delay the diagnosis of a condition that requires early recognition and immediate treatment.

Once a haematoma is recognised, the wound should be explored immediately. If a delay is anticipated or if airway jeopardy is a risk, skin incision and the closure of the strap muscles should be done at the bedside, and the haematoma evacuated. The patient should then be returned to the operating theatre, as soon as possible, to control the bleeding.

Unilateral Recurrent Nerve Palsy

Thyroid and parathyroid surgery accounts for a significant number of unilateral recurrent nerve paralysis, and surgeons must have intimate knowledge of the course of the recurrent laryngeal nerves and treat them carefully during surgery. While the use of electrical devices to monitor or stimulate the nerve during surgery is recommended, the most important method of avoiding injury to the nerve is a thorough knowledge of the anatomy of the region and a meticulous surgical technique.

Injury to the recurrent nerve is rarely appreciated during surgery. Even in the early postoperative period, unilateral vocal cord paralysis may not be clinically evident. The paralysed cord tends to drift to the lateralised position, and the injury becomes apparent eventually. A routine inspection of the vocal cords following thyroid and parathyroid surgery is advocated to ensure early diagnosis and patients should be informed early on to minimise the likelihood of subsequent litigation. Once the diagnosis of a unilateral cord paralysis has been made, the treatment should be outlined. Asymptomatic or minimally symptomatic patients may warrant only close observation.

Conversely, aphonic patients with severe aspiration may need immediate interventions. Patients with mild vocal complaints are the most difficult to treat as the prognosis of recovery of the traumatised recurrent laryngeal nerve should be determined. The use of laryngeal electromyography (LEMG) is helpful; it tests the electromechanical activity of the thyroarytenoid and cricoarytenoid muscles using percutaneous monopolar electrodes. Rehabilitation may be expectant or temporised by the use of injection medialisation; autologous fat to augment the lateralised vocal cord may be all that is required. The fat may persist for a length of time, between three months to several years. Unfortunately this absorption is unpredictable and further procedures may be necessary.

Patients who remain with a paralysed vocal cord after six or more months will benefit from a medialisation thyroplasty. Those with a persistent posterior chink on phonation or with vocal cord height differences may require an additional arytenoid adduction procedure to improve voice quality.

Bilateral Vocal Cord Paralysis

Thyroidectomy remains a common cause of immediate breathing difficulty postoperatively. The bilateral injury may be evident immediately or may not be clinically present for up to several hours after extubation. If the patient develops stridor during extubation or in the recovery room, flexible laryngoscopy is performed and the diagnosis is confirmed. At this point, a decision will need to be made on the immediate management of the patient's airway. If the nerves are considered to "mildly" traumatised, a course of steroids may be given over a period of days and the patient extubated at a later time. A tracheostomy is more likely to be performed and the expectant recovery period is a few weeks to months. The recovery may be predicted by the use of LEMG. If voluntary movement of the vocal cords does not return after nine months or if the data reveals that recovery is unlikely, a definitive procedure can be planned. Many patients are adverse to the idea of a permanent tracheostomy. The surgical goal of static procedures is to rehabilitate the patient with bilateral vocal cord paralysis while finding the delicate balance between airway, voice and aspiration. Dynamic procedures aim at reinnervating the function of the laryngeal abductors, by ansa hypoglossi-omohyoid neuromuscular pedicle transfer to the posterior cricoarytenoid muscle.

Hypoparathyroidism

Hypoparathyroidism is one of the most common and most serious complications from thyroid and parathyroid surgery. It can result from inadvertent surgical removal of the parathyroid glands or by compromising their vascular supply. Fortunately, in most instances postoperative hyperaparathyroidism is a temporary condition. However, when it is permanent, the patient is committed to lifelong symptomatic treatment with calcium, and/or Vitamin D. To avoid this complication, the surgeon must make every effort to preserve one or more viable parathyroid glands, particularly while performing a total or subtotal thyroidectomy.

Clinical manifestations of hypocalcaemia may appear between 1–7 days after surgery. The symptoms and signs of hypocalcaemia result from increased neuromuscular excitability caused by low levels of ionised calcium. The initial symptoms consist of perioral parasthesia, tingling of the extremities, and anxiety. At this stage, tetany can be induced by diagnostic manoeuvres, such as controlled hyperventilation, tapping the facial nerve over the stylomastoid area (Chvostek Sign) or occluding the arterial blood supply to the arm for three minutes (Trousseau Sign). If hypocalcaemia is not treated, the patient will develop potentially life-threatening manifestations, such as carpopedal spasm, tetanic seizures, and laryngeal spasm.

As soon as the patient becomes symptomatic, a blood sample should be tested for ionised calcium and phosphate levels after which calcium should be given intravenously. Because most of these patients require extra calcium for several weeks, oral supplements should be initiated as soon as it is feasible. If normal calcium levels cannot be maintained with the recommended doses of oral calcium, oral therapy with Vitamin D should be instituted. Consultation and management with an endocrinologist should be recommended.

REFERENCES

1. Kern EB. (2003) The preoperative discussion as a prelude to managing a complication. *Arch Otolaryngol Head Neck Surg* **129**: 1163–1165.
2. Rosenthal EL, Dixon SF. (2003) Free flap complications: when is enough, enough? *Curr Opin Otyolaryngol Head Neck Surg* **11**: 236–239.
3. Hunt PM, Burkey BB. (2002) Use of local and regional flaps in modern head and neck reconstruction. *Curr Opin Otolaryngol Head Neck Surg* **10**: 249–255.
4. Robbins KT, Favrot S, Hanna D, Cole R. (1990) Risk of wound infection in patients with head and neck cancer. *Head Neck* **12**: 143–148.
5. Simo R, French G. (2006) The use of prophylactic antibiotics in head and neck oncological surgery. *Curr Opin Otolaryngol Head Neck Surg* **14**: 55–61.
6. Johnson JT, Yu VL. (1989) Role of aerobic gram-negative rods, anaerobs, and fungi in wound infection after head and neck surgery: implications for antibiotic prophylaxis. *Head Neck* **11**: 27–29.
7. Johnson JT, Bloomer WD. (1989) Effect of prior radiotherapy on postsurgical wound infection. *Head Neck* **11**: 132–136.
8. Klussmann JP, Knoedgen R, Wittekindt C *et al.* (2002) Complications of suspension laryngoscopy. *Ann Otol Rhinol Laryngol* **111**: 972–977.
9. Gaut A, Williams M. (2000) Lingual nerve injury during suspension microlaryngoscopy. *Arch Otolaryngol Head Neck Surg* **126**: 669–671.
10. Lai ATY, Chow TL, Lee DTY, Kwok SPY. (2003) Risk factors predicting the development of complications after foreign body ingestion. *Br J Surg* **90**: 1531–1535.
11. Fernandez FF, Richter A, Freudenberg S *et al.* (1999) Treatment of endoscopic oesophageal perforation. *Surg Endosc* **10**: 962–966.
12. Bradley PJ. (1997) Tracheostomy and the obstructed airway. In: Hibbert J (ed), *Scott-Brown's Diseases of the Ear, Nose and Throat*, 6th edn. (Butterworths, London, Boston), Chapter X.
13. Gender EM, Ferlito A, Shaha AR *et al.* (2003) Complications of neck dissection. *Acta Otolaryngol* **123**: 795–801.

14. Hehar SS, Bradley PJ. (2001) Management of chyle leaks. *Curr Opin Otolaryngol Head Neck Surg* **9**: 120–125.
15. Porto DP, Adams GL, Foster C. (1986) Emergency management of carotid artery rupture. *Am J Otolaryngol* **7**: 213–217.
16. O'Quin RJ, Lakshminarayan S. (1982) Venous air embolism. *Arch Intern Med* **142**: 2173–2176.
17. Chandawarkar RY, Cervino AL, Pennington GA. (2003) Management of iatrogenic injury to the spinal accessory nerve. *Plast Reconstr Surg* **11**: 611–619.
18. Makitie AA, Irish J, Guillane PJ. (2003) Pharyngocutaneous fistula. *Curr Opin Otolaryngol Head Neck Surg* **11**: 78–84.
19. Bradley PJ. (2001) Consent to treatment and major salivary gland surgery. *ENT News* 55–59.
20. Fewins J, Simpson CB, Miller FR. (2003) Complications of thyroid and parathyroid surgery. *Otolaryngol Clin N Am* **36**: 189–206.
21. Sood S, Quraishi MS, Bradley PJ. (1998) Frey's syndrome and parotid surgery. *Clin Otolaryngol* **23**: 291–301.

Chapter 8

COMPLICATIONS OF CARDIOTHORACIC SURGERY

Joanna Chikwe and Thanos Athanasiou

By its very nature cardiothoracic surgery is associated with several life threatening complications, as well as many common and major complications. This chapter describes the complications associated with cardiothoracic surgery in three sections, general, cardiac and thoracic.

1. GENERAL COMPLICATIONS

Respiratory Compromise

A thoracotomy causes more Respiratory Compromise than a median sternotomy. The additional, specific respiratory problems of subsequent operation, e.g., lung resection, and cardiopulmonary bypass, are discussed below. Following thoracic surgery pulmonary dysfunction is maximal for 24 hours postoperatively.[1] Seventy two hours later, the vital capacity may be less than 50% of the preoperative values,[2] and takes two weeks to return to normal. The total lung compliance falls by 25%, and dead space is increased. Atelectasis is present in over 50% of the patients and is associated with increased intra-pulmonary shunts, and raised pulmonary vascular resistance. Consequently, these patients may have a PaO_2 of less than 7.5 kPa, on room air. The factors contributing to these changes can be classified as pre, intra and postoperative.

Smoking, recent respiratory infection, respiratory disease, commonly obstructive airways disease, and obesity are the main preoperative risk factors for postoperative respiratory dysfunction. The vast majority of patients under-going cardiac surgery and lung have a history of smoking. Chronic smokers almost invariably have evidence of chronic obstructive airways disease. Exer-tional dyspnoea, sputum production or wheeze is associated with increased postoperative pulmonary complications, and a third of these patients will have pulmonary complications requiring additional therapy. By giving up smok-ing eight weeks or more before surgery, some of the chronic changes in the bronchopulmonary tree are reduced and the rate of pulmonary complications decreases to less than 15%; pulmonary complications probably increase in patients who stop smoking less than eight weeks before surgery. A recent res-piratory infection is an indication for cancelling non-emergency cardiac and lung resection surgery, because increased or purulent secretions can lead to atelectasis, pneumonia, bronchial plugging and eventual occlusion of smaller endotracheal tubes requiring reintubation. These patients are almost invari-ably elderly; resting PaO_2 decreases linearly with age and patients over 75 years are at greater risk of pulmonary problems.

Obesity increases the risk of postoperative atelectasis. In a morbidly obese patient, sleep apnoea and chronic atelectasis may lead to pulmonary hyperten-sion, which contributes to postoperative respiratory insufficiency. Pulmonary hypertension is also present in up to 25% of the patients undergoing mitral valve surgery.

The choice of incision, opening the pleura and handling the lungs, and the use of cardiopulmonary bypass have a major impact on respiratory func-tion postoperatively. Both median sternotomy and thoracotomy are associ-ated with decreased lung capacities postoperatively; left lower lobe collapse occurs in over 50% of on-pump coronary bypass patients. The increased pain associated with a thoracotomy further predisposes patients to atelectasis: an epidural is key to improving postoperative respiratory function. The pleura may be opened deliberately or inadvertently during surgery, and although the evidence is mixed as to whether this increases the risk of postoperative atelectasis and effusions, increased handling of the lung is probably detrimental. Damage to either the phrenic nerve while opening the chest, harvesting the internal mammary artery, creating a window in the pleura, or using topical cooling results in phrenic nerve paresis (temporary or permanent) which has a significant impact on respiratory function postoperatively.

Narcotics, opioid analgesics and sedatives further depress ventilation. Anticholinergics dilate the airways, increasing the dead space. Inotropes and catecholamines with α activity increase pulmonary vascular resistance while β-blockers cause bronchoconstriction. The use of non-humidified oxygen, including during continous positive airway pressure (CPAP) predisposes to mucous retention and plugging. Before routine use of low molecular weight heparin, acute pulmonary embolism was an important cause of postoperative respiratory dysfunction following lung resection for malignancy, particularly in elderly patients.

chest infection

The reported incidence of pneumonia following cardiothoracic surgery varies from 2–20%.[2] This reflects the variation in diagnostic criteria. A history of cough with purulent sputum or purulent secretions aspirated from the ET tube, suggests chest infection. The diagnosis is confirmed by the presence of pyrexia, bronchial breath sounds, reduced air entry, leucocyte neutrophila, raised C-reactive protein and signs of consolidation on the chest X-ray. A sputum culture may yield sensitivities of causative organisms. In the dyspnoeic, hypoxic patient arterial blood gases are required to guide immediate management.

There is no evidence to confirm that prophylactic physiotherapy helps prevent chest infection after surgery. The single most important intervention is to prevent patients with active chest infections from undergoing surgery. Any elective patient with a current cough (dry or productive), temperature, clinical signs of chest infection, neutrophilia, or suspicious chest X-ray should be deferred for a fortnight and reassessed. Patients who are active smokers, or have stopped smoking within the last six weeks, chronic obstructive pulmonary disease (COPD), obesity, prolonged ventilation, aspiration, particularly after stroke are associated with increased risk of chest infection. Physiotherapy aids patients with a cough to expectorate sputum and prevent mucus plugging. Effective analgesia is important to allow patients to cough.

The definitive treatment is antibiotics: empirical antibiotic use varies among institutions but oral ciprofloxacin provides adequate Gram-positive and Gram-negative cover until the organism sensitivities are known. If aspiration pneumonia is suspected, intravenous cefuroxime and metronidazole should be used. For patients requiring oxygen (PaO_2 < 8.0 kPa in room air), humidifying it reduces the risk of mucus plugs, and makes secretions easier to shift. Continuous positive airways pressure (CPAP) can be used to improve basal collapse. The hypoxic, tachypnoeic, tiring patient on maximal respiratory support should be reviewed urgently by an anaesthetist for elective re-intubation and ventilation.

pulmonary embolism

Postoperative pulmonary embolism (PE) is rare.[3] In cardiac patients bypass results in residual heparin effect, haemodilution, thrombocytopaenia, and platelet dysfunction; and low molecular weight heparin and TED stockings are being increasingly used. Off-pump coronary cases receive a large dose of heparin and DVT prophylaxis intraoperatively; patients undergoing lung resections routinely receive DVT prophylaxis. The 30 day mortality of acute massive PE is about 40%,[4] about 10% of deaths occuring within the first hour, and up to 80% within the first two hours. The mortality of surgical intervention is up to 70% for patients requiring CPR or mechanical circulatory support preoperatively. The operative mortality of stable patients is about 30%.

PE is incorrectly diagnosed in almost 75% of patients. The differential diagnosis includes acute myocardial infarction, aortic dissection, septic shock, chest infection, haemothorax and pneumothorax. Massive PE is when there is haemodynamic compromise, or when over 30% of the pulmonary vasculature is compromised. Its clinical features include symptoms of dyspnoea, pleuritic or dull chest pain, and signs including tachypnoea, tachycardia, hypotension, and elevated jugular venous pressure. The patient may have risk factors for or clinical evidence of deep vein thrombosis (DVT). Bedside tests are, however, unhelpful in diagnosis: an ECG may show right ventricular strain pattern (S1, Q3, T3) but this is neither a specific nor a sensitive test. Transthoracic or transoesophageal echocardiography shows right ventricular dilatation, tricuspid regurgitation, and right atrial or right ventricular thrombus. PaO_2 is usually low along with low $PaCO_2$, and a chest X-ray may show consolidation and effusion early on.

Pulmonary angiography, spiral CT, and VQ scanning are diagnostic.[5] VQ scans have a near 100% sensitivity and low specificity in the diagnosis of acute major PE; the results are given as high, intermediate or low probability of PE. Pneumonia, atelectasis and previous PE also cause ventilation-perfusion mismatches. Pulmonary angiography is the gold standard investigation for acute PE. The associated mortality is 0.2%, and it should not be carried out in haemodynamically unstable patients. While contrast spiral CT has a sensitivity of 80–90% and a specificity of 95%, subsegmental emboli, are frequently not picked up. Magnetic resonance imaging (MRI) has a specificity of 80% and a sensitivity of 77%, and is superior to CT scans in identifying sub-segmental emboli. However, limited availability and high cost means that MRI is not a routinely used modality.

If the patient is haemodynamically unstable, emergency pulmonary embolectomy should be considered, and CPR and extracorporeal life support may be indicated. For patients with a large PE and no contraindications (which include recent surgery) thrombolysis is the definitive management. Ward management involves sitting the patient up and administering 100% O_2. Severely compromised patients may require intubation. Heparin should be given as a bolus of 5,000 u intravenously followed by an infusion titrated to maintain an APTR (activated partial thromboplastin ratio) of 1.8–2.5. Low molecular weight tinzaparin is licensed for use in acute PE, and has the same efficacy as unfractionated heparin but without the requirement for repeated APTT (activated partial thromboplastin time) checks. If the patient is not scheduled for further surgery, warfarin therapy is commenced. The indications for emergency pulmonary thromboembolectomy include a definite diagnosis of acute massive PE and life-threatening circulatory insufficiency, a large right atrial or ventricular thrombus, and contraindicated or unsuccessful thrombolysis.

Exacerbation of COPD

The incidence of moderate to severe COPD in cardiac surgical patients is about 5%, going up to 10% in patients undergoing lung resection. Most studies show that mild to moderate COPD is not associated with a significant increase in postoperative complications, mortality or length of stay.[2] Severe

COPD and preoperative steroid use has an associated mortality of up to 20% following cardiothoracic surgery, with significantly poorer medium and long-term outcomes. This is primarily a clinical diagnosis; most patients have a history of preoperative COPD, and present with increasing dyspnoea, sputum and wheeze. Patients are tachypnoeic with reduced air entry, oxygen saturations and PaO_2.

All patients on preoperative β-agonist inhalers must routinely be prescribed regular postoperative nebulisers (saline 5 ml prn, salbutamol 2.5–5 mg qds prn and becotide 500 mcg qds prn). β-blockers may safely be recommenced, but extra caution must be exercised in starting them for the first time in patients with asthma or severe COPD. In hypoxic patients with COPD, maximal oxygen, by CPAP if necessary, must be provided and blood gases monitored: oxygen must NOT be restricted initially for fear of reducing hypoxic respiratory drive, as hypoxic cardiac arrest is a far more important complication than problems due to hypercapnia.

Pleural effusion

Up to half of the patients undergoing cardiothoracic surgery develop pleural effusions, which may be unilateral or bilateral.[6] Internal mammary artery (IMA) harvesting is associated with a higher rate of ipsilateral pleural effusions — up to 75% of patients are affected. It is unclear whether pleurotomy at the time of IMA harvest, or using pedicled rather than skeletonised IMA increases the risk of pleural effusion. Dyspnoea, pleuritic chest pain, decreased air entry, dullness to percussion and elevated C-reactive protein, and leucocytosis suggest pleural effusion. It may be difficult to distinguish between consolidation and effusion on a chest X-ray, but a meniscus sign is suggestive of pleural effusion and an air-fluid level is diagnostic of a hydropneumothorax. If in doubt, an ultrasound will quantify the size of the effusion and locate a safe area and direction for drainage.

Small pleural effusions can be treated with increasing diuretic therapy (frusemide 40–80 mg od). Large pleural effusions (more than 3–4 cm deep on ultrasound) should be drained with a pigtail catheter if they occur late postoperatively, or a formal chest drain if they occur early because they are likely to be predominantly blood and clots. Patients with residual pleural effusions post-thoracotomy should be treated with caution because there are frequent adhesions that make drain insertion hazardous. In this situation, drains should be inserted under ultrasound guidance. The drain must be left inside until less than 100 ml drains in 24 hours.

Major Haemorrhage

Approximately 5% of the patients undergoing median sternotomy for cardiac surgery,[7] and 1–2% of those undergoing thoracotomy for lung resection surgery require re-exploration for major haemorrhage in the early postoperative period. The morbidity associated with this is substantial, due to re-sedation, re-intubation, massive transfusion, and repeat surgery. The risk factors for major haemorrhage can be classified as pre-, intra- and postoperative. The preoperative risk factors include medication such as aspirin, clopidogrel, warfarin, thrombolytics, and abciximab, bleeding diathesis, age, prior sternotomy, and infective endocarditis. The intra-operative risk factors include surgical technique, bypass causing platelet dysfunction, thrombocytopaenia and fibrinolysis, and residual heparin effect. The postoperative risk factors include dilutional coagulopathy from excessive administration of synthetic colloid or crystalloid, massive transfusion with red cells, hypothermia, and uncontrolled hypertension.

Mediastinal bleeding is normally greatest in the hours immediately following surgery, tailing off to near zero over 6–12 hours. While bleeding varies depending on a number of peri-operative factors, the acceptable rates of bleeding are up to 2 ml/kg/hour for the first 2–3 hours, up to 1 ml/kg/hour for the next three hours and less than 0.5 ml/kg/hour by the end of 12 hours post-closure. Excessive haemorrhage refers to mediastinal drainage outside these parameters. In the presence of haemodynamic instability suggesting ongoing loss that is not confirmed by excessive mediastinal drainage, a chest X-ray may reveal a large haemothorax.

If bleeding is torrential, or the patient is haemodynamically unstable, an emergency resternotomy is indicated. Otherwise, the priority is volume replacement and identification and correction of any coagulopathy. Blood is the logical choice to replace on-going blood loss. A colloid is given to maintain mean arterial pressures of 70–75 mm Hg, and central venous pressures of 8–10 mmHg. Platelets are administered to maintain the platelet count at $>100^9$/L or higher if the patient was on preoperative anti-platelet medication including aspirin or clopidogrel. Protamine should be given to counter-act any residual heparin effect, FFP to correct elevated APTT or APTR at approximately 5–10 ml/kg, and cryoprecipitate to achieve fibrinogen levels of 1–2 mg/L (10 bags will raise fibrinogen by about 0.6 mg/L).

It is important to avoid hypothermia; infusion warmers should be used where large volumes of cold fluid are being administered. The patient's core temperature must be maintained at 37°C because hypothermia sup-presses coagulation mechanism and platelet function. Hypertension must be controlled with adequate sedation and intravenous glyceryl trinitrate (GTN) infusions. Pethidine is used to treat shivering. Urgent resternotomy should be considered if the bleeding rate does not taper after the coagulopathy is treated, for over 400 ml blood loss in one hour, or if the total mediastinal drainage is greater than 2 L.

Complications of Thoracic Incisions

Currently, the advantages of conventional sternotomy and thoracotomy far outweigh the disadvantages. These incisions provide excellent access to all areas of the chest wall, pleural cavity and mediastinum, facilitating cardiac and aortic surgery as well as major pulmonary resection. They are readily extended into the neck and abdominal regions. The complications associated with thoracic incisions are listed in Table 1.

Deep sternal wound infection

The Centre for Disease Control and Prevention defines deep sternal wound infection (DSWI) as infection involving tissue deep to the subcutaneous lay-ers accompanied by positive cultures, macroscopic or histological evidence, symptomatology or pus.[8] Its incidence is reported in 0–5% with an asso-ciated mortality of up to 50%.[6] Because up to 75% of wound infection is present after discharge from hospital, the incidence of DSWI is frequently underreported. The risk factors may be classified as pre-, intra- and postoper-ative. The preoperative risk factors include age, diabetes, obesity, smoking, steroid therapy, and COPD. The intraoperative risk factors include para-median sternotomy, bilateral pedicled mammary artery harvest, prolonged surgery, and poor surgical technique (including excessive bone wax and cautery

Table 1.   Complications of Thoracic Incisions

Incision	Complications
All major thoracic incisions	Immediate • Respiratory Compromise • Trauma to underlying viscera, and neurovascular structures Early • major haemorrhage, requiring resternotomy/rethoracotomy • Superficial wound infection Late • Chronic pain syndromes, scarring
Median sternotomy	Immediate • Brachial plexus, phrenic nerve injury Early • Deep sternal wound infection, mediastinitis • Sternal dehiscence Late • Chronic osteomyelitis • sternal instability • Incisional hernia • Prominent sternal wires requiring removal • Keloid, hypertrophic scarring
Posterolateral thoracotomy	Immediate • Major air leak, pneumothorax • Brachial plexus and peripheral nerve injury Early • Prolonged air leak, effusion • Deep wound infection, empyema Late • Seroma • Chronic pain, paraesthesia • Herniation lung

Table 1.   (*Continued*)

Incision	Complications
Anterior thoracotomy	Immediate
	• Respiratory Compromise
	Early
	• Wound infection, empyema
	Late
	• Chronic pain, paraesthesia
Thoracoabdominal	
Mediastinoscopy	Immediate
	• Injury to neck vessels, thyroid, trachea
	• Laryngeal nerve palsy
	• Wound infection
VATS	Immediate
	• Trauma to intercostal neurovascular bundle, underlying lung
	• Brachial plexus injury
	• Major air leak
	• Conversion to conventional thoracotomy
	Early
	• Wound infection
	Late
	• Port site recurrence
	• Port site herniation
Redo incision	As for individual incision but with greatly increased risk of trauma to underlying structures, and major haemorrhage

to the periosteum, inaccurate placement of sternal wires and poor aseptic technique). The postoperative risk factors include re-sternotomy for bleeding, multiple transfusions, mediastinal bleeding, prolonged ventilation and impaired nutrition.

The main diagnostic criteria are fever, leucocytosis, positive blood cultures, and serous or purulent discharge from the wound or wound dehiscence. A sternal "click" (palpable movement in the sternum on coughing, or shaking the head) suggests sternal instability, which is frequently associated with infection in the early postoperative period. A pericardial effusion in the presence of sepsis may suggest mediastinitis. A chest X-ray may show fractured or migrating sternal wires, and a CT may reveal non-union, retrosternal pus, osteomyelitis, and in severe cases, a pericardial effusion.

The prevention of DSWI is important, and there are several aspects to prophylaxis. The preoperative measures include weight reduction in obese patients, reducing steroid therapy as far as possible, optimising respiratory function, screening for and treating methicillin-resistant *Staphylococcus aureus* (MRSA). Shaving patients in the anaesthetic room instead of the night before on the ward results in lower numbers of skin organisms. The operative measures include meticulous aseptic and operative technique; excessive cautery to the sternal periosteum and the application of bone wax must be avoided. Leg and sternal wound instruments should be maintained separately because sharing increases the incidence of *E. coli* sternal wound infection. Postoperatively, appropriate antibiotic prophylaxis (normally three doses of a broad spectrum cephalosporin) are administered, with one dose given on induction to ensure peak blood levels by the time of incision. Hygiene is extremely important postoperatively, and washing hands between patients is mandatory (alcohol rinse has been shown to be more effective than soap and water at reducing cross-infection).

A cough lock may reduce pain and the acute impact of dehiscence. Intravenous antibiotics should be started early, as soon as wound and blood cultures have been taken, and adjusted to bacterial sensitivities. Vacuum dressing has been shown to reduce the risk of a DSWI developing into mediastinitis. Surgical debridement and rewiring may be necessary, and is never undertaken lightly. Patients may have multiple organ dysfunction as a result of sepsis, and friable tissue, and surgery often takes place when adhesions are maximal (4–6 weeks postoperatively). The principles are the same as for elective re-sternotomy. The patient must be administered appropriate antibiotics on induction. Devitalised tissue is debrided back to bleeding margins, including the sternal edges, which should be undermined sufficiently to place sternal wires. All pus is evacuated from the pericardium, while paying great care to the anastomotic lines, since they may be involved in infection. Pus and bone must be sent for culture to guide the treatment and detect osteomyelitis. Where primary closure cannot be achieved due to multiple extensive debridements, the options include pectoralis major advancement flaps, transrectus abdominus muscle (TRAM) flaps and rarely omental flaps; plastic surgeons should be involved. There are many alternative primary closures, such as standard closure, betadine washout, Robicek closure, sternal bands, irrigation systems, mass sutures and none have been proved superior.

Superficial wound infection

The Centre for Disease Control and Prevention defines superficial wound infection (SWI) as infection involving only the skin and subcutaneous tissue along with purulent drainage, positive cultures, or symptoms.[8] The incidence of superficial sternal wound infection is about 3–5%, superficial saphenous vein harvest site infection, up to 25%, and superficial radial wound harvest site infection, about 5%. The diagnosis is usually based on local cellulitis or discharge. Wound swabs and blood should be sent for culture.

An SWI can normally be managed conservatively. Broad-spectrum antibiotics are started empirically and adjusted as soon as bacterial sensitivities are known. Sternal and radial artery wound infections are most commonly caused by Gram-positive organisms, while leg wound infections are caused predominantly by Gram-negative organisms. A minority of cases may present superficial collections of pus, and any fluctuant areas should be incised and drained. Deeper wounds, including superficial collections that have been incised and drained, or those producing large volumes of exudate should be treated with a vacuum dressing until they become superficial areas of granulation tissue. The patient should be aggressively monitored for any signs of DSWI.

Sternal instability and sterile dehiscence

Sterile sternal instability and dehiscence, which has an incidence of 1–2%, is usually due to poor surgical technique, or "cheese-wiring" of the sternal wires through a soft, osteoporotic sternum.[6] The patient complains of excessive chostochondral pain and "clicking" on movement, and instability may be palpated when the patient coughs. These may be managed either conservatively with prophylactic antibiotics and support dressings, or with elective sternal rewiring. If it does not become infected, an unstable sternum eventually forms a cartilaginous flexible union or pseudoarthrosis. An unstable sternum is a risk factor for prolonged ventilation and chest infections in the postoperative period.

Sternal dehiscence

sternal dehiscence presents similarly to abdominal wound dehiscence with serosanguinous discharge from the wound 3–5 days postoperatively and an increase in the white cell count, usually preceding the sudden opening up of the wound on coughing or straining. The patient should be helped back into bed, reassured and given appropriate opiate analgesia. The wound should be covered with sterile saline soaked gauze, and the swabs sent for culture. Most patients should be taken back to the theatre for debridement and re-wiring. Occasionally, if wires have cheese-wired through soft sternums in patients with major comorbidity, management is with vacuum dressings and cough-locks.

Hypertrophic and Keloid scars

Midline incisions have a tendency to form raised, red hypertrophic scars. Keloid scars (where the lumpy scar tissue exceeds the margin of the scar) are commonest in patients of African descent. There is no known way of avoiding these unsightly scars, apart from attempting to minimise the length of the sternotomy incision, or considering submammary incisions. Topical silicone gel dressings worn every day for several months will reduce the prominence of hypertrophic scars, but they can relapse when the dressings are abandoned. Keloid scars do not respond to surgical excision, but referral to a plastic surgeon is indicated if the patient is unhappy with the cosmetic result, as steroid injections may offer some improvement.

sternal wires

Sometimes patients, especially if they are very thin, complain of prominent sternal wires. If the sternum is stable, these wires may be removed, under a general anaesthetic with appropriate monitoring because of the risk of unexpected re-sternotomy. If the patient is unhappy with just one or two wires mark them with the patient preoperatively, and remove through stab incisions.

Incisional hernias

Approximately 5% of median sternotomy incisions are complicated by incisional hernias,[9] usually located in the linear alba below the xiphoid process. The preoperative risk factors include obesity, malnutrition and COPD. The intraoperative factors include failure to approximate the edges of the rectus muscle and sheath, and the use of absorbable sutures. The postoperative factors include wound infection, pulmonary complications and constipation associated with straining. The diagnosis is clinical, usually in the out-patient clinic, a few months to years later; the hernia appears as a soft midline swelling that is reducible, reappearing on coughing or standing erect. They are usually painless although large hernias may be associated with a dragging sensation. Any change in bowel habit, local tenderness, irreducibility or colicky abdominal pain, nausea and vomiting are suggestive of incarcerated bowel, and the hernia should be treated as a surgical emergency. Incisional hernias should normally be repaired to prevent sequelae, such as bowel obstruction. The margins of the linea alba should be identified, and the hernia sac mobilised and reduced entirely. The linea alba should then be repaired with non-absorbable sutures or a mesh, such as marlex or gore-tex.

Incisional lung hernias are rare, but their exact incidence is unknown because of the diagnostic challenge that they present. They occur as a result of dehiscence from a thoracotomy incision, or failure to approximate the intercostal muscles and ribs. Anterior herniation is more common than posterior because the rib spaces are wider, and the chest musculature is less well developed. The diagnostic features include pain along the distribution of the affected intercostal nerves, which may be difficult to distinguish from intercostal neuralgia. The hernia is almost spongy to palpation and maximal during Valsalva manoeuvres, and CT is normally diagnostic. Lung hernias less than 5 cm in size, which are minimally symptomatic may be managed conservatively. Larger, symptomatic hernias, or those increasing in size should be repaired. The treatment options include mobilising the dehisced muscle layers with primary reapposition, flaps based on muscle, fascia or periosteum, and prosthetic material such as gore-tex or marlex mesh.

Peripheral nerve injuries

Brachial plexus injury

This is caused indirectly by sternal retraction, and directly by trauma while placing central lines. It can also be due to excessive traction on the upper arm while positioning the patient for posterolateral thoracotomy and VATS procedures. Branchial plexus injury presents as paraesthesia and weakness in the C8–T1, and in severe cases, in the C6–C7 distribution. The formal diagnosis is by electromyogram (EMG) studies. It can be avoided by placing the sternal retractor as caudally as possible and opening it slowly. The treatment involves physiotherapy, with referral to a pain service for chronic pain which does not respond to analgesia.

Horner's syndrome

Horner's syndrome comprises ptosis, meiosis, anyhydrosis and enopthalmosis resulting from damage to the sympathetic nerve supply to the eye, at any stage in its journey from the central nuclei and spinal cord to post-ganglionic fibres via the stellate ganglion. Inadvertent damage during central line placement, carotid endarterectomy, harvest of the proximal IMA, damage to the stellate ganglion during sympathectomy, and stroke are some of the causes of this syndrome. Its treatment is symptomatic.

Recurrent laryngeal nerve palsy

This may occur as a result of IMA harvesting, trauma to the arch of the aorta, e.g. from cannulating or during aortic arch surgery, trauma to the nerve in the neck from internal jugular vein cannulation, pressure injury from a malpositioned endotracheal cuff, and cold injury. It presents as hoarseness and breathlessness after extubation, and patients should be examined by an ENT surgeon.

Phrenic nerve palsy

This is discussed below.

Sympathetic dystrophy (radial and saphenous nerves)

Injury to these nerves when harvesting conduit may result in paraesthesia (over the anatomical snuff box in radial nerve injury and over the medial malleolus and ankle in saphenous nerve injury). Occasionally it is associated with increasing pain, swelling and trophic changes (hair loss, shiny skin). Sympathetic dystrophy is difficult to treat; it may respond to NSAIDs such as ibuprofen, regular analgesia, or amitryptilline for intractable neuropathic pain.

Ulnar nerve injury

The failure to protect the arms with padding, intra-operatively may lead to ulnar nerve paresis from pressure injury to the nerve as it passes around the medial epicondyle of the elbow.

2. COMPLICATIONS OF CARDIAC SURGERY

Complications Post-cardiotomy

Low cardiac output

A satisfactory cardiac output is the aim of postoperative cardiovascular management. Cardiac output is the volume of blood ejected by the heart per minute and is equal to heart rate multiplied by stroke volume (the volume of blood ejected by the heart per beat). Cardiac index is the cardiac output adjusted to take into account the size of the patient, and is a more accurate reflection of the cardiac function. If cardiac output measurements are available (pulmonary artery catheter or transoesophageal Doppler) a cardiac index of $>2.5 \, l/min/m^2$ is satisfactory. In its absence, a mean arterial pressure of 70–80 mmHg, with a urine output of 1 ml/kg/hour, base deficit of <2, skin temperature of 36.5–37.5°C, and palpable pedal pulses (if present preoperatively) mean that the cardiac index is greater than $2.5 \, l/min/m^2$. The causes of low cardiac output and hypoperfusion states can be classified as causes of reduced stroke volume, and reduced heart rate (outlined in the section on arrhythmias).

The stroke volume depends on preload, afterload and contractility. Preload is a measure of the wall tension in the left ventricle at the end of diastole, but is difficult to quantify directly. Central venous pressure (CVP), pulmonary artery wedge pressure (PAWP), and left atrial pressure (LAP) (sometimes referred to as "filling pressures") are indirect measures of preload. The preload can be optimised by administering a colloid to increase it or looping diuretics to decrease it, aiming for an RAP of 12–16, a PAWP of 10–14, or an LAP of 12–16. Patients with chronic mitral regurgitation, and hypertrophied ventricles (aortic stenosis, mitral stenosis, HOCM) require higher filling pressures, occasionally greater than 20 mm Hg. Excessive preload is deleterious for a number of reasons: it increases ventricular wall tension which exacerbates ischaemia as myocardial oxygen demand is increased and myocardial perfusion is decreased, and leads to pulmonary oedema, splanchnic congestion and potentially cerebral oedema. The failure of filling pressures to rise with adequate volume may be due to vasodilatation or capillary leak. It is sometimes necessary to vasoconstrict a patient with a small amount of noradrenaline (4 mg in 250 ml of 5% dextrose at 0.03–0.06 mcg/kg/min) to achieve a satisfactory preload.

Afterload is a measure of the left ventricle wall tension during systole. It is determined by preload, which establishes the maximum 'stretch', and the resistance against which the heart must eject, which is a function of systemic vascular resistance (SVR), vascular compliance, mean arterial pressure, and any left ventricular outflow tract pressure gradient. SVR, which usually reflects the amount of peripheral vasoconstriction, is a commonly used indirect measurement of afterload. Excessively high or low afterload is deleterious. Patients with good cardiac outputs (CI > 2.5) and hypotension as a result of peripheral vasodilatation are treated with vasoconstrictors such as noradrenaline (4 mg in 50ml at a rate of 0.03–0.3 mcg/kg/min). The afterload is raised in the hypovolaemic patient because of reflex vasoconstriction; it may be corrected with careful volume infusion. Hypothermia is a common cause of raised SVR postoperatively. The patient has to be kept warm using blankets, and infusion warmers, if large volume transfusions are required. A variety of vasodilators can be used to lower the SVR: GTN (200 mg in 250 ml at a rate of 1–20 ml/hour) is commonly used in most units as it has a beneficial effect on myocardial perfusion, in addition to peripheral vasculature; SNP is a particularly potent vasodilator that is reserved as a second line adjunct in the control of hypertension, because its beneficial effect on myocardial perfusion is not as high as GTN. There are a number of inotropes with vasodilatory properties that reduce the afterload. These are milrinone, dopexamine, dobutamine and dopamine in decreasing order of ability to reduce the afterload and they should be considered in the context of low cardiac output.

Contractility is a measure of the strength of myocardial contraction at a given preload and afterload. The mean arterial pressure and cardiac output are the commonly used indirect measures of contractility. Compliance is a measure of the distensibility of the left ventricle in diastole, with stiff, hypertrophied ventricles having low compliance. Left centricular end-diastolic pressure (LVEDP), which may be measured at preoperative cardiac catheterisation or estimated by preoperative echo, is an indirect measure of compliance. Contractility can be increased through two mechanisms. The fast acting mechanism is important in clinical practice, and involves an increase in Ca^{2+} uptake by myocytes. This occurs through increased stimulation of α_1 and β_1 adrenergic receptors, or via direct effect on electrolyte concentrations. The second process is less important in immediate postoperative care as it takes place over several weeks, and results in up-regulation of ATP-ase receptors, which has a similar effect on myocyte electrolyte concentration gradients. Positive inotropes include sympathetic nerve stimulation (both mechanisms), adrenaline (α_1 and β_1 adrenergic agonist), noradrenaline (weaker α_1 and β_1 adrenergic agonist), dopamine (weaker α_1 and β_1 adrenergic agonist), dobutamine (very weak α_1 and stronger β_1 adrenergic agonist), ephedrine (weak α_1 and β_1 adrenergic agonist), metaraminol (strong α_1 and weak β_1 adrenergic agonist), enoximone and milrinone (increases Ca^{2+} influx by inhibiting inactivation cAMP), digoxin (inhibits Na/K ATPase to raise intracellular Ca^{2+}), calcium (increases Ca^{2+} influx).

Cardiac tamponade

Tamponade may present as acute haemodynamic compromise within hours of surgery as a result of mediastinal bleeding, or insidiously days to weeks after surgery. Occasionally patients present with acute symptoms following the removal of epicardial pacing wires, or mediastinal drains. This is characterised by progressive hypotension (often present despite increasing inotrope administration), tachycardia (in patients that have not been administered β-blockers), raised CVP, and pulsus paradoxus. The patient may be confused, and show signs of peripheral shut down. Hypotension normally results in oliguria, and subsequent symptoms of fluid overload and renal impairment. Non-specific signs include muffled heart sounds and pericardial rub. Most patients have small pericardial effusions postoperatively which normally resolve without causing cardiac tamponade. In about 5% of patients these effusions increase in size, and may cause tamponade. Late tamponade, caused by a chronic bleed, late rupture of suture lines or pericarditis, may present with ill-defined symptoms such as malaise, lethargy, chest discomfort, and anorexia with or without the classical findings of acute tamponade. A postero-anterior chest X-ray may reveal an enlarged cardiac silhouette. Echocardiography is diagnostic; trans-oesophageal echocardiography has much greater sensitivity and specificity than trans-thoracic.[10] The location of the effusion and the depth (in cm) should be described. Anything greater than 2 cm is significant, although large chronic effusions may not cause tamponade, while small acute ones may. Cardiac tamponade is present if there is right ventricular diastolic collapse. The patient may be resuscitated with volume and inotropes as a temporizing measure. The definitive management is re-exploration, which may be through a sub-xihphoid approach with TOE guidance to confirm that the entire effusion has been drained, or under direct vision through a re-sternotomy.

Pericarditis

Pericarditis post-cardiotomy (also known as post-pericardiotomy and Dressler's syndrome) affects about 5% of patients, and is more common in young patients. It may occur within a week of surgery or be delayed by several months. The classical symptoms are constant chest pain that is sore rather than dull, pyrexia and a pericardial rub; malaise, lethargy, myalgia and arthralgia are also often present. White cell count, C-reactive protein and erythrocyte sedimentation rate are often high and pericardial and/or pleural effusions may be noted on chest radiography and echocardiography. On a 12-lead ECG, ST segments are elevated concave upwards in all leads. The symptoms are usually controlled with oral non-steroidal antiinflammatory drugs such as ibuprofen 400 mg tds for six weeks. Oral prednisolone has been used successfully in cases refractory to non-steroidal drugs. The associated pericardial effusions which develop in a minority of patients should be treated as appropriate (see below).

Pericardial effusion

In most patients, pericardial effusions occur postoperatively but resolve without causing cardiac tamponade. In about 5% of the patients these effusions increase in size. An asymptomatic pericardial effusion may be detected on a routine chest X-ray, appearing as an enlarged and globular cardiac silhouette. Echocardiography is diagnostic. If the patient is not haemodynamically compromised by cardiac tamponade these effusions may be treated by starting or increasing diuretic therapy. Hypoalbuminaemia should be corrected by addressing nutritional requirements and prescribing protein supplements or nasogastric feeding. Cardiac tamponade must be actively excluded and if present, treated aggressively.

Constrictive pericarditis

Constrictive pericarditis occurs in about 0.5% of cardiotomies, and is a late sequalae of up to half the cases with the post-cardiotomy syndrome. Over a period of few months to years, haemorrhagic pericarditis progresses to a thickened, fibrotic, frequently calcified pericardium that causes chronic cardiac tamponade. Other risk factors include mediastinal irradiation and postoperative haemopericardium. Constrictive pericarditis may be asymptomatic for years. Fatigue progresses to effort dyspnoea, hepatomegaly and ascites with peripheral oedema, and rarely, orthopnoea and paroxysmal nocturnal dyspnoea. The symptoms include increased jugular venous pressure (JVP), Kussmaul's sign, pulsus paradoxus, systolic retraction in the left parasternal region and "pericardial knock." Salt and water retention is a key feature. Calcification is present in 40% on the chest X-ray, with enlarged cardiac silhouette in 30%, while the echocardiography reveals that with inspiration the right ventricle fills supra-normally but the left underfills because of left deviation of the septum. Echocardiography will also detect thickened pericardium and pericardial effusion. Cardiac catheterisation shows equalisation of LVEDP and RVEDP, a dip plateau pattern in the ventricular filling pressure curve, and a prominent "y" descent in the JVP. Chronic constrictive pericarditis may be managed medically with diuretics. Surgical pericardiectomy has a 5-year survival rate of 65%; 5% of patients have persistent symptoms of heart failure postoperatively. The operative mortality is 2–3%.

Arrhythmias

Over a third of the patients develop supraventricular arrhythmias postoperatively, because of changes in automaticity and conduction.[11] They are an important cause of postoperative complications including low cardiac output syndrome, especially in patients with hypertrophic left ventricle or poor ventricular function, embolic stroke and other ischaemic phenomena. A number of common factors contribute to arrhythmias, and these must be rapidly excluded before instituting the specific treatments described below. The causes of arrhythmias can be classified as pre-, intra- and postoperative.

Postoperative arrhythmias are more common in older patients. Patients with pre-existing atrial fibrillation usually revert to atrial fibrillation even if their initial rhythm after bypass is sinus rhythm. Preoperative heart block and ventricular dysrhythmias are often exacerbated postoperatively. Mitral valve disease is associated with an enlarged left atrium, and this predisposes patients to atrial arrhythmias. Patients with dilated left ventricle (ischaemic cardiomyopathy, decompensated valvular heart disease), hypertrophic left ventricle (aortic stenosis, hypertensive cardiomyopathy) are more prone to ventricular dysrhythmias.

Poor intraoperative cardioprotection including ineffective cooling, inadequate cardioplegia, incomplete electromechanical arrest, and ventricular distension predispose to postoperative arrhythmias. The surgical procedure has an important role in the incidence and nature of postoperative arrhythmias. Incomplete myocardial revascularisation predisposes to postoperative ventricular and supraventricular arrhythmias. Any damage to the conduction pathways during decalcification and suturing of mitral or aortic valve annulus, atriotomy, or ventriculotomy may result in a temporary or permananent heart block. Ineffective de-airing and exclusion of debris from the circulation predisposes to arrhythmias. There is a 3–4% incidence of complete heart block requiring permanent pacemaker insertion after aortic valve replacement.

Postoperative causes of arrhythmias can be classified as cardiovascular, respiratory, electrolyte, drug and metabolic, systemic, vagal and mechanical. The cardiovascular causes include myocardial ischaemia secondary to incomplete revascularisation, coronary vasopasm, conduit kinking or occlusion, hypoxia or high myocardial oxygen demand. A failure in valve repair or prosthesis, hypovolaemia, pulmonary artery catheter, and less commonly, central venous catheter insertion, intracardiac pacing wires, endocarditis and pericarditis are also arrhythmogenic. The respiratory causes of arrhythmias include hypoxia, hypercapnia, acidosis, endotracheal tube irritation, pneumothorax, atelectasis, and pneumonia. Furthermore, hyperkalaemia, hypokalaemia, hypomagnesemia, and hypocalcaemia may exacerbate or cause arrhythmias. Drug withdrawal or toxicity, in particular β-blockers, digoxin, calcium channel blockers, bronchodilators, tricyclic antidepressants and alcohol may result in arrhythmias. Adrenaline and dopamine are particularly arrhythmogenic. The common metabolic causes of arrhythmias include hyper- and hypothyroidism, and hypoglycaemia. The systemic causes of arrhythmias include fever, hypothermia, anxiety and pain; bradycardia is common when the patient is asleep. Vagal stimulation can cause arrhythmias. The sources of vagal stimulation include nasogastric tube insertion, gastric dilation, intubation, nausea and vomiting. The mechanical causes of postoperative arrhythmias include pericardial collections, tamponade, tension pneumothorax, and rarely, cold fluids injected into right atrium via the central line.

The investigation and treatment of arrhythmias following cardiac surgery follows the same broad principles employed in general medicine and surgery. It is important to diagnose and treat the underlying reversible causes listed above. The major, potentially reversible causes of postoperative ventricular arrhythmias that must be actively detected and treated include myocardial ischaemia, and electrolyte abnormalities, particularly hypokalemia. Relative hypokalemia is a common factor: KCl infusions are given centrally to maintain serum K+ at 4.5–5.0 mmol/L. The choice of anti-arrhythmic is often dictated by ventricular function. In patients with poor left ventricular function, or who are inotrope dependent, negative inotropes such as β-blockers or amiodarone should be avoided in favour of a positive inotrope such as digoxin. Bradycardia that results in low cardiac output states and refractory to treatment of the underlying cause can be managed by using chronotropes including adrenaline, dopamine, dopexamine, isosprenaline and atropine, or appropriate pacing if epicardial wires are *in situ*.

Hypertension

Once antihypertensive infusions such as GTN and propofol are discontinued, and myocardial function recovers from the insult of surgery, blood pressure normally returns to preoperative levels. Most patients have high blood pressure preoperatively, controlled with a variety of oral medication including anti-anginals, most of which are discontinued in the peri-operative period. Hypertension develops in most patients by Day 3 postoperatively if appropriate drugs are not started. To treat it, preoperative anti-hypertensives are restarted at a lower dose. Anti-anginals such as GTN preparations, isosorbide mononitrate, or nicorandil are normally discontinued. Angiotensin converting enzyme inhibitors (ramipril 2.5–10 mg od po nocte) are routinely started in most patients for secondary prevention, and used in those with poor left ventricular function to reduce the afterload. ACE-II inhibitors (losartan 40 mg bd po) are used in patients with a problematic dry ACE-inibitor cough. ACE-inhibitors are not restarted in patients with hypotension or impaired renal function, but this can be reviewed in the outpatient environment. Patients in whom the radial artery has been used as conduit, or total arterial revascularisation has been performed are usually started on a Ca channel blocker (diltazem 60 mg tds po for six weeks) to prevent vasospasm. In patients with tachyarrhythmias and good left ventricle function, β-blockers are the first line treatment for hypertension, but Ca channel blockers can also work well.

Complications of Cardiopulmonary Bypass (CPB)

These include the complications of cannulation, namely aortic dissection, air embolism, and inferior vena cava laceration, as well as those resulting from passage of blood through the non-endothelial circuitry. Changes in temperature, acid-base balance, haemodilution, non-pulsatile flow, drugs, circulating volume and the mechanics of bypass all contribute to the dysfunction of blood constituent cascades and whole organ systems.

Aortic dissection

Aortic dissection from aortic cannulation has an incidence of about 0.3%.[12] It is usually recognised at aortic cannulation. It is characterised by intimal haematoma with bleeding at a distance from the cannula site, blood does not rise up the aortic cannula on cannulation, and blood does not flow normally on removing the tubing clamp. The patient becomes profoundly hypotensive with low right atrial pressure, ischaemic changes develop on the ECG, there is "no swing" on connecting the arterial line with the aortic cannula, there are low systemic pressures confirmed by the perfusionist and palpation, high line pressures on infusing prime via the aortic cannula, and venous return is poor. If the transoesophageal echocardiography shows a dissection flap, emergency repair of the dissection, usually with an interposition graft, is required in addition to the planned surgery. Bypass must be stopped immediately, and the venous line clamped. The aortic cannula should be placed into the right atrium so that volume can be given rapidly. The surgeon must proceed to femoral-caval bypass immediately, and occasionally, to cannulation of the distal arch. When recognised intraoperatively, the survival from aortic dissection is about 80%.[3]

IVC laceration

The IVC may be lacerated by the passage of the venous cannula, attempts at snaring the cavae, or dissection during redo surgery. Intrapericardial tears are obvious from venous haemorrhage into the pericardial sling, classically after the bypass has been terminated. Intra-abdominal tears result in poor venous return, low systemic and filling pressures, and loss of volume from the bypass circuit requiring volume replacement. The management of iatrogenic tears of the IVC during cardiac surgery is not well described. Attempts at primary repair frequently result in extending the tear, or unacceptable narrowing of the vessel, and patch repairs with pericardium or saphenous vein graft are recommended. Intra-abdominal tears pose a challenge, and endovascular stents have been used to manage it.

Air embolism

Air can enter the heart from the operative field, the pump or from anaesthetic lines. Fatal air embolism can occur from amounts as small as 0.25 ml/kg entering the left side of the heart and the coronary and cerebral circulation. Although right-sided air embolism is better tolerated in the absence of patent foramen ovale, it can lead to severe pulmonary hypertension. Surgical sources of air include aortic cannulation, cardiotomy for valve surgery, entraining air with aggressive right superior pulmonary vein venting, and entraining air from an opened left coronary artery while venting the aortic root. Air tends to collect in the left atrium, in the right superior pulmonary vein, and within the trabeculae of the left ventricle, which explains the rationale for standard de-airing techniques. Air embolism from the CPB circuit can occur if the CPB reservoir empties, and a fundamental safety principle is to maintain the volume of the reservoir by interrupting bypass if necessary. Accidental disconnects, punctures, taps open to air, oxygenator or vacuum assist malfunction can potentially result in air embolism. Treatment depends on the severity and timing. Coronary air embolism is best managed by continuing CPB, with appropriate pinching of the aorta distal to the aortic cannula to increase coronary perfusion pressures for a few minutes. Hypothermia, retrograde coronary and cerebral perfusion and de-airing procedures are useful adjuncts. Ventilating the patient with 100% oxygen and decreasing cerebral oxygen demand by packing the patient's head in ice may also help. If air embolism occurs before or after CPB with cardiac arrest, the patient must be placed with the head down in the left lateral position and CPR instituted. Drug therapy is first aimed at increasing the mean arterial pressure to "flush" air through to the venous circulation, and limit tissue damage with steroids, diuretics, antiplatelet agents, anticonvulsants and barbiturates. The surgical procedure should be completed regardless of the timing. Compression in a hyperbaric chamber and ventilation with 100% oxygen is the definitive management, but poses logistical challenges.

Cardiovascular complications

The cardiovascular system undergoes the greatest physiological stresses during both bypass and beating heart surgery. Myocardial compliance falls because of myocardial oedema, and higher filling pressures are required to generate the same stroke volume. Contractility is impaired as a result of myocardial oedema, metabolic derangements, myocardial stunning and ischaemia (caused by coronary artery and arterial conduit spasm, air and particulate emboli, manipulation of the heart post-bypass, periods of hypoperfusion during transfer and factors affecting gas exchange). Myocardial function continues to decline for 6–8 hours postoperatively as a result of ischaemia-reperfusion injury, before returning to the baseline. Hypothermia is common as it is difficult to keep up with heat loss from an open chest in the theatre. It is detrimental as it predisposes to ventricular arrythmias, coagulopathy and metabolic acidosis, and raises the afterload, thereby increasing myocardial oxygen demand. However, the high systemic vascular resistance (SVR) helps maintain mean arterial pressures until the patient is rewarmed. It is vital to ensure that adequate volume replacement and if necessary, inotropic support are provided to avoid hypotension during rewarming. Patients may "over-shoot" to temperatures above 37.5°C because of abnormalities in the central thermoregulation resulting in a pronounced peripheral vasdilatation and hypotension associated with a poorer neurological outcome. Vasodilatation and capillary leak indicate a progressive requirement for volume resuscitation to achieve satisfactory filling pressures that must be balanced against volume overloading, which has a particularly deleterious effect on the respiratory function.

Respiratory complications

In addition to pulmonary complications resulting from thoracotomy and sternotomy incisions, the pulmonary function may be further compromised by bypass. Pulmonary oedema is caused by the activation of complement[13] and sequestration of neutrophils in the pulmonary vasculature where they mediate the increase in capillary permeability, which is compounded by the fluid shifts described above. Cardiopulmonary bypass reduces the effect of natural surfactant, compounding the effects of general anaesthetic and median sternotomy that predispose to pulmonary dysfunction. It also increases shunts, reduces compliance and functional residual volume, and can cause adult respiratory distress syndrome. Other factors contributing to pulmonary problems following bypass include pre-existing pulmonary oedema, post-perfusion lung syndrome, administration of protamine, anaphylaxis (from protamine, antifibrinolytics and other drugs), intrapulmonary shunts, mechanical factors such as pneumothorax, haemothorax and obstruction of the tracheobronchial tree by blood or mucous plugs. Being supine further reduces the functional residual capacity. The fluid shift into the interstitial space, exacerbated by fluid overloading the vasodilated patient during rewarming in an attempt to maintain mean arterial pressures, further impairs oxygenation.

The administration of protamine can cause a number of adverse reactions, grouped into three main types by the Horrow classification. Type I is hypotension from rapid administration, Type II includes anaphylactic reactions, which are further subdivided into IIa or true anaphylaxis, IIb or immediate anaphylactoid, and IIc or delayed anaphylactoid reactions, and Type III comprising catastrophic pulmonary vasoconstriction.

Renal complications

Cardiopulmonary bypass results in major changes in fluid distribution and renal function, moderated by pharmacological agents employed primarily for haemodynamic support. The importance of correct fluid management cannot be overstated: it is the difference between a satisfactory postoperative course and one complicated by multi-system failure. Most patients arrive in the ICU in a state of total body sodium and water overload, which becomes more pronounced with the additional volume given as the patient warms and vasodilates, even though the patient may have a relatively depleted intravascular volume. Haemodilution, microemboli, catecholamines, low perfusion pressure, diuretics, hypothermia, aprotinin and haemolysis impair the renal function. Acute renal impairment has an incidence of 5–10% following bypass while impairment requiring new dialysis has an incidence of 0.5%.[14]

Central nervous system complications

Neurological disorders following cardiac surgery have been categorised into Type I (cerebral death, non-fatal stroke, new transient ischaemic attack) and Type II (new intellectual deterioration or seizures).[15] The incidence of major neurological events ranges from 1–5% postoperatively, and is associated with increased mortality and morbidity. Type II neurocognitive dysfunction is more common than Type I, with evidence suggesting its incidence to be as high as 60% depending on the testing method used.

The risk factors for stroke include age (in patients >80 years the risk of cerebrovascular accident (CVA) is 5–10% compared to under 1% in patients under 65 years without other risk factors), diabetes, previous history of stroke or transient ischaemic attack (increases risk threefold), carotid artery atherosclerosis, perioperative hypotension, calcified ascending aorta and aortic valve, left sided mural thrombus, cardiotomy, long duration of cardiopulmonary bypass, postoperative atrial fibrillation and failure to administer postoperative antiplatelet therapy.

The causes of stroke can be broadly divided into embolic, haemorrhagic, hypoxic and hypoperfusion. The embolic causes include microemboli, debris from the operative field, mural thrombus, debris from valve excision, particularly calcified aortic valve, septic emboli from endocarditis, trauma to the aorta from cannulation and clamping, air embolism, and carotid atheroma. Cerebral haemorrhage occasionally results from heparinisation on bypass and postoperative warfarinisation. Cerebral hypoperfusion may result from carotid and vertebral artery stenosis, dissection, hypotension, circulatory arrest (long period or insufficient cooling), and raised intra-cranial pressure. Stroke may result from profound hypoxia before, during or after bypass.

The single most important preoperative intervention is to identify significant carotid artery disease. All patients with a previous history of stroke or transient ischaemic attack (TIA), or with a carotid bruit should undergo duplex ultrasonography of the carotids. Some surgeons duplex all patients over the age of 80, or those with severe extra-cardiac arteriopathy. The risk of stroke from carotid endarerectomy is 3.5%, and from cardiac surgery following endarterectomy is 4%.[16] Patients with a stenosis of their internal carotid artery of <75% have a greater risk of stroke from carotid endarterectomy than from cardiac surgery alone, and their carotid disease should be left untreated. Patients with a stenosis of >75% but <99% of their internal carotid artery, and a history of TIA or stroke have a lower risk of stroke if they undergo carotid endarterectomy (or stenting in suitable subjects). While stenting is performed before surgery, carotid endarterectomy before cardiac surgery carries a perioperative risk of myocardial infarction (MI) of 5–7%, and after cardiac surgery, carries a 5–7% risk of perioperative cerebrovascular accident (CVA). The operative technique measures include a careful selection of aortic cannulation sites. This can be guided by an intraoperative ultrasound of the ascending aorta, which identifies diseased plaques at risk of embolisation, and is much more accurate than digital palpation. Meticulous removal of debris from the operative field in open heart (especially aortic valve) surgery, exclusion or air from all arterial lines, and thorough de-airing is a key part of stroke prevention. "No touch" technique in coronary artery bypass grafting has been shown to reduce stroke rates to <1%.[17] Systemic cooling provides additional cerebral protection. Limiting the use of pump suction reduces microemboli. Postoperative preventive measures include routine aspirin (and clopidogrel after carotid endarterectomy) and blood pressure control.

The aim is to establish a definitive diagnosis, a cause to guide appropriate secondary prevention, and a baseline of function to help plan long-term rehabilitation, or withdrawal of therapy. A full neurological examination (cognitive function, cranial nerves, and tone, power, reflexes and sensation in all four limbs) must be carried out. Modern contrast head CT will show infarcts within two hours (older scanners may not pick up lesions until they are 2–3 days old). It is important to distinguish between haemorrhagic and ischaemic CVA (one in 10 are hemorrhagic) as the management of each is entirely different. MRI is necessary to image brainstem lesions. Haemorrhagic stroke (including subarachnoid and subdural haemorrhage and intracranial bleeds) should be suspected if there is a history of head injury, or major coagulopathy. CT confirmation of diagnosis should be obtained urgently because early neurosurgical management may be indicated. If the patient is being war-farinised for a mechanical valve prosthesis, the risk of causing an embolic event by reversing anticoagulation (with Vit. K, FFP or clotting factors) is less than 0.02% for each day that the patient is not anticoagulated.[18] The risk of re-bleeding is greatest within the first 24 hours; anticoagulation should be stopped, and coagulopathy corrected. It can be restarted within 1–2 weeks if the patient is stable. Cardiothoracic patients are not candidates for thrombolysis. Antiplatelet therapy reduces the risk of a serious vascular event in high-risk patients by a quarter, the risk of non-fatal myocardial infarction by one third, and non-fatal cerebrovascular event by one quarter.[19]

Gastrointestinal complications

Serious gastrointestinal complications occur in 1–2% of patients following cardiac surgery. Peptic ulceration is a response to stress, not CPB *per se*. The increased permeability of gut mucosa leads to endotoxin translocation adding to the inflammatory response, and pancreatitis and mild jaundice are not uncommon. Gut ischaemia may be caused by emboli or hypoperfusion. About a quarter of patients develop mild hepatic dysfunction. Fulminant hepatic failure occurs in 0.1%.

Activation of blood constituents

Plasma protein systems

CPB activates five plasma protein systems: the contact system, the intrinsic and extrinsic coagulation pathways, and the complement and fibrinolytic cascades.[20] When blood encounters the non-endothelialised surfaces of the CPB circuit and the operative field, plasma proteins are instantly adsorbed onto the surface to produce a protein layer that varies with the material and the duration of exposure. A dynamic is established between the circulating and adsorbed proteins. Heparin-coated circuits change the reactivity of adsorbed proteins but do not reduce thrombogenicity. The contact system (factors XII, XI, prekalikrein and kinogen) is activated by non-endothelial surfaces, which in turn activates the intrinsic coagulation pathway, the complement pathway and neutrophils. Activated factor XI initiates the intrinsic coagulation pathway, which eventually converts prothrombin to thrombin, and fibrinogen to fibrin providing a major stimulus to coagulation during bypass. Tissue factor produced by the damaged tissue surfaces of the wound triggers the extrinsic coagulation pathway by activating Factor VII. Factor XIIa, produced by the contact pathway, activates C1 of the classic complement pathway, augmented by the alternative complement pathway that predominates during CPB, to produce anaphylotoxins. These increase capillary permeability, alter the vasomotor tone, impair cardiac function, activate neutrophils, mast cells and platelets, and mediate cell and platelet lysis. Thrombin produced by the activation of the coagulation cascade stimulates endothelial cells to produce tissue plasminogen activator, which cleaves plasminogen to plasmin resulting in progressive fibrinolysis.

Cellular systems

CPB activates five cellular systems, which mediate systemic inflammation.[20] Platelet activation via the glycoprotein IIb/IIIa receptor complex by heparin, thrombin, complement, plasmin, platelet activating factor, hypothermia and adrenaline results in a decrease in platelet numbers and function, and is a major cause of postoperative bleeding. Although dilution decreases neutrophil counts during CPB, activation by complement, kallikrein, Factor XIIa, and interleukin 1B results in their accumulation in the lungs where they mediate increased capillary permeability and interstitial oedema. Monocytes are activated more slowly than other cellular elements by complement, endotoxins and contact with the CPB circuitry, producing tissue factor, cytokines and conjugating with platelets. Lymphocytes including B-lymphocytes, natural killer cells, and T-helper cells are collectively reduced by CPB, reducing γ-interferon production, phagocytosis and the response to infection for days. Endothelial cells do not circulate, but produce tPA in response to circulating thrombin, activating the fibrinolytic pathway.

Haemostatic complications

Bleeding and thrombotic complications associated with CPB are related to activation of platelets and plasma proteins, protamine and heparin. Bleeding times do not return to normal for 4–12 hours following bypass. Disseminated intravascular coagulation (DIC), and heparin-induced thrombocytopaenis (HIT) and thrombosis (HITT) are rare complications from heparinisation for bypass. Anti-fibrinolytics such as aprotinin have been used to reduce bleeding postoperatively.

Endocrine complications

The combined stressors of surgery, hypothermia, CPB, and non-pulsatile flow trigger a hormonal stress response. The levels of cortisol, adrenaline and noradrenaline rise during bypass and along with blood glucose, remain in this elevated state for at least 24 hours. Circulating T3 falls below the normal range. The release of numerous vasoactive substances in addition to those described above, results in "physiological and biochemical chaos".

Complications of Coronary Artery Bypass Surgery

Myocardial ischaemia

Myocardial ischaemia following cardiac surgery may be caused by several factors. The technical reasons include incomplete revascularisation (less common now due to increased surgical experience), and conduit kinking, which results from grafts left too long or oriented poorly. Vasopasm of coronary arteries, or arterial conduits may occur spontaneously or as a response to vasoconstrictors such as noradrenaline. Early graft thrombosis suggests a technical problem; grafts that are kinked, under tension because they are too short, or were traumatised during harvesting are more prone to thrombosis. Its causes include the failure to administer standard anti-platelet medication postoperatively, and rarely a hypercoagulable state. Endarterctomised vessels are more prone to thrombosis than vessels with an intact endothelium. In coronary steal an unligated large first intercostal "steals" the flow from the left internal mammary artery, and this phenomenon is a debatable cause of postoperative ischaemia. Trauma to native coronaries at or near the annulus during valve surgery may result in occlusion from a proximal dissection, thrombus, embolus or obstruction of the coronary ostia by the valve strut. Hypotension, dysrhythmia, hypoxaemia, and profound anaemia are systemic causes of myocardial ischaemia.

The history, particularly of chest discomfort brought on by exertion and relieved by GTN, must be recorded. If radial artery grafts were used, the patient should be prescribed Ca channel blockers. Physiotherapists may report bradycardia on exercising. A 12-lead ECG will confirm the presence of myocardial ischaemia. Cardiac enzymes (CK^{MB} and Troponin I and T) are normally raised postoperatively, but serial measurements showing a continued rise suggest ongoing myocardial damage. Echocardiography may show new regional wall abnormalities in the territory of the affected coronary artery. The definitive investigation is cardiac catheterisation to identify coronary obstruction.

Medical treatment is the mainstay in patients with poor native vessels where incomplete revascularisation was the only viable surgical strategy and there is no evidence that grafts have occluded acutely. Such patients should be restarted on an infusion of GTN, and administered aspirin. Preoperative anti-anginal medication should be restarted. In patients with ischaemic changes refractory to medical management, without percutaneous or surgical revascularisation strategy the insertion of an intra-aortic balloon pump should be considered. The indications for emergency angiography should be discussed with a cardiologist.

Perioperative myocardial infarction

Primary MI is defined as either ST segment elevation, or raised troponin accompanying symptoms suggestive of acute coronary syndrome. While acute graft occlusion causes postoperative infarcts, up to 80% of post-operative infarcts are supplied by patent grafts.[22] In these cases, the causes of infarction include incomplete revascularisation, inadequate myocardial protection, emboli and vasospasm. Perioperative MI is difficult to diagnose because the patient may be unable to provide an adequate history, or distinguish between cardiac and non-cardiac chest pain, and because cardiac enzymes are usually raised postoperatively. Postoperative ECG contain many non-specific changes, and the new heart block may mask the ST segment changes. MI is suggested by haemodynamic compromise associated with ST segment elevation, new Q waves (new T wave inversion is a common finding in postoperative ECGs) and a significant increase in CK^{MB} or troponin beyond usual postoperative levels. Echocardiography may show new regional wall abnormalities in the territory of the affected coronary artery. Management options are the same as those outlined for myocardial ischaemia, but reflect the fact that this group of patients may be extremely unwell and at risk of multi-system failure. Freedom from MI is 94% at five years, and 73% at 15 years.

Late recurrent angina, MI and reintervention

Angina recurs in 40% of the patients by 10 years postoperatively.[23] The highest rates of recurrence are at three months, related to incomplete revascularisation and early graft occlusion, and three years, because of the progression of coronary disease and graft stenosis. Patients who experience recurrent angina, however, have similar survival rates to those that remain symptom free. The use of the left internal mammary artery (LIMA) as a conduit results in much better long-term graft patency rate which correlates to improved freedom from symptoms. Non-risk-adjusted freedom from reintervention following coronary artery bypass grafts (CABG) is 97% after five years, 89% at 10 years, and 72% at 15 years. Vein graft atherosclerosis is the commonest cause of reintervention, followed by progression of native vessel disease. Increased use of LIMA to LAD (left anterior descending) anastomoses has reduced the frequency of reoperation and lengthened the interval between the first and the second coronary operation. The other main risk factor for reoperation is younger age.

Postoperative progression of native vessel disease

The high-grade stenoses in native vessels tend to progress whether they are proximal or distal to the anastomoses.[25] In contrast, low grade stenoses distal to the anastomoses do not do so, although some evidence suggests that the opposite is true if the graft is non-functioning. In non-grafted arteries, 25–50% of lesser stenosis progress within five years.[25] In vessels that were disease free at the time of reoperation, new lesions will be detected in 15% at five years.[26]

Complications of Valve Surgery

The incidence of specific complications varies according to prosthesis type (see Table 2).

Infective endocarditis

Infective endocarditis complicates 0.2–0.5% of mechanical valve replacements within 30 days of surgery, 2% at five years and 1% per annum thereafter.[27] The figures for tissue valves are similar, but slightly less at 30 days. A septic screen consisting of blood, urine, sputum, and wound swabs for culture should be carried out in any valve patient with a temperature greater than 37.5°C more than three days postoperatively. The standard advice regarding antibiotic prophylaxis for invasive procedures should be adhered to from the first day following surgery and not just after discharge: for example, bladder catheterisation should be covered by one dose of gentamicin 120 mg im. Any potential

Table 2.   Overview of the Complications of Valve Surgery

Complication	Mechanical Valve	Bioprosthetic Valve
Infective endocarditis	0.5% within 30 days, 2% at five years	0.2% within 30 days, 2% at five years
Prosthesis failure	Negligible	Aortic 30% at 15 years, mitral 60% at 15 years
Bleeding problems	7% of patients will have a major bleeding episode p.a. Mortality 1.3% p.a. Thrombosis: 95% of cases	If on aspirin, patients over 65 years have 0.2–0.4% incidence of GI bleeding at five years Thrombosis: 5% of cases
Heart block	13% transient, 2% permanent, uncommon in MVR	13% transient, 2% permanent, uncommon in MVR
CVA and death	No difference	No difference

source of bacteraemia should be treated aggressively, because infective endo-carditis can result from venflon cellulitis, superficial wound infections, urinary and respiratory tract infections and most commonly, from infections related to arterial and central venous catheters. The Duke criteria are 95% specific with a 92% negative predictive value.[7]

Duke diagnostic criteria for infective endocarditis

Definite: 2 major OR 1 major + 3 minor OR 5 minor
Possible: 1 major + 1 minor OR 3 minor

Major criteria

Blood culture (*Strep. viridans, Strep. bovis*, HACEK, *Staph. aureus, enterococci* with no primary focus from two separate cultures OR persistent positive cul-tures > 12 hours apart OR all three or majority of four separate cultures positive drawn over the space of > 1 hour).

Echocardiographic evidence: Oscillating intracardiac mass in the absence of alternative explanation OR abscess OR new regurgitant lesion OR new partial dehiscence of prosthetic valve.

Minor criteria

Predisposition/fever >38°C/embolic phenomena/blood culture or echocardiographic evidence not meeting major criteria.

Choosing the right time to operate is difficult; the surgeon must balance the possibility of eradicating infection with medical treatment and optimizing major comorbidity, taking into account that these patients are often extremely unwell, and liable to deteriorate irreversibly. The indications for surgery in native valve endocarditis (e.g. post-mitral or tricuspid valve repair, aortic homograft or autograft replacement) include acute MR with heart failure or AR, fungal endocarditis, evidence of annular or aortic abscess, sinus, or aneurysm, or new onset conduction disturbances, failure of medical management (persistent valve dysfunction and evidence of sepsis after 7–10 days of antibiotic therapy), or recurrent emboli after antibiotic therapy. The indications for surgery in prosthetic valve endocarditis (not homograft or autograft) include heart failure with prosthetic valve dysfunction, early prosthetic endocarditis (less than two months after surgery), fungal endocarditis, *Staphylococcal* endocarditis not responding to antibiotics, Gram-negative organisms, paravalvular leak, anular or aortic abscess, sinus, fistula, or aneurysm, or new onset conduction disturbances, vegetations on the prosthesis, or persistent sepsis despite antibiotics. Surgery should be delayed for 5–10 days after central neurological events. The goal of surgery is to remove infected tissue and drain abscesses, reverse haemodynamic abnormalities, and restore cardiac and vascular architecture. Transoesophageal echo is critical while planning surgery, which may involve drainage of abscesses, debridement of necrotic tissue, closure of acquired defects such as ventricular septal defect, ring abscess, fistulae and aneurysms, in addition to valve repair and replacement.

Paraprosthetic leak

Incidental paraprosthetic leaks occur in about 5% of aortic valve replacements and 10–20% of mitral valve replacements.[28] Paraprosthetic leaks within 30 days of surgery are usually the result of either the sewing ring being poorly seated within a calcified, irregular annulus or a suture cutting out of the annulus. Wash jets, the regurgitant jets typical of the valve mechanism, may be mistaken for paravalvular leaks. Late paravalvular leaks are usually associated with endocarditis, in which case they almost always require surgical repair following treatment with antibiotics. High velocity paravalvular leaks may cause haemolysis that may be severe enough to indicate valve replacement. If neither haemolysis nor infective endocarditis is present, the management of the leak depends on the degree of haemodynamic compromise; small leaks that do not progress can be treated conservatively for many years.

Prosthesis failure

Structural problems, not associated with thrombosis, endocarditis, haemolysis or haemorrhage, may necessitate valve replacement. Structural failure of mechanical valves is rare: the few valves that have had a higher than expected incidence of problems, such as the silver coated sewing ring of the Silzone valve, have been withdrawn. Of patients with aortic bioprostheses, 65% are free from structural failure at five years, compared to 53% for mitral bioprostheses.[28] Patients are reviewed annually, either by the cardiologists or cardiothoracic surgeons, with a transthoracic echo to identify and monitor valve failure. The indications for surgery for structural failure of a bioprosthesis are the same as for regurgitant lesions of native valves.

Valve thrombosis

Valve thrombosis is rare in the appropriately anticoagulated patient. Its incidence in patients with tissue valves and appropriately anticoagulated patients with mechanical valves is the same, at 0.1–5.7% per patient per year.[29] The most common cause of valve thrombosis is inadequate anticoagulation because of poor compliance, changes in other medication and illness, which is why 95% of cases occur in mechanical valves. Mechanical mitral valves are affected in over 60% of cases while mechanical aortic valves affected in 30% of cases. Smaller diameter aortic valves are affected more commonly than the larger valves. Patients with prosthetic valve thrombosis may present with pulmonary oedema, poor peripheral perfusion and systemic embolisation, but the most common scenario is acute hemodynamic compromise. Thrombi (>5 mm) that are not obstructing the valve orifice or mechanism may be treated with formal anticoagulation alone, but larger thrombi require thrombolysis, which is fast replacing surgery as treatment.

Complete heart block

Most surgeons routinely place temporary epicardial pacing wires as up to 20% of the patients undergoing isolated mitral or aortic valve replacement suffer transient heart block postoperatively. Heart block normally settles after three or four days as haematoma and oedema resolve, but prolonged heart block should be discussed with a cardiologist in case a permanent pacemaker is indicated. Two to three percent of aortic valve surgery patients will require permanent pacemaker insertion[30]; this is a day case procedure and should not delay discharge, but should be postponed until the INR is <1.5. The preoperative risk factors for permanent pacemaker insertion are not well defined but probably include preoperative heart block and heavily calcified valves.

Early and late mortality

Early mortality is due to cardiac failure, usually within a few days of operation. The higher mortality in patients undergoing bioprosthetic mitral valve replacement is related to their preoperative comorbidity, including age. Overall survival (including hospital deaths) after aortic valve replacement is approximately 75% at five years, 60% at 10 years, 40% at 15 years.[31] Survival can be described in terms of hazard phases. The early, rapidly declining hazard phase (short-term survival) is dominated by perioperative mortality. It gives way to an intermediate-term survival phase about six months after the operation where the death rate remains steady at approximately 1% p.a. into the longer term. The risk factors for late mortality are advanced age, mitral valve regurgitation, (ischaemic > non-ischaemic), enlarged left ventricular and left atrial dimensions, NYHA class III or IV, and increased operative and ischaemic time.

Reoperation for any reason

The risk of reoperation after mitral valve surgery is 5% at five years[31]; bioprostheses have a late rising hazard function. Freedom from reoperation after repair at 5–10 years ranges from 80–98%, largely related to the degree of mitral regurgitation in the early postoperative period.

Complications of Thoracic Aortic Surgery

Paraplegia from spinal cord ischaemia affects up to 20% of the patients undergoing surgery on the descending aorta.[32] The blood supply to the spinal cord is from vertebral and radicular arteries (segmental branches of the thoracic and abdominal aorta). In its lower segments the spinal cord depends on the radicular arteries. The great radicular artery (artery of Adamkiewicz) usually present at T12–L2 frequently provides the entire arterial supply for the lower two-thirds of the cord. Strategies to minimise the risk of spinal cord ischaemia include surgical techniques, hypothermia, intraoperative cerebrospinous fluid withdrawal, and pharmacological adjuncts. Most surgeons attempt to preserve and reimplant large radicular arteries, particularly below T10. Some surgeons monitor the somatosensory and motor evoked potentials (SSEP and MEP respectively) which provide a better indication of the anterior cord function, clamping intercostals vessels sequentially and dividing them only if no change in SSEP is seen after 10 min of clamping. It is important to minimise the ischaemic time by maintaining perfusion of vessels downstream of the distal graft anastomosis, and by preventing hypotension. Whole body hypothermia offers some protection to ischaemic injury. The most important principle is the reduction of spinal cord temperature during the ischaemic period; surface and intrathecal cooling have been used in addition to whole body cooling. Intra-operative withdrawal of cerebrospinous fluid is designed to increase perfusion pressure of the cord, by increasing the difference between intracramial and arterial pressures. There is little evidence to support this technique, which also runs the important risk of intrathecal bleeding leading to paraparesis. Pharma-cological adjuncts include corticosteroids, sodium thiopental, prostaglandin E, and a variety of oxygen free radical scavengers. These are not used routinely as they have not shown any significant difference in the outcome.

3. COMPLICATIONS OF THORACIC SURGERY

Complications of Lung Resection for Malignancy

Death and recurrence

The operative mortality for lung resection for bronchogenic malignancy has steadily improved. While the mortality rates in retrospective reviews published 30 years ago ranged from 5–10% for lobectomy, and 14–19% for pneumonec-tomy, these have dropped to 1.2–1.5% and 3.2–10% respectively, in studies published within the last 10 years.[33] Age is a risk factor, with patients below 65 years having a significantly lower mortality. Another important risk factor is a history of ischaemic heart disease. The causes of operative death include respiratory failure and pneumonia, bronchopleural fistula, cardiac failure, and rarely haemorrhage.

The five-year survival rate is 60–70% for patients undergoing resection of Stage 1 adenocarcinoma, 50% for Stage IIa, and 25% for Stage IIb. The results for squamous cell carcinoma are 83%, 64%, and 53% respectively. Recurrence is associated with a median survival of 18 months.[33]

Bronchopleural fistula and empyema

A bronchopleural fistula is a large communication between the bronchi and the pleural space. It is usually associated with sepsis in the form of an empyema, because the bronchial tree is colonised with bacteria. The incidence of bronchopleural fistula following resection for bronchogenic malignancy cited in the literature ranges between 1–5%[34]; the mortality associated with it may be as high as 30%.[34] The preoperative risk factors include advanced age, malnutrition, steroids, and neo-adjuvant radiotherapy. The intraoperative risk factors include a devascularised stump or anastomosis, as well as incomplete margins at the bronchial stump. The postoperative risk factors include wound infection. It is extremely important not to devascularise the bronchial margins; the normal practice is to reset the bronchus as close as possible to the trachea or main bronchus without compromising the lumen, and without excessive perihilar dissection. The optimum method of stump closure and anastomosis are subject to debate but pedicled flaps of pericardial or pleural fat, or intercostal muscle applied to the bronchial stump or anastomosis are an effective way of preventing suture line break down and the formation of a bronchopleural fistula in high risk cases.

Classically, bronchopleural fistulas present 7–10 days postoperatively, and occasionally weeks to months after surgery. Patients present with fever, purulent secretions that may be worse when lying on the contralateral side, persistent large or worsening air leak and or pleural collection, and occasionally subcutaneous emphysema. Inflammatory markers are raised, and chest radiography shows a collection, often with a fluid level. Following pneumonectomy a decrease (rather than the steady increase normally observed postoperatively) in the fluid level as a result of air entering the pleural space and some fluid leaving it via the bronchial tree is pathognomonic of a bronchopleural fistula. While bronchoscopy may identify large fistulas, or dehiscence of the anastomosis, small fistulas or leaks may only be detected as local movement of secretions, or as a small area of inflammation or granulation tissue.

The treatment of bronchopleural fistula depends on the aetiology, size and timing of the fistula. Intercostal drain insertion is important to drain the empyema, relieving any air leak, reducing sepsis and preventing further aspiration of pus into the bronchial tree. However, radiological guidance is required if lung adhesions are suspected from the chest radiograph. Up to a third of small, early fistulae that are not due to residual local tumour, occurring in otherwise healthy patients, close spontaneously with the insertion of an intercostal drain. Large fistulae, and those associated with incomplete resection margins, wound infection, large air leaks and those not responding to conservative management require surgical repair. Completion pneumonectomy may be unavoidable if resection of the bronchial stump compromises the lumen of the remaining bronchus. The empyema is evacuated, parenchymal cortex, if any, is removed from the remaining lung to encourage full expansion, and a pedicled vasularised flap (normally of intercostal muscle) is sutured round the new anastomosis. Successful VATS treatment of early bronchopleural fistula has also been described. Some surgeons elect to obliterate the empyema space using myoplasty and thoracoplasty. A range of irrigation techniques have also been employed, such as the Claggett technique. Here, the pleural space is irrigated with antibiotics, packed with sterile gauze to encourage granulation tissue, and a rib space resected to leave an open thoracostomy. The packing is removed after a few days or weeks, the cavity filled with antibiotic solution, and the thoracostomy closed surgically. This technique is successful in two thirds of patients with empyema.

Prolonged air leak

Prolonged air leak is defined as one lasting more than seven days postoperatively. Clinically, the under water seal bubbles continuously; if the air leak is small the underwater seal only bubbles on forced expiration e.g. coughing. Most patients have a small degree of air leak from the lung parenchyma, usually from dissection in the lung fissures that may have been adherent or obliterated, and from parenchymal resection lines. The bronchial stump or anastomosis is checked prior to closure for a gross air leak, which is addressed at the time of surgery. Small air leaks normally close spontaneously within two to five days of surgery. Large air leaks result from problems at the bronchial stump or anastomosis, inadvertent trauma to the bronchial tree, large bullae, or large surface area of raw lung parenchyma commonly after redo-thoracotomy or decortication. These are normally persistent and if identified intraoperatively need definitive management. Air leaks from the bronchial stumps or anastomoses are addressed by placing additional sutures at the site of air leak. Pedicled flaps, pericardial or pleural flaps, and occasionally intercostal muscle sutured to the bronchial stump or anastomosis are useful adjuncts for preventing and treating major air leaks postoperatively, and are used routinely by some surgeons. There are several fibrin-based glues designed for topical application over areas of raw parenchyma that help reduce postoperative air leak. Large or burst bullae should be resected. Automatic stapled suture lines are preferred for resection of lung parenchyma, including incomplete fissures as they minimise air leak.

Postoperatively, air leaks are treated by encouraging lung expansion (see the section on "Intrapleural Space" below) for apposition of lung surfaces. It is vital to check for obvious extra-pleural sources of air leak, including the drain site, drain position, all drain connections, the underwater seal, and suction. Occasionally, the drain entrains air from outside the pleural cavity, either because the drain hole is too large (in which case additional mattress sutures should be replaced around the drain site) or because the intercostal drain holes are no longer fully inside the pleura (in which case the drain must be removed immediately and another one sited if appropriate).

Occasionally, it may be felt that the air leak is being exacerbated by the drain holes lying immediately above the source of air. In this case, reducing suction, or pulling the drain back a few centimetres may be useful. Additional drains may be placed under radiological guidance. If these measures fail to address the problem, the patient should be re-explored, and the source of the air leak repaired surgically as described above. Talc slurry pleurodesis is employed for patients with persistent air leaks who are considered too frail to tolerate further surgery: a suspension of talc, local anaesthetic and saline is injected using an aseptic technique into the intercostal drain, and the patient rolled around to distribute the mixture throughout the pleural space. This is done to encourage an inflammatory reaction causing the lung to adhere to the chest wall, reducing air leaks; this technique should not be employed in patients requiring surgical re-exploration. For air leaks that fail to respond to these measures one option is to retain the intercostal drain, but trimming it and replacing the underwater seal with a one-way Heimlich flutter valve. This can be managed in the outpatient area if the pleural space does not increase off suction. There is however, a substantial risk of empyema resulting from prolonged presence of an intercostal drain, and this option is usually considered only in patients who have undergone surgery for palliative reasons.

Complications of bronchial and tracheal resections

Sleeve resections are associated with a higher mortality and morbidity than a simple lobectomy with an operative mortality approaching 7.5%.[35] Local recurrence is as high as 10%. Ischaemia or dehiscence of the bronchial anastomosis leading to bronchopleural fistula affects 3–5% of the patients. Suspected anastomotic dehiscence should be investigated bronchoscopically (some centres perform this as a routine postoperative procedure). Any evidence of failure of the anastomosis is an indication for re-exploration and repair. Excessive granulation tissue may form at the site of the anastomosis and may be removed bronchoscopically. Anastomotic strictures may respond to bronchoscopic dilatation with solid bougies or balloon dilators. If the anastomotic problems are impossible to address during reoperation, completion pneumonectomy is recommended.

Complications of Oesophageal Resection and Reconstruction

Death and recurrence

Operative mortality for resection in the case of oesophageal malignancy is inversely proportional to the surgeon's experience and centre activity.[36] Mortality rates in retrospective reviews ranged between 0–17.3%.[36] Patient risk factors include the inability to carry out normal daily activities or do active work, pulmonary, cardiac or hepatic dysfunction, and tumour location. No difference in operative mortality or long term survival has been demonstrated between the transhiatal and transthoracic approaches. The commonest cause of operative death is sepsis, usually from anastomotic failure, followed by respiratory failure and MI. The recurrence rate following macroscopically curative resection is approximately 50% at five years, with over 80% of recurrences occurring within 24 months of surgery, and 60% occurring in patients with stages 3 or 4 disease.[37] In patients with recurrence within two years, 50% survival was less than nine months, compared to over one year in patients with later recurrence.

Anastomotic complications

Anastomotic leak is the most important complication of oesophageal resection, and the single largest cause of postoperative mortality. The primary aetiology is ischaemia from inadequate preservation of local and regional blood supply during mobilisation. The site of the anastomosis, which may be cervical or thoracic depending on the type of oesophagectomy, dictates both the likelihood of anastomotic dehiscence, the presentation and the associated morbidity. Intrathoracic anastomoses have a dehiscence rate of approximately 10%, compared to closer to 20% for cervical anastomoses. [38] The mortality associated with leakage from intrathoracic anastomoses is as high as 75% compared to 20–30% for cervical dehiscence.[38] Contained thoracic leaks are usually heralded by a pleural effusion or pneumothorax associated with sepsis. They may be investigated with gastrograffin contrast and CT studies. Small anastomotic leaks may heal spontaneously if the lung is completely expanded (effectively buttressing the anastomosis), and insertion of an intercostal drain may be all that is required. Persistent leaks are managed by direct repair or with pedicled flaps via thoracotomy or thorascopic approaches. Cervical leaks present with cellulitis and surgical emphysema, and are investigated in the same manner as thoracic leaks. The wound should be reopened. Leaks contained within the neck fascial compartments may be treated conservatively, but if there is evidence of mediastinitis, surgical exploration, debridement and repair is indicated. Both cervical and thoracic anastomotic leaks may present as septic shock associated with purulent drainage in the first 48 hours postoperatively. The aetiology is ischaemia followed by gastric necrosis with surgical exploration, resection of the ischemic stomach, and stoma formation being the only option for treatment; the mortality rate is high. Clinically silent leaks may be detected through routine contrast studies, and percutaneous drainage and parenteral nutrition are the recommended treatment, unless the patient deteriorates requiring surgical drainage.

Anastomotic strictures occur in up to 20% of oesophagectomy patients.[40] Strictures formed early in the postoperative period are due to inflammatory changes associated with wound healing while those forming late are usually related to local recurrence or chronic reflux oesophagitis. They present with progressive dysphagia or odynophagia. Any investigation in the early postoperative period centres on defining the anatomy, whereas detection of anastomotic recurrence in late strictures mandates gastrogaffin swallow, contrast enhanced CT, and eosophagoscopy along with biopsy. Most strictures respond to dilatation, which is associated with a <5% rate of oesophageal perforation. Resection is an option for persistent strictures in otherwise fit individuals without evidence of recurrence.

Functional disorders

There are two types of "dumping" syndrome. Early dumping results from rapid transit of high molecular weight solids into the jejunum resulting in hyperglycaemia, and transit of water down the osmotic gradient into the bowel lumen. It affects up to 20% of patients, [40] and presents with nausea, vomiting diarrhoea, faintness and dyspnoea within minutes of ingesting a meal. Late dumping is caused by reactive hypoglycaemia, and patients present with dizziness, breathlessness and nausea. Both syndromes may improve with time. Eating smaller meals frequently; avoiding dairy products, high carbohydrate meals, and excessive fluid intake with meals; and anti-diarrhoeal agents are helpful.

The converse problem, delayed gastric emptying, may be due to vagal denervation, torsion and compression, pressure differences between the intrathoracic neo-stomach and the abdominal duodenum, and mucosal oedema. These patients are at risk of regurgitation, reflux, and aspiration pneumonia acutely, along with stricture formation and malnutrition in the longer term. Erythromycin improves gastric emptying but gastric outlet obstruction may require pyloroplasty.

Complications of Anti-reflux Surgery

Mortality

Anti-reflux surgery is associated with a mortality rate of less than 1%, and low complication rates.[41] The recurrence of reflux, or complete failure of the procedure to prevent it is one of the commonest complications and varies from 5–20% in the literature. The aetiology includes incorrect diagnosis (particularly, the failure to recognise motility disorders preoperatively) as well as technical failures. The preferred treatment is medical therapy because redo-surgery is associated with higher associated failure, morbidity and mortality.

Iatrogenic injury

Damage to adjacent structures, particularly the spleen when dividing the short gastric arteries, and the left lobe of the liver during mobilisation, results in significant postoperative bleeding in less than 5% of the patients.[41] Intraoperative splenectomy has an incidence of about 1%. Bile leaks, diaphragmatic injury, and intra-abdominal abscesses, which occur as a result of injury to the stomach or bowel have been reported in up to 5% of patients. If identified intraoperatively, such injuries must be addressed immediately as the mortality associated with unrecognised visceral perforation during anti-reflux surgery may be as high as 15%. Conservative management with total parenteral nutrition of such leaks, identified postoperatively may be successful, but deteriorating clinical picture mandates surgical intervention.

Fistula formation

Internal fistulas between the wrap and the oesophagus result from excessive tension in the sutures that fix the fundoplication to the oesophagus, unrecognised intraoperative visceral perforation, local ischemia and sepsis. They present with dyspepsia refractory to medical therapy, and are best identified on contrast swallow studies. The definitive treatment is surgical repair of the fistula. External fistulas occur through similar mechanisms to internal fistulas, although they are significantly less common. The definitive management is normally surgical reconstruction.

Paraoesophageal herniation

Herniation of the fundoplication wrap through the oesophageal hiatus has an incidence of 1–2%.[41] The risk factors include large hiatus hernia and a laparoscopic approach, and the common cause is the failure to adequately approximate the right and left crura. Herniation usually presents late with new onset dysphagia, epigastric discomfort and early satiety. Investigations include gastrograffin swallow studies, and the treatment of choice is re-exploration and repair.

Functional problems

Gas bloating which is associated with flatulence is one of the most common postoperative problems, and is due to a combination of vagal denervation, reducing gastric motility and air swallowing. It presents with symptoms of early satiety and epigastric discomfort, which usually improve with time, and promotiliants for immediate symptom control. Long-term problems with diarrhoea and dumping syndromes usually improve without specific intervention over time.

Dysphagia may occur early or late postoperatively, reflecting the multiple causes. Early dysphagia, which affects over half the patients, reflects postoperative local oedema or haematoma, both of which resolve relatively rapidly. A fundoplication that is excessively tight or malpositioned normally requires operative reintervention. Late dysphagia may represent stricture formation as a result of previous reflux, and is managed by repeated dilatation. The development of oesophageal carcinoma must be actively excluded by contrast swallow studies, contrast enhanced CT, oesophagoscopy and biopsy. Complete gastric inlet obstruction is rare and is normally due to the same causes as early dysphagia.

Complications of Mediastinal Surgery

Resection of anterior mesiastinal masses

The resection of thymoma and other invasive mediastinal masses may result in damage to either phrenic nerve, the left recurrent laryngeal nerve, the thoracic duct, and major vascular structures. The complications associated with these injuries are described below.

Thymectomy, which is carried out to treat myasthenia gravis and thymoma, is normally performed via a median sternotomy, and sometimes via limited upper sternotomy, VATS and transcervical approaches. In thymectomy for myasthenia gravis, up to 50% of the patients will be in remission at 20 years following surgery (compared with 20%, one year postoperatively), and up to 90% will be in partial remission.[42] The complete removal of the thymus is a key factor in achieving remission, but rates of incomplete resection are not well documented in the literature. Postoperative respiratory failure is the second most important complication, affecting up to 5% of patients, who may be electively ventilated postoperatively to avoid this problem. Careful preoperative planning including optimising medical therapy, plasmapheresis, careful titration of anaesthetic agents, and avoidance of neuromuscular blockade are key to preventing respiratory failure postoperatively. Postoperative respiratory failure can be managed with reintubation and ventilation. The complications due to myasthenia gravis including opthalmoplegia, ptosis, dysphagia, dysarthria, and skeletal muscle weakness, may also appear postoperatively.

Mediastinocopy and mediastinotomy

The morbidity and mortality of mediastinoscopy is low, with complications in less than 2% of patients and no deaths in a series of 1000 cases.[43] The most important complication is haemorrhage usually resulting from overly vigorous blunt dissection or inadvertent biopsy of a major vascular structure such as the aorta, pulmonary trunk, superior vena cava, azygous, or innominate artery. Small tears and venous bleeding can normally be controlled by direct packing and pressure, but a significant damage to vascular structures requires thoracotomy and surgical repair. Rarely, tears in the pulmonary trunk or posterior aorta may be inaccessible without cardiopulmonary bypass, and damage to the distal right or left pulmonary artery impossible to address without pneumonectomy. Atherosclerotic embolisation from the aortic arch, or ischaemia from compression of the innominate artery may cause stroke. Oesophageal or bronchial perforations are uncommon and may not be recognised intraoperatively; however, after the patient has been discharged, they may present with sepsis, pleural effusion or surgical emphysema. Both injuries require surgical repair at the time of surgery if recognised intraoperatively, or postoperatively.

Thorascopic sympathectomy

This procedure has a low complication rate. The most common complications include failure to divide the sympathetic structures resulting in the persistence of symptoms postoperatively, inadvertent injury of the stellate ganglion resulting in Horner's syndrome postoperatively, and injury to the brachial plexus. Compensatory sweating, classically in the trunk, axillae and groin, and gustatory sweating affect a minority of patients postoperatively.

Endoscopy and Stenting

The incidence of oesophageal perforation during diagnostic and therapeutic endoscopy has reduced from 0.03% and 0.3% in 1976 to less than 0.01% and

0.2% respectively,[44] although it is higher in pneumatic dilatation for achalasia. The diagnosis of oesophageal perforation relies on a high index of clinical suspicion. Asymptomatic suspected perforation, post-procedural pneumothorax, pneumopericardium and free intra-abdominal air, should be investigated with water-soluble contrast swallow studies. A repeat endoscopy may identify lesions following negative swallow studies and is preferred over contrast CT to localise the perforation. Patients with contained small perforations, no distal obstruction, and no evidence of clinical sepsis may respond to conservative management with parenteral nutrition, fluid resuscitation, broad-spectrum antibiotics, proton pump inhibitors and prokinetic agents. Surgical repair, which is indicated in patients who do not fall into this group, is usually carried out via a thoracotomy, and involves primary repair in layers if oesophageal mucosal edges are healthy, a variety of pedicled tissue flaps to support any repair, or resection and oesophagogastric anastomosis which has a significant mortality. Decortication of the pleural space is frequently necessary.

Oesophageal stents have an associated mortality as high as 50% although the incidence of perforation is less than 5%.[44] Misplacement of the stent distal or proximal to the obstructing tumour occurs in up to 15%, and its management involves the placement of additional stents rather than stent removal, which can cause significant injury. Stent migration occurs in up to a third of patients; if this is distal, into the stomach or small intestine, endoscopic or surgical removal is necessary to avoid the risk of perforation. Tumour overgrowth occurs in over a third of patients and is managed with laser or diathermy, or stent insertion. Airway obstruction is a risk in stenting very proximal tumours. It may be possible to insert a tracheal or bronchial stent to address this. Haemorrhage from erosion of the stent into major vascular structures including the aorta and pericardium may be massive and fatal. Upper gastro-intestinal bleeding post-stent insertion must be investigated endoscopically; if there is evidence of erosion immediate removal may be required.

General Thoracic Complications

Intrapleural space

Intrapleural spaces develop when the lung fails to fill the pleural cavity after collapse or resection. The intrapleural space is normally obliterated by re-expansion of the remaining lung, mediastinal shift particularly post-pneumonectomy, narrowing of the intercostal spaces, and elevation of the ipsilateral hemidiaphragm. The failure of these mechanisms to obliterate the pleural space is due to poor compliance of the residual lung (which may be due to intra-parenchymal problems such as atelectasis, or extra-parenchymal problems such as incomplete removal of cortex during decortication for empyema), persistent air leaks, and occasionally mediastinal fibrosis. This occurs in approximately a third of pulmonary resections. Of these persistent pleural spaces, approximately three quarters will undergo spontaneous resolution, while half the remainder resolve with insertion of an intercostal drain. Of those that persist, half result in empyema.

Postoperative pleural spaces may be prevented by a careful placement of large gauge pleural drains at the apex and base of the lung to optimise drainage of fluid and air. In extensive resections a pleural space is anticipated, some surgeons elect to perform a phrenic nerve crush, which results in elevation of the ipsilateral hemidiaphragm at the expense of its function. Thoracoplasty, where a subperiosteal resection of the first two to three ribs is performed, reduces the apical pleural space. The principle of pneumoperitoneum, which is not widely performed, is to elevate the diaphragm obliterating the pleural space by insufflating 1500 ml of air into the peritoneum.

The treatment of postoperative pleural space includes encouraging lung expansion using physiotherapy and early mobilisation, and the generation of non-invasive mechanical and physiological positive pressure using continuous positive airway pressure and birding. The prevention of mucus retention is key; oxygen should be humidified wherever possible, saline and bronchodilator nebulizers should be given regularly, and adequate analgesia and chest physiotherapy should be employed to maximise cough effectiveness. Intercostal drains are routinely placed on high flow low pressure suction at −2 to −3 kPa. If there is no air leak and the lung is fully inflated, it is discontinued after 48 hours, just before the drain removal. However, if the lung fails to re-expand fully, the thoracic suction may be increased slowly up to −5 kPa. Persistent pleural spaces may be treated conservatively if small and not associated with air leaks or infection. Large persistent pleural spaces normally require serial chest X-rays, and elective thoracoplasty is no longer performed for these. The treatment of empyema and persistent air leak is described above.

Surgical emphysema

This is the presence of subcutaneous air. Air enters the soft tissues usually from a major intra-thoracic air leak through a wound, or occasionally entrained from outside the chest wall. Clinically, there is swelling which is "crunchy" to touch and crackly on auscultation. Swelling may be localised to drain or wound site, but in severe cases it extends rapidly across the trunk, over the neck, face and both limbs. The patient may be unable to open his eyes because of the swelling, and the voice has a characteristic nasal sound because of swelling in the soft tissues of the pharynx (occasionally severe enough to compromise the upper airway). With the exception of airway compromise, which may require intubation, the management of surgical emphysema is directed at locating the source of the air leak and treating it. Chest radiography should be performed urgently to look for simple or tension pneumothorax. With appropriate repositioning or insertion of a new intercostal drain surgical emphysema normally resolves over the course of five to ten days, and is not usually associated with adverse sequelae.

Chylothorax

Chylothorax occurs following less than 0.5% of lung resections for bronchogenic carcinoma, and in up to 3% of oesophagectomies.[45] It is more common after pneumonectomy, when compared with lobectomy or segmentectomy. The aetiology is usually intraoperative injury to the thoracic duct or its tributaries. The resection of large proximal tumours, extensive lymphadenectomy and dissection around the left main bronchus and left oesophageo-tracheal groove, and redo-surgery increase the risk of injury. The injury may be noticed intraoperatively, as milky fluid accumulates slowly in the operative field. The injury should ideally be repaired and if this is not possible, both ends of the duct should be ligated. Postoperatively persistent sero-sanguinous pleural drainage greater than 500 ml per day is suggestive of a chylous leak. If the patient is not eating normally, the fluid may be clear rather than the classical milky colour. Fluid triglyceride greater than 110 mg/dL has a 99% specificity and sensitivity for chyle.

The management is initially conservative. Large gauge intercostal drains are mandatory for effective drainage of the pleural space. The patient should be placed on a no-fat, medium chain triglyceride diet. Conservative management is successful in a third to half of the cases within 10–14 days. A chyle leak refractory to conservative management should be ligated or repaired surgically as it predisposes to infection, and has an adverse impact on nutritional status. The standard approach is ligation of the thoracic duct near the diaphragm, which can be carried out via a low left or right thoracotomy or a laparotomy. Thoracoscopic approaches are used increasingly frequently.

Bronchovascular fistula

Fistula formation can occur between bronchial or tracheal resection margins and bronchiolar or pulmonary branch arteries, or brachiocephalic artery. Bronchovascular fistula formation following sleeve resection is rare, and can be largely avoided by wrapping the bronchial anastomosis with a pedicled tissue flap. It is characterised by a "herald bleed" presenting as haemoptysis, followed by a catastrophic bleed, which rapidly compromises the airway. Haemoptysis following sleeve lobectomy should be investigated with urgent bronchoscopy, which may show active bleeding or obvious dehiscence but more commonly reveals only granulation tissue. Surgical repair is indicated in this instance. The anaesthetic management of an actively bleeding bronchovascular fistula involves selective intubation of the contralateral bronchus.

Tracheoinnominate fistulas complicate less than 1% of tracheostomies and tracheal resections but have a high associated mortality. Its presentation is similar to that of bronchovascular fistulas with a herald bleed preceding the catastrophic main bleed. It may be possible to obtain digital control of the innominate artery via a tracheal stoma by inserting a finger into the stoma and compressing the artery against the manubrium. The definitive management is surgical repair.

Cardiac herniation

Cardiac herniation complicates less than 1% of pulmonary resections, but if undiagnosed, is associated with a mortality rate as high as 50%.[46] Herniation is associated with an intrapericardial pneumonectomy. The contents of the middle mediastinum herniate through the pericardial defect into the ipsilateral chest cavity following a change in position, raised contralateral positive pressures (positive pressure ventilation, coughing, extubation) or decreased ipsilateral negative pressures (excessive suction applied to intercostal chest drain). The patient presents acute hypotension, raised jugular venous pressure and displacement of the apex beak to the operated side. The right-sided displacement causing obstruction of the superior vena cava may be associated with cyanosis of the head, neck and upper limbs. Chest radiography shows displacement of the heart. The closure of pericardial defects, either using synthetic patches or direct closure, prevents this complication and is probably mandatory following right-sided pneumonectomy. The treatment involves urgent re-exploration, restoration of the heart to its normal anatomical position and closure of the pericardial defect as above.

Lobar torsion

Lobar torsion during or after lung resection results from rotation of the residual lung on its bronchovascular pedicle. This leads to an obstruction of the pulmonary venous return, lobar oedema, consolidation and eventually infarction. Lobar torsion most commonly affects the right middle lobe after a right upper lobectomy if the horizontal fissure is very well developed. It occurs in less than 1% of cases post-lobectomy, but is associated with a mortality rate approaching 20%.[47] Torsion may be recognised intraoperatively, and routinely assessing how easily the lung inflates and inspecting the bronchovascular pedicle is good practice. The pedicle should be completely untwisted and the lung secured in the correct position. Unrecognised torsion presents insidiously postoperatively. Clinical findings may be limited to pyrexia in the early postoperative period. Early chest radiography may show lobar collapse and consolidation, abrupt termination of the bronchial air pattern and hilar displacement. Over the following postoperative days, patients develop signs of sepsis, eventually associated with purulent discharge and a large air leak from the pleural drains. Urgent flexible bronchoscopy is usually diagnostic: a "fish-mouth" bronchus that permits passage of the scope to reveal normal distal airways but collapses on scope withdrawal is pathognomonic. If the lung has infarcted, its management consists of resection of the lobe and any portion of residual lung with compromised viability. In contrast, if the lung is viable, it is simply untwisted and resutured in place.

REFERENCES

1. Kouchoukos NT, Blackstone EH, Doty DB, Hanley FL and Katp RB. (2003) Postoperative care. In: *Kirklin/Baratt-Boyes Cardiac Surgery*, 3rd edn. (Churchill Livingstone, Elsevier), pp. 195–253.
2. Bojar RM. (2005) Respiratory management. In: *Manual of Perioperative Care in Adult Cardiac Surgery*, 4th edn. (Blackwell Science), pp. 293–339.
3. Josa M, Siouffi SY, K Silverman AB, *et al.* (1993) Pulmonary embolism after cardiac surgery. *J Am Coll Cardiol* **21**: 990–996.
4. Shammas N. (2000) Pulmonary embolus after coronary artery bypass surgery: a review of the literature. *Clin Cardiol* **23**: 637–644.
5. Fedullo PF, Tapson VF. (2003) The evaluation of suspected pulmonary embolism. *N Engl J Med* **349**: 1247–1256.
6. Little AG. (2004) *Complications in Cardiothoracic Surgery. Avoidance and Treatment* (Futura Publishing Co. Inc., USA).
7. *Fifth National Adult Cardiac Surgical Database Report.* (2003) The Society of Cardiothoracic Surgeons of Great Britain and Ireland. Compiled by Keogh BE, and Kinsman R. (Dendrite Clinical Systems Ltd., 2004).
8. Mangram AJ, Horan TC, Pearson ML. Guidelines for the prevention of surgical site infection (1999). *Infect Control Hosp Epidemiol* **20**: 247–278.
9. Davidson BR, Bailey JS. (1986) Incisional herniae following median sternotomy incisions: their incidence and aetiology. *Br J Surg* **73**: 995–996.
10. Price S, Prout J, Jaggar SI, Gibson DG, Pepper JR. (2004) Tamponade following cardiac surgery: terminology and echocardiography may both mislead. *Eur J Cardiothorac Surg* **26**: 1156–1160.
11. Creswell LL, Schuessler RB, Rosenbloom M, Cox JL. (1993) Hazards of postoperative atrial arrhythmias. *Ann Thorac Surg* **56**: 539–549.
12. Still RJ, Hilgenberg AD, Akins CW, Daggett WM, Buckley MJ. (1992) Intraoperative aortic dissection. *Ann Thorac Surg* **53**: 374–379.
13. Chenoweth DE, Cooper SW, Hugli TE, Stewart RW, Blackstone EH, Kirklin. (1981) Complement activation during cardiopulmonary bypass: evidence for generation of C3a and C5a anaphylatoxins. *N Engl J Med* **304**: 497–503.
14. Conlon PJ, Stafford-Smith M, White WD, *et al.* (1999) Acute renal failure following cardiac surgery. *Nephrol Dial Transplant* **14**: 1158–1163.
15. Roach GW, Kanchuger M, Mangano CM, *et al.* (1996) Adverse cerebral outcomes after coronary bypass surgery. *N Engl J Med* **335**: 1857–1863.
16. Eagle KA, Guyton RA, Davidoff R, *et al.* ACC/AHA 2004 guideline update for coronary artery bypass graft surgery: a report of the American College of Cardiology/American Heart Association Task Force on Practice Guidelines

(Committee to Update the 1999 Guidelines for Coronary Artery Bypass Graft Surgery). American Heart Association Web Site. Available at: http://www.americanheart.org/presenter.jhtml?identifier=9181.

17. Lev-Ran O, Braunstein R, Sharony R, *et al.* (2005) No-touch aorta off-pump coronary surgery: the effect on stroke. *J Thorac Cardiovasc Surg* **129**: 307–313.

18. Crawley F, Bevan D, Wren D. (2000) Management of intracranial bleeding associated with anticoagulation: balancing the risk of further bleeding against thromboembolism from prosthetic heart valves. *J Neurol Neurosurg Psych* **69**: 396–398.

19. Antithrombotic Trialists' Collaboration. (2002) Collabarative met-analysis of andomised trials of antiplatelet therapy for prevention of death from myocardial infarction, and stroke in high risk patients. *Br Med J* **324**: 71–86.

20. Menasche P, Edmunds LH. (2003) Extracorporeal circulation. The inflammatory response. In: Cohn LH, Edmunds H (eds), *Cardiac Surgery in the Adult*, 2nd edn (McGraw Hill).

21. Iyer VS, Russell WJ, Leppard P, *et al.* (1993) Mortality and myocardial infarction after coronary surgery: a review of 12,003 patients. *Med J Aust* **159**: 166.

22. Brindis TG, Brundage BH, Ullyot DJMcKay CW, Lipton MJ, Turley K. (1984) Graft patency in patients with coronary artery bypass operation complicated by perioperative myocardial infarction. *J Am Coll Cardiol* **3**: 55–62.

23. Sergeant P, Blackstone E, Meyns B. (1998) Is return of angina after coronary artery bypass grafting immutable, can it be delayed, and is it important? *J Thorac Cardiovasc Surg* **116**: 440.

24. Sergeant P, Blackstone E, Meyns B, Stockman B, Jashiri R. (1998) First cardiological or cardiosurgical reintervention for ischaemic heart disease after primary coronary artery bypass grafting. *Eur J Cardiothorac Surg* **14**: 480.

25. Guthaner DF, Robert EW, Alderman EL Wexler L. (1979) Long term serial angiographic studies after coronary artery bypass surgery. *Circulation* **60**: 250.

26. Palac RT, Meadows WR, Hwang MH, *et al.* (1981) Progression of coronary artery disease in medically and surgically treated patients 5 years after randomisation. *Circulation* **64**: II17.

27. Mylonakis E, Calderwood SB. (2001) Infective endocarditis in adults. *N Engl J Med* **345**: 1318–1331.

28. Hammermeister KE, Sethi GK, Henderson WG, Oprian C, Kim T, Rahimtoola S. (1993) A comparison of outcomes in men 11 years after heart-valve replacement with a mechanical valve or bioprosthesis: veterans affairs cooperative study on valvular heart disease. *N Engl J Med* **328**: 1289–1296.

29. Vongpatanasin W, Hillis LD, Lange RA. (1996) Prosthetic heart valves. *N Engl J Med* **335**: 407–416.

30. Limongelli G, Duccsheschi V, D'Andrea A, *et al.* (2003) Risk factors for pacemaker implantation following aortic valve replacement: a single centre experience. *Heart* **89**: 901–904.

31. Blackstone EH, Kirklin JW. (1985) Death and other time related events after valve replacement. *Circulation* **72**: 753.

32. von Oppell UO, Dunne TT, De Groot MK, Zilla P. (1994) Traumatic aortic rupture: twenty year meta-analysis of mortality and risk of paraplegia. *Ann Thorac Surg* **58**: 585.

33. Ahanger AC, Shabir S, Dar AM, *et al.* (2003) Early operative mortality after surgical treatement of bronchogenic carcinoma. *IJCTVS* **19**: 174–177.

34. Wright CD, Wain JC, Mathisen DJ, Grillo HC. (1996) Post-pneumonectomy bronchopleural fistula after sutured bronchial closure: incidence, risk factors and management. *J Thorac Cardiovasc Surg* **112**: 1367–1371.

35. Tedder M, Ansadt MP, Tedder S, *et al.* (1992) Current morbidity, mortality and survival after bronchoplastic procedures for malignancy. *Ann Thorac Surg* **54**: 387–391.

36. Begg CB, Cramer LD, Hoskins WJ, *et al.* (1998) Impact of hospital volume on operative mortality for major cancer surgery. *JAMA* **280**: 1747–1751.

37. Osugi H, Takemura M, Higashino M, *et al.* (2003) Causes of death and pattern of recurrence after esophagectomy and extended lymphadenectomy for squamous cell carcinoma of the thoracic esophagus. *Oncol Rep* **10**: 81–87.

38. Muller JM, Erasmi H, Stelzner M, *et al.* (1990) Surgical therapy of oesophageal carcinoma. *Br J Surg* **77**: 845–857.

39. Wong J, Cheung H, Lui R, Fan YW, Smith A, SIu KF. (1987) Esophagogastric anastomosis performed with a stapler: the occurrence of leakage and stricture. *Surgery* **101**: 408–410.

40. De Leyn P, Coosemans W, Lerut T. (1992) Early and late functional results in patients with intrathoracic gastric replacement after oesophagectomy for carcinoma. *Eur J Cardiothorac Surg* **6**: 79–84.

41. Urschel JD. (1993) Complications of antireflux surgery. *Am J Surg* **65**: 68–70.

42. Masaoka A, Yamakawa Y, Niwa H, *et al.* (1996) Extended thymectomy for myasthenia gravis patients: a 20 year review. *Ann Thorac Surg* **62**: 853–859.

43. Luke WP, Pearson PG, Todd TR, *et al.* (1986) Prospective evaluation of mediastinoscopy for assessment of carcinoma of the lung. *J Thorac Cardiovasc Surg* **91**: 53–56.

44. Low DE. (2004) Complications of esophageal surgery. In: Little AG (ed), *Complications in Cardiothoracic Surgery. Avoidance and Treatment* (Blackell Futura), pp. 390–404.

45. Cerfolio RJ, Allen MS, Deschamps C, Trastek VF, Pairolero PC. (1996) Postoperative chylothorax. *J Thorac Cardiovasc Surg* **112**: 1361–1365.

46. Deiraniya AK. (1974) Cardiac herniation following intrapericardial pneumonectomy. *Thorax* **29**: 545–552.

47. Schuler JG. (1973) Intraoperative lobar torsion producing pulmonary infarction. *J Thorac Cardiovasc Surg* **65**: 951.

Chapter 9

COMPLICATIONS OF VASCULAR SURGERY

Christopher N. Compton, Navyash Gupta
and Michel S. Makaroun

Medical comorbidities in vascular surgery patients are prevalent, and any clinician involved in the care of such a patient population should be familiar with the diagnosis, treatment and prevention of medical complications. A detailed history and physical, thoughtful preoperative planning and testing are the most valuable measures used to prevent both medical and surgical complications. Choosing the appropriate procedure for a patient and avoiding unnecessary invasive tests are paramount. Early recognition and treatment of the complications associated with vascular surgery can lead to a reduction in morbidity and mortality.

RENAL COMPLICATIONS

Renal dysfunction is a common morbidity of both vascular surgery and preoperative angiographic evaluation. Fluid shifts and haemodynamic lability during aortic surgery, direct ischaemia and embolisation during renal reconstruction or angioplasty, and radiocontrast nephropathy may all contribute to kidney failure. In addition, 5 to 15% of vascular surgery patients have pre-existing renal dysfunction.[1] Many modalities have been proposed for the prevention and treatment of renal failure in these settings. There is likely more folklore than fact regarding the optimal management of vascular surgery patients at increased risk for renal dysfunction.

Radiocontrast administration is a well-documented cause of renal dysfunction. Contrast-induced nephropathy occurs in less than 2% of the general population,[2] but the incidence of clinically significant contrast-induced renal failure among diabetic patients with pre-existing renal insufficiency is as high as 8.8%.[3] Contrast exposure is the third leading cause of new acute renal failure in hospitalised patients.[4] The mortality rate for hospitalised patients developing contrast nephropathy is 34% versus 7% for age and comorbidity-matched patients who received intravenous contrast without developing renal impairment.[5] Angiography is an essential part of the evaluation of patients for many vascular operations, and its use is inherent in endovascular procedures. However, non-invasive diagnostic modalities can often be substituted for angiography, with similar diagnostic utility. Postoperative confirmation of renal artery bypass graft patency as well as screening for occlusive mesenteric ischaemia can be performed with duplex, avoiding the risk of contrast nephropathy. Rarely is preoperative angiography required prior to carotid endarterectomy or aortic aneurysm repair.

The pathogenesis of contrast nephropathy appears to be related to both a direct toxic effect on the epithelial cells of the renal tubules and renal medullary ischaemia.[6] The choice of contrast agent appears to influence the risk of contrast nephropathy. There is evidence that CO_2 angiography has less nephrotoxicity than iodinated contrast agents.[7] However, CO_2 angiography has limitations in defining the anatomy of large diameter vessels, such as the aorta or inferior vena cava (IVC), and in high-resistance vascular beds, such as the tibial vessels in patients with poor runoff. Cerebral arteries should not be studied with CO_2.[8] Rudnick *et al.*, published a randomised, prospective trial comparing a non-ionic contrast medium, Iohexal, to Diatrizoate Meglumine for coronary angiography. In patients with baseline serum creatinine $>1.6\,mg/dL$, the risk of contrast nephropathy is 3.3 times greater with the ionic contrast than that with Iohexal.[9] Gadolinium has also shown promise as a less nephrotoxic alternative to contrast dye.[10]

Several agents have been suggested for the prevention of contrast — associated nephropathy, including hydration, furosemide, mannitol, low-dose dopamine, aminophylline, atrial natriuretic peptide, acetylcysteine, alprostadil and captopril, although only hydration is widely accepted.[11] A randomised prospective trial comparing 0.45% saline IV hydration versus saline plus either furosemide or mannitol revealed that the administration of mannitol or furosemide was less effective at preventing contrast-induced nephropathy than saline hydration alone.[12] The administration of captopril for three days, starting just prior to coronary angiography decreases the risk of the development of nephrotoxicity by 79% and results in a mean increase of GFR by 13 mL/min versus a decrease of 9.6 mL/min for patients with diabetes mellitus randomised to a control group.[13]

The *New England Journal of Medicine* published a randomised, prospective trial in 2000, comparing IV hydration and the oral administration of acetylcysteine to IV hydration alone for patients with chronic renal insufficiency undergoing CT scans with IV contrast. Patients in the treatment arm were administered 600 mg of oral acetylcysteine twice daily on the day prior to, and on the day of, the exam. In the treatment group, 2% of patients experienced an increase in serum creatinine 48 hours post-contrast administration versus 21% of patients in the control arm, which reached statistical significance.[14] Although the results of other studies have been variable, a meta-analysis of seven randomised controlled trials comparing acetylcysteine and hydration with hydration alone for the prevention of contrast nephropathy corroborated the benefit of acetylcysteine.[15]

It seems reasonable that for patients undergoing angiography who have pre-existing renal insufficiency, IV hydration 12 hours before and after the procedure, the use of low-osmolar, non-ionic contrast and the administration of acetylcysteine before and after the procedure are warranted. Patients on metformin should not take the medication for approximately 48 hours or after contrast administration until the absence of renal failure is documented. Witholding metformin is based on reports of lactic acidosis precipated by contrast nephropathy in patients taking the medication.[16]

Renal failure complicates 6% of elective abdominal aortic aneurysm (AAA) repairs[17] and approximately 20% of patients undergoing the repair of ruptured AAA.[18] After thoracoabdominal aortic aneurysm repair, Crawford reported a need for dialysis in 5% of patients with normal preoperative serum creatinine levels and 17% of patients with preoperative creatinine levels greater than

2 mg/dL.[19] Postoperative renal failure carries a significant increase in mortality. Sixty-six percent of patients requiring dialysis after elective AAA died, although renal function recovered in 70% of survivors after a mean of 18 days.[20]

The pathophysiology of perioperative renal dysfunction is likely to be multifactorial. Renal injury may be from hypoperfusion, toxic effects of medication, free radicals or embolisation. Fluid shifts and haemodynamic lability during aortic surgery result in decreased renal perfusion. Renal failure is most likely to occur with suprarenal aortic surgery, but even after infrarenal aortic cross clamping, renal blood flow has been shown to decrease by 40%.[21] Embolisation may occur during open aortic surgery as well as endovascular treatment of the aorta or renal arteries. Renal artery embolisation was detected postoperatively in 13/174 patients receiving aortic endografts at the University of Ulm in Germany.[22] Ramirez et al.[23] noted cholesterol emboli at autopsy in 30% of patients who died within six months after undergoing aortography and 25.5% of patients who died within six months after undergoing coronary angiography. In contrast, the incidence of cholesterol embolism was 4.3% in age-matched controls who had not undergone a previous invasive vascular procedure. Thurlbeck and Castleman[24] found significant cholesterol emboli in the renal arteries of 77% of patients who died after the repair of abdominal aortic aneurysms. Some have advocated using a "no touch" technique during renal artery stenting by placing a second 0.035-inch J-wire within the guide catheter during cannulation of the renal artery. This helps prevent the tip of the guide from rubbing against the aortic wall.[25]

During aortic surgery, there are six basic approaches used to provide renal protection[26]:

1. *Maintaining adequate renal O_2 delivery*
   Adequate cardiac output should be ensured by maintaining preload and inotropic support, if necessary. Appropriate oxygen-carrying capacity with haemoglobin should be provided. Minimising aortic cross-clamp time is vital. Stoney et al., found a 10-fold increase in risk in postoperative renal dysfunction when suprarenal aortic cross-clamp time was greater than 50 minutes, compared to 30 minutes or less, and the risk of even transient, marginal elevations in creatinine are extremely rare when the suprarenal aorta is clamped for 25 minutes or less.[27]

2. *Suppressing renovascular vasoconstriction*

   Providing adequate preload is most important. Angiotensin-converting enzyme inhibitors have been shown to have a beneficial effect.[28]

3. *Renovascular vasodilatation*

   Fenoldopam administration at 0.1 mcg/kg/min in patients undergoing infrarenal aortic aneurysm repair demonstrated a significant improvement in postoperative creatinine levels and renal function compared to patients randomised to a placebo.[29] Compared to a control group receiving placebo, patients undergoing elective thoracoabdominal aneurysm repair and receiving fenoldopam at 0.05 mcg/kg/min had a significantly more rapid return of renal blood flow after cross-clamping, shorter ICU stay, shorter hospital stay and demonstrated trends towards decreased mortality and need for dialysis, despite the fact that the control group was significantly younger and had less co-morbidities.[30] There is no experimental evidence to support the use of dopamine for the preservation of renal function. In addition to its action on DA1 receptors, dopamine has agonistic effects on DA2 and alpha1 adrenergic receptors, both of which mediate vasoconstriction. Two large randomised placebo controlled multicentre trials failed to demonstrate the beneficial role of dopamine in the prevention of renal failure.[31,32] In contrast, fenoldopam stimulates post-synaptic, peripheral DA1 receptors, selectively. It has been shown to increase renal blood flow, urine output and natriuresis.[33]

4. *Maintaining tubular flow*

   Adequate preload is the most important. Mannitol is postulated to increase tubular flow by acting as an osmotic diuretic, increasing renal blood flow, as well as minimising reperfusion injury by scavenging free radicals.[34] Although mannitol has been of significant benefit for the function of renal allografts,[35] the evidence for prevention of renal failure during aortic surgery is scarce.

5. *Decreasing renal cellular O_2 consumption*

   Mild cooling of the kidneys should be considered when extended periods of renal ischaemia are anticipated. Animal studies have demonstrated a significant benefit of cooling to 35°C on renal function with a model of renal ischaemia of 45 minutes duration.[36] Oschner[37] described a technique for renal preservation during suprarenal aortic cross-clamping. A solution consisting of 2,500 U of heparin and 100 mL of 20% mannitol in 500 mL of Lactated Ringer's solution is cooled to 4°C. 500 mL of the perfusate is delivered to the kidneys by infusing the isolated aortic segment containing the renal arteries just after cross-clamping or 100 mL is infused directly into the renal artery ostia. Coselli *et al.*[38] demonstrated a statistically significant decrease in postoperative renal dysfunction after the repair of Type II thoracoabdominal aneurysms in patients receiving selective renal perfusion of cold crystalloid solution compared to patients randomised to receiving selective perfusion of normothermic blood.

6. *Attenuating reperfusion injury*

   Ischaemia-reperfusion injury liberates reactive oxygen species which can mediate free radical damage. Reactive oxygen species (ROS) are potent oxidising and reducing agents that directly damage cellular membranes by lipid peroxidation. In addition, ROS stimulate leukocyte activation and chemotaxis by activating plasma membrane phospholipase A_2 to form arachidonic acid, an important precursor for eicosanoid synthesis (e.g. thromboxane A_2 and leukotriene B_4).[39] Preliminary studies have shown some benefit from treatment with antioxidants. For patients undergoing elective infrarenal aortic aneurysm repair, treatment with Allopurinol, vitamins E and C, N-acetylcysteine and mannitol yielded a significantly higher creatinine clearance than patients randomised to standard treatment.[40]

CARDIAC COMPLICATIONS

Despite improvements in anaesthetic techniques and patient management, coronary artery disease remains the principal cause of both early and late mortality after peripheral vascular operations.[41] Up to 40% of perioperative deaths after aortic reconstruction are cardiac in origin.[42] By performing routine coronary angiograms in 1000 consecutive peripheral vascular patients, Hertzer and colleagues found severe-correctable or severe-inoperable coronary artery disease in 36% of patients with aortic aneurysms, 28% of those with lower extremity ischaemia, and 32% of those with cerebrovascular disease. Only 8% of patients in that series had normal coronary arteries.[43]

The rationale for cardiac evaluation prior to planned vascular surgery is to determine which patients are at risk for perioperative cardiac events, and to intervene when possible to decrease the risk of perioperative cardiac complications. This logic assumes that there is a reliable method to determine cardiac risk, that cardiac diagnostic testing and interventions themselves are low risk, and that intervention provides a protective effect. Krupski found that 38% of patients subjected to extensive preoperative assessment of cardiac risk had adverse events indirectly or directly related to their cardiac evaluation.[44] Previous coronary angioplasty or CABG does not eliminate the potential for perioperative MI. When comparing patients undergoing vascular surgery with or without prior cardiac revascularisation, Back *et al.*[45] found that having a CABG within the last five years or PTCA within two years provided a moderate benefit over patients who had not undergone revascularisation. No patients with recurrent symptoms and who had undergone CABG for more than five years or PTCA less than two years prior had adverse outcomes. However, remote revascularisation (CABG > 5 years; PTCA > 2 years) was independently associated with operative mortality.

To evaluate the long-term outcomes (five-year survival) and cost-effectiveness of selective coronary revascularisation before major vascular surgery, Glance[46] compared four different methods of cardiac evaluation prior to vascular surgery. Patients either proceeded directly to surgery or were screened using one of three possible preoperative screening strategies. In the first strategy, all patients were screened with a dipyridamole-thallium test. In the second strategy, all patients underwent coronary angiography. The third strategy, selective screening, first divided patients into high-, intermediate-, and low-risk groups using clinical criteria. High-risk patients underwent preoperative angiography. Intermediate-risk patients were screened non-invasively, and low-risk patients proceeded directly to surgery without further testing. Proceeding directly to vascular surgery resulted in the poorest five-year survival rate (77.4%) compared with preoperative risk stratification followed by selective coronary revascularisation, routine non-invasive testing (86.1%), selective testing (86.0%), and routine angiography (87.9%; p = 0.00). The incremental cost-effectiveness ratio for selective testing was significantly lower than for routine angiography ($44,800/years of life saved (YLS) vs $93,300/YLS; p < 0.02). Routine non-invasive testing was not found to be cost-effective. Thirty-day mortality was the same for all four strategies (p = 0.84). The authors concluded that selective screening before vascular surgery may improve five-year survival and be cost-effective, and that neither routine non-invasive testing nor routine angiography appears to be cost-effective compared with currently accepted medical therapies.

The American Heart Association has published recommended guidelines for preoperative cardiac evaluation.[47] Based on these a guidelines, a reasonable approach is as follows[48]:

Cardiac stress imaging should be done in patients with low functional status and intermediate (stable angina, prior MI or congestive heart failure [CHF], or diabetes mellitus) or minor (age >70 years, abnormal electrocardiogram [EKG], rhythms other than sinus, previous stroke, or severe hypertension) clinical risk factors. Coronary angiography is generally performed for recurrent ischaemic symptoms after previous CABG or PTCA, presence of major clinical risk factors (recent MI <3–6 months, unstable angina, or decompensated CHF), reversible defects involving moderate or large regions of left ventricular wall during stress imaging, or the presence of clinical variables justifying angiography according to recent ACC/AHA practice guidelines.[49] Primary or secondary (after previous revascularisation) coronary interventions by CABG or PTCA were considered in patients with significant (>70%) stenoses or occlusions responsible for cardiac symptomatology and/or abnormal stress imaging results.

In addition to the proper screening of patients prior to surgery, pharmacotherapy in the perioperative period has been shown to significantly decrease the incidence of adverse cardiac events. The administration of clonidine 90 minutes prior to the induction of anaesthesia for vascular surgery decreases the incidence of perioperative cardiac ischaemic events from 39% to 24% (p < 0.01).[50] Treatment with bisoprolol, a selective B_1 antagonist, one week prior to elective vascular surgery in high-risk patients decreased the incidence of cardiac death from 17% to 3.4% (p < 0.02), and non-fatal myocardial infarction from 17% to 0% (p < 0.001).[51] Likewise, the administration of atenolol prior to the induction of anaesthesia in high risk patients undergoing non-cardiac surgery reduced the overall mortality at six months postoperatively from 8 to 0% (p < 0.001), over the first year from 14 to 3% (p = 0.005), and over two years from 21 to 10% (p = 0.019).[52] Based on these studies, perioperative beta-blockade has become the standard of care in vascular surgery patients who do not have an absolute contraindication to its administration. Despite previous concerns regarding beta-blockade in patients with co-morbidities such as COPD, diabetes, and heart failure, very few patients have an absolute contraindication to receiving beta-blockers. Selective Beta$_1$ adrenergic antagonists have even been shown to decrease mortality in patients with chronic congestive heart failure.[53] Absolute contraindications are as follows[54]:

- Asthma (active or recent)
- COPD (moderate or severe with reversible obstruction)
- Decompensated heart failure (even after optimising medical therapy)
- Heart block (second- or third-degree block without pacemaker)
- Sick sinus syndrome
- Symptomatic bradycardia
- Symptomatic hypotension

GI Complications

Ischaemic colitis is a well-documented complication after aortic surgery. Its incidence ranges from 2%[55] for elective AAA repair and 7%[56] for ruptured repairs if the diagnosis is made clinically, to 4.5%[57] and 60%[58] for elective and ruptured repairs, respectively, if routine endoscopy is performed. Mortality associated with the development of ischaemic colitis is twice that of unaffected patients.[59] The involved area of the colon is confined to the sigmoid in 63% and the left hemicolon in 32% of patients. And pancolitis is seen in 6% of patients and the rectum may also be affected.[60] Early recognition of postoperative ischaemic colitis is important to allow for the institution of supportive measures. Warning symptoms include bloody or Haemoccult-positive diarrhoea, especially in the early postoperative period increased fluid requirements, fever of uncertain aetiology, unexplained leukocytosis or thrombocytopenia, abdominal distention and acidosis.[61]

Findings suspicious for colonic ischaemia on physical exam should prompt investigation with flexible sigmoidoscopy. This procedure may be done rather expeditiously at the bedside and has a high level of reliability. Brandt *et al.*[62] found that findings on sigmoidoscopy performed for clinical signs of ischaemia in patients who had undergone the repair of ruptured AAAs correlated very well with clinical outcome. All patients with normal examinations or those showing only haemorrhagic mucosa were confirmed by either subsequent clinical course or autopsy. Patients felt to have clear full-thickness ischaemia on initial or follow-up sigmoidoscopy had findings confirmed at immediate laparotomy. There was a 67% mortality associated with full-thickness necrosis in this series.

Treatment of ischaemic colitis in the postoperative setting depends on its severity. Patients who have signs of peritonitis or uncorrectable acidosis should undergo laparotomy followed by resection of the involved segment of the colon with construction of colostomy or ileostomy. A primary anastamosis in this setting should be avoided. Milder forms of colitis may be treated supportively. Approximately50%ofpatientswillrespondtoconservativetreatment.[63]Adequate haemodynamicparametersshouldbemaintainedandhydration,bowelrestwith nasogastric decompression, and intravenous antibiotics should be instituted.

Multiple factors have been suggested to contribute to postoperative colonic ischaemia. The colon has been shown to sustain a disproportionate decrease in perfusion during periods of diminished cardiac output.[64] The inferior mesenteric artery is noted to be patent in only 25 to 50% of patients undergoing AAA repair.[65] This may make the colon more susceptible to ischaemia during periods of hypotension or decreased flow, especially in watershed regions. Watershed areas are described between the SMA and IMA circulation (Griffiths' point) and the IMA and hypogastric circulation (Sudeck's point). Ischaemic colitis resulting from atheroemboli during AAA repair via a patent IMA has also been described.[66]

The state of the inferior mesenteric artery at the time of operation, and the utility of reimplanting patent IMAs is controversial. Some series have documented no difference in the incidence of ischaemia between patients with or without patent IMAs, as well as no difference between patients undergoing reimplantation of the IMA versus ligation.[67,68] In contrast, Zelenock and colleagues[69] prospectively studied 100 consecutive patients undergoing elective or urgent aortic reconstruction, in whom a strategy of aggressive colonic and direct pelvic revascularisation was implemented. By routine endoscopy they found an incidence of colonic ischaemia of only 3% and none of the cases were transmural, nor required resection. Despite differences of opinion regarding the relevance of the IMA in colonic ischaemia, all IMA ligations during aortic reconstruction should be performed at the origin, to minimise the disruption of collateral vessels.

Prosthetic Graft Infection

Elective vascular surgery procedures are considered clean. Fortunately, prosthetic graft infections in this setting are rare, but when they occur, they lead to significant morbidity and mortality. The risk of infection varies with the position of the graft, with the incidence of infection for aortic grafts confined to the abdomen being 0.5 to 1%, for aortofemoral grafts 1.5 to 2%, and for infrainguinal grafts that originate in the groin up to 6%.[70] Wound contamination by skin organisms at the time of surgery is the primary mode of infection,[71] but haematogenous seeding of grafts has also been reported.[72] There has been a shift in the types of microbiologic agents identified in recent years. Previously, *Staphylococcus aureus* was the etiology of over half of all vascular graft infections.[73] Currently, *Staphylococcus epidermidis* accounts for 60% of all prosthetic infections.[74] Late infection of an apparently well-incorporated graft may occur one month to several years after surgery due to the indolent nature of *S. epidermidis* graft involvement.[75]

The presentation of a prosthetic vascular infection may be highly variable depending on the organism involved and the location of the infection. Graft infection at the groin may present with cellulitis or draining purulence. Aortic graft infection is more difficult to diagnose, and may manifest with fevers, leukocytosis, or generalised malaise. The diagnostic test of choice when the diagnosis is unclear remains controversial. A duplex exam is a good initial test for groin and lower extremity bypass grafts. The presence of perigraft fluid outside the immediate postoperative period is suggestive of infection. The presence of fluid three months, or gas seven weeks, postoperatively on duplex scanning is abnormal.[76] CT imaging of the abdomen may be performed to identify periaortic infection (Fig. 1). Accessible fluid collections may be sampled under CT-guidance in equivocal cases. CT has a sensitivity

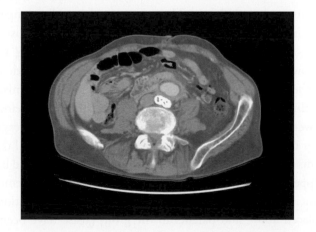

Fig. 1.   Infected aortic prosthesis with gas-containing fluid collection.

of 94% and specificity of 85% when the criteria of perigraft fluid, perigraft soft-tissue attenuation, ectopic gas, pseudoaneurysm, or focal bowel wall thickening are used.[77] In the early postoperative period, signs of graft infection can be difficult to differentiate from normal postoperative changes and adjunctive tests may be necessary. Perigraft air is rare beyond one week after surgery, but is not pathognomonic of graft infection until 4–7 weeks after surgery.[78,79] Technetium white blood cell scans have shown promise in diagnosing early graft infections or those without significant clinical findings. In a group of 97 patients with suspected aortic graft infection, including 32 patients with non-specific symptoms, mTc-HMPAO-labelled leukocyte scanning revealed a sensitivity of 100% and an accuracy of 96.9%.[80] The major limitation of tagged leukocyte scanning is the incidence of false positives, especially early in the postoperative period.

Prevention of graft infection is of the utmost importance. Perioperative antibiotics are mandatory. In 1978 Kaiser *et al.* documented the efficacy of cefazolin to prevent surgical wound infection in vascular surgery when compared to placebo.[81] The infection rate was 0.9% in the cefazolin group and 6.8% in the placebo group. Based on its low toxicity and broad antimicrobial activity, cefazolin should be the antibiotic of choice in patients undergoing vascular procedures. The exceptions are patients who are allergic to cefazolin, in hospitals with high incidence of oxacillin-resistant strains and patients who have had recent oxacillin-resistant infections, in which case vancomycin should be the prophylactic agent of choice. Prophylactic antibiotics should be given 30 to 60 minutes prior to incision. Prophylactic antibiotics should not be continued longer than 24 hours. There is no evidence that longer regimens decrease the infection rate, but have been shown to increase cost.[82] In addition to a pre-surgical scrub, the choice of hair removal timing and method has been shown to affect wound infection rates. In a study to determine the optimal method of hair removal, over 1000 patients were randomised to either shaving or clipping, in the morning of surgery or the night before. Patients who underwent hair removal by clipping on the morning of surgery had significantly fewer infections than any other method. It was estimated that for each 1000 patients treated, a savings of approximately $270,000 could be realised if the AM clipper method replaced shaving for preoperative hair removal.[83] The choice of incision may also influence the rate of wound infection. Oblique incisions placed above and parallel to the groin crease have been shown to have a significantly lower risk of infection than those placed vertically across the groin crease.[84] Any perioperative factor that can be controlled should be used to reduce the risk of infection.

Although autogenous lower extremity grafts, which are exposed due to infection, but are intact, may be salvaged by local wound debridement and coverage with rotational or free muscle flaps, however, the treatment of infected prosthetic grafts is significantly more complicated. The principles of management of infected aortic prosthetic grafts are as follows[85]:

1. *Total excision of the infected graft* as a nidus for continued bacterial sepsis; to prevent propagation of arterial wall infection with resultant pseudoaneurysm formation or rupture.
2. *Wide and complete debridement* of devitalised and infected tissue. Most importantly, the aortic stump must be debrided back to healthy tissue, even when proximal control is difficult. The fibrotic graft bed must also be debrided.
3. *Maintain or establish vascular flow to the distal bed.* The optimal method of achieving this is controversial, but preservation of perfusion is vital to prevent lower extremity, pelvic and colon ischaemia.
4. *Institute intensive and prolonged antibiotic coverage* to control sepsis and prevent secondary infection of newly placed graft.

The options for treatment include:

1. Extra-anatomic bypass (EAB) in conjuction with infected graft removal, whether simultaneously, sequenced before or after removal of infection, or as a staged procedure. The gold standard for aortic graft infection is EAB followed by aortic graft removal several days later, as a staged procedure. The superficial and profunda femoral arteries can be approached laterally with prosthetic graft to avoid infection in the groin, if necessary. One of the major concerns about placement of an EAB prior to removal of graft infection is reinfection of the new conduit. The risk of reinfection of newly placed prosthetic conduits in this setting is low, reported to be 4.5%.[86] The staged approach reduces the physiological stress placed on the patient, and is associated with decreased length of stay, less blood loss,[87] and reduced mortality.[88] The major limitation with this technique is the patency rate of the extra-anatomic bypass. Primary and secondary patency rates for axillo-femoral-femoral bypass of 75 and 100% respectively at 41 months have been reported.[89] When the

popliteal artery is used for the anastamosis, secondary patency rates decrease to 33% at 12 months.[90] Aortic stump rupture (ASR) is the most devastating complication associated with this approach. Rates of ASR vary from 0 to 40%,[91,92] although in recent series with double layer monofilament closure and adequate debridement, ASR rates of 2% should be expected.[93] Generally it is recommended that the aortic stump be buttressed with a tongue of omentum to prevent this complication.

2. *In situ* reconstruction with autogenous conduit. Reconstruction of arterial flow in the setting of aortic graft infection can be performed with the greater saphenous vein or the superficial femoral-popliteal vein (SFPV). The theory behind this treatment modality is that the autogenous vein is resistant to infection, is durable long-term, and provides an in-line method of bypass in patients who cannot undergo EAB for technical reasons. One major limitation of this procedure is the fact that it is not staged, and results in extensive operative time. The group at the University of Texas Southwestern[94] has the most experience with SFPV reconstruction in the setting of aortic infection. They consider significant medical co-morbidities, such as unstable angina, and the presence of extensive bleeding from aortoenteric fistula, to be contraindications to this procedure. The SFPV is an excellent size match for the aorta, alleviating the need to leave an aortic stump. In their most recent series, the mean operative time was 7.9 hours, operative mortality was 7.3%, lower extremity paresis in 7.3%, compartment syndrome in 12%, and major amputation in 5%. Notably, 13% required compression stockings for long-term venous insufficiency. Autogenous venous reconstruction may be a valuable option for patients who cannot undergo extra-anatomic bypass. However, those who have less experience with this technique may have difficulty duplicating the results of the group in Dallas.

3. *In situ* reconstruction with prosthetic conduit. The replacement of infected aortic grafts with standard polyester conduits is of historical interest only. The Mayo clinic reported a reinfection rate of 29% when untreated; *in situ* polyester conduits were used to treat aortic graft infection.[95] The rate of reinfection decreased to 11% when rifampin-soaked grafts were used. Untreated polyester grafts combined with rifampin do not show durable antimicrobial activity because of the rapid loss of drug concentrations in and around the graft site.[96] Coating the prosthesis with collagen enables the graft to provide antimicrobial activity and demonstrate *in vitro* resistance to *Staphylococcus aureus*

infection for up to three weeks.[97] Others[98] have reported similar outcomes after aortic replacement with rifampin-bonded prostheses. More recently,[99] silver-coated polyester grafts have shown an advantage over rifampin-bonded conduits, with a recurrent infection rate of 3.7% over mean follow-up of 16.5 months. The possible advantages of *in situ* reconstruction with prosthetic graft include ready availability of conduit, absence of aortic stump after reconstruction, and resistance to degradation. However, the high rate of reinfection precludes this method from becoming the treatment of choice, even with antibiotic releasing prostheses.

4. *In situ* reconstruction with homograft. Despite the discouraging results of using aortic homografts to treat aortic aneurysms prior to the availability of synthetic grafts, there has been a resurgence in interest for their use in replacing infected aortic grafts. This is due to their ready availability, and perceived resistance to infection. In the modern era, aortic homograft replacement of infected aortic prostheses has been associated with graft complications in 26% of patients during long-term follow-up, including three cases of aortic stump sepsis and one graft enteric fistula within the first year postoperatively.[100] More recently, results from the United States cryopreserved aortic allograft registry have demonstrated graft-related complications such as persistent infection, graft limb occlusion, haemorrhage and pseudoaneurysm formation in 20% of patients over a mean follow-up of 5.3 months.[101] Based on current results, the use of aortic allografts in the setting of infection cannot be advocated, except as a temporary bridge to definitive repair in patients who cannot undergo extra-anatomic bypass and do not have suitable autogenous conduits.

5. Partial removal of infected graft material. Partial graft removal has been proposed to treat prosthetic graft infection while significantly reducing morbidity compared to complete resection. It may be applied to proximal infections from aortoenteric fistulas, as well as graft limb involvement from infection at the groin level. After the removal of non-incorporated, infected portions of the graft an interposition graft is placed for proximal infections; for infected graft limbs, an autogenous or prosthetic conduit may be used to bypass to the groin level. The premise of this modality is that the presence of graft incorporation and the lack of organisms on intraoperative gram stain of incorporated portions reliably rule out infection. However, evidence in the literature would indicate otherwise. This approach is associated with a rate of persistent or recurrent infection of 35%.[102,103] This option is only likely to be successful

with isolated segments of graft infection and those caused by low virulent bacteria.

Although limb salvage is the major concern in patients with infected lower extremity bypass grafts, the significant risk of mortality is inherent, as well. Calligaro reported a 23% mortality and 15% amputation rate for patients undergoing complete excision of infected peripheral prosthetic grafts.[104] Because of these risks, other less aggressive measures have been advocated to treat lower extremity graft infection. The current options to treat lower extremity graft infection include:

1. Total removal of infected graft and lower extremity amputation. This method is best suited for patients with irreversible ischaemia or those who are too unstable to undergo bypass.
2. Total removal of infected graft and replacement with autogenous venous conduit. This is the treatment of choice when the limb would be threatened without bypass, but is still salvageable. Because of its resistance to infection, venous conduits may be placed through a previously infected tissue bed, provided that adequate debridement of infected or necrotic tissue has been performed. Tissue coverage of the vein graft is mandatory. Options include rotational muscle flaps, free flaps or skin flaps.
3. Total removal of infected graft without immediate bypass. If the original operation was performed for claudication, removal of the infected graft may not result in a threatened limb. If this is the case, after adequate debridement and the repair or oversewing of the native artery, wound care may be performed until the tissue bed is clean, and a new graft placed several weeks later.
4. Conservative treatment, consisting of partial graft removal, with subsequent interposition grafting or complete graft preservation combined with secondary wound closure or immediate soft tissue coverage. If the anastomotic sites are intact and the graft is patent, and an intervening segment of the graft is infected, it may be removed with the subsequent placement of an interposition graft. Veith[105] and associates have advocated conservative treatment in infected lower extremity vein grafts with intact anastomoses. They achieved a 19% mortality and 8% amputation rate in survivors using this methodology. Of the patients treated without soft tissue coverage, 20% developed anastomotic haemorrhage, prompting

the authors to advocate tissue coverage in patients undergoing graft preservation. The Mayo Clinic[106] retrospectively compared patients with lower extremity autogenous and prosthetic graft infections who underwent partial or total graft excision to those undergoing drainage, debridement, and total graft preservation with soft tissue coverage. Patients treated without graft excision had a significantly higher limb salvage rate (p = 0.012) than those undergoing partial or total graft excision; there was no difference in mortality rates between the two groups.

To summarise, infected lower extremity grafts are more amenable to conservative treatment than infected aortic prostheses. However, a patent graft and intact anastamoses are required for a trial of graft salvage. Soft tissue coverage, preferably in the form of a muscle flap, should be employed in all cases.

PARAPLEGIA

Paraplegia is one of the most devastating complications of aortic surgery. The complete pathophysiology has not been elucidated, and the risk varies widely based on the location and nature of the surgery. The incidence of postoperative paraplegia ranges from 0.25%[107] for abdominal aortic aneurysm repair to as high as 16% for elective thoracoabdominal aneurysms (TAAAs).[108] The incidence is even higher for ruptured TAAA repair.[109] Of all TAAAs, type II carry the highest risk of paraplegia or paraparesis.[108] Knowledge of the vascular anatomy of the spinal cord is imperative.

The anterior spinal artery arises from the anastomosis of two branches from the intracranial vertebral arteries. It travels in the anterior sulcus of the spinal cord and extends from the level of the olivary nucleus to the conus medullaris. It supplies the ventral surface of the medulla and the anterior two thirds of the spinal cord. The artery is continuous in the upper cervical region. However, in the segments inferior to the upper cervical region, it consists of anastomosing branches from the anterior radicular arteries.

The two posterior spinal arteries most commonly arise from the vertebral arteries. However, in some instances, they arise from the PICA. There are contributions from numerous posterior radicular arteries that form an anastomotic network on the posterior surface of the spinal cord. These arteries supply the posterior one third of the spinal cord. The anterior and posterior spinal arteries join in an anastomotic loop at the conus medullaris.[110]

The different regions of the spinal cord receive an unevenly distributed blood supply. The upper cervicothoracic region between C1 and T2 is richly vascularised by the anterior spinal artery in the most superior segments, and radicular arteries in the lower cervical and upper thoracic segments. The artery of the cervical enlargement is the most important of these radicular arteries. There are a number of radiculomedullary arteries that feed the posterior spinal arteries. The intermediate or midthoracic portion of the cord between T3 and T8 is poorly vascularised by intercostal arteries. There are a limited number of segmental feeders to the posterior spinal arteries. In the lower or thoracolumbosacral region, there is again a rich vascular supply through the radiculomedullary branches of the intercostal and lumbar arteries. One important artery is the great anterior radicular artery of Adamkiewicz (ARM). There are numerous posterior radicular arteries at this level.[110] The ARM is the most substantial contributor to these. Dissection of cadavers shows that 70% of ARMs originate from intercostal or lumbar arteries on the left side frequently at the level of T8 to L1,[111] and the origin of the ARM can vary from T7 to L4.[112] The ARM may be successfully localised preoperatively by angiography, but this knowledge does not necessarily prevent the risk of postoperative paraplegia.[113]

Arterial branches of the hypogastric arteries and middle sacral arteries, and, in particular, the iliolumbar artery seem also to contribute to the extrinsic circulation of the lower spinal cord.[114] The iliolumbar artery may be an important collateral circulation contributor since complete graft replacement of the thoracic and abdominal aorta without reimplantation of the intercostal and lumbar arteries has been performed without postoperative neurological complications.[115] In addition, ligature or endovascular occlusion of one or both of the hypogastric arteries, which give rise to the iliolumbar and lateral sacral arteries, has resulted in spinal cord ischaemic injury.[114]

Although paraplegia after aortic surgery occurs in even the most experienced hands, optimising factors that can be controlled allows for an improved outcome. Results of TAAA repair have steadily improved over time and several strategies have been proposed to decrease the risk of postoperative paraplegia. Stanley Crawford is generally credited with ushering TAAA repair into the modern era. The use of left heart bypass for distal aortic perfusion and

CSF drainage are considered the standard of care currently, and have helped decrease the rate of paraplegia post-TAAA to 10% or less in some series.[116]

Animal experiments have shown that in the setting of aortic cross-clamping, the combination of increased cerebrospinal fluid pressure and decreased arterial pressure results in diminished spinal cord perfusion.[117] By lowering the spinal fluid pressure the incidence of paraplegia after descending aortic occlusion was decreased, but when CSF pressure equalled or exceeded distal aortic pressure, paraplegia occurred uniformly. In a randomised, prospective trial, Coselli[118] found a significant benefit to CSF drainage during the repair of TAAAs, decreasing the paraplegia rate from 13.0% to 2.6%.[118] The technique for CSF drainage is described below.

Patients are placed in the right lateral decubitus position, and a 5F silicone lumbar catheter is introduced into the subarachnoid space at the L3 or L4 intervertebral space via a Tuohy needle. The catheter is connected to a pressure transducer and a drainage set that includes a 75-mL graduated cylinder and a 500-mL drainage bag. The transducer's zero point is set while level with the patient's spine. The CSF pressure is monitored continuously during surgery and the early postoperative period. Cerebrospinal fluid is allowed to freely drain with gravity whenever CSF pressure exceeds 10 mm Hg. In patients without a spinal cord deficit, the drain is removed on postoperative day 2. In the presence of a neurologic injury, however, the catheter is kept in place beyond two days.

Left heart bypass has also been shown to reduce the incidence of paraplegia after TAAA repair.[119] The rationale behind distal aortic perfusion is to provide retrograde blood flow to the spinal cord through lumbar and intercostal arteries, as well as through distal collaterals. Passive or centrifugal pumps may be used. Centrifugal pumps are used preferentially because they can maintain distal pressures at 60 mm Hg, and can avoid the complications of air embolism. In animal studies, distal aortic perfusion was associated with lumbar gray matter spinal cord blood flow more than double that in animals with CSF drainage alone.[120]

Sequential aortic clamping should be used in conjunction with left heart bypass. This technique involves cross-clamping a short proximal segment of the descending aorta after left heart bypass is completed. The proximal anastamosis is performed first, while distal perfusion is maintained. The proximal clamp is then moved below the proximal anastamosis to restore perfusion to the left subclavian artery. The distal clamp is then moved just proximal to the celiac axis to allow for reimplantation of the intercostal vessels. The clamps can then be moved down sequentially during the reimplantation of the visceral and renal vessels.

The intercostal and lumbar arteries between T9 and L1 should be preserved and reimplanted when possible. Reimplanation can be achieved with a button anastomosis or a Carrel patch. Cambria *et al.* have found that the sacrifice of intercostal vessels between T9 and L1 was associated with an odds ratio of 6:1 of developing spinal cord ischaemic complications.[121]

Complications of Endovascular Therapy

Much enthusiasm has surrounded endovascular therapy in recent years, largely based on the prospect of providing an alternative to open surgery which causes less of a physiological insult to patients and results in decreased morbidity and mortality. However, endovascular therapies have their own inherent complications which must be taken into account when counselling patients about the relative benefits of minimally invasive therapy.

Complications of endovascular therapy are divided into those related to the access sites and those from stent-grafts, themselves. Intuitively, one might believe that wound infections occur more commonly after endovascular treatment of AAA than open repair because of the use of groin incisions for access. However, the rate of endograft infection is significantly lower than that of open AAA grafts (0.4% versus 1.3%).[122] As mentioned previously, shaving should be done with electric clippers on the morning of surgery to minimise infection risk. Both micro- and macroembolisation may occur during endograft placement. Massive micro-embolisation after endovascular AAA repair has a reported incidence of between 4 and 17%, often resulting in mortality.[123] Microembolisation will often manifest as colonic ischaemia, whereas macroembolisation may result in lower extremity ischaemia. Although some have suggested distal clamping during endovascular manipulation as a means of preventing embolisation, in reality, distal clamping prevents distal embolisation, but increases the risk of renal and/or visceral embolisation.[124] To avoid these complications, open repair should be performed for aneurysm with large amount of proximal thrombus. In those cases with a high risk of embolisation, but when endovascular therapy is necessary, the use of the brachial artery for wire placement may decrease the incidence of embolisation. Attention to preoperative CT scan images should allow for choosing the least diseased iliac artery for endograft access, and thereby decrease the chances of access site complications.

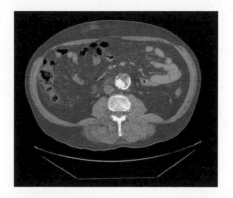

Fig. 2. CT scan of Type II endoleak with perigraft flow of contrast.

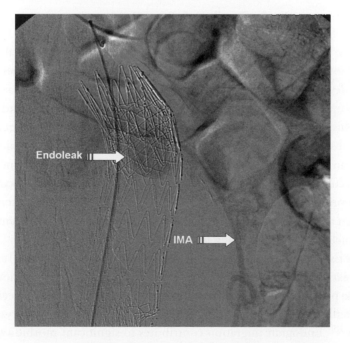

Fig. 3. Type II endoleak from IMA.

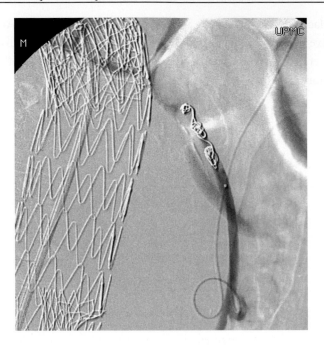

Fig. 4.   Type II endoleak from IMA s/p coiling.

Acute iliac limb occlusion after endovascular aneurysm repair is not uncommon. The rate of limb occlusion is device-specific, and is highest for the Ancure device (11% at 12 months),[125] a device that is no longer available for use. Unsupported grafts appear to be at increased risk for kinking and thrombosis. This result as an early complication from the improper measurement of graft limbs or as a late complication from graft migration. Femoral-femoral bypass can be used to treat graft limb occlusion, but is not without morbidity. Endovascular methods have been successful in opening graft limb occlusions. Both thrombolysis[126] and mechanical thrombectomy via sheath placement[127] have been reported. After thrombus removal, endovascular stent placement can often ameliorate the underlying lesion responsible for thrombosis.

The risk of graft migration is relatively small (3.6% at 12 months) and does not appear to be related to the specific device used.[128] Proximal fixation is presumed to play a role. Preoperative anatomic characteristics have not been found to be predictive of postoperative graft migration,[129] nor has aneurysm neck dilation.[130] Endograft migration contributes to significant morbidity, resulting in open repair in 20% of patients, and rupture in 10–15% of patients.[131]

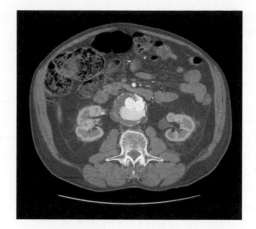

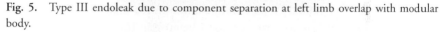

Fig. 5.   Type III endoleak due to component separation at left limb overlap with modular body.

Endoleaks are a unique complication of endovascular grafting (Figs. 2–5). They result from the flow of blood from the vascular lumen to the aneurysm sac due to the lack of proximal or distal fixation (Type I), from retrograde perfusion of the aneurysm sac from the inferior mesenteric or lumbar arteries (Type II), from a defect in the graft material or disconnection of components (Type III), leakage of blood through pores in the graft material (Type IV), or from an indeterminate source (Type V). The rate of endoleaks after endograft placement ranges from 7.1% at two years for Cook Zenith device,[132] to 13.9% at four years for AneuRx device,[133] and 20% at two years for Gore Excluder endograft.[134]

REFERENCES

1. Clark NJ, Stanley TH. (1994) Anaesthesia for vascular surgery. In: Miller RD (ed), *Anaesthesia* (Churchill Livingstone, New York), pp. 1851–1895.
2. Berg KJ. (2000) Nephrotoxicity related to contrast media. *Scand J Urol Nephrol* **34**: 317–322.
3. Parfrey PS, *et al.* (1989) Contrast material-induced renal failure in patients with diabetes mellitus, renal insufficiency, or both. A prospective controlled study. *N Engl J Med* **320**: 143–149.
4. Hou SH, *et al.* (1983) Hospital acquired renal insufficiency: a prospective study. *Am J Med* **74**: 243–248.

5. Levy EM, *et al.* (1996) The effect of acute renal failure on mortality: a cohort analysis. *J Am Med Assoc* **275**: 1489–1494.
6. Barrett BJ. (1994) Contrast nephrotoxicity. *J Am Soc Nephrol* **5**: 125–137.
7. Hawkins IF, Jr. (1994) CO2 digital angiography: a safer contrast agent for renal vascular imaging? *Am J Kidney Dis* **24**: 685–694.
8. Spinosa DJ, *et al.* (2002) Gadolinium-based contrast agents in angiography and interventional radiology. *Radiol Clin North Am* **40**: 694–710.
9. Rudnick MR, *et al.* (1995) Nephrotoxicity of ionic and nonionic contrast media in 1196 patients: a randomised trial. The Iohexol Cooperative Study. *Kidney Int* **47**: 254–261.
10. Rieger J, *et al.* (2002) Gadolinium as an alternative contrast agent for diagnostic and interventional angiographic procedures in patients with impaired renal function. *Nephrol Dial Transplant* **17**: 824–828.
11. Mueller C, *et al.* (2002) Prevention of contrast media-associated nephropathy: randomised comparison of two hydration regimens in 1620 patients undergoing coronary angioplasty. *Arch Intern Med* **162**: 329–336.
12. Solomon R, *et al.* (1994) Comparison of saline, mannitol and furosemide to prevent acute decreases in renal function induced by radiocontrast agents. *N Engl J Med* **331**: 1416–1420.
13. Gupta RK, *et al.* (1999) Captopril for prevention of contrast-induced nephropathy in diabetic patients: a randomised study. *Indian Heart J* **51**: 521–526.
14. Tepel M, *et al.* (2000) Prevention of radiographic-contrast-agent-induced reductions in renal function by acetylcysteine. *N Engl J Med* **343**: 180–184.
15. Rainer B, *et al.* (2003) Acetylcysteine for prevention of contrast nephropathy: meta-analysis. *Lancet* **362**: 598–603.
16. Murphy SW, *et al.* (2000) Contrast nephropathy. *J Am Soc Nephrol* **11**: 177–182.
17. Diehl JT, *et al.* (1983) Complications of abdominal aortic reconstruction. An analysis of perioperative risk factors in 557 patients. *Ann Surg* **197**: 49–56.
18. Gloviczki P, *et al.* (1992) Ruptured abdominal aortic aneurysm: repair should not be denied. *J Vasc Surg* **15**: 851.
19. Crawford ES, *et al.* (1986) Thoracoabdominal aortic aneurysms: preoperative and intraoperative factors determining immediate and long-term results of 605 patients. *J Vasc Surg* **3**: 389–404.
20. Braams R, *et al.* (1999) Outcome in patients requiring renal replacement therapy after surgery for ruptured and non-ruptured aneurysm of the abdominal aorta. *Eur J Vasc Endovasc Surg* **18**: 323–327.
21. Gopalan PD, Burrows RC. (2003) Critical care of the vascular surgery patient. *Crit Care Clin* **19**: 109–125.
22. Gorich J, *et al.* (2002) *J Endovasc Ther* **9**: 180–184.

23. Ramirez G, *et al.* (1978) Cholesterol embolisation: a complication of angiography. *Arch Intern Med* **138**: 1430–1432.

24. Thurlbeck WM, Castleman B. (1975) Atheromatous emboli to the kidneys after aortic surgery. *N Engl J Med* **257**: 442–447.

25. Feldman RL, *et al.* (1999) No-touch technique for reducing aortic wall trauma during renal artery stening. *Catheter Cardiovasc Intervent* **46**: 245–248.

26. Sheinbaum R, *et al.* (2003) Contemporary strategies to preserve renal function during cardiac and vascular surgery. *Rev Cardiovasc Med* **4**: S21–S28.

27. Wahlberg E, *et al.* (2002) Aortic clamping during elective operations for infrarenal disease: the influence of clamping time on renal function. *J Vasc Surg* **36**: 13–18.

28. Gupta RK, *et al.* (1999) Captopril for prevention of contrast-induced nephropathy in diabetic patients: a randomised study. *Indian Heart J* **51**: 521–526.

29. Halpenney M, *et al.* (2002) The effects of fenoldopam on renal function in patients undergoing elective aortic surgery. *Eur J Anaesth* **19**: 32–39.

30. Sheinbaum R, *et al.* (2003) Contemporary strategies to preserve renal function during cardiac and vascular surgery. *Rev Cardiovasc Med* **4**: S21–S28.

31. Chertow GM, *et al.* (1996) Is the administration of dopamine associated with adverse or favourable outcomes in acute renal failure? *Am J Med* **101**: 49–53.

32. Kadieva VS, *et al.* (1993) The effect of dopamine on graft function in patients undergoing renal transplantation. *Anaesth Analg* **76**: 362–365.

33. Lokhandwala MF. (1987) Preclinical and clinical studies on the cardiovascular and renal effects of fenoldapam, a DA-1 receptor agonist. *Drug Dev Res* **10**: 123–134.

34. Magovern GJ, Jr, *et al.* (1984) The mechanism of mannitol in reducing ischaemic injury: hyperosmolarity or hydroxyl scavenger? *Circulation* **70**(Suppl 1): 91–95

35. Van Valenberg PLJ, *et al.* (1987) Mannitol as an indispensable constituent of an intraoperative hydration protocol for the prevention of acute renal failure. *Transplantation* **19**: 4140–4142.

36. Pelkey TJ, *et al.* (1992) Minimal physiologic temperature variations during renal ischaemia alter functional and morphologic outcome. *J Vasc Surg* **15**: 619–625.

37. Oschner JL, *et al.* (1984) A technique for renal preservation during suprarenal abdominal aortic operations. *Surg Gynaecol Obstet* **159**: 388–390.

38. Koksoy C, *et al.* (2002) Renal perfusion during thoracoabdominal aortic operations: cold crystalloid is superior to normothermic blood. *Ann Thorac Surg* **73**: 730–738.

39. Toyokuni S, *et al.* (1999) Reactive oxygen species-induced molecular damage and its application in pathology. *Pathol Int* **49**: 91–102.

40. Wijnen MH, *et al.* (2002) Can renal dysfunction after infra-renal aortic aneurysm repair be modified by multi-antioxidant supplementation? *J Cardiovasc Surg* **43**: 483–488.

41. Krupski WC, *et al.* (2002) Preoperative cardiac risk management. *Cardiovasc Surg* **10**: 415–420.

42. Galland RB. (1998) Mortality following elective infrarenal aortic reconstruction: a joint vascular research group study. *Br J Surg* **85**: 633–636.

43. Hertzer NR, *et al.* (1984) Coronary artery disease in peripheral vascular patients: a classification of 1000 coronary angiograms and results of surgical management. *Ann Surg* **199**: 223–233.

44. Krupski WC, *et al.* (2002) Preoperative cardiac risk management. *Cardiovasc Surg* **10**: 415–420.

45. Back MR, *et al.* (2002) Limitations in the cardiac risk reduction provided by coronary revascularisation prior to elective vascular surgery. *J Vasc Surg* **36**: 526–533.

46. Glance LG. (1999) Selective preoperative cardiac screening improves five-year survival in patients undergoing major vascular surgery: a cost-effectiveness analysis. *J Cardiothorac Vasc Anaesth* **13**: 265–271.

47. Eagle KA, *et al.* (1996) Guidelines for perioperative cardiovascular evaluation for non-cardiac surgery. Report of the American College of Cardiology/American Heart Association task force on practice guidelines. *Circulation* **93**: 1278–1317.

48. Back MR, *et al.* (2002) Limitations in the cardiac risk reduction provided by coronary revascularisation prior to elective vascular surgery. *J Vasc Surg* **36**: 526–533.

49. Scanlon PJ, *et al.* (1999) ACC/AHA guidelines for coronary angiography: executive summary and recommendations. *Circulation* **99**: 2345–2357.

50. Stuhmeier KD. (1996) Small, oral dose of clonidine reduces the incidence of intraoperative myocardial ischaemia in patients having vascular surgery. *Anaesthesiology* **4**: 706–712.

51. Poldermans D, *et al.* (1999) The effect of bisoprolol on perioperative mortality and myocardial infarction in high-risk patients undergoing vascular surgery. *N Engl J Med* **341**: 1789–1794.

52. Mangano DT, *et al.* (1996) Effect of atenolol on mortality and cardiovascular morbidity after noncardiac surgery. *N Engl J Med* **335**: 1713–1720.

53. Heidenreich PA, *et al.* (1997) Effect of beta-blockade on mortality in patients with heart failure: a meta-analysis of randomised clinical trials. *J Am Coll Cardiol* **30**: 27–34.

54. Howard PA. (2000) Optimising beta-blocker use after myocardial infarction. *Am Fam Physician* **62**: 1771–1772.

55. Longo W, *et al.* (1996) Ischaemic colitis complicating abdominal aortic aneurysm surgery in the US veterans. *J Surg Res* **60**: 351–354.

56. Welling R, *et al.* (1985) Ischaemic colitis following repair of ruptured abdominal aortic aneurysm. *Arch Surg* **120**: 1368–1370.

57. Bast T, *et al.* (1990) Ischaemic disease of the colon and rectum after surgery for abdominal aortic aneurysm: a prospective study of the incidence and risk factors. *Eur J Vasc Surg* **4**: 253–257.

58. Hagihara PF, *et al.* (1979) Incidence of ischaemic colitis following abdominal aortic reconstruction. *Surg Gynaecol Obstet* **149**: 571–573.

59. Piotrowski JJ, *et al.* (1996) Colonic ischaemia: the Achilles heel of ruptured aortic aneurysm repair. *Am Surg* **62**: 557–561.

60. Van Damme H, *et al.* (2000) Ischaemic colitis following aortoiliac surgery. *Acta Chir Belg* **102**: 216–218.

61. Toursarkissian B, Thompson RW. (1997) Ischaemic colitis. *Surg Clin North Am* **77**: 461–470.

62. Brandt CP, *et al.* (1997) Flexible sigmoidoscopy: a reliable determinant of colonic ischaemia following ruptured abdominal aortic aneurysm. *Surg Endosc* **11**: 113–115.

63. Piotrowski JJ, *et al.* (1996) Colonic ischaemia: the Achilles heel of ruptured aortic aneurysm repair. *Am Surg* **62**: 557–561.

64. Bulkey GB, *et al.* (1983) Effects of cardiac tamponade on colonic haemodynamics and oxygen uptake. *Am J Physiol* **244**: 604–612.

65. Piotrowski JJ, *et al.* (1996) Colonic ischaemia: the Achilles heel of ruptured aortic aneurysm repair. *Am Surg* **62**: 557–561.

66. Bayne SR, *et al.* (1994) A rare complication in elective repair of an abdominal aortic aneurysm: multiple transmural colonic infarcts secondary to atheroemboli. *Ann Vasc Surg* **8**: 290–295.

67. Piotrowski JJ, *et al.* (1996) Colonic ischaemia: the Achilles heel of ruptured aortic aneurysm repair. *Am Surg* **62**: 557–561.

68. Van Damme H, *et al.* (2000) Ischaemic colitis following aortoiliac surgery. *Acta Chir Belg* **102**: 216–218.

69. Zelenock GB, *et al.* (1989) A prospective study of clinically and endoscopically documented colonic ischaemia in 100 patients undergoing aortic reconstructive surgery with aggressive colonic and direct pelvic revascularisation, compared with historic controls. *Surgery* **106**: 771–780.

70. Seeger JM. (2000) Management of patients with prosthetic vascular graft infection. *Am Surg* **66**: 166–177.

71. Cruse PE, Foord R. (1980) A 10-year prospective study of 62,939 surgical wounds. *Surg Clin North Am* **69**: 27–40.

72. Edmiston CE, *et al.* (1989) Coagulase-negative staphylococcal infections in vascular surgery: epidemiology and pathogenesis. *Infect Control Hosp Epidemiol* **10**: 111–117.

73. Liekwig WG, Greenfield L. (1977) Vascular prosthetic infections. *Surgery* **81**: 335–342.

74. Hicks RCJ, Greenhalgh RM. (1997) The pathogenesis of vascular graft infection. *Eur J Vasc Endovasc Surg* **14** (Suppl A): 5–9.

75. Wilson SE. (2001) New alternatives in the management of infected vascular prostheses. *Surg Infect* **2**: 171–177.

76. Orton DF, *et al.* (2000) Aortic prosthetic graft infections: radiologic manifestations and implications for management. *Radiographics* **20**: 977–993.

77. Low RN, *et al.* (1990) Aortoenteric fistula and perigraft infection: evaluation with CT. *Radiology* **175**: 157–162.

78. Qvarfordt PG, Reilly LM, Mark AS, *et al.* (1985) Computed tomographic assessment of graft incorporation after aortic reconstruction. *Am J Surg* **150**: 227–231.

79. O'Hara PJ, *et al.* (1984) Natural history of periprosthetic air on computerised axial tomographic examination of the abdomen following aortic aneurysm repair. *J Vasc Surg* **1**: 429–433.

80. Liberatore M, *et al.* (1997) Aortofemoral graft infection: the usefulness of 99mTc–HMPAO-labelled leukocyte scan. *Eur J Vasc Endovasc Surg* **14**(Suppl): 27–29.

81. Kaiser AB, *et al.* (1978) Antibiotic prophylaxis in vascular surgery. *Ann Surg* **188**: 283–289.

82. Scher KS. (1997) Studies on the duration of antibiotic administration for surgical prophylaxis. *Am Surg* **63**: 59–62.

83. Alexander JW, *et al.* (1983) The influence of hair-removal methods on wound infections. *Arch Surg* **118**: 347–352.

84. Chester JF, *et al.* (1992) Vascular reconstruction at the groin: oblique or vertical incisions? *Ann R Coll Surg* **74**: 112–114.

85. Bunt TJ. (2001) Vascular graft infections: an update. *Cardiovasc Surg* **9**: 225–233.

86. Reilly LM. (2002) Aortic graft infection: evolution in management. *Cardiovasc Surg* **10**: 372–377.

87. Reilly LM, *et al.* (1987) Improved management of aortic graft infection: the influence of operation sequence and staging. *J Vasc Surg* **5**: 421–431.

88. Seeger JM, *et al.* (1999) Influence of patient characteristics and treatment options on outcome of patients with prosthetic aortic graft infection. *Ann Vasc Surg* **13**: 413–420.

89. Seeger JM, *et al.* (2000) Long-term outcome after treatment of aortic graft infection with staged extra-anatomic bypass grafting and aortic graft removal. *J Vasc Surg* 32: 451–461.

90. Seeger JM, *et al.* (1999) Influence of patient characteristics and treatment options on outcome of patients with prosthetic aortic graft infection. *Ann Vasc Surg* 13: 413–420.

91. Peck JJ, Eidemiller LR. (1992) Aortoenteric fistulas. *Arch Surg* 127: 1191–1194.

92. Yeager RA, *et al.* (1990) Improving survival and limb salvage in patients with aortic graft infection. *Am J Surg* 159: 466–469.

93. Yeager RA, *et al.* (1999) Improved results with conventional management of infrarenal aortic infection. *J Vasc Surg* 30: 76–83.

94. Valentine JR, Clagett GP. (2001) Aortic graft infections: replacement with autogenous vein. *Cardiovasc Surg* 9: 419–425.

95. Young RM, *et al.* (1999) The results of *in situ* prosthetic replacement for infected aortic grafts. *Am J Surg* 178: 136–140.

96. Powell TW, *et al.* (1983) A passive system using rifampin to create an infection-resistant prosthesis. *Surgery* 94: 765–769.

97. Chervu A, *et al.* (1991) Efficacy and duration of anti-staphylococcal activity comparing three antibiotics bonded to Dacron vascular grafts with a collagen release system. *J Vasc Surg* 13: 897–901.

98. Hayes PD, *et al.* (1999) *In situ* replacement of infected aortic grafts with rifampin-bonded prostheses: the Leicester experience (1992 to 1998). *J Vasc Surg* 30: 92–98.

99. Batt M, *et al.* (2003) *In situ* revascularisation with silver-coated polyester grafts to treat aortic infection: early and midterm results. *J Vasc Surg* 38: 983–989.

100. Kieffer E, *et al.* (1993) *In situ* allograft replacement of infected infrarenal aortic prosthetic grafts. *J Vasc Surg* 17: 349–356.

101. Noel AA, *et al.* (2002) Abdominal aortic reconstruction in infected fields: early results of the United States cryopreserved aortic allograft registry. *J Vasc Surg* 35: 847–852.

102. Becquemin JP, *et al.* (1997) Aortic graft infection: is there a place for partial graft removal? *Eur J Vasc Endovasc Surg* 14(Suppl A): 53–58.

103. Miller JH. (1993) Partial replacement of an infected arterial graft by a new prosthetic polytetrafluoroethylene segment: a new therapeutic option. *J Vasc Surg* 17: 546–558.

104. Calligaro KD, *et al.* (1994) Selective preservation of infected prosthetic arterial grafts: analysis of a 20-year experience with 120 extracavitary infected grafts. *Ann Surg* 20: 461–471.

105. Calligaro KD, *et al.* (1992) Management of infected lower extremity autologous vein grafts by selective graft preservation. *Am J Surg* **164**: 291–294.

106. Cherry KJ, *et al.* (1992) Infected femorodistal bypass: is graft removal mandatory? *J Vasc Surg* **15**: 295–303.

107. Szilagyi DE, *et al.* (1978) Spinal cord damage in surgery of the abdominal aorta. *Surgery* **83**: 38–56.

108. Svenson LG, *et al.* (1993) Experience with 1509 patients undergoing thoracoab-dominal aortic operations. *J Vasc Surg* **17**: 357–368.

109. Rampoldi V, *et al.* (1995) Ruptured aneurysms of the thoracoabdominal aorta: a case series. *Panminerva Med* **37**: 123–128.

110. Goetz CG. (2003) *Textbook of Clinical Neurology*, 2nd edn. (Elsevier).

111. Koshimo T, *et al.* (1999) Does the Adamkiewicz artery originate from large segmental arteries? *J Thorac Cardiovasc Surg* **117**: 898–955.

112. Dommise GF. (1974) The blood supply of spinal cord. *J Bone Joint Surg* **56**: 225–235.

113. Williams MG, *et al.* (1991) Angiographic localisation of spinal cord blood supply and its relationship to postoperative paraplegia. *J Vasc Surg* **13**: 23–35.

114. Juvonen T, *et al.* (2002) Strategies for spinal cord protection during descend-ing thoracic and thoracoabdominal aortic surgery: up-to-date experimental and clinical results — a review. *Scand Cardiovasc J* **36**: 136–160.

115. Pokela R, *et al.* (1989) Surgery of thoracoabdominal aneurysms. *Eur J Cardio-thorac Surg* **3**: 456–463.

116. Safi HJ, Bartoli S, Hess KR, *et al.* (1994) Neurologic deficit in patients at high risk with thoracoabdominal aortic aneurysms: the role of cerebral spinal fluid drainage and distal aortic perfusion. *J Vasc Surg* **20**: 434–444.

117. Miyamoto K, Ueno A, Wada T. (1960) A new and simple method of preventing spinal cord damage following temporary occlusion of thoracic aorta by draining the cerebrospinal fluid. *J Cardiovasc Surg* **1**: 188–197.

118. Coselli JS, *et al.* (2002) Cerebrospinal fluid drainage reduces paraplegia after thoracoabdominal aortic aneurysm repair: results of a randomised clinical trial. *J Vasc Surg* **35**: 631–639.

119. Coselli JS, LeMaire SA. (1999) Left heart bypass reduces paraplegia rate after thoracoabdominal aortic aneurysm repair. *Ann Thorac Surg* **67**(Suppl): 1931–1934.

120. Elmore JR, *et al.* (1992) Spinal cord injury in experimental thoracic aortic occlu-sion: investigation of combined methods of protection. *J Vasc Surg* **15**: 789–799.

121. Cambria RP, *et al.* (2000) Epidural cooling for spinal cord protection dur-ing thoracoabdominal aneurysm repair: a five-year experience. *J Vasc Surg* **31**: 1093–1102.

122. Fiorani P, *et al.* (2003) Endovascular graft infection: preliminary results of an international enquiry. *J Endovasc Ther* **10**: 919–927.

123. Thompson MM, *et al.* (1997) Microembolisation during endovascular and conventional aneurysm repair. *J Vasc Surg* **25**: 179–186.

124. Lipsitz EC, *et al.* (1999) Should initial clamping for abdominal aortic aneurysm repair be proximal or distal to minimise embolisation? *Eur J Vasc Endovasc Surg* **17**: 413–418.

125. Ouriel K, *et al.* (2003) Endovascular repair of abdominal aortic aneurysms: device-specific outcome. *J Vasc Surg* **37**: 991–998.

126. Amesur NB, *et al.* (2000) Endovascular treatment of iliac limb stenoses or occlusions in 31 patients treated with the Ancure endograft. *J Vasc Intervent Radiol* **11**: 421–428.

127. Milner R, *et al.* (2003) A new endovascular approach to treatment of acute iliac limb occlusions of bifurcated aortic stent grafts with an exoskeleton. *J Vasc Surg* **37**: 1329–1331.

128. Ouriel K, *et al.* (2003) Endovascular repair of abdominal aortic aneurysms: device-specific outcome. *J Vasc Surg* **37**: 991–998.

129. Lee JT, *et al.* (2002) Stent-graft migration following endovascular repair of aneurysms with large proximal necks: anatomical risk factors and long-term sequelae. *J Endovasc Ther* **9**: 652–664.

130. Kalliafas S, *et al.* (2002) Stent-graft migration after endovascular repair of abdominal aortic aneurysm. *J Endovasc Ther* **9**: 743–747.

131. Kalliafas S, *et al.* (2002) Stent-graft migration after endovascular repair of abdominal aortic aneurysm. *J Endovasc Ther* **9**: 743–747.

132. Sternbergh WC, *et al.* (2004) Influence of endograft oversizing on device migration, endoleak, aneurysm shrinkage, and aortic neck dilation: results from the Zenith multicentre trial. *J Vasc Surg* **39**: 20–26.

133. Zarins CK, *et al.* (2003) The US AneuRx clinical trial: six-year clinical update 2002. *J Vasc Surg* **37**: 904–908.

134. Kibbe MR, *et al.* (2003) The Gore Excluder US multicentre trial: analysis of adverse events at two years. *Sem Vasc Surg* **16**: 144–150.

Chapter 10

COMPLICATIONS OF SURGERY OF THE UPPER GASTROINTESTINAL TRACT

Colleen B. Gaughan, Alexander A. Parikh and John M. Daly

INTRODUCTION

Advances in diagnostic studies, operative techniques, and perioperative management of diseases of the upper gastrointestinal tract have led to an overall reduction of morbidity and mortality for surgery of the oesophagus, stomach and duodenum.[1–4] Nevertheless, the unique anatomy of the upper gastrointestinal tract, traversing three body regions (neck, thorax and abdomen) in close association with the lungs, heart, diaphragm, liver and pancreas, places these other vital organs at risk when resection, replacement, or repair of the oesophagus, stomach, or duodenum is attempted. Futhermore, patients with upper gastrointestinal malignancies pose a particular challenge to the surgeon when attempting a resection for cure or palliation. Many factors that are necessary for a successful surgery are compromised in this population leading to increased postoperative morbidity and mortality.[5] The tumour itself may cause

333

proximal intestinal obstruction leading not only to nutritional deficiencies but also causing metabolic derangements and electrolyte disorders. The association of upper gastrointestinal tract cancers with smoking and alcoholism may lead to cardiovascular and pulmonary risks that must be anticipated and managed in the perioperative period.[6,7] In this chapter, the authors review the most common complications of surgery of the upper gastrointestinal tract, focusing on their recognition and treatment.

ESOPHAGUS

Surgery for Cancer of the Oesophagus

Oesophageal cancer usually presents insidiously, with its first symptoms presenting as dysphagia, at a time when the disease may have already progressed beyond resection. Resectability rates are modest (54–69%), and more than 50% of patients will have unresectable or metastatic disease at the time of presentation.[8–10] For patients with resectable disease, the five-year survival rate is 5–20% with an operative mortality of 4–10%.[11–13] The average rates of major morbidity for patients undergoing oesophageal resection for cancer are 27% for patients without preoperative chemoradiation therapy and 37% for patients with preoperative chemoradiation therapy.

Transhiatal vs transthoracic oesophagectomy for cancer

The two major operative strategies for oesophageal resection for cancer are the tranhiatal and transthoracic approach. No randomised series has demonstrated a clear superiority of one technique of oesophagectomy over another. However, in a recent report from the University of Amsterdam, the transhiatal approach was associated with lower peri-operative morbidity and mortality, but no significant difference in overall survival.[14] It was noted, in this study, however, that there was a trend toward improved five-year survival in the transthoracic oesophagectomy group. Theoretically, the authors proposed that this could be due to the more extensive lymphadenectomy performed with the transthoracic oesophagectomy, with more thorough staging, or more thorough extirpation of the disease. Another reason for the reduced survival in the transhiatal group could be due to the fact that these patients were less compliant with postoperative adjuvant therapy regimens than the transthoracic group.

Haemorrhage

There is a greater risk of bleeding associated with the transhiatal approach to oesophagectomy due to blunt dissection.[15] The small arterial branches that feed the oesophagus directly from the aorta or bronchial arteries are rarely the source of major haemorrhage. The greater risk is the tearing of venous structures, such as the azygous vein. This can result in catastrophic haemorrhage, requiring the packing of the mediastinum and rapid conversion to a thoracotomy to control haemorrhage. There is also a risk of delayed haemorrhage from the short branches that feed the oesophagus directly from the aorta, the short gastric vessels, or from an unrecognised splenic injury.

Tracheobronchial injury

Bronchoscopy should be performed preoperatively if the tumour's location or stage are concerning for airway involvement, such as those with upper or mid-thoracic tumours. In the transthoracic approach to oesophagectomy, the airways are at risk due to the need to place an endoluminal bronchial blocker or dual lumen endotracheal tube for deflation of the right lung during the surgery. The airways may be damaged during the placement or adjustment of these tubes or during the dissection of the oesophagus and nodal basin along the trachea. During the transhiatal approach, the airway may be injured during the blunt dissection of the oesophagus anteriorly or laterally. Although this is a commonly feared complication of oesophagectomy, its actual incidence is low, and there is no difference in the rate of major airway injury according to the type of oesophagectomy undertaken.[16]

Recognition of tracheobronchial injury may be difficult with transhiatal oesophagectomy. Subtle signs include low exhaled tidal volumes, odour of anaesthetic fumes, decreased peak airway pressures, and bubbling from the operative field.

In the event of an intraoperative tracheal or bronchial injury, the first priority should be achieving adequate ventilation and airway control. Methods for managing ventilation during the operation are to convert to single lung ventilation or to intubate the tracheobronchial tree distal to the injury using fibre-optic endoscopic guidance. The oesophagectomy should be completed and the airway repaired at the end of the procedure. Defects greater than 1 cm require repair with a vascularised pedicle, such as an intercostals or pericardial flap, or mediastinal fat. Defects less than 1 cm may be closed primarily, but should be buttressed with a vascularised pedicle, or even the conduit used for oesophageal substitute.

Pneumothorax

A pneumothorax is rarely a significant problem during the transthoracic approach to oesophagectomy. A tube thoracostomy is used to drain the chest postoperatively, and if necessary, a primary repair of a tear of the parietal pleura is possible.

A pneumothorax is a common complication of a transhiatal oesophagectomy.[15] Recognition is crucial so that aspiration of the chest cavity or tube thoracostomy may be performed at the end of the procedure. A chest radiograph should be performed postoperatively regardless of the approach chosen to assess for pneumothorax, pneumomediastinum, and to confirm placement of the chest tubes and nasogastric tubes.

Recurrent laryngeal nerve injury

Unfortunately, injury to the recurrent laryngeal nerve is usually not apparent until after the patient has recovered sufficiently to demonstrate the defect through either hoarseness of voice or dysphagia. Injury may occur during the mobilisation of the cervical oesophagus in transhiatal oesophagectomy or during the blunt dissection in the chest. Traction injuries are usually self-limited, but may take several months to resolve.[17] In a recent study from the University of Hong Kong, patients were prospectively followed after oesophagectomy.[18] All patients underwent postoperative laryngoscopy to document the rate of recurrent laryngeal nerve palsy. In this series, 13.3% of patients were found to have vocal cord weakness. Half of these patients experienced only transient symptoms and 20% were asymptomatic. These figures are higher than those reported in other series. However, this series was the first to document postoperative laryngoscopy for all patients prospectively, and implies that recurrent laryngeal nerve palsy is more common than previously thought.

If airway compromise occurs as a result of previous contralateral injury, tracheostomy and a cord medialisation procedure should be performed. We advocate preoperative direct laryngoscopy for any patient with a history of neck surgery or injury or a history of radiation to the neck.

Cardiovascular complications

During blunt dissection of the lower third of the oesophagus with a transhiatal oesophagectomy, compression of the left atrium and/or elevation of the left ventricle can result in bradycardia and hypotension, due to arrhythmias and decreased venous return. This may not be well tolerated in elderly patients or in individuals with cardiac, pulmonary, or renal disease. Maintenance of adequate filling pressures and normalisation of electrolytes can minimise these effects. Although these effects usually resolve with the withdrawal of the surgeon's hand from the mediastinum, it is important to co-ordinate the progress of the operation with the anaesthesiologist to avoid any prolonged episodes of hypotension.

Pulmonary complications

Pulmonary complications are the leading causes of morbidity and mortality after oesophagectomy, and are more common with a transthoracic approach.[18–23] Risk factors include advance age, COPD, malnutrition, history of severe gastrooesophageal reflux, neoadjuvant therapy, and operative blood loss greater than 1000 mL. Prevention of pulmonary complications and improved postoperative intensive care unit management has led to decreased morbidity and mortality associated with oesophagectomy over the last 20 years.[4,18,21]

Optimisation of preoperative nutrition has never been proven to benefit oesophagectomy patients, but modification of other risk factors, such as abstinence from cigarette smoking[21,24] and participation in a pulmonary rehabilitation programme[21] have demonstrated improved survival. The use of epidural anaesthesia and appropriate perioperative antibiotics decreases the rate of perioperative pneumonia.[15,25] Postoperatively, nasogastric tube decompression, aspiration precautions, and early extubation and mobilisation all help to prevent postoperative atelectasis and pneumonia. Early flexible bronchoscopy should be performed if signs of a pneumonic process manifests to aid in managing secretions and exclude tracheobronchial injuries. Tracheostomy is indicated if mechanical ventilation is required for more than one week for patients unable to be weaned from support.

Gastrooesophageal or oral regurgitation that can lead to aspiration occurs in about 30% of oesophagectomy patients with a cervical anastomosis.[15,18,26]

Supportive care is the mainstay, in addition to patient education to eat smaller but more frequent meals, and to avoid the recumbent position after eating.

Anastomotic leak

The complications of ischaemia, leak, and stricture are closely related, and the relationship among them is poorly understood. The prevalence of anastomotic leak following oesophagectomy varies from 6.3–23% in reported series.[15,27–33] Anastomotic leak is more likely to occur in patients who are malnourished, have had preoperative radiation therapy, have tension at the anastomosis, or have co-morbid conditions requiring preoperative treatment, such as diabetes, congestive heart failure and chronic obstructive pulmonary disease.[34] Approximately half of all anastomotic leaks will heal with a stricture that later requires dilatation.[29,34] Cervical anastomosis and use to the distal stomach for anastomosis were also associated with benign stricture formation.[35]

Hand-sewn versus stapled anastomosis

In a study from the University of Hong Kong, the two techniques of stapled versus hand-sewn intrathoracic anastomosis were compared prospectively.[36] This study found that there was no difference in the rates of anastomotic leak between the two techniques. However, there was a significantly higher rate of anastomotic stricture in the stapled anastomosis group. This result has been supported in many trials, including a metanalysis of the randomised trials by Beitler in 1998,[37] concluding that the two techniques have equivalent leak rates, but that there is a higher rate of stricture with the stapled anastomosis (Table 1). It has been noted that neither technique addresses the problem of conduit ischaemia, the foremost cause of postoperative anastomotic leaks.

Transhiatal versus transthoracic technique

There is no difference in the rate of anastomotic leaks according to which technique of oesophagectomy is chosen, according to large series.[14,36] However, the mortality rates of an anastomotic leak in the neck are lower (20% vs 60%) than leaks within the thoracic cavity. Generally, it is felt that a cervical anastomotic leak is less morbid and easier to manage by opening the neck wound to allow drainage. When anastomotic leaks occur, they do so most commonly on

Table 1. Trials Comparing Hand-Sewn versus Stapled Anastomotic Technique

	Anastomotic Leak		Anastomotic Stricture	
	Hand-Sewn	Stapled	Hand-Sewn	Stapled
Law et al.[36]*	1.6%	4.9% (NS)	9.7%	40% (p = 0.0003)
Orringer et al.[29]	10–15%	2.7%	N/A	N/A
Singh et al.[33]	23%	6% partial mechanical 3% total mechanical (p < 0.05)	58%	19% partial mechanical 18% total mechanical (p < 0.05)
Beitler and Urschel[37]	8%	9% (NS)	16%	27% (p < 0.024[†]
	11%	6% (p < 0.0001)	16%	31% (p < 0.0001)[‡]

*Prospective randomised trial.
[†]Meta-analysis of randomised trials.
[‡]Meta-analysis of non-randomised trials.

the third to fifth postoperative day, manifested by fever, leukocytosis, crepitus, and increased wound drainage and erythema. Patients who develop a leak from a cervical anastomosis usually respond well to drainage so long as the oesophageal conduit is viable. The cervical incision should be opened widely to drain. Attempts to repair the defect are unnecessary, as systemic sepsis rarely occurs. Computed tomography of the neck and chest may be helpful in determining if there is mediastinal contamination which can be managed with directed drainage. Nearly all cervical anastomotic leaks will heal with local wound measures, however, if mediastinitis and sepsis results, a diverting oesophagectomy may be performed. One-third to one-half of patients with cervical anastomotic leaks will develop an anastomotic stricture requiring repeated dilatation.[15,27,29]

Disruption of an intrathoracic anastomosis and subsequent mediastinitis is a common cause of death after oesophagectomy. The leak rate for intrathoracic anastomosis has been reported to be from 6–22%, with the lower leak rates achieved in high volume, experienced centres. The mortality rate of a thoracic oesophageal anastomotic leak is 20–60%, accounting for 9–40% of all perioperative deaths for this procedure.[4,38] Although most patients with an intrathoracic anastomotic leak do survive, their hospital course is long and complicated, leaving them prone to noscomial infections and complications from prolonged immobility. In a study by Wong in 2001, the anastomotic leak rate accounted for 9% of deaths after transthoracic oesophagectomy. This study demonstrated an improvement in the death rate for oesophagectomy that was accounted for by better critical care and prevention of postoperative pulmonary complications. There was no change in the rate of anastomotic leak over this study time period.[4]

Intrathoracic anastomotic leaks usually present after the 7th postoperative day with unexplained fever, leukocytosis, compromised respiratory status and sepsis. Without prompt, adequate treatment, death from sepsis and organ failure is likely. Re-exploration should be performed through the same thoracic incision. Small defects may be locally repaired, but if large defects are present, the goal of operative therapy should be the creation of a controlled fistula and wide drainage of the area to control sepsis. If the oesophageal conduit is not viable, all necrotic tissue must be debrided, and the ends closed with the gastric remnant returned to the abdomen and a diverting cervical oesophagostomy performed. Reconstruction is performed later, after the patient has recovered from the initial episode of sepsis. It is imperative that a feeding jejunostomy is placed to allow for enteral feedings. The early detection of intrathoracic anastomotic leaks is pertinent to the patient's survival; this has led some authors to advocate obtaining gastrograffin swallowing studies as early as the first postoperative day. However, recent studies suggest that this test is neither sensitive nor specific enough to be useful for screening.[39]

Some anastomotic leaks may not be clinically apparent, but are detected on routine postoperative contrast studies, most commonly performed on the fifth to seventh postoperative day. If the patient is asymptomatic, and the radiographic leak is small (<1 cm), and well-drained, it may be treated conservatively with the withholding of oral feeding and repeat radiographic examination in five to seven days.[40] This again highlights the importance of a distal enteric feeding tube. Larger leaks should be drained operatively as they may lead to the formation of tracheoesophageal fistula or mediastinitis, even if the patient is asymptomatic.

Due to the high incidence of anastomotic leaks in oesophageal surgery and the associated morbidity and mortality associated with those leaks, much attention has been paid to the methods of preventing anastomotic breakdown. Preoperatively, carious or abscessed teeth should be removed or repaired to minimise the severity of an infection from anastomotic disruption caused by swallowing oral bacteria. With either the transhiatal or transthoracic approach, and either a stapled or hand-sewn anastomotic technique, meticulous dissection and mobilisation are necessary to achieve a tension-free anastomosis. Proper preparation of the oesophageal replacement is essential for a viable conduit. Preservation of the right gastroepiploic and, if possible, the right gastric arteries for a stomach conduit, of the marginal artery from the middle colic artery for a colonic interposition, as well as the prevention of twisting or kinking of the vascular pedicle is paramount to ensure adequate blood supply. Preservation of the fundus, rather than the cardia of the stomach, allows the maximal length of the conduit to achieve a tension-free anastomosis. If the oesophageal hiatus is repaired, it should be left loose enough, such that the surgeon's hand could reach into the posterior mediastinum, to prevent venous congestion of the vascular pedicle. Postoperatively, a nasogastric tube should be placed to prevent distension of the oesophageal replacement.

Conduit necrosis is fatal in up to 50% of cases.[41,42] A recent study from McMaster University in Ontario, Canada, reported that the independent risk factors associated with mortality from an oesophageal leak were gastric necrosis and the need for operative intervention.[42] They also noted a trend toward increased mortality in patients that presented with an anastomotic leak within the first week of surgery. They did not make a distinction between cervical and intrathoracic anastomotic leaks, as they found them to be nearly equally fatal. Prompt re-exploration after a short period of resuscitation with resection of all devitalised tissue and the creation of a diverting oesophagostomy is necessary for conduit necrosis. The surgeon should have a high degree of suspicion for conduit necrosis if the patient experiences sepsis within the first five days after surgery. Reconstruction is performed several months later, and a feeding jejunostomy is used for enteral nutrition in the interim.

Conduit obstruction

Anastomotic strictures occur in 5–42% of patients regardless of the type of conduit chosen or approach used. Risk factors for the development of an anastomotic stricture include obesity, conduit ischaemia and anastomotic leak. The most common presenting symptom of a stricture is postoperative dysphagia, usually within six months of operation. Diagnosis is by endoscopy, and most patients can be managed by endoscopic dilatation. Care should be taken when dilating oesophagojejunal or oesophagocolonic anastomoses, as these are thinner walled organs and more prone to perforation. Strictures that are resistant to endoscopic therapy, those that are associated with a chronic oesophageal-cutaneous fistula, or jejunal or colonic strictures may require surgical intervention. A variety of stricturoplasty techniques exist, and their detailed description is out of the realm of this chapter. Nevertheless, it is very uncommon for these techniques to be used because of the success of endoscopic therapy. Occasionally, carefully selected patients with persistent strictures may be able to perform their own dilatations at home.

Other causes of conduit obstruction include obstruction at the oesophageal hiatus caused by a hiatal repair that is too constricting or caused by placing the conduit in a retrosternal position. Using the retrosternal position may be necessary in reoperative surgery, as the previous posterior mediastinal conduit may be left *in situ*. The retrosternal placement of a conduit requires the creation of a neohiatal opening, and resection of the clavicular head, manubrium and costal cartilage of the first rib to prevent obstruction.

If the oesophageal hiatus is made too wide, small bowel herniation may result, causing intestinal obstruction. Operative intervention is necessary to prevent strangulation and usually can be accomplished through the abdomen. The oesophageal hiatus should be closed enough to permit the surgeon's hand into the posterior mediastinum and the oesophageal replacement should be anchored to the hiatus.

Retention of food and secretions in the oesophageal conduit is poorly understood. Maintenance of the pleural envelopes during transhiatal oesophagectomy may aid in preventing functional obstruction as it maintains the conduit in straight alignment in the mediastinum. Anchoring of the conduit in the mediastinum during transthoracic oesophagectomy may achieve the same result. Adequate pyloromyotomy or pyloroplasty are other preventive techniques. Functional obstruction is usually treated medically with dietary precautions and prokinetics. Endoscopic dilatation of the pylorus may also aid in the resolution of a functional obstruction. Vagal sparing oesophagectomy, in early oesophageal cancer, has been advocated as a means of preserving both the secretory and reservoir function of the gastric conduit after oesophagectomy. It has been shown to preserve normal gastric emptying in 70% of patients.[43]

Chylous leak

Chylous leak occurs in 1–3% of all oesophagectomies.[44] Risk factors include prior radiation therapy, midthoracic tumours, and prior intrathoracic surgery. It usually presents on the fifth postoperative day, with excessive serous chest tube drainage (>800 mL/day) or in the left neck. The diagnosis can be established by feeding the patient cream and watching for the change in the colour of the chest tube output. High volume leaks will not close spontaneously and require operative ligation to avoid immunologic and nutritional depletion.[44] Enteral nutrition should be stopped and total parenteral nutrition started. In cases of small volume leaks (<400 mL/day) longer term TPN (two weeks) may result in closure.

If injury to the thoracic duct is suspected intraoperatively, an attempt at ligating the thoracic duct should be made. Some surgeons routinely oversew the thoracic duct just above the right diaphragm to prevent chylous leak. Approach to the thoracic duct can be gained via the right chest incision or a right video assisted thoracoscopic surgery may be performed. If the thoracic duct cannot be visualised, ligating the loose areolar tissue between the oesophagus and thoracic spine will usually suffice. Percutaneous embolisation and blockage of the retroperitoneal lymphatic vessels is a novel therapy that may be useful in critically ill patients with medically uncontrollable chylothorax.[45]

Complications of neoadjuvant therapy

Between 85–95% of patients at the time of surgical therapy for oesophageal cancer will have lymph node involvement. Neoadjuvant therapy, in the form of chemoradiation therapy, given before surgery may increase resectability and aid in controlling systemic disease. In two randomised controlled trials, there was a survival advantage to combined modality preoperative therapy (Table 2).[46–49] However, the survival benefit of neoadjuvant therapy for oesophageal cancer is still being debated. In addition, there is concern that preoperative chemoradiation therapy may lead to an increased rate of postoperative complications. Initial studies of preoperative radiation therapy for oesophageal cancer did report an increased rate of pulmonary complications postoperatively, however more recent investigations have shown that chemoradiation therapy is well tolerated and not associated with an increased rate of postoperative complications.[50] In a study by Rice *et al.*, elderly patients were found to have increased

Table 2. Randomized Trials of Preoperative Combined Modality Therapy versus Surgery Alone

	Chemoradiation Therapy Protocol	Resection Rate	Operative Mortality	Median Survival	Survival
Walsh *et al.*[47]	Surgery	100%	4%	11 mth	3 yr: 6%
	CDDP/5-FU + 40 Gy	88%	8%	16 mth	3 yr: 32%
Bossett *et al.* (EORTC)[48]	Surgery	Not available	4%	18.6 mth	5 yr: 25%
	CDDP + 37Gy	Not available	12.3%	18.9 mth	5 yr: 25%
Urba[49]	Surgery	90%	2%	17.5 mth	3 yr: 16%
	CDDP/VBL/5-FU + 45Gy	90%	7%	17 mth	3 yr: 30%

rates of atrial fibrillation and blood transfusion postoperatively, but not to have increased pulmonary, neurologic, cardiac or renal complications.[51] Prognostic benefit of preoperative chemoradiation therapy has only been demonstrated in patients who respond to preoperative therapy and undergo a complete surgical resection. Post-chemoradiation therapy pathologic stage has been found to be an independent predictor of survival.[52] Chemoradiation therapy may be the sole therapy chosen for patients whose operative risk is prohibitive. Complications of chemoradiation therapy itself are usually related to the close association of the oesophagus to other vital organs, and the difficulty in excluding these organs from the radiation field. These complications include pneumonitis, pericarditis, myocarditis, oesophageal stricture (40%), fistula formation and spinal cord damage. Myelosuppression and anaemia have also been reported as systemic complications of neoadjuvant therapy. Radiation therapy is contraindicated in the presence of a tracheoesophageal fistula. Radiation therapy as a sole therapy for oesophageal cancer is considered a palliative therapy because of the high rates of tumour recurrence.

Antireflux Surgery

Intraoperative complications

Intraoperative complications of antireflux operations are rare. The overall mortality rate ranges from 0.3% to 1%.[53] Inadvertent injuries to the spleen or perforation of the oesophagus, although rare, are well described complications with potentially life-threatening sequelae. Capsular tears of the spleen with persistent bleeding have been reported in 3–7% of abdominal antireflux operations.[53] Most of these tears can be controlled with tamponade or electrocautery. According to a 2003 review of the Washington state discharge database and the Health Care Utilisation Project database, splenectomy was performed in 2.7% of antireflux operations from 1992–1997.[54]

Accidental perforation of the oesophagus is a more serious complication, as it may not be easily recognised at the time of operation. An unrecognised, untreated oesophageal perforation is felt to be uniformly fatal. Perforation of the oesophagus during antireflux surgery is most likely to occur during reoperative surgery or while mobilising the oesophagus or attempting to pass an instrument around the oesophagus posteriorly. The primary repair of a perforated oesophagus without reinforcement is usually inadequate and prone to dehiscence. Some authors have therefore advocated reinforcing the primary repair with the gastric fundus wrap in the fundoplication, using it as a serosal patch. Reported incidence of oesophageal perforation during antireflux surgery in the above series was 1.1%.[54]

The most common complication of an antireflux operation is dysphagia. Preoperative oesophageal manometry may help in determining which patients are at risk for postoperative dysphagia by identifying patients with impaired oesophageal motility. The type of antireflux surgery chosen is less important in determining the outcome of antireflux surgery than carefully selecting the patient preoperatively and performing a thorough preoperative diagnostic workup.[55] Postoperative dysphagia may be treated with endoscopic dilatation, or the wrap may need to be taken down.

Failed antireflux operation

The principles of antireflux surgery are common for the many types of antireflux operations that exist:

- To reduce the gastro-oesophageal junction into the abdomen to restore at least 1.5 to 2 cm of abdominal oesophagus.
- To narrow the oesophageal hiatus posteriorly to prevent the creation of an iatrogenic paraesophageal hernia.

- To restore the lower oesophageal sphincter mechanism by creating a high pressure zone in the distal oesophagus with the fundoplication.

The failure of an antireflux surgery usually results from the violation of any one of these principles. Postoperative heartburn was found to be the best predictor of failed antireflux surgery in a series by Pellegrini.[56] An intrathoracic fundoplication, herniation, may result from either the failure to restore an adequate length of oesophagus into the abdomen or the failure to adequately close the diaphragmatic hiatus. Some authors advocate anchoring the oesophagus to the abdominal side of the hiatus to prevent herniation of the wrap into the chest. Herniation of the fundoplication may occur as a result of the failure to recognise a scarred and foreshortened oesophagus that may have required additional thoracic mobilisation or an oesophageal lengthening procedure. An intrathoracic fundoplication is at risk for ischaemia, ulceration and perforation. Re-exploration and investigation of the cause of operative failure should be undertaken as soon as the problem is discovered to prevent these sequelae. When re-exploring for a failed reflux operation, an alternative approach may be chosen (such as a transthoracic, if the first operation was transabdominal) to avoid the extensive adhesions that may be encountered. An antireflux procedure that does not allow for eructation or vomiting may be caused by the technical error of making a fundic wrap too tight or by using the cardia of the stomach as opposed to the fundus in creating the wrap. The fundic wrap should be "floppy," allowing easy passage of the surgeon's finger between the wrap and the oesophagus. Using the cardia instead of the fundus for the wrap will not allow for the receptive relaxation of the wrap during deglutition, and will lead to symptoms of dysphagia and gas bloat.

Functional digestive disturbances

Dysphagia is common postoperatively, and a sensation of fullness experienced by patients is usually caused by oedema at the fundic wrap. Fortunately, this usually resolves spontaneously. Prokinetic drugs, avoidance of the supine position after meals, and taking smaller meals more frequently may help in managing the symptoms caused by postoperative oedema. Many patients with severe reflux disease often swallow air to relieve their reflux symptoms before surgery. These patients may need education to stop this habit postoperatively, as it may lead to gastric distension and pain postoperatively. The gas bloat syndrome is usually caused by a fundic wrap that is too tight, that does not allow eructation, resulting in painful gastric distension and hyperflatulence. The fundic wrap in this case should be revised. Gastric emptying should also be evaluated as a pyloroplasty or pyloromyotomy may be indicated. Patients with ineffective oesophageal motility on preoperative studies may not tolerate a Nissen fundoplication, and may experience postoperative dysphagia. A Nissen fundoplication provides an outflow resistance of approximately 20 mmHg to the oesophagus; if the musculature of the oesophagus is not strong enough to propel a bolus against this resistance, the patient will experience dysphagia. These patients may be better served with a partial fundoplication.

Surgery for achalasia/oesophageal myotomy

Oesophageal myotomy for achalasia has a success rate of 95% in relieving the symptoms of achalasia. Complication rates are low, and are similar to those encountered for antireflux surgery. Insufficient myotomy, oesophageal perforation, perioesophageal scarring and gastro-oesophageal reflux oesophagitis are the most common complications of an operation for achalasia. Unrecognised oesophageal perforation is a potentially life-threatening complication, and has been previously discussed in the section on antireflux surgery. With an increased length of follow-up, the success rate of oesophageal myotomy decreases. Dysphagia and perioesophageal scarring present early, usually within three years of operation. Conversely, gastro-oesophageal reflux oesophagitis is a common complication and can occur up to 10 years postoperatively. An antireflux procedure may become necessary to control symptoms, and potentially prevent progression of the metaplasia to adenocarcinoma. Some authors have advocated performing a partial fundoplication at the time of the oesophageal myotomy.[57,58] With the advent of improved laparoscopic techniques, the thoracic approach to oesophageal myotomy has become less popular.[58] Patients report less discomfort and less dysphagia with the laparoscopic approach compared to the thoracic approach. There have been no randomised prospective trials comparing oesophageal myotomy without fundoplication to myotomy with fundoplication via either a thoracic or laparoscopic approach.

STOMACH AND DUODENUM

Although the number of surgical procedures performed for peptic ulcer disease has declined substantially over the last few decades, they are still being performed. However, they are now performed for complicated or recurrent disease only, since the advent of treatment for *H. pylori* infection and the further development of gastric acid suppression therapy. These patients tend to be older, with more comorbid conditions. Currently, the indications for surgical therapy for peptic ulcer disease include the failure of medical therapy to heal the ulcer after 12 weeks of acid suppression therapy and the treatment for *H. pylori* infection. Another indication for surgery would be the failure of medical therapy for an ulcer that initially responded to treatment. And lastly, surgery is indicated any time malignancy cannot be excluded as the cause of ulceration. The choice of operation depends upon the type of peptic ulcer. The surgical procedure of choice for a type I ulcer is a distal gastrectomy, including the ulcer with either a Bilroth I or II reconstruction. An alternative for this type of ulcer is a local excision of the ulcer and selective vagotomy. Type II and III ulcers require an acid suppressing operation and resection of the ulcer. The procedure of choice is antrectomy and vagotomy with either a Bilroth I or II reconstruction. A vagotomy and pyloroplasty may be performed for duodenal ulcers, if the ulcer is proven to be non-malignant. A type IV ulcer can present a difficult problem for resection. Procedures range from a distal gastrectomy with extension along the lesser curvature to include the ulcer (Pauchet, Shoemaker procedures), a portion of oesophageal wall with the lesser curvature (Csendes procedure), to a total or near total gastrectomy. It is also possible to leave the ulcer *in situ* in the setting of extensive inflammation and perform an antrectomy and vagotomy. Multiple biopsies must be taken of the ulcer to confirm that it is not malignant.

Gastric Cancer

Overall, the incidence of gastric cancer worldwide is declining, although the incidence of proximal gastric cancers are on the rise. Operative morbidity and mortality for gastric cancer have also declined considerably in the last two decades. Improvements in perioperative care , more aggressive lymphadenectomy and staging, and advancements in adjuvant therapy for gastric cancer have led to improvements in long-term survival. Although curative resection is the treatment of choice for gastric cancer, there is debate about the extent of lymphadenectomy that should be performed. In Japan, where there is an aggressive screening programme for early gastric cancer, the rates of survival after gastric cancer resection are much higher than in the West. The Japanese Research Society for the Study of Gastric Cancer has standardised lymph node dissection for gastric cancer, and advocate extensive lymph node dissection (either D2 or D3[59]). In two randomised trials in the West comparing D1 and D2 dissections, the rate of in-hospital mortality and short-term morbidity were higher with D2 dissection.[60] In addition, follow-up of these studies did not demonstrate any long-term improvement in survival or any decrease in the rate of relapse among patiens who underwent a D2 lymph node dissection.[61]

Anastomotic Leak

Patients with anastomotic leaks usually present with abdominal pain, tachycardia, fever, distension and leukocytosis after the fifth postoperative day. Contrast-enhanced computed tomography and water-soluble contrast upper GI series are diagnostic. Small leaks may be managed non-operatively if they are adequately drained, and may heal spontaneously while the patient is supported using TPN. However, if there is any doubt about the adequacy of drainage, most patients will benefit from re-exploration with irrigation of the peritoneal cavity, decompression of the leaking segment, and wide drainage of the area of spillage. The defect at the anastomosis may also be directly intubated for drainage. A distal feeding jejunostomy tube should also be placed at this time, if the patient is haemodynamically stable, to permit enteral nutrition while the leak heals.

Duodenal Stump Dehiscence

Duodenal stump suture/staple line dehiscence is a disastrous complication with an incidence of 1.1% and a mortality rate of 0.6%. This complication occurs most commonly after emergent surgery for a duodenal ulcer or for a bleeding gastric ulcer with or without malignancy. Its incidence after planned resection for gastric cancer is rare. In the majority of cases, the leak is due to a technical error and failure of the suture or staple line. Other factors may contribute to the breakdown of the duodenal stump, such as the obstruction of the afferent loop, pancreatitis, and inflammation of the duodenum at the time of surgery. Patients usually present during the first week after surgery with epigastric pain, fever, tachycardia, and a deterioration in the patient's condition.

Complications of duodenal stump dehiscence include peritonitis and sepsis, pancreatitis, fistula formation, and abscess formation. Wide drainage of an inflamed duodenal stump with a duodenostomy tube for decompression may prevent suture line dehiscence or assist in creating a controlled fistula in the presence of a leak. Management of a stump dehiscence may warrant re-exploration with irrigation of the peritoneal cavity and the placement of drains in the retroperitoneum, but the guiding principle to follow in these cases is to adequately drain the area, rather than attempting to repair the inflamed duodenum. Close attention must be paid to fluid and electrolyte management, TPN should be administered, or the patient may be fed enterally if a distal feeding tube is placed. Closure should occur in two to three weeks.

Pancreatitis/Gallstones

Acute pancreatitis is usually caused by direct trauma to the pancreas during the operation. Treatment is non-operative, except in the case of necrotising pancreatitis or the creation of a pancreatic fistula.

Gallstones may be caused by dennervation of the gall bladder during truncal vagotomy. Prophylactic cholecystectomy is generally not supported during gastric surgery. However, if the gall bladder appears abnormal, is known to contain stones, or future attempts at reoperation will be prohibitively difficult, cholecystectomy should be performed.

Delayed Gastric Emptying/Gastric Stasis

Delayed gastric emptying is common after gastric surgery. It may be due to gastric motor dysfunction or mechanical obstruction. Reoperation for delayed gastric emptying is often difficult and hazardous. The inflammation and adhesions experienced postoperatively are intense in the first six weeks, which is usually when the patient's symptoms become apparent. If the patient's symptoms can be temporised by the placement of a decompressing G tube and a distal jejunal feeding tube for enteral nutrition, the patient should be nursed through this period unless there is a high grade mechanical obstruction demonstrated.

During this period, some patients will resolve their symptoms, obviating the need for surgery.

Patients typically present with nausea, vomiting, bloating, epigastric pain, and weight loss. The first goal is to rule out mechanical obstruction. This can be done with a CT scan, an upper GI series or endoscopy. If oedema is seen, the patient should be treated conservatively. Once mechanical obstruction is ruled out, medical treatment with prokinetic agents can then ensue, and is successful in most cases when the cause of delayed gastric emptying is post-surgical. Prolonged gastroparesis that is refractory to medical treatment following hemi-gastrectomy is best treated with completion gastrectomy and the creation of an oesophageal-jejunal anastomosis with a jejunal J pouch. Success rates for this operation have been reported to be 68–87% for the resolution of symptoms.[62–64] Patients may be considered for a gastric pacemaker, if they are found to have an underlying motility disorder, but the results are varied.[65]

Roux syndrome

Following a distal gastrectomy with Roux-en-Y gastrojejunostomy, a small percentage of patients will present with nausea, vomiting, and symptoms similar to delayed gastric emptying. An endoscopy may show bezoar formation, dilation of the gastric remnant, and dilation of the Roux limb. A gastric emptying scan shows delayed solid and liquid emptying. Motility studies demonstrate propulsive waves toward the stomach in the Roux limb. The disordered motility probably occurs in all patients who have a Roux-en-Y procedure, however, only a subset of patients experience these symptoms, possibly due to concomitant disordered gastric motility. Patients with a large gastric remnant and truncal vagotomy experience this syndrome more often. Treatment consists of prokinetic agents and acid suppression therapy, and possibly surgical therapy to diminish the size of the gastric remnant. If gastric motility is severely disordered, a total gastrectomy may be necessary. The dilated Roux limb should also be resected and another Roux-en-Y constructed with a Roux limb that is at least 40 cm long. This will alleviate the symptoms in approximately 70% of cases.

Dumping Syndrome

As many as 25% of post-gastrectomy patients experience some degree of dumping syndrome postoperatively. It is thought to be due to the ablation of the pylorus, and the loss of regulation of the osmolarity of food entering the small bowel. This occurs after any surgical technique that ablates the pyloric valve, such as pyloromyotomy, pyloroplasty, gastric resection with Bilroth I or II or Roux-en-Y reconstruction, as well as oesophagectomy and total gastrectomy.

Early dumping occurs 15–30 minutes after eating, resulting from a rapid egress of gastric contents into the proximal small bowel. Symptoms include nausea, cramping, diarrhoea, light-headedness, diaphoresis and palpitations. Diagnosis is usually clinical, based on symptoms, although a gastric emptying scan will demonstrate the rapid emptying of the stomach. It is usually managed by the modification of dietary habits, such as taking smaller meals and avoiding concentrated carbohydrates. Octreotide is also useful in managing symptoms, especially diarrhoea, probably by inhibiting the effects of the gut hormones responsible for the symptoms such as VIP, pancreatic polypeptide, motilin, peptide YY and glucagon.

Late dumping, or alimentary hypoglycemia, occurs in 2% of post-gastrectomy patients. Symptoms are vasomotor in character: weakness, sweating, dizziness, flushing and confusion. These symptoms usually occur several hours after eating, and are associated with hypoglycemia. The presence of hyperosmolar food delivered to the small intestine initially overstimulates the secretion of enteroglucagon, resulting in hyperglycemia and the excessive secretion of insulin in the immediate post-prandial period. The rapid entry of glucose into cells stimulated by the excessive stimulation of insulin results in hypoglycemia and hypokalemia. Patients alternate between states of hyperglycemia and hypoglycemia, and will self-treat their hypoglycemic episodes with a sugar-containing snack to relieve their symptoms. Approximately 80% of patients will resolve this pattern over several months, however, dietary modification with the avoidance of hyperosmolar carbohydrates and treatment with octreotide to suppress the release of enteroglucagon can alleviate symptoms.

In patients with persistent dumping syndrome (symptoms longer than one year), a surgical therapy should be considered. The goal is to slow gastric emptying into the jejunem or duodenum. Surgical options include either conversion of a Bilroth II anastomosis to a Roux-en-Y gastrojejunostomy or a Henley jejunal interposition for a Bilroth I anastomosis may be appropriate.

Post-vagotomy Diarrhoea

Although diarrhoea may occur in the short term for many patients, long-term persistence of diarrhoea occurs in less than 1% of patients. Some patients will experience acquired lactase deficiency after gastric resection, but others may manifest with a syndrome of post-vagotomy diarrhoea. Post-vagotomy diarrhoea is thought to be due to the loss of autonomic control of intestinal motility. The malabsorption produced by the rapid intestinal transit time results in steatorrhoea, and malnutrition and metabolic derangements develop, such as hypokalemia, hypocalcemia, and hypomagnesemia. Hypokalemia may be associated with cardiac arrhythmias, while hypocalcemia and hypomagnesemia may result in osteopenia. Unlike dumping syndrome, the symptoms of diarrhoea are not related to the osmolarity of meals or the rate of gastric emptying. The rapid passage of bile salts into the colon inhibits water resorption, contributing to dehydration. Cholestyramine, a bile adsorbing resin, has been used with some success in controlling the diarrhoea, although it does not address the dysmotility as a causal factor. Antimotility agents and smooth muscle relaxants have varied success. Dietary modifications such as limiting liquids with meals, and limiting carbohydrates and dairy products also have some degree of success. For patients with persistent diarrhoea, surgical therapy may be considered. Conversion to a Roux-en-Y gastrojejunostomy if the patient has had a previous Bilroth I or II procedure, or the interposition of a reversed 10 cm segment of jejunem 100 cm distal to the ligament of Treitz may slow intestinal transit time. Results of the jejunal interposition procedure are varied, and may lead to bacterial overgrowth and functional obstruction.

Bile Reflux Gastritis

Bile acids in contact with gastric mucosa for prolonged periods of time may erode the protective mucosal barrier leading to ulceration and metaplasia. Symptoms occur in the early post-prandial period and are related to gastritis and ulceration: epigastric pain, nausea and bilious vomiting. The symptoms may develop months or years after the initial operation. Patients will frequently avoid eating and thus acquire nutritional deficiencies and lose weight. Acid suppression therapies are ineffective. Diagnosis is made by a combination of having a high index of suspicion, endoscopy demonstrating diffuse gastritis, and a nuclear gastric emptying scan that demonstrates a delay in gastric emptying. These studies also demonstrate enterogastric reflux, however, this may be found in normal subjects without symptoms. Treatment is with a combination of mucosal protective agents (sucralfate, aluminum hydroxide) and bile adsorbents (cholestyramine) with prokinetic agents. Surgical therapy is aimed at diverting the bile flow from the stomach. Options include the conversion of a Bilroth I or II to a Roux-en-Y gastrojejunostomy with a long (60 cm) afferent limb, a Henley jejunal interposition (70–100% successful for the diversion of bile from the stomach), or a Braun enteroenterostomy (100% successful for bile diversion). For patients who have persistent symptoms of bile reflux gastritis despite these manoeuvres, a near total or total gastrectomy may be necessary. Despite the diversion of bile flow from the stomach or even total gastrectomy, these patients are rarely left asymptomatic after surgical therapy.

Afferent Loop Syndrome

Afferent loop syndrome is caused by a stricture or kinking of the afferent loop of a Bilroth II anastomosis, preventing the flow of bile from reaching the food in the afferent limb. Care must be taken in the construction of the afferent limb to avoid too much redundancy that may lead to kinking, or in a retrocolic approach to create a mesenteric defect that is too small and obstructs the afferent limb. This may present early after the operation due to technical errors or late after the operation as a result of adhesions. Symptoms may include right upper quadrant or epigastric pain, post-prandial pain, followed by vomiting of clear bile not associated with food. Bacterial overgrowth in the afferent limb may produce leukocytosis and fever. The patient is at risk for ascending cholangitis and haemorrhagic pancreatitis if untreated. Diagnosis is made by clinical history and radiographic studies such as CT scan or upper GI series that demonstrates a dilated afferent limb. Treatment is conversion to a Bilroth I anastomosis, if able, or conversion to a Roux-en-Y gastrojejunostomy with the afferent loop connected to the Roux loop approximately 60 cm distal to the gastrojejunostomy to prevent bile reflux. A vagotomy is necessary to prevent marginal ulceration.

Marginal/Recurrent Ulceration

The most common etiology of marginal ulceration after gastrectomy is a retained vagus nerve or retained antrum on the duodenal stump after distal gastrectomy. Diagnosis is made endoscopically. Endoscopic spraying of a congo red solution may reveal areas where vagal innervation is intact and ulceration may occur due to the presence of acid. Retained antrum bathed in the alkaline bath of duodenal contents will produce gastrin without the negative feedback of acid to suppress it. The elevated gastrin level will be suppressed by a secretin stimulation test, thus distinguishing it from gastrinoma. A "Meckel's scan," a 99mTc sulphur colloid scan, will also demonstrate the retained antrum adjacent to the duodenum.

Management of complications of marginal ulceration can be treated endoscopically with electrocautery of a bleeding ulcer, medically with acid suppression, or surgically with completion antrectomy via an abdominal approach or vagotomy via either an abdominal or transthoracic approach. In patients who have had distal gastrectomy for cancer, the perianastomotic gastric ulcers should be biopsied to exclude recurrence of malignancy.

Anaemia and Nutritional Abnormalities

Loss of the acidic environment in the proximal gastrointestinal tract makes the absorption of iron less efficient resulting in iron deficiency anaemia. In addition, bypassing of the duodenum, such as in a Roux-en-Y gastrojejunostomy limits the absorptive area for iron.

Vitamin B12 is absorbed by its association with intrinsic factor produced by the parietal cells of the stomach. Its absorption is also favoured by an acidic stomach environment. Vitamin B12 deficiency results in megaloblastic anaemia.

Gastric surgery also disturbs calcium and vitamin D metabolism. Calcium absorption occurs primarily in the duodenum, which may be bypassed. Fat malabsorption may result in chelation of calcium and excretion in stool. Vitamin D may be poorly absorbed due to diarrhoea and steatorrhoea caused by increased intestinal transit time after vagotomy. Vitamin D and calcium deficiencies may result in osteopenia and osteomalacia. This may present as musculoskeletal complaints and fractures years after gastric operation. Bone density should be studied and the patient treated with calcium and vitamin D supplementation. Prevention of these complications can be accomplished with patient education about these vitamin and mineral deficiencies, dietary modification and nutritional supplementation, and the monitoring of blood counts and bone density of high risk patients.

CONCLUSIONS

The complexity of surgery of the upper gastrointestinal tract is apparent upon review of the possible complications. Not only is the anatomy challenging, but the physiologic properties of these organs are also complex. Their function profoundly affects the daily life and well-being of the patient. The tenets of a thorough preoperative evaluation, meticulous surgical technique and vigilant postoperative surveillance for complications are all necessary for a successful operation. Improvements in diagnostic modalities, surgical advancements, and perioperative care and management have decreased the rate of postoperative complications for these surgeries over the last 20 years.

REFERENCES

1. McCulloch P, Ward J, Tekkis PP. (2003) Mortality and morbidity in gastro-oesophageal cancer surgery: initial results of ASCOT multicentre prospective cohort study. *BMJ* **327**(7425): 1192–1197.
2. Crookes PF, Incarbone R, Peters JH, *et al.* (1995) A selective therapeutic approach to gastric cancer in a large public hospital. *Am J Surg* **170**(6): 602–605.
3. Swisher SG, Hunt KK, Holmes EC, Zinner MJ, McFadden DW. (1995) Changes in the surgical management of oesophageal cancer from 1970 to 1993. *Am J Surg* **169**: 609–614.
4. Whooley BP, Law S, Murthy SC, *et al.* (2001) Analysis of reduced death and complication rates after oesophageal resection. *Ann Surg* **233**(3): 338–344.
5. Bozzetti F, L.C., Gavazzi C, Bidoli P, *et al.* (1998) Nutritional support in patients with cancer of the oesophagus: impact on nutritional status, patient compliance to therapy and survival. *Tumor* **84**(6): 681–686.
6. Engel LS, Chow WH, Vaughan TL, *et al.* (2003) Population attributable risks of oesophageal and gastric cancers. *J Natl Cancer Inst* **95**(18): 1404–1413.
7. Castellsagué X, Munoz N, De Stefani E, *et al.* (1999) Independent and joint effects of tobacco smoking and alcohol drinking on the risk of oesophageal cancer in men and women. *Int J Cancer* **82**(5): 657–664.
8. Coia LR, Minsky BP, Berkey BA, *et al.* (2000) Outcome of patients receiving radiation for cancer of the oesophagus: results of the 1992–1994 patterns of care study. *J Clin Oncol* **18**(3): 455.

9. Eloubeidi MA, Wallace MB, Hoffman BJ, *et al.* (2001) Predictors of survival for oesophageal cancer patients with and without celiac axis lymphadenopathy: impact of staging endosonography. *Ann Thorac Surg* 72(1): 212–219.

10. Enzinger PC, Mayer RJ. (2003) Oesophageal cancer. *N Engl J Med* **349**(23): 2241–2252.

11. Berger AC, Farma J, Scott WJ, *et al.* (2005) Complete response to neoadjuvant chemoradiotherapy in oesophageal carcinoma is associated with significantly improved survival. *J Clin Oncol* **23**(19): 4330–4337.

12. Ellis FH, Jr, Heatley GJ, Krasna MJ, *et al.* (1997) Oesophagogastrectomy for carcinoma of the esophagus and cardia: a comparison of findings and results after standard resection in three consecutive eight-year intervals with improved staging criteria. *J Thorac Cardiovasc Surg* **113**(5): 836–848.

13. Kaklamanos IG, Walker GR, Ferry K, *et al.* (2003) Neoadjuvant treatment for resectable cancer of the oesophagus and the gastrooesophageal junction: a meta-analysis of randomised clinical trials. *Ann Surg Oncol* **10**(7): 754–761.

14. Hulscher JBF, Van Sandick JW, de Boer AG, *et al.* (2002) Extended transthoracic resection compared with limited transhiatal resection for adenocarcinoma of the oesophagus. *N Engl J Med* **347**(21): 1662–1669.

15. Orringer MB, Marshall B, Iannettoni MD. (1999) Transhiatal oesophagectomy: clinical experience and refinements. *Ann Surg* **230**: 392–400.

16. Hulscher JBF, ter Hofstede E, Kloek J, *et al.* (2000) Injury to the major airways during subtotal oesophagectomy: incidence, management, ans sequelae. *J Thorac Cardiovasc Surg* **120**: 1093–1096.

17. Masamichi B, Shimada M, Nakano S, *et al.* (1999) Does hoarseness of voice from recurrent nerve paralysis after oesophagectomy for carcinoma influence patient quality of life? *J Am Coll Surg* **188**(3): 231–236.

18. Law SM, Wong KH, Kwok KF, *et al.* (2004) Predictive factors for postoperative pulmonary complications and mortality after oesophagectomy for cancer. *Ann Surg* **240**(5): 791–800.

19. Fang W, Kato H, Tachimori Y, *et al.* (2003) Analysis of pulmonary complications after three-field lymph node dissection for oesophageal cancer. *Ann Thorac Surg* **76**(3): 903–908.

20. Mariette C, Taillier G, Van Seuningen I, Triboulet JP. (2004) Factors affecting postoperative course and survival after en bloc resection for oesophageal carcinoma. *Ann Thorac Surg* **78**(4): 1177–1183.

21. Ferguson MK, Durkin AE. (2002) Preoperative prediction of the risk of pulmonary complications after oesophagectomy for cancer. *J Thorac Cardiovasc Surg* **123**(4): 661–669.

22. Ferguson MK. (1999) Preoperative assessment of pulmonary risk. *Chest* 115(90002): 58S–63.
23. Avendano CE, Flume PA, Silvestri GA, *et al.* (2002) Pulmonary complications after oesophagectomy. *Ann Thorac Surg* 73(3): 922–926.
24. Bains M. (1997) Complications of abdominal right-thoracic (Ivor Lewis) oesophagectomy. *Chest Surg Clin N Am* 7(3): 587–598.
25. Flisberg P, Tornebrandt K, Walther B, Lundberg J, Pain relief after oesophagectomy: thoracic epidural analgesia is better than parenteral opioids. *J Cardiothorac Vasc Anaesth* 15: 282–287.
26. Ludwig DJ, Thirlby RC, Low DE. (2001) A prospective evaluation of dietary status and symptoms after near-total oesophagectomy without gastric emptying procedure. *Am J Surg* 181: 454–458.
27. Iannettoni MD, Whyte RI, Orringer MB. (1995) Catastrophic complications of the cervical esophagogastric anastomosis. *J Thorac Cardiovasc Surg* 110(5): 1493–1501.
28. Dimick JB, Upchurch GR, Iannettoni MD, Orringer MB. (2004) National trends in outcomes for oesophageal resection. *Ann Thorac Surg* 79(1): 212–216.
29. Orringer MB, Marshall B, Iannettoni MD. (2000) Eliminating the cervical oesophagogastric anastomotic leak with a side-to-side stapled anastomosis. *J Thorac Cardiovasc Surg* 119(2): 277–288.
30. Crestanello JA, Deschamps C, Cassivi SD, *et al.* (2005) Selective management of intrathoracic anastomotic leak after oesophagectomy. *J Thorac Cardiovasc Surg* 129(2): 254–260.
31. Briel JW, Tamnankar AP, Hagen JA, *et al.* (2004) Prevalence and risk factors for ischaemia, leak and stricture of oesophageal anastomosis: gastric pull-up versus colon interposition.[see comment]. *J Am Coll Surg* 198(4): 536–541; discussion 541–542.
32. Urschel JD, Bennett WF, Miller JD, Young JE. (2001) Handsewn or stapled oesophagogastric anastomoses after oesophagectomy for cancer: meta-analysis of randomised controlled trials. *Dis Oesophag* 14(3-4): 212–217.
33. Singh D, Maley RH, Santucci J, *et al.* (2001) Experience and technique of stapled mechanical cervical oesophagogastric anastomosis. *Ann Thorac Surg* 71(2): 419–424.
34. Honkoop P, Siersema PD, Tilanus HW, *et al.* (1996) Benign anastomotic strictures after transhiatal oesophagectomy and cervical oesophagogastrostomy: risk factors and management. *J Thorac Cardiovasc Surg* 111(6): 1141–1148.
35. Law S, Suen DJ, Wong KH, *et al.* (2005) A single-layer, continuous, hand-sewn method for oesophageal anastomosis: prospective evaluation in 218 patients. *Arch Surg* 140(1): 33–39.

36. Law S, Chu KM, Wong J. (1997) Comparison of hand-sewn and stapled oesophagogastric anastomosis after oesophageal resection for cancer: a prospective randomised controlled trial. *Ann Surg* **226**(2): 169–173.
37. Beitler AL, Urschel JD. (1998) Comparison of stapled and hand-sewn oesophagogastric anastomoses. *Am J Surg* **175**(4): 337–340.
38. Whooley BP, Wong J. (2000) Intrathoracic oesophageal anastomosis: is it worth the risk? *Aust NZ J Surg* **70**(9): 677–680.
39. Tirnaksiz MB, Deschamps C, Allen MS, Johnson DC, Pairolero PC. (2005) Effectiveness of screening aqueous contrast swallow in detecting clinically significant anastomotic leaks after oesophagectomy. *Eur Surg Res* **37**(2): 123–128.
40. Sauvanet A, Baltar J, Le Mee J, Belghiti J. (1998) Diagnosis and conservative management of intrathoracic leakage after oesophagectomy. *Br J Surg* **85**(10): 1446–1449.
41. Cassivi S. (2004) Leaks, strictures and necrosis: a review of anastomotic complications following oesophagectomy. *Sem Thorac Cardiovasc Surg* **16**(2): 124–132.
42. Urschel KA, Alanezi K, Urschel JD. (2004) Mortality secondary to oesophageal anastomotic leak. *Ann Thorac Cardiovasc Surg* **10**(2): 71–75.
43. Banki F, Mason RJ, DeMeester SR, *et al.* (2002) Vagal-sparing oesophagectomy: a more physiologic alternative. *Ann Surg* **236**(3): 324–335; discussion 335–336.
44. Merigliano S, Molena D, Ruol A, Zaninotto G, *et al.* (2000) Chylothorax complicating oesophagectomy for cancer: a plea for early thoracic duct ligation. *J Thorac Cardiovasc Surg* **119**(3): 453–457.
45. Cope C, Kaiser LR. (2002) Management of unremitting chylothorax by percutaneous embolisation and blockage of retroperitoneal lymphatic vessels in 42 patients. *J Vasc Interv Radiol* **13**(11): 1139–1148.
46. Naughton P, Walsh TN. (2004) Multimodality therapy for cancers of the oesophagus and gastric cardia. *Exp Rev Antican Therap* **4**(1): 141–150.
47. Walsh TN, Noonan N, Holywood D, *et al.* (1996) A comparison of multimodal therapy and surgery for oesophageal adenocarcinoma. *N Engl J Med* **335**(7): 462–467.
48. Bossett J-F, Gignoux M, Triboulet JP, *et al.* (1997) Chemoradiotherapy followed by surgery compared with surgery alone in squamous-cell cancer of the oesophagus. *N Engl J Med* **337**(3): 161–167.
49. Urba S. (1997) Combined-modality treatment of oesophageal cancer. *Oncology* **11**(9 supplement): 63–67.
50. Tabira Y, Okuma T, Kondo K, Yoshioka M, *et al.* (1999) Does neoadjuvant chemotherapy for carcinoma in the thoracic oesophagus increase postoperative morbidity? *Jap J Thorac Cardiovasc Surg* **47**(8): 361–367.

51. Rice DC, Correa AM, Vaporciyan AA, *et al.* (2005) Preoperative chemoradiotherapy prior to oesophagectomy in elderly patients is not associated with increased morbidity. *Ann Thorac Surg* **79**(2): 391–397.

52. Chirieac LR, Swisher SG, Ajani JA, *et al.* (2005) Posttherapy pathologic stage predicts survival in patients with oesophageal carcinoma receiving preoperative chemoradiation. *Cancer* **103**(7): 1347–1355.

53. Finlayson SR, Laycock WS, Birkmeyer JD. (2003) National trends in utilisation and outcomes of antireflux surgery. *Surg Endosc* **17**(6): 864–867.

54. Flum DR, Koepsell T, Heagerty P, Pellegrini CA. (2002) The nationwide frequency of major adverse outcomes in antireflux surgery and the role of a surgeon's experience, 1992–1997. *J Am Coll Surg* **195**(5): 611–618.

55. Zaninotto G, Molena D, Ancona E. (2000) A prospective multicentre study on laparoscopic treatment of gastro-oesophageal reflux disease in Italy: type of surgery, conversions, complications and early results. Study group for the laparoscopic treatment of gastro-oesophageal reflux disease of the Italian Society of Endoscopic Surgery (SICE). *Surg Endosc* **14**(3): 282–288.

56. Eubanks TR, Omelanczuk P, Richards C, Pohl D, Pellegrini CA. (2000) Outcomes of laparoscopic antireflux procedures. *Am J Surg* **179**(5): 391–395.

57. Khajanchee YS, Kanneganti S, Leatherwood AE, *et al.* (2005) Laparoscopic Heller myotomy with Toupet fundoplication: outcomes predictors in 121 consecutive patients. *Arch Surg* **140**(9): 827–834.

58. Luketich JD, Fernando HC, Christie NA, *et al.* (2001) Outcomes after minimally invasive oesophagomyotomy. *Ann Thorac Surg* **72**(6): 1909–1913.

59. Sano T, Sasako M, Yamamoto S, *et al.* (2004) Gastric cancer surgery: morbidity and mortality results from a prospective randomised controlled trial comparing D2 and extended para-aortic lymphadenectomy — Japan Clinical Oncology Group Study 9501. *J Clin Oncol* **22**(14): 2767–2773.

60. Bonenkamp JJ, Songun I, Hermans J, Sasako M, *et al.* (1995) Randomised comparison of morbidity after D1 and D2 dissection for gastric cancer in 996 Dutch patients. *Lancet* **345**(8952): 745–748.

61. Bonenkamp JJ, Hermans J, Sasako M, *et al.* (1999) Extended lymph-node dissection for gastric cancer. *N Engl J Med* **340**(12): 908–914.

62. Forstner-Barthell AW, Murr MM, Nitecki S, Camilleri M, *et al.* (1999) Near-total completion gastrectomy for severe postvagotomy gastric stasis: analysis of early and long-term results in 62 patients. *J Gastrointest Surg* **3**(1): 15–21.

63. Farahmand M, Sheppard BC, Deveney CW, Deveney KE, Crass RA. (1997) Long-term outcome of completion gastrectomy for nonmalignant disease. *J Gastrointest Surg* **1**(2): 182–187.

64. Eckhauser FE, Conrad M, Knol JA, Mulholland MW, Colletti LM. (1998) Safety and long-term durability of completion gastrectomy in 81 patients with postsurgical gastroparesis syndrome. *Am Surg* **64**(8): 711–716.

65. Mason RJ, Lipham J, Eckerling G, *et al.* (2005) Gastric electrical stimulation: an alternative surgical therapy for patients with gastroparesis. *Arch Surg* **140**(9): 841–848.

Chapter 11

COMPLICATIONS OF COLORECTAL SURGERY

Paul B. Boulos and Austin O'Bichere

INTRODUCTION

It is imperative that surgeons performing open or laparoscopic colorectal procedures are familiar with the risks involved. The potential benefit of surgery should be measured against the morbidity associated with pre-existing conditions not related to the primary disease and which may jeopardise the surgical outcome. Complications are related to the patient's fitness, the operative procedure, surgical technique and anaesthesia. Therefore the surgeon's role, besides careful patient selection and preoperative optimisation of pre-existing medical conditions, extends to a level of knowledge and technical skill that should minimise early and late morbidity.

This chapter draws attention to frequently encountered complications associated with colorectal surgery that, with awareness, could be prevented and describes their management. Laparoscopy related complications are discussed in another chapter.

SMALL BOWEL OBSTRUCTION

bowel obstruction within the postoperative period (within 30 days) is due to paralytic ileus or mechanical obstruction. It is crucial for management that distinction is made between the two types of obstruction.

Paralytic ileus is invariable after abdominal surgery and is due to reflex inhibition of normal peristalsis. It is painless and lasts for a few days but is prolonged by intra-abdominal sepsis or bleeding, visceral injury, immobility and some medications (ganglion blocking agents, atropine, diuretics).

Mechanical bowel obstruction that occurs early in the postoperative period is commonly caused by fibrinous adhesions before they become organised by the invasion of fibroblasts and sprouting capillaries to form permanent fibrous adhesions. It is less frequently a result of internal herniation, volvulus, anastomotic oedema, intraperitoneal haematoma or abscess.

Clinical Presentation

The cardinal features of intestinal obstruction are pain, vomiting, abdominal distension and constipation.

Paralytic ileus is painless initially, but with progressive intestinal dilatation the patient experiences abdominal discomfort that develops into constant pain if the intestine is ischaemic from excessive distension. By contrast mechanical obstruction gives rise to central and colicky pain that may be associated with borborygmus. The pain is eased by vomiting, which with prolonged obstruction is excessive and the vomitus is faeculent. If the patient had been on unrestricted oral intake constipation is late to develop as bowel movement will continue until the distal segment empties.

In paralytic ileus the abdomen is diffusely distended whereas in mechanical obstruction the degree of distension is dependent upon the duration of obstruction and on the level of obstruction, and therefore on the length of bowel involved, and whether the obstruction is partial or complete. The presence of free intra-peritoneal fluid from intestinal leak, bleeding or ascites increases the distension. The abdomen can feel tense and is tympanitic, but tenderness and guarding may not be evident unless the bowel is ischaemic from gross distension or strangulation, or if there is an abscess or inflammatory mass although may not be easily palpable in a grossly distended abdomen. The bowel sounds are absent in paralytic ileus, but are hyperactive and high-pitched in mechanical obstruction coinciding with attacks of colic. However with prolonged mechanical obstruction the bowel sounds may become infrequent and are tinkling as the bowel becomes paralytic and dilated.

The degree of dehydration reflects on the severity of obstruction and signs of sepsis may be due to strangulation, ischaemia or an inflammatory process that precipitated the obstruction.

Management

An erect plain abdominal film confirms the diagnosis by demonstrating a dilated small intestine with air-fluid levels but does not distinguish between paralytic and mechanical obstruction. The absence of air in the colon is indicative of complete mechanical bowel obstruction whereas in paralytic ileus the colon may also be involved and is air-distended. The initial management is conservative and includes bowel rest (nil by mouth), intestinal decompression (by nasogastric tube aspiration), resuscitation (intravenous fluid and electrolyte replacement) and monitoring (clinical assessment, haemodynamic measurements, and hourly urine output, blood count, C-reactive protein, arterial gases, urea and electrolytes).

An ultrasound or CT scan is essential in mechanical obstruction and in non-resolving paralytic ileus particularly if associated with signs of sepsis or when it develops after return of bowel activity as this may herald the onset of an intra-abdominal complication. The choice between ultrasound or CT scan depends on convenience, availability and expertise. An abdominal ultrasound scan distinguishes between the types of obstruction by identifying hyperactive from adynamic bowel segment and transition from dilated to collapsed intestine. It defines intra-abdominal complications by detecting free or localised fluid or gas collection indicative of an intestinal leak or bleeding and by outlining visceral and intraperitoneal inflammatory changes. An abdominal CT scan with or without contrast is more precise in defining these changes and is of better diagnostic value when an ultrasound scan is equivocal as gaseous distension interferes with ultrasonographic imaging.

An intra-abdominal abscess or infected fluid is drained percutaneously under ultrasound or CT scan guidance and an inflammatory mass is treated with intravenous antibiotics while monitoring the patient's clinical progress. This treatment may be sufficient for paralytic ileus or mechanical obstruction to resolve spontaneously provided there is no persistent underlying sepsis from an ischaemic or injured bowel or dehisced anastomosis when laparotomy becomes necessary.

In the absence of clinical and radiological signs of an intra-abdominal complication, paralytic ileus is likely to resolve with conservative management. In mechanical obstruction, unless the obstruction is partial, laparotomy should be considered if there is no improvement within 48 hours or earlier if obstruction is progressing. The presence of abdominal signs, fever, a markedly elevated white cell count ($>18.0 \times 10^9$/L), a base deficit and absent bowel sounds are suggestive of strangulation. An abdominal CT scan with oral contrast or a water soluble contrast follow through is helpful in confirming mechanical obstruction before proceeding with laparotomy, when a period of conservative management has failed, especially in high risk patients. The passage of flatus or liquid stool, diminishing abdominal distension and nasogastric aspirates and the return of bowel sounds are reliable clinical indicators of resolving obstruction which can be confirmed by abdominal X-rays.

Laparotomy is carried out under prophylactic broad-spectrum antibiotics to prevent the translocation of bacteria through the bowel wall and to minimise the consequences of contamination from inadvertent or planned enterotomy. The surgical procedure involves the division of adhesions and bands, release of internal herniation, reduction of a volvulus, resection or proximal diversion of a narrowed anastomosis or an inflammatory mass. In order to facilitate abdominal closure the bowel contents are milked retrogradely into the stomach and drained via a nasogastric tube or by suction via an enterotomy.

HAEMORRHAGE

Haemorrhage is either *primary* or *secondary*. *Primary* bleeding at the time of surgery or in the immediate postoperative period is the result of poor surgical technique and the failure to achieve satisfactory haemostasis, although clotting disturbance from massive transfusion and restoration of blood pressure with fluid replacement or drug therapy are contributing factors. *Secondary* haemorrhage occurring 7–10 days after surgery is attributed to a dislodged blood clot, dissolution of ligature material or erosion of a vessel due to intra-abdominal infection.

Clinical Presentation

Haemorrhage may present with subtle signs or with shock depending on the site and rate of blood loss. Mild acute blood loss is characterised by cold, clammy skin and decreased capillary refill of more than two seconds due to cutaneous vasoconstriction, tachycardia and orthostatic hypotension. With greater blood loss overt hypotension and oliguria develop. An abdominal examination is helpful if there is progressive distension. The output in drains can be misleading because the drains are often blocked with clot when there is active haemorrhage. It is important to note that acute haemorrhage does not immediately reduce the haematocrit level; serial haematocrit measurements will show precipitous fall after fluid resuscitation.

Management

This includes immediate infusion with an isotonic crystalloid solution through large bore peripheral or central vein cannulas while a blood sample is obtained for cross-matching. The adequacy of volume replacement is assessed by the urinary output (0.5–1.0 ml/kg/hr) and central venous pressure measurements. Every patient with major postoperative haemorrhage should have platelet count, prothrombin time (PT) and partial thromboplastin time (PTT) measurements. When these parameters are abnormal fibrinogen and fibrin degradation products are also measured. In a patient with a healthy liver, reaction to blood transfusion and disseminated intravascular coagulopathy are likely causes. Continued haemodynamic instability despite therapy with fluid and blood products and the correction of clotting abnormalities is an absolute indication for surgical intervention.

Bleeding from poor haemostasis is preventable with care in some frequently encountered situations:

Anterior abdominal wall

When performing abdominal stomas, transverse or paramedian abdominal incisions, the epigastric vessels that lie deep in the longitudinal plane of the rectus abdominis muscles may be injured. The cut arterial ends may retract into the muscle belly and bleeding may not be apparent until it manifests later in the postoperative period with an abdominal wall haematoma and bruising.

Intraperitoneal

When mobilising the colon named blood vessels can be injured: the gonadals and rarely the inferior vena cava when the right colon is freed from its peritoneal attachment and reflected medially; the paraduodenal vessels if the hepatic flexure is mobilised too far medially; traction on the splenic flexure of the colon during its mobilisation with undue care especially if tethered by congenital or aquired adhesions from previous surgery can cause a capsular tear, lacerations of the splenic pulp or the hilum; the gastroepiploic vessels when the omentum is removed en bloc with the transverse colon.

Mesentry

The mesenteric vessels when severed can be difficult to control in inflamed or thickened mesentry as in active Crohn's disease or ongoing intraperitoneal sepsis when a transfixation stitch of the cut ends is more secure than ligation. When a mesenteric vessel is injured and retracts or a ligature slips blood may only escape between the mesenteric peritoneal leaves below the line of resection forming a haematoma that can compress the mesenteric vessels causing segmental ischaemia. Incising the mesenteric peritoneum decompresses the haematoma and haemorrhages can be controlled with electorcautery and spurting arteries are under-run. The adjacent bowel should be inspected for its viability.

Pelvis

When there is locally advanced or recurrent cancer, previous pelvic surgery or radiotherapy, complicated diverticular or Crohn's disease, pelvic dissection of the rectum should be performed cautiously. Rarely a middle sacral artery over the sacral promontory or a left common iliac vein is injured at the start of the pelvic dissection. Patients with portal hypertension with large and numerous retroperitoneal vessels are at particular risk of bleeding.

The lower pelvic side walls may cause significant bleeding when the pelvic fascia is pulled medially by fibrosis or tumour tethering leading to dissection outside the fascia that may injure the internal iliac vessels. Dissection along the correct plane is avascular down to the lateral ligaments which when divided without clamping or ligation, seldom bleed significantly.

Presacral haemorrhage is sometimes unavoidable when the presacral fascia that overlies the high pressure anterior venous plexus is disrupted if thin and friable or is densely adherent to the mesorectal fat. Presacral haemorrhage can also occur from injury to the anterior presacral plexus or basivertebral veins during the placement of rectopexy sutures. Significant haemorrhage can occur if the basivertebral veins are divided at the level of the lower sacral foramina. These veins communicate with the internal vertebral venous system, a large valve-less venous system that communicates with the inferior vena cava. The rapid blood loss associated with this injury is related to high hydrostatic pressure in the depth of the pelvis accentuated in the lithotomy position, which increases venous pooling within the pelvis. In most instances bleeding can be controlled by packing, suture ligation, clips or cautery, but these will be ineffective if the basivertebral veins are injured at the sacral foramina because these large veins retract into the sacral foramina when bone wax or thumbtacks are employed to occlude the foramina and arrest the bleeding.

Perineal

Haemorrhage may occur following open packing of the perineal wound to treat uncontrolled bleeding from the pelvis (usually presacral) or from the divided levator muscles. Packing is usually removed after 48 to 72 hours if the patient remains haemodynamically stable and is not showing signs of ongoing bleeding. Early postoperative perineal bleeding or when changing the pack demands a careful search for any underlying cause that may require re-exploration to control the haemorrhage.

Anal canal

Some bleeding is expected after anorectal surgery but excessive bleeding within the first 48 hours is usually related to incomplete ligation of a vascular pedicle, a slipped ligature or unrecognised bleeding vessel that had been compressed by the retractors. Delayed haemorrhage is caused by sloughing of a ligature by trauma at defaecation and local suppuration.

GASTROINTESTINAL FISTULA

This is an abnormal communication between the gastrointestinal tract and the skin or another viscus. The presence of a fistula in the postoperative period almost always denotes an anastomotic leak. Other causes are an inadvertent enterotomy during the division of adhesions, retraction and mesenteric injuries with resultant bowel ischaemia, and injury to the bowel during closure of the abdominal wall. In the absence of ischaemia or total disruption of an anastomosis these fistulas are expected to close in the early postoperative period (<30 days).

Clinical Presentation

This is easily recognisable when intestinal fluid appears in a drain placed at surgery. Otherwise signs of sepsis that include oliguria, tachycardia, fever, hypotension and leukocytosis may precede the appearance of enteric or faecal contents draining from a surgical wound or a drain. Abdominal signs are infrequent and present as cellulitis around the incision wound and less frequently diffuse or localised tenderness and guarding depending on whether intestinal fluid had also dispersed freely or remained localised in the peritoneal cavity.

Management

Nearly all enterocutaneous fistulas heal spontaneously by conservative measures aimed at reducing intestinal secretions, avoiding bowel obstruction distal to the fistula site, promoting skin healing and maintaining nutritional support, fluid and electrolyte balance. Small bowel fistulas particularly proximal jejunal fistulas are more problematic than distal fistulas because usually the fluid output is high (>500 mls/24 hr) and is rich in electrolytes and pancreatic enzymes and bile. It is therefore useful that a fistula is evaluated by imaging to determine its location and length, the presence or absence of a local abscess and to exclude distal obstruction, by instilling contrast via the cutaneous fistulous opening complemented by small or large bowel contrast studies and CT scanning.

Oral intake is restricted while nutrition is provided by Total Parentral Nutrition (TPN) delivered through a central line although elemental diet is preferred and is appropriate in patients with low output or colocutaneous fistulas. Electrolytes measurements are performed regularly and replacement adjusted according to the losses. Other measures include protective skin barriers, enema or suppositories to prompt bowel evacuation, Somatostatin analogues and H2 antagonists or Proton Pump inhibitors given to reduce gastrointestinal secretions and fistula output.

Surgical intervention is indicated once the patient's condition is optimised in the presence of diffuse peritonitis. Otherwise sepsis with no evidence of peritonitis is managed with intravenous broad-spectrum antibiotic therapy that is modified according to blood cultures. A CT scan of the abdomen and pelvis with guided percutaneous drainage if abdominal or pelvic abscess is detected. This may have to be repeated whenever the patient shows signs of sepsis during the course of conservative management.

The effectiveness of treatment is determined by reduction in the daily measured volume of fistula fluid output. Distal obstruction, an adjacent abscess, inflammatory bowel disease, radiation damage, malignancy at the site of fistulisation, exposed intestinal mucosa or epithelialisation of the fistula tract and persistent sepsis are predictors of a less favourable outcome. However conservative management is worth pursuing as it has beneficial effects on the patient's overall fitness and allows intra-abdominal inflammation to subside reducing the hazards of re-exploration.

The indications for surgical intervention are peritonitis, persistent sepsis and failed conservative treatment. The surgical procedure should take into account the patient's metabolic status (anaemia and hypoalbuminaemia), the extent of intra-abdominal contamination, the nature of the fistula and underlying intestinal disease. Under optimal conditions fistulas are excised with the involved segment of intestine with primary anastomosis with or without proximal diversion. Alternatively the excised bowel ends are exteriorised as a stoma and mucus fistula and occasionally a diversion stoma proximal to the fistula can be sufficient as in anastomotic leaks.

ANASTOMOTIC DEHISCENCE

Anastomotic leakage from the small or large bowel is one of the most feared complications because it increases morbidity and mortality. The risk of leakage is higher in anastamoses below the peritoneal reflection than those located intraperitoneally. Clinically insignificant leaks identified radiologically with water soluble contrast enemas have been reported to be three to four times

higher than clinically apparent leaks. The risk of leakage from a low anastomosis within 6 cm from the anal verge is higher and routine temporary
faecal diversion has been advocated. A proximal diverting stoma to protect
a low pelvic or technically inadequate anastamosis does not alter the risk of
dehiscence but ameliorates the septic effects of the leak.

Besides the location of the anastomosis several factors that include technical and intrinsic patient factors contribute to impaired healing and should be
taken into account to minimise the risk of anastomotic dehiscence. Technical
factors are ischaemia or oedema at the bowel ends, tension on the anastomosis,
inadequate closure of anastomosis, and generalised or localised sepsis near the
anastomosis. Patient factors are anaemia, malnutrition, high dose of steroids or
other immunosuppressant agents, poor bowel preparation, co-existent medical illness, previously irradiated bowel or active inflammatory bowel disease at
the anastomosis and distal obstruction to an anastomosis.

Clinical Presentation

This depends on the site and size of the leak which may not be clinically
evident or manifest with sepsis with or without abdominal signs. Pyrexia,
tachycardia, oliguria and prolonged ileus are suggestive signs; abdominal pain
and tenderness or guarding is variable. A leak that had been walled off by
adjacent organs and omentum to form an abscess located commonly under the
diaphragm (subphrenic) may herald respiratory infection and the patient may
complain of shoulder tip pain and hiccoughs; or in the pelvis (pelvic) causing
diarrhoea. An abscess may manifest at a later time with discharge through the
abdominal incision or as an enterocutaneous fistula. A significant leak will
cause faecal peritonitis and circulatory failure leading to multiorgan failure.

Management

Diagnosis of anastomotic dehiscence by clinical examination is feasible in
colorectal anastomoses if it lies within the reach of the examining finger and
the defect is large. Leukocytosis and intestinal organisms isolated on blood
cultures are suggestive but the diagnosis relies on a CT scan with intravenous,
oral and rectal contrast material, showing extravasation of contrast from the
intestine, free intra-abdominal fluid or an abscess. A water-soluble contrast

enema is used to evaluate the integrity of a colorectal anastomosis but is less useful for more proximal anastomoses because the contrast becomes too dilute to accurately define the anastomosis which may be disrupted further by air distension. A barium enema should be avoided because of the morbidity of barium peritonitis.

Asymptomatic leaks demonstrable radiologically are infrequent as contrast enemas are not performed routinely although they are sometimes detectable as peri-anastomotic air fluid filled collection on an abdominal CT scan obtained for an unrelated reason. The leak in this clinical circumstance is of no clinical consequence and will heal spontaneously.

A symptomatic leak is treated by broad-spectrum intravenous antibiotic therapy and bowel rest, maintaining nutrition by TPN or elemental diet, and an abscess or intraperitoneal collection. A percutaneous drainage of pelvic abscess may be accessible via a trans-rectal or a trans-vaginal approach or through the anastomosis in low extra-peritoneal anastomotic leaks. Associated intestinal fistula is managed as described previously. A conservative approach is continued provided the patient does not remain septic.

Failed conservative management or a leak with peritonitis demands re-exploration after the patient is resuscitated. Repair of the anastomosis should not be attempted because the tissues are friable and in the presence of intra-abdominal sepsis is certain to fail. A proximal diversion preserves the anasto-mosis and is particularly preferred in low extra-peritoneal anastomosis and the appearances on a preoperative contrast enema or the operative findings suggest a small leak. Diversion is acceptable in an early postoperative leak while the bowel is still clean. It is inadvisable, when the leak is late after the patient had resumed oral intake because the leak will remain a source of persistent sepsis; a safer option is to excise the anastomosis and exteriorise the bowel ends as a stoma and distal mucus fistula although its reversal is more demanding than the reversal of a diversion stoma.

ANASTOMOTIC STRICTURE

Anastomotic strictures are infrequent in intraperitoneal colonic anastomoses and usually occur with low colorectal and ileoanal anastomoses due to tis-sue ischaemia, anatomic leak, local sepsis and proximal diversion prevent-ing stretching of the anastomosis by passing stool, irrespective of whether a sutured or stapled anastomosis had been carried out. Strictures from recurrent carcinoma or inflammatory bowel disease develop much later after surgery. Symptoms of a significant stricture are constipation, frequent and small bowel movements, and abdominal distension. A patient who had a proximal diversion with the primary procedure will exhibit these symptoms after closure of the stoma. It is prudent that prior to closure of a stoma that an anastomosis is not only evaluated for evidence of a leak by a contrast study but also for its patency by ensuring that a 19 mm sigmoidoscope can be passed through the anastomosis. A low and soft stricture is easily dilated digitally, more proximal or rigid strictures are dilated with a rigid sigmoidoscope, Hegar's dilators or gum-elastic bougies under anaestheisa, or endoscopic balloon dilatation under sedation. A symptomatic stricture not responding to these measures requires resection.

Small bowel anastamoses narrow initially due to oedema related to surgical trauma or a localised perianastomotic inflammation from a small leak. This is of no significance although it is probably a cause of postoperative intestinal obstruction that occasionally complicates small intestinal resection and resolves on conservative treatment. Otherwise small bowel anastomotic strictures apart from recurrent Crohn's disease is unusual and must be attributed to poor surgical technique.

VISCERAL INJURY

Mobilisation of the colon and rectum, and minor anorectal surgery can damage other viscera as a result of close anatomical proximity and tethering by the primary pathological process particularly cancer, Crohn's disease and diverticulitis. Damage is unavoidable when an organ is involved with the primary colonic disease. Awareness of the hazard involved demands cautious dissection to avoid or minimise the extent of the injury and alertness to the consequences of such an event. One should be familiar with structures that are particularly vulnerable and the means of avoiding and dealing with the damage, and as with all complications early identification is the key to minimising morbidity.

Clinical Presentation and Management

Stomach

The stomach does not frequently encroach onto the field of dissection unless it is involved with the colonic disease and usually at its distal end, when sleeve or partial resection might be necessary to free the diseased colon. While the stomach has a rich blood supply it is essential that the arterial arcade formed by the left and right gastric epiploic arteries along its greater curvature is not damaged while mobilising or excising the omentum. The omentum is approached distal to the arcade and dissection should proceed keeping the arcade under vision. Laceration or ischaemia of the stomach wall should be easy to identify and repaired in two layers of absorbable suture or is excised with a linear stapler and over-run with interrupted sutures as appropriate.

A leak from the stomach should be considered in a patient with post-operative sepsis if the surgical procedure was in the region of, or involved, the stomach. Conservative management is not advocated unless a leak demonstrated with a contrast study is small, or draining freely via a drainage catheter that had been placed at surgery or under imaging guidance with no evidence of intra-abdominal collection on a CT scan. Otherwise urgent intervention and closure of the defect is necessary.

Duodenum

The duodenum, particularly its second and third parts, can be damaged with overzealous mobilisation of the hepatic flexure and undue care if the duodenum is not carefully freed from the mesentry of the colon. The duodenum should be clearly identified, isolated and inspected for partial or full thickness seromuscular tears and perforations which are easily repaired in a standard manner. With large defects usually as part of a primary excisional procedure, the duodenum is mobilised along its lateral and posterior borders as far as its medial attachment to the pancreas to allow a two-layer tension-free repair, a repair around a T-tube or Foley catheter to create a controlled fistula, or a Roux en Y loop (end to side) anastomosis to the duodenal defect. Injury at the pancreatic border of the duodenum or involvement of the pancreas requires the expertise of a pancreatic surgeon as pancreatico-duodenectomy might be necessary.

A missed injury present with peritonitis, which is a surgical emergency, or as a fistula via a drainage tube that can be managed conservatively, provided the patient is not septic, the output is low and there is no intra-abdominal collection on a CT-scan. However, early surgical intervention is usually advocated especially if a contrast study demonstrates a large duodenal leak. The choice of surgical procedures is similar to elective repair although the size of the defect, tethering and friability of the tissues by surrounding inflammation should determine the safest option.

Small intestine

Adhesions from previous laparotomies increase the risk of inadvertent entero-tomy and serosal tears. The small bowel is at risk when the abdomen is opened through an old incision. When possible the abdomen is opened through an area not previously operated on, otherwise the fascia is incised carefully through the least indurated part of the wound. Mobilisation of the small bowel is most difficult if performed 10 to 30 days after a previous laparotomy because of the density of tissue inflammation; repeat laparotomy is best avoided during this time. Filmy adhesions can be gently pulled apart and denser adhesions are divided with blunt-tipped scissors or electrocautery, dissection is kept close to the small bowel to avoid damage to other organs. Seromuscular tears with substantial muscle damage or with mucosa protruding through the defect are repaired. When suture closure is insufficient or if a tear is wide and the bowel viability is endangered by damage to its mesentry, the segment of bowel should be resected after mobilisation to ensure a tension-free anastomosis. The small bowel distal to an anastomosis or repair should be mobilised and any potential adhesion or obstructing band divided to avoid a suture line leak.

An undetected injury or a leak from a repair or an anastomosis will manifest with peritonitis or intra-abdominal abscess, or enterocutaneous fistula and are managed as described previously.

Pancreas

The tail of the pancreas which is in close contact with the splenic hilum can be injured if splenectomy is necessitated because of disease involvement or injury during mobilisation of the splenic flexure of the colon. It is safer if the tail of the pancreas is divided with a linear stapler when it is densely adherent to the spleen or is involved in the disease process or has been bruised during dissection. When mobilising the splenic flexure of the colon and when the lesser sac is entered to free the transverse colon adhesions should be divided carefully to free the mesocolon from the surface of the pancreas. This approach, when carefully performed, rarely damages the pancreas.

In the postoperative period following a procedure in the proximity of, or involving, the pancreas, unexplained abdominal pain or excessive fluid in a drainage tube containing high amylase levels in the fluid or serum are diagnostic of traumatic pancreatitis or a pancreatic fistula. Conservative treatment with total parentral nutrition or elemental diet and limiting oral intake is successful in most instances. Antibiotics are administered if there are features of sepsis. CT-monitoring and percutaneous drainage may be required to prevent intra-abdominal collection although a pancreatic abscess is a rare complication.

Spleen

It is essential to regard splenic injury as a high risk of colonic surgery because invariably mobilisation of the splenic flexure is a pre-requisite for left-sided colonic resection to increase distal length for tension-free rectal or anal anastomosis. A high splenic flexure, congenital or acquired adhesions from previous surgery, desmoplastic adherence and a large tumour in the splenic flexure, extensive diverticulosis, splenomegaly and difficult exposure because of a patient's body habitus are factors that call for caution. Splenic injury may occur during traction on the splenic flexure of the colon or omentum resulting in tears of the splenic capsule, parenchyma or hilum commonly along the lower and medial poles of the spleen where most of the pericolonic, peritoneal and omental attachments lie.

Splenic injury could be avoided. When resecting a tumour in the region of the splenic flexure, by entering the lesser sac and ligating the omental vessels from medial to lateral, the omentum and colon can then be freed from the lower pole of the spleen. When mobilising the splenic flexure to create length, the splenic attachments are approached from the medial and lateral directions, the omentum is mobilised off the splenic flexure of the colon and the spleen, and the colon is freed.

With capsular tears, a combination of electrocautery, various haemostatic agents and packing is sufficient in most instances. Should the bleeding continue other local methods are applied such as clipping individual bleeding vessels, figure of eight sutures, or segmental ligation of the hilar vessels. Splenectomy rather than conservation may be unavoidable if these measures fail or there is need to limit the operation time.

Missed injury is realised in the postoperative period by abdominal disten-sion, excessive blood in the drainage tube and haemodynamic instability when emergency splenectomy is required.

Ureter

The ureters are particularly vulnerable during five manoeuvres: medial mobil-isation of the sigmoid colon, ligation of the inferior mesenteric artery, rectal mobilisation adjacent to the sacral promontory, division of the lateral liga-ments and reperitonealisation of the pelvis. It is essential that the ureters are identified by carefully mobilising the colon from its congenital adhesions and separating its mesentry from the posterior peritoneum that overlies the ureters and the gonadal vessels. In complex cases a sling is placed around the ureters so that it is in constant view during dissection. Ureteric stents aid in intra-operative identification of the ureters; although they do not prevent injury they allow earlier recognition and prompt repair of the injury. Urethral stents are particularly recommended in severe inflammatory conditions including previous colonic or rectal surgery or radiotherapy and large pelvic masses. Stents may be placed preoperatively or intra-operatively via a cystoscope or intra-operatively through a cystotomy. When an injury is suspected methy-lene blue dye administered intravenously is seen extravasating at the site of the injury, fluid boluses with frusemide causes diuresis with distension and peristalsis of the ureter; alternatively an intraoperative intravenous urogram is performed.

Injuries to the ureter include devascularisation, crush, transection and avulsion. Dissection should always be lateral to the abdominal ureter because its blood supply is medial, and medial to it in the pelvis because the blood supply is lateral. A devascularised ureter may appear discoloured and lack peristalsis, and if recognised the ureteric edges are trimmed and primary anastomosis of the spatulated ends is carried out with a ureteric stent in place. A transected ureter is treated similarly. Ligation and crush injury are treated with the release of the clamp or ligature and the placement of a ureteric stent for 7 days. While these injuries can be handled by the colorectal surgeon a urologist should be involved especially in injuries of the pelvic ureters.

In the postoperative period ureteric injury due to a combination of obstruction and urinary leak causes pyrexia, abdominal pain, distension and tenderness, and secondary paralytic ileus. Ureteric injury should be considered if the urine output is low and there is excessive clear fluid drainage if a tube had been placed at surgery. The nature of the fluid is determined by comparing its content of protein, urea and creatinine with serum. An ultrasound by demonstrating an obstructed kidney or free fluid in the intra-abdominal cavity aids diagnosis, but an intravenous urography determines the nature of the injury although sometimes a retrograde pyelogram may also be necessary. If there is incomplete obstruction a retrograde double J stent is placed, and if this fails, or is not feasible, a percutaneous nephrostomy tube is placed to preserve renal function until delayed definitive repair is planned.

Bladder

The bladder is exposed to injury at exploration with a lower incision of an abdomen with adhesions from previous surgery. A cystotomy in the anterior surface of the bladder is easily closed with two layers of absorbable suture, and a catheter is left to drain the bladder for 7 days. Injury to the posterior bladder can occur when mobilising an inflammatory or neoplstic recto-sigmoid mass or during perineal excision of the rectum. The repair is more demanding especially if the injury is at the base of the bladder when a urologist should be involved because of the risk of damaging the ureters during the repair. This can be carried out from inside the bladder through an anterior cystotomy, whereby ureteric stents are passed retrogradely to ensure their patency.

Injuries undetected will manifest as vesicoperineal fistula or enterovesical fistula. Veiscoperineal fistula is recognised by urine leakage through the perineal wound. The diagnosis is confirmed by a cystogram. Small fistulas may close with urethral or suprapubic catheter drainage for a minimum duration of 6 weeks and up to 6 months in an irradiated bladder before surgical repair is considered. Enterovesical fistulas are associated with abscess formation and present with pnematuria, faecaluria and recurrent urinary tract infection. Surgical intervention includes drainage of the abscess, excision of the fistula tract, closure of the bladder and diversion of the faecal stream.

Anal sphincters

The anal sphincters are exposed to damage during commonly performed anorectal procedures especially if they are not performed judiciously in patients with Crohn's disease.

The internal sphincter is damaged if division during sphincterotomy extends beyond the level of the dentate line or the length of the fissure in females and during haemorrhoidectomy or the excision of large skin tags if the haemorrhoidal tissue or the skin tag is not freed from the internal anal sphincter before its excision. Anal dilatation has been employed to reduce internal anal sphincter tone for the treatment of anal fissures and haemorrhoids but this is associated with sphincter disruption and is an obsolete procedure. Similarly excessive stretching of the internal anal sphincter by anal retraction during transanal procedures and insertion of the circular stapler can result in its damage.

The external anal sphincter is also vulnerable to damage during the above procedures but is particularly at risk when anal fistulas in elderly patients and in women with previous episiotomies or obstetric sphincter injury, and high complex fistulas, are treated by primary fistulotomy or fistulectomy. A staged approach with seton placement using silastic catheters, vascular loops, rubber bands or a heavy silk thread is advocated.

Treatment for soiling and leakage includes bulking agents and biofeedback therapy. Once damaged it is impossible to repair the internal anal sphincter. Overlapping sphincteroplasty for external anal sphincter injury improves continence in the majority of patients although improvement is not long-term.

GENITOURINARY COMPLICATIONS

Other than operative trauma genitourinary complications comprise voiding and sexual dysfunction related to neurological damage during a pelvic dissection which might be unavoidable particularly in a resection for carcinoma. However with knowledge of the pelvic anatomy, surgical technique can be refined, exercising caution where nervous structures are particularly vulnerable, hence minimising the risk of these complications and improving the quality of life.

Applied pelvic neuroanatomy

Innervation of the distal genitourinary tract is comprised of sympathetic, parasympathetic and somatic nerves. The sympathetic nerves arise from T1–2 to L3 via the thoracolumbar trunk, the superior hypogastric plexus lies anterior to the aorta at the origin of the inferior mesenteric artery. During high ligation of the inferior mesenteric artery, the superior hypogastric plexus is vulnerable and should be avoided. The hypogastric plexus descends in front of the left common iliac artery and at the level of the sacral promontory splits into the left and right hypogastric nerves where by following the free edge of the mobilised sigmoid colon the plain between the mesorectum and the hypogastric nerves is entered where they are easily identifiable and are within view as mesorectal dissection proceeds when mobilising the rectum. The hypogastric nerves run along the pelvic side walls lateral to the rectum and medial to the ureters and iliac vessels. Parasympathetic nerves known as nervi eregentes arise from S2–4 and join the hypogastric nerves to form the inferior hypogastric plexus or pelvic plexus which is adherent to the pelvic wall by surrounding tissue and is usually away from the surgical planes but is still at risk during wide ligation of the lateral stalks. The pelvic plexus that now contains sympathetic, parasympathetic and visceral afferent fibres, descends laterally and converges anteriorly in the area of the prostate gland or vagina, where it is vulnerable during anterior rectal mobilisation. It innervates the base of the bladder and proximal urethra, and in males the prostate gland and the seminal vesicles. Somatic innervation is by the pudendal nerve from the sacral plexus (S2–4) which divides into the inferior rectal, perineal and penile or clitoral branches that provide sensory innervation to the penis and clitoris, and motor supply to the striated external anal and urethral sphincter.

Voiding dysfunction

The parasympathetic nerve supply is responsible for bladder contraction, the sympathetic nerve supply allows relaxation of the bladder wall and contraction of the bladder neck while the perineal branch of the pudendal nerve supplies the striated external urethral sphincter.

Early complications are recognised on removal of the urinary catheter and include urinary retention, infection and incontinence due to posterior bladder displacement after abdomino-perineal excision of the rectum, neurologic injury and pre-existing outlet obstruction precipitated by epidural anaesthesia, central narcotic anaesthesia, prolonged bed rest and alpha agonist and anticholinergic medication. Recatheterisation, antibiotics, withdrawing drugs that contribute to urine retention and trial of alpha-adrenergic blockers (to inhibit sympathetic stimulation and improve detrusor function and relax the bladder neck) are effective simple measures.

Patients with urinary symptoms that continue longer than 6 weeks after surgery should undergo urodynamic studies to determine the nature of the injury and differentiate it from a simple outlet obstruction requiring prostatectomy. The parasympathetic nerve supply is the component of innervation frequently injured by transection of the nerve supply or neuropraxia, rarely is the sympathetic nerve damaged. While bladder function may return after unilateral injury or neuropraxia, with bilateral nerve transection clean intermittent catheterisation will be required indefinitely as no drugs consistently improve bladder function.

Sexual dysfunction

This is more common in males than females because of the anatomical relationship of the rectum to the nerves responsible for sexual function and better understanding of the male sexual response and disorders that follow pelvic surgery. Women suffer decreased libido, difficulty with orgasm and most commonly dyspareunia. Male dysfunction includes erectile difficulty, retrograde ejaculation and total impotence. Erection is parasympathetically mediated via the pelvic plexus and is governed by impulses that travel along the nervi eregentes, while ejaculation is under sympathetic control and damage will result in retrograde ejaculation. Sexual dysfunction is more likely with increased age and resection for cancer than inflammatory bowel disease where dissection is close to the rectal wall and perineal excision is performed in the intersphincteric plane.

STOMA COMPLICATIONS

Despite care when constructing a stoma by the preoperative marking of its site and technical detail, complications may still arise. Complications are more frequently encountered in unplanned stomas, in obese patients, in the elderly, and with longer follow-up. Stoma siting does limit problems related to the appliance and consequently the skin, and is best performed before surgery with the patient standing, sitting and supine so that a site is selected that is visible to the patient and does not interfere with clothes and belts, and is away from bony prominences, skin folds and scars.

Clinical Presentation and Management

Some but not all complications are more likely to occur in the postoperative period although for other reasons they may arise later when other complications also develop.

Early Complications

Skin problems

Skin irritation is more common in patients with ileostomy than with a colostomy because of the poor adherence of the appliance and exposure of the skin to the stoma effluent, usually the result of flush or a retracted stoma, an improperly placed stoma and allergy to adhesive materials on the bag. The liquid effluent from a right-sided or transverse colostomy will cause skin irritation because the appliance does not allow a watertight seal around the flat stoma.

With strict hygiene, skin barriers and local antimicrobials the majority of these skin problems are manageable unless the stoma is defective and is revised. Pyoderma gangrenosum can occur around the stoma in patients with inflammatory bowel disease and should not be confused with simple irritation as it requires treatment with steroids and other anti-inflammtory agents.

Necrosis

This is the result of skeletonisation of the terminal bowel and inadequate abdominal wall opening particularly if the mesentery is thickened with fat or inflammation. A change to a purple colour of a stoma is more likely to be due to ischaemia rather than to venous engorgement or submucosal haematoma if the stoma does not feel warm and there is no arterial ooze from the mucosa on pin-prick. The level of necrosis should be determined by examining the stoma with a paediatric proctoscope or a flexible endoscope as this influences management.

If viable tissue is present above the fascial plane a conservative approach is adopted. For an ileostomy this demands particular attention to the appliance and to skin care when the spout sloughs and the stoma is flush with the skin. The long-term result of superficial necrosis is stenosis when the stoma can be revised by local exploration. Necrosis below the fascia and therefore intra-peritoneally requires immediate exploratory laparotomy. If there is concern about recurrent necrosis because of tension or body wall thickness, a loop-end stoma or divided-end-loop stoma should be constructed in order to avoid skeletonisation of the bowel.

Retraction

Tension on the stoma, improper construction or siting and ischaemia are responsible factors. An abdominal opening that is wider than the bowel lumen causes tension on the mucocutaneous sutures which break and the stoma separates from the skin. This is more likely to occur when forming a colostomy than an ileostomy, and is an emergency if the colostomy recedes into the peritoneal cavity. Otherwise colostomy retraction is not as clinically significant as retraction of an ileostomy as with flush stoma the appliance adheres poorly and the skin is damaged by intestinal effluent. Stoma retraction may occur as a late complication if a patients gains excessive weight.

Local revision involves measures to secure the ileostomy spout eversion and these include bidirectional seromyotomies to induce fibrosis, sutures to include the bowel edge, serosa at skin level and the skin edge, sutures between the serosa and fascia around the stoma, stapling the everted stoma with a bladeless linear cutting stapling instrument.

Colostomy refashioning may demand mobilisation of the splenic flexure of the colon or even division of the inferior mesenteric artery at its origin in the obese patient to prevent tension on the colostomy.

Obstruction

This is commonly due to food bolus obstructing an oedematous newly fashioned ileostomy. Stenosis complicating ischaemia is a common cause of colostomy and ileostomy obstruction. The obstruction resolves spontaneously or by saline irrigation of the ileostomy through a Foley catheter and a careful dilatation with the finger or graduated dilators can be attempted in a stenosed stoma. Only if these measures fail to relieve obstruction, refashioning the stoma is considered and this will probably require re-exploration as at this early stage local revision can be technically difficult and not safe because of inflammation and odema at the site of the stoma.

Late Complications

Prolapse

Ileostomy prolapse is rare and is usually associated with parastomal hernia, and is more common in obese patients. Repair requires refashioning of the ileostomy with local repair of the parastomal hernia which is rarely successful in the long term.

Colostomy prolapse is also not common and is associated with parastomal hernia, but is seen more frequently in paraplegic patients who had a stoma for constipation, rectal prolapse, incontinence and in right sided or transverse colostomies. The prolapse which is an intussusception of the proximal bowel is easily reducible and patients learn how to reduce their own prolapse. Elective treatment is to excise the redundant colon with local repair of the parastomal hernia if present and if the prolapse recurs, resiting the stoma or colectomy with ileostomy might be required.

Hernia

Parastomal hernia is the commonest complication among patients with stomas. Obesity, chronic respiratory disease, and a predilection to other abdominal hernias are predisposing factors. There is no evidence that a stoma through the rectus muscle reduces the risk of a parastomal hernia.

A parastomal hernia is repaired if it is causing psychological stress, interfering with the adherence of the appliance, causing pain from intestinal incarceration or obstruction, associated with prolapse or is cosmetically unacceptable. Local repair may involve suture approximation of the defect with or without mesh reinforcement and if this fails, resiting of the stoma might be necessary.

Stenosis

This is commonly due to ischaemic superficial necrosis at the time the stoma was formed. Stenosis and fistulation can be a manifestation of recurrent Crohn's disease. Obstructive symptoms and difficulty with the appliance are the main reasons for revision of the stoma. Local revision is feasible at least 3 months after the initial procedure as fibrosis becomes established and the tissue planes are better defined to allow exteriorisation of a fresh segment of the bowel for fashioning a new stoma. However in Crohn's disease the extent of the disease should be defined with a barium study as a laparotomy might be more appropriate.

Fistulation

This usually follows subcutaneous infection which can be avoided by keeping the size of the abdominal wall opening to the size of the bowel and preserving the subcutaneous fat, in order not to create a potential dead space for haematoma and infection, and by not suturing the serosa to the fascia especially in Crohn's disease. Recurrent Crohn's disease in the efferent limb to a stoma can fistulate through the stoma.

Pain around the stoma, discharge, poor adherence of the appliance and skin irritation are reasons for local revision of a stoma that might involve proximal bowel resection in Crohn's disease or resiting of the stoma if the skin and subcutaneous tissues are inflamed.

Complications of Stoma Closure

The closure of a stoma has its morbidity and should not be delegated to an inexperienced surgeon. The main complications are intestinal leak and intestinal obstruction.

A leak is either from the suture line or unrecognised inadvertent intraperitoneal damage to the bowel from traction or sharp injury while freeing the stoma through a narrow abdominal aperture. It is therefore safer to extend the incision or convert to a standard laparotomy if the stoma is densely adherent. A leak often manifests as an enterocutaneous fistula than with peritonitis.

Intestinal obstruction is due to oedema or stenosis at the anastomosis and is more common with ileostomy than colostomy closure because of the narrower lumen of the bowel. When the intestinal ends are judged to be narrow, side-to-side anastomosis is easily performed with a linear stapler and provides a wider lumen than an end-to-end anstomosis.

In either complication, conservative management is adopted before surgical intervention is considered.

SEPSIS

In abdominal operations signs of sepsis in the postoperative period after ruling out extra-abdominal causes are either due to wound or intra-abdominal infection.

Wound infections

Wound infection depends on the size and virulence of the bacterial inoculum, local wound environment and the host organism defenses. Risk factors for wound infection are operations on the abdomen, operations lasting more than 2 hours, and a clean or dirty operation. Therefore the patient's general condition is optimised, tissue damage is avoided and contamination prevented by mechanical bowel preparation and prophylactic systemic antibiotics.

Wounds at high risk of infection should be left open and packed until delayed primary closure is carried out once the wound has filled with healthy granulation tissue and there is minimal exudate and no pathogenic organisms are isolated on wound culture. Otherwise the wound is left to heal by secondary intention.

A closed wound that shows erythema, tenderness or exudates, is managed by removing the sutures or staples, and any purulent material is drained and the wound dressed appropriately. If there is fascial dehiscence the wound is debrided and closed with retention sutures with the option to limit the closure to the abdominal wall leaving the skin and fat layers open for local dressings. Antibiotics are prescribed according to bacteriological analysis.

The most serious wound infections are the necrotising soft tissue infections because of associated mortality and should be suspected, in the case of unusually severe pain in the incision, spreading erythema, oedema or crepitus when a clinical microbiologist should be involved. This is an emergency that requires prompt debridement with the excision of all necrotic tissue to the margins of viable tissues. Initial broad spectrum antibiotic therapy is with penicillin, aminoglycoside or clindamycin until tissue cultures are available. These patients usually require repeated debridements, prolonged intensive wound care and subsequently skin grafting.

Perineal wound infection

This is associated with closure rather than with open packing of the perineal wound especially when excision of the rectum is complicated by faecal contamination. Treatment is by opening the wound and local care. However the wound might not heal and if it remains unhealed for more than six months it is then defined as a perineal sinus. Although soft tissue excision is more extensive for cancer than for inflammatory bowel disease where the levators and the external anal sphincters are preserved by performing intersphincteric excision, persistent perineal sinuses are more common with inflammatory bowel disease or when rectal excision is performed after radiation therapy.

With pelvic floor and sphincter muscle repair, the reconstituted anal canal creates tension on the perineal incision that is responsible for skin ischaemia and necrosis, wound disruption and infection. It is safer to carry out partial closure of the wound and rely on healing by secondary intention for complete healing.

Intra-abdominal infection

This should be suspected if the patient exhibits fever, prolonged ileus, abdominal pain or leucocytosis. Abdominal examination for tenderness or an intra-abdominal mass is limited by the abdominal incision. Ultrasonography in the postoperative period is hampered by the wound, dressings and drainage tubes and is unhelpful in surveying the abdomen and pelvis for fluid or gas collections especially if there is intestinal gas distension from ileus.

Abdominal and pelvic CT is the investigation of choice and it allows the placement of a percutaneous catheter for the drainage of abdominal or pelvic abscesses avoiding the morbidity of surgical drainage, although it might not be as successful in complex abscesses. The organisms usually isolated include facultative gram negative bacilli, aerobic gram negative bacilli, obligate and aerobic organisms and enterococci or other faecal streptococci. A combination of an antianaerobe plus aminoglycoside or a third generation cephalosporin is recommended, but it may have to be modified according to culture results. The effectiveness of treatment is determined by the resolution of the signs of sepsis within 48 hours and diminution in the size of the abscess on repeated CT scans. Otherwise re-exploration should be considered.

Abscesses and enteric fistulas associated with anastomotic dehiscence are managed as described already. Dehiscence of the rectal stump after Hartmann's or subtotal colectomy for acute fulminating colitis can be the cause of pelvic sepsis unless the rectal stump had been exteriorised as mucus fistula, although a mucus fistula can be the source of infection if it retracts into the pelvis. Instillation of contrast material into the rectum may confirm extravasation from the apex of the rectal stump, which can be successfully managed by percutaneous drainage of the abscess and catheter irrigation of the rectal stump to evacuate residual faecal material. It is prudent that the rectal stump is always washed out at the time of the primary operation.

ABDOMINAL COMPARTMENT SYNDROME

Abdominal compartment syndrome (ACS) is a potentially fatal consequence of increased intra-abdominal pressure related to the prolonged exposure of the bowel and massive intravenous fluid replacement associated with conditions that colorectal surgeons frequently encounter namely intra-abdominal haemorrhage, pelvic fractures, intestinal obstruction and colonic cancer. Prolonged unrelieved elevation of intra-abdominal pressure can cause pulmonary compromise, renal impairment, cardiac failure, shock and death.

Pathophysiology

Oliguria is often the first evidence of excessive intra-abdominal pressure attributed to renovascular rather than ureteric compression from occlusive pressure on the inferior vena cava and renal veins, and to a lesser extent direct pressure on the renal arteries as well as direct extrinsic pressure on the kidneys.

Ventilation is impeded from compromised inspiration because the lungs are compressed. Progressive increase in the peak inspiratory pressure is required to maintain tidal volume. Hypercarbia and potentially fatal respiratory acidosis may develop. Elevated $pCO2$ and rising peak inspiratory pressures are signs of significant abdominal pressure.

Pressure on the inferior vena cava reduces cardiac return while the heart pumps against increased aortic and peripheral vascular resistance. Cardiac output is diminished, and cardiovascular failure and shock are terminal events.

Compression on the inferior vena cava leads to peripheral venous stasis causing severe oedema of the lower extremities and potential for thrombosis and pulmonary embolism.

Diagnosis and Treatment

Postoperative ACS develops within the first 24 hours. Oliguria manifests within 12 hours after surgery. Renal scan, renogram and excretory urograms are likely to be normal. Intravesical pressure measurement is the most useful and it corresponds with the intra-abdominal pressure when the patient is in the supine position, but is less accurate when the patient is in the Trendelenburg or reversed Trendelenburg position. In most critically ill patients a Foley catheter is already in place, which can be connected to a water manometer via a three-way stopcock. A pressure above 25 mmHg should cause concern because when prolonged the risk of renal failure is considerable especially in patients with compromised renal function. Hypovolaemic and seriously ill patients are at risk of ACS at even lower pressure when other clinical parameters should also be considered. Re-opening the abdomen to release the mounting pressure in the abdominal cavity before irreversible damage occurs is life-saving.

It is preferable that ACS is anticipated and prevented. During a protracted surgical procedure intravesical and/or ventilatory pressures are helpful measurements and if wound closure is difficult, the wound is left open. A variety of materials are used for temporary cover of the bowel, including sterilised plastic material fashioned from intravenous or irrigation fluid bags termed "Bogota bag." A staged abdominal repair is deferred until the patient has recovered.

CONCLUSION

This account is not by any means comprehensive, but it provides an overall insight into common postoperative complications associated with colorectal surgery and highlights preventive measures that rely on sensible judgement in decision-making, caution and technical skill. Complications due to functional disturbance are related to the nature of the procedure; they are not within the theme of this chapter and should be taken into account when considering the overall morbidity.

Chapter 12

COMPLICATIONS OF MAJOR HEPATOBILIARY SURGERY

David J. Reich, Hoonbae Jeon,
Jorge A. Ortiz and Cosme Manzarbeitia

In this chapter, the authors seek to describe the various complications that may occur during or after major hepatobiliary surgery, to provide treatment options, and to discuss perioperative steps that minimise the risk of these problems. The authors try to provide a broad coverage of what has been learned by leading hepatobiliary surgeons, and also to share our personal experience in this field. The topics covered include complications related to procedures routinely performed by hepatobiliary surgeons, including hepatic resection, biliary resection for malignancy and radiofrequency ablation (RFA). Complications of cholecystectomy, common bile duct exploration and other biliary procedures for benign disease, the domain of the general surgeon, are not covered in this chapter.

Several developments in the 1990s have led to a significant improvement in results after major hepatobiliary surgery. Perhaps most importantly, there are a growing number of hepatobiliary surgeons, many of whom work as part of experienced liver transplant and hepatobiliary surgical teams. There is increasing communication and collaboration among these groups, even at a global level, that facilitates learning. Patients benefit from hepatobiliary surgeons' increased focus on liver anatomy and physiology. For example, the better understanding of these disciplines gleaned from living donor and other reduced size liver transplant procedures has been applied to non-transplant resectional techniques. As more cutting edge hepatobiliary surgery is performed, more effective equipment for imaging, resection and ablation continues to be invented, including magnetic resonance imaging (MRI) vascular studies and cholangiography, laparoscopic ultrasonography, the cavitron ultrasonic surgical aspirator (CUSA), the harmonic scalpel, more versatile stapling devices, RFA, and so on. Paralleling these surgical advances, has been a finer understanding of coagulation and the development of a wide array of haemostatic agents that have led to reduced morbidity from hepatobiliary surgery. Complementing all these advances are further improvement in the fields of anaesthesia and critical care. The aforementioned progress has greatly facilitated the safer performance of increasingly aggressive hepatobiliary surgery and has made it possible to offer valuable surgical therapy to more patients afflicted with diseases of the liver and bile ducts.

COMPLICATIONS OF HEPATIC RESECTION

The general approach to major hepatobiliary resection used by groups in the United States, Europe and Asia is similar, and includes careful selection of patients, care by a highly experienced and skilled surgical team, preoperative radiological evaluation, and an attempt at minimal blood transfusion. A recent nationwide study in the United States demonstrated that procedure volume is an important predictor of mortality after major hepatobiliary resection.[1] Strict adherence to operative principles is the most important strategy for the prevention of complications. Local complications such as bleeding, necrosis, biliary fistula and sepsis can be prevented to a large degree by precise application of modern techniques of liver surgery.

Results of Hepatic Resection

As a result of the aforementioned advances, the current mortality rate after major hepatobiliary resection even in cirrhotic patients is less than 1% at

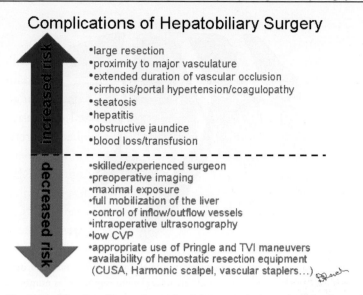

Complications of Hepatobiliary Surgery

increased risk
- large resection
- proximity to major vasculature
- extended duration of vascular occlusion
- cirrhosis/portal hypertension/coagulopathy
- steatosis
- hepatitis
- obstructive jaundice
- blood loss/transfusion

decreased risk
- skilled/experienced surgeon
- preoperative imaging
- maximal exposure
- full mobilization of the liver
- control of inflow/outflow vessels
- intraoperative ultrasonography
- low CVP
- appropriate use of Pringle and TVI maneuvers
- availability of hemostatic resection equipment
  (CUSA, Harmonic scalpel, vascular staplers…)

Fig. 1. Depiction of various factors that either increase or decrease the risk of complications following hepatobiliary resection.

some large centres.[2–8] Prior to the 1990s, this mortality rate was reported as being 3% to 8%.[2,9] Interpreting mortality rates for hepatobiliary resection is not straightforward because there are multiple variables that can potentially effect patient outcomes, including the nature of the resection (i.e. the amount of resected hepatic parenchyma, the surface area of the transection plane, and proximity of the lesion to major vasculature); the underlying condition of the hepatic parenchyma (i.e. the presence of steatosis, hepatitis, cirrhosis, and/or obstructive jaundice); and technical aspects of the surgery (i.e. the amount of intra-operative blood loss and transfusion, the duration of vascular occlusion, and the skill and experience of the surgeon). The distribution of these factors varies among case series from different centres. Thus, reports of morbidity and mortality rates after major hepatobiliary resection should be cautiously interpreted. Figure 1 depicts various factors that either increase or decrease the risk of complications following hepatobiliary resection.

Anatomic and Technical Principles of Hepatic Resection

A surgeon's knowledge of liver anatomy is critical in ensuring good outcomes after hepatobiliary surgery (Fig. 2). The liver has segmental subdivisions in its

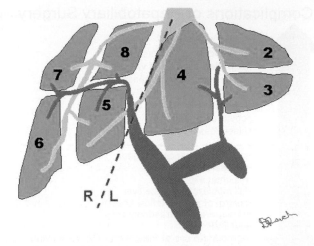

Fig. 2. Appreciation of the hepatic anatomy is critical for the safe conduct of hepatobiliary resection. The liver can be divided into four sectors and eight segments (as numbered), which are each supplied by separate branches of the portal vein (darker blue). These sectors are each separated by an hepatic vein (lighter blue). Cantlie's line (red) marks the plane in which the middle hepatic vein runs, and defines the resection margin for right and left hepatic lobectomies.

internal architecture and a variety of anatomical variations in the vasculature and biliary system exist from individual to individual. Therefore, it is advisable to obtain a detailed road map of the patient's hepatic vascular anatomy via computed tomography (CT) scan or MRI prior to major resection. At present, liver resection is based on precise knowledge of the natural lines of division of the liver.[10] One can gain an appreciation for the segmental anatomy of the liver by studying the corrosion cast model of the liver created by injecting resin into the portal vein, hepatic arteries and bile ducts. The liver can be divided into four sectors and eight segments, which are each supplied by separate branches of the portal vein. These sectors are each separated by an hepatic vein.[11] Cantlie's line marks the plane in which the middle hepatic vein runs. Intraoperative ultrasonography is an integral tool for navigating the internal landmarks of hepatic segmental anatomy in modern hepatic surgery.[12] Theoretically, resection of any of the eight segments or any combination of segments is possible,[13] under ultrasonographic guidance[14] or via the extra-glissonian approach.[15]

During the infancy of modern hepatobiliary surgery, the thoracoabdominal incision was almost exclusively used in order to maximise exposure of the operative field. However, since the introduction of costal arch retractors that are fixable to the operating table, most cases are done via the abdominal approach, which is associated with less postoperative morbidity. Strong costal arch retractors such as Stieber or Thompson retractors allow for adequate exposure of the suprahepatic or retrohepatic vena cava, which is the most difficult area to expose. A bilateral subcostal incision with a midline extension toward the sternum ("Mercedes incision") is the standard incision for most major hepatobiliary procedures. Some surgeons still use variants of the thoracoabdominal incision, which provide an easier approach to the dome of the liver and less mobilisation of the right side of the liver.[16]

Special attention is required during the transverse (or oblique) stage of the Mercedes incision to open the abdominal wall all the way to the posterior axillary line, aiming at the tip of the 10th rib, so that the rib cage can be elevated enough to visualise the hepatic dome and suprahepatic vena cava. Typically, it is wise to expose the suprahapatic vena cava and hepatic veins after division of the coronary ligament, prior to resection. Maximal exposure with stable retraction of the rib cage, full mobilisation of the liver from its ligamentous attachments to the diaphragm and retroperitoneum, and identification of inflow and outflow vascular structures are essential to safely perform major hepatobiliary resection.

Vascular Occlusion Techniques for Hepatic Resection

In 1902, Pringle wrote that blood loss from the injured liver could be arrested by occlusion of the portal triad.[17] Continuous or intermittent inflow occlusion can be performed safely up to one hour in the normothermic patient. Intermittent clamping has been shown to be better tolerated by the hepatic parenchyma than continuous clamping in animal models and human subjects.[18–20] Fifteen minutes of inflow occlusion and five minutes of reperfusion resulted in less ischaemia-reperfusion injury during the period of ischemic preconditioning.[19–21] With inflow occlusion, the hepatic parenchyma is perfused by less oxygenised blood from the hepatic veins, which ameliorates ischaemia-reperfusion injury secondary to clamping.[22] The Pringle manoeuvre is generally recommended for major hepatic resections.[23] However, severely fibrotic or steatotic parenchyma does not tolerate the ischaemic insult of inflow occlusion. Resection of such liver tissue may be performed without the Pringle manoeuvre, using an assortment of technologically advanced haemostatic dissecting instruments, including ultrasonic and hydrojet dissectors. Inflow occlusion is also avoided with graft hepatectomy for living-donor liver transplantation, in which case it is necessary to protect both the liver graft and the donor's liver remnant from ischaemia during the parenchymal transection. In summary, the Pringle manoeuvre is easy, quick and effective for the reduction of blood loss and the maintenance of haemodynamic stability, and it avoids injury to the hepatic parenchyma.

In the case of massive hepatic resection for a large tumour or a tumour in close proximity to the confluence of hepatic veins or the vena cava, total vascular isolation (TVI), which arrests inflow and outflow, may be necessary to prevent excessive bleeding or air embolism.[24] To decrease excessive venous pooling in the lower body that results from cross-clamping of the vena cava, the supraceliac aorta may be clamped at the same time or a venovenous bypass may be instituted. Even with the significant changes in cardiac output and systemic vascular resistance, adequate systemic blood pressure and pulmonary artery wedge pressure can be maintained in the absence of severe acidosis.[25] Theoretically, the surgical field should be completely bloodless with this manoeuvre. However, back bleeding from the adrenal vein or other retroperitoneal collateral vessels is possible. To achieve complete haemostasis, it is necessary to mobilise the caudate lobe of the vena cava. Aggressive fluid resuscitation and invasive haemodynamic monitoring are required because of the decreased venous return from caval clamping. Anaesthetic management and the management of postoperative morbidity can be difficult.[26] For these reasons, TVI is restricted to selected cases.[27,28] To avoid the shortcomings of TVI, a technical modification of the procedure that does not occlude the vena cava, but achieves haemostasis of hepatic venous tributaries, is also feasible.[29]

Division of the Hepatic Parenchyma

The most essential component of dividing the hepatic parenchyma is the selective destruction of hepatocytes, while initially preserving the fibre-rich blood vessels and bile ductules. After being exposed, the blood vessels and bile ductules can be ligated or cauterised in the plane of resection. Several techniques and devices have been used to divide the hepatic parenchyma, but there is no consensus on which method is superior. The traditional method, the so-called finger fracture technique, is seldom used in the current era except in the case of traumatic laceration of the liver.[30] Finger fracture involves significant haemorrhage, which in turn makes it difficult to locate the correct anatomical plane of dissection. The clamp crushing technique, which is a refined version of the finger fracture technique, is widely used, safe and effective. The surgeon uses a haemostatic clamp to selectively crush the soft hepatic parenchyma, while avoiding the tubular blood vessels and bile ductules within. These are then discretely clipped or ligated. Ligation of tiny blood vessels and bile ductules is not only time consuming, it is also ineffective, resulting in incompletely controlled structures that may become a source of postoperative bleeding or bile leakage. Therefore, the surgeon must be flexible in making decisions about when to use titanium clips, suture ligation or electrocautery, depending on the situation.

The CUSA, Harmonic Scalpel and Hydro Jet are technologically advanced dissecting instruments that can facilitate haemostatic liver resection. Vibration of the piezoelectric unit at the tip of the CUSA destroys tissue, while irrigating and aspirating debris from the operative field.[31] The CUSA handpiece may be armed with monopolar electrocautery to facilitate haemostatic dissection.[32] The Harmonic Scalpel uses ultrasonically activated shears for haemostatic tissue dissection. The hydro jet dissector (Jet Cutter) uses a high-pressure water stream to selectively destroy hepatic parenchyma.[33,34] When using these devices it is important to minimise transmission of energy to the same spot for a prolonged period of time in order to avoid vascular injury. The tip of the device should be kept in continuous oscillatory motion, perpendicular to the resection plane when using the CUSA and Harmonic Scalpel, and parallel to the resection plane when using the water jet. By using the CUSA, Harmonic Scalpel or Hydro Jet, inflow occlusion can be avoided, thus minimising hepatic ischaemia. They provided haemostatic cutting and are not associated with increased risk of postoperative bleeding, bile leak, or abscess formation at the cut margins. Use of a vascular stapler for hepatic resection can also aid in minimising blood loss and reducing the need for inflow occlusion. Regardless of which resection techniques and devices are used, it is important to minimise the amount of tissue ischaemia along the resection plane. Mattress suturing of the resection margin is no longer recommended because of the resultant tissue necrosis.

Haemorrhage from Hepatic Resection

Table 1 lists the various complications that can occur after hepatobiliary resection. In earlier years, liver resection was associated with a high risk of significant haemorrhage. This limited the performance of safe surgery. More recently, a better understanding of the hepatic surgical anatomy, improved vascular imaging techniques, refined anesthetic management, and the development of technologically advanced dissecting equipment have significantly improved the ability to perform hepatobiliary surgery haemostatically. Certainly, hepatobiliary surgical patients require adequate correction of any underlying coagulopathy and/or thrombocytopenia, with the infusion of fresh frozen plasma, cryoprecipitate, and/or platelets.

Intraoperative bleeding

Intraoperative haemorrhage is one of the most significant risk factors for postoperative complications. Therefore, the following methods of reducing intraoperative blood loss deserve close attention. During routine right hepatic resection, complete mobilization of the liver is necessary before beginning the parenchymal transection. When the right hepatic lobe is rotated medially, control of the right hepatic vein outside of the liver is possible, which helps to reduce the amount of intraoperative blood loss.[35,36] Introduction of this controlled hepatectomy technique in the 1950s[37] and its revival in the 1980s[38] has significantly contributed to reduced blood loss and decreased morbidity from major hepatobiliary resection. By combining this approach with the Pringle

Table 1.   Complications of Hepatobiliary Resection

- intraoperative hemorrhage
- postoperative hemorrhage
- acute hepatic failure
- subacute hepatic insufficiency
  (ascites, encephalopathy, jaundice, GI bleed)
- bile leak
- sepsis
- abscess
- biliary stricture
- hepatic artery pseudoaneurysm
- arteriovenous fistula
- renal failure

manoeuvre, the surgeon can eliminate bleeding from the transected hepatic parenchyma, except for back bleeding from hepatic venous tributaries.

Traditionally, patients were prepared for hepatobiliary resection by intentional volume overloading in anticipation of intraoperative blood loss. However, maintaining a low (<8 cm H_2O) intraoperative central venous pressure (CVP) has proven to be a simple way to reduce bleeding during parenchymal transection without TVI.[39,40] Simply lifting the mobilised liver a few centimetres can help to reduce back bleeding from hepatic venous tributaries. Again, it is important to mobilise the liver so that the surgeon can easily visualise and manipulate the transection plane with the left hand. Use of manoeuvres such as the reverse Trendelenberg position to elevate the liver above the right atrium, or partial banding of the infrahepatic vena cava to decrease venous return have been tried by several groups to decrease blood loss from hepatic veins. However, a recent study failed to demonstrate that the use of either of these manoeuvres decreased the pressure gradient between the hepatic veins and superior vena cava.[41] One should also note that manipulating a CVP too low can lead to the development of an air embolism.

Venous bleeders from the transected plane should be temporarily controlled with light finger pressure before being permanently controlled with fine sutures. The natural response of placing a suction tip against venous bleeders should be avoided as it results in further blood loss. The author's preference is to locate small venous bleeders on the transected plane by intermittently flushing the surgical field with saline and placing the suction cannula in the dependent portion of the operating field. Until reasonable haemostasis has been achieved, the pace of the transection should be slowed or even stopped.

Detachment of the hepatic ligamentous structures and rotation of the liver can be impossible in the setting of a large tumour on the right side. Since intraoperative iatrogenic rupture of an hepatocellular carcinoma is associated with increased intraoperative blood loss and intraperitoneal extrahepatic recurrence, extreme care should be taken during right lobe mobilisation in the presence of a large tumour.[42] In this situation, an alternative may be parenchymal transection without hepatic mobilisation. This technique is known as the anterior approach or retrograde hepatectomy.[43] By minimising manipulation of the liver parenchyma and rotation of the hepatoduodenal ligament, this approach minimises compromised blood flow to the liver, thus preserving remnant liver function.[44] A drawback of the anterior approach is the risk of massive back bleeding from the deeper plane of parenchymal transection; without prior mobilisation of the right lobe of the liver and the tumour, the hepatic lobe cannot be lifted up and compressed manually.

Postoperative bleeding

The most common cause of postoperative bleeding is the dislodgement of a ligature or clip from a divided venous tributary or hepatic arterial branch. Whenever a large-calibre vein such as the portal vein or an hepatic vein is divided, the stump should be ligated with a trans-fixed suture or over-sewn with vascular suture because the thin wall and short stump of these veins do not securely hold suture. When cauterising a resected plane with monopolar cautery or an argon beam coagulator, one should be careful to avoid burning the ligatures. Coating the raw surface of the resection plane with topical haemostatic agents may decrease postoperative bleeding and bile leakage. Fibrin sealants represent an improvement over conventional topical agents because they contain components that actively form clots.[45,46]

Even after the achievement of a completely dry hepatic resection surface, it is not uncommon to encounter postoperative bleeding in the patient with cirrhosis, portal hypertension and hypersplenism. Minimal postoperative bleeding in a haemodynamically stable patient can be observed and treated with the transfusion of fresh frosen plasma and platelets. However, the surgeon must maintain a low threshold for surgical re-exploration, otherwise clot induced fibrinolysis and consumptive coagulopathy will develop and exacerbate haemorrhage. Even if re-exploration fails to identify a focus of significant haemorrhage, lavage of the clots reverses the fibrinolytic cascade and is often in and of itself effective at stopping the bleeding.

Even if there is no ongoing haemorrhage, the patient with a large haematoma after hepatic resection should usually be taken to the operating room for haematoma evacuation and peritoneal lavage. Haematomas not only harbour bacteria and lead to the development of intra-abdominal abscess, but also become a source of bilirubin overload in the remnant liver. Imaging studies are indicated in the face of prolonged unconjugated hyperbilirubinemia after hepatobiliary resection to exclude a collection of blood in the abdominal cavity.

Haemorrhage from an arterial pseudo-aneurysm is an unusual complication that can occur in the setting of intra-abdominal abscess or leakage from the biliary anastomosis. Bleeding from a pseudo-aneurysm can occur abruptly and is often fatal. Nonetheless, vigilant monitoring for this complication is warranted because the gross rupture of a pseudo-aneurysm often follows prodromal signs and symptoms such as increased abdominal or back pain, fever, leukocytosis, and/or haemobilia from a herald bleed.[47] Surgery should be reserved for patients in whom transarterial embolisation or stenting fails or is not feasible.[48,49] Even after successful haemostasis with an interventional radiologic procedure, hepatic failure and sepsis can develop as a result of ischaemic damage to the liver. The absence of collateral arterial vessels is a relative contraindication to transarterial embolisation.[48]

Bile Leakage and Fistula Formation after Hepatic Resection

Unlike bleeding, bile leakage at the time of surgery is not easily detected without vigilant visual inspection of the operative field. The principal source of bile leakage is the transected liver surface, although major biliary injury or insufficiency of a biliary anastomosis are other possible sources. Leakage of bile from the transected surface is important to detect intraoperatively, otherwise it has a high likelihood of leading to intra-abdominal abscess. The most important way to prevent postoperative bile leakage is to meticulously manage the transected liver surface. Even when bile leakage is minimal it can still be detected intraoperatively by searching for bile staining on a fresh sponge compressed against the transected surface. Although a prospective, randomised trial showed no benefit from trying to decrease bile leakage by injecting a solution through the cystic duct and then closing leaking areas, this technique can sometimes be helpful.[50] The routine placement of drains after elective hepatic resection continues to be a source of debate.[51,52] Proponents of drain placement argue that it is safe and lessens the risk of septic complications after a bile leak. Opponents cite the risks of ascending infection and patient discomfort. For patients with chronic parenchymal disease, it is probably best to avoid drain placement after hepatic resection, considering the risk of ascites accumulation and infection.[53]

Patients with a bile leak typically present with signs and symptoms of an intra-abdominal abscess and may be jaundiced. Ultrasound or CT scan of the abdomen localises the biloma. Most biliary leakage after hepatic resection can be managed non-surgically by percutaneous drainage of the extrahepatic collection and the administration of antibiotics empirically and then appropriately guided by culture results. An hepatobiliary (99m)Tc-iminodiacetic acid (HIDA) scan may help to qualify the magnitude of a leak. Endoscopic retrograde cholangiopancreatogram (ERCP) confirms integrity of the major bile ducts, and sphincterotomy decompresses the biliary tree and facilitates leak closure. Operative intervention is more likely to be required if a leak emanates from a major duct injury, such as a severed accessory or aberrant duct, or from an anastomosis.[54,55] Ducts smaller than 4 cm can usually be ligated or clipped. Larger ones require biliaryenteric bypass.

Hepatic Decompensation and Liver Failure after Hepatic Resection

Even though the maximum extent of liver resection that is compatible with good postoperative outcome remains unclear, it is generally believed that as much as 70% (three of four sectors) of the liver can be safely resected if there is no parenchymal disease. The total liver volume can be calculated based on the patient's body surface area.[56,57] However, the relative contribution of each segment to the total liver volume is variable.[58] Therefore, for precise anatomic planning for massive hepatic resection a CT scan or MRI is necessary.[59]

The liver with underlying damage from cirrhosis or obstructive jaundice has a diminished capacity for regeneration. In these situations, meticulous evaluation of baseline liver function as well as anatomical planning of the resection is critical. The indocyanine green (ICG) clearance test is the most widely accepted test for the preoperative evaluation of functional hepatic reserve.[60–63] ICG clearance is used to determine the optimal extent of resection in patients with chronic liver disease.[64]

Although hepatic resection has been considered the gold standard for the treatment of primary hepatic tumours, in the era of liver transplantation this approach should be reserved for patients without decompensated cirrhosis. The evolution of techniques of segmental liver resection has led to the ability to achieve better tumour clearance while preserving function of the remnant liver, particularly relevant to patients with compensated cirrhosis.[65] The width of the resection margin does not appear to influence the rate of postoperative recurrence of hepatocellular carcinoma.[66] When resecting hepatocellular carcinoma from the cirrhotic liver, preserving hepatic parenchyma and minimising manipulation of the remnant liver are more important than achieving wider resection margins.

Preoperative portal vein embolisation (PVE) has been used to induce compensatory hypertrophy of the liver remnant after resection. PVE has been successfully used prior to elective hepatic resection for hepatocellular carcinoma in the cirrhotic liver, cholangiocarcinoma in the jaundiced liver, and metastatic carcinoma in the normal liver.[67-74] A recent prospective randomised trial demonstrated that PVE is only beneficial for hepatic resection in patients with chronic liver disease.[75] This procedure is still recommended as a preoperative adjunct, even for resection of a normal liver when the anticipated remnant liver volume will be smaller than 30% of the original volume.[76] An advantage is that portal venous pressure can be measured during PVE, which is important because a significant elevation of portal venous pressure is associated with an increased risk of decompensation of liver function after hepatic resection.[77]

Although acute hepatic failure can occur, most patients experiencing hepatic dysfunction following liver resection will manifest subacute hepatic insufficiency with only mild, transient hyperbilirubinemia and possibly ascites and/or encephalopathy, lasting up to a few weeks. Some will suffer variceal haemorrhage. Ascites is particularly common in the face of malnutrition or extensive lymphatic dissection. When the more acute hepatic failure occurs, signs are rarely evident in the intraoperative period. Typically, a relatively "normal" first 48–72 postoperative hours, in which the patient is often extubated and seems to be faring well, is followed by progressive elevation of liver enzymes, prothrombin time (PT), and bilirubin, and the development of encephalopathy. If untreated, this condition can progress to frank coma, uncorrectable coagulopathy, hepatorenal syndrome with oliguria, multisystem organ failure, and eventual death. Early recognition of liver failure is essential, so that monitoring of liver enzymes, lactate and clotting parameters should be done frequently after major liver resection. Ultrasonography and/or reoperation to ensure patency of the hepatic vasculature and to exclude torquing of the remnant liver may be life-saving. Replacement of blood products should be done with care so as not to overtransfuse, which can lead to portal vein or hepatic artery thrombosis. Early, aggressive therapy of oliguria with fluid and colloid replacement should be guided by the monitoring of haemodynamic parameters with a pulmonary artery (PA) catheter. Volume overload will aggravate oedema in the remnant liver and decrease the chance of recovery. Management of encephalopathy may require reintubation for airway protection. Salvage liver transplantation may be appropriate in rare instances of liver failure after major resection, but only if there was no prohibitive tumour burden.

COMPLICATIONS OF RESECTION FOR BILIARY MALIGNANCY

Considering that the majority of patients undergoing major hepatobiliary resection for biliary malignancy are in the seventh or eighth decades of their lives and therefore have a higher incidence of medical comorbidity, the risk of hepatic resection and the best type of resection for each individual patient needs to be weighed against the survival benefit. Figure 1 and Table 1 relate to resection for biliary malignancy, just as they do to hepatic resection.

Preoperative Planning

A histologically negative resection margin is the most favourable prognostic variable for bile duct carcinoma.[78] To achieve this goal with proximal bile duct or gall bladder carcinomas, concomitant hepatic resection may be necessary in addition to resection of the extrahepatic bile duct with regional lymphadenectomy. The necessity of preoperative biliary decompression in patients with malignant obstructive jaundice remains controversial and is not uniformly recommended.[79,80] However, for bile duct carcinoma in the hepatic hilum that requires major hepatic resection, preoperative decompression of the biliary tree decreases infectious complications from underlying cholangitis and improves the regenerative capacity of the liver parenchyma.[81,82]

Due to the proximity of the portal vein and hepatic artery to malignant lesions, detailed preoperative imaging is extremely important for staging. An arteriogram and portal venogram as well as a cholangiogram are essential to plan for resection of hilar cholangiocarcinoma.[83] MRI cholangiogram and MRI angiogram may be adequate instead of conventional ERCP and angiogram. The nature and extent of tumour invasion should be evaluated in detail when planning the resection. Portal venous inflow and bile flow are important for the maintenance of liver cell size and mass.[84,85] Segmental or lobar atrophy may result from portal venous occlusion or biliary obstruction.[86]

Appreciation of the anatomical distortions on preoperative imaging is important to individualise the treatment strategy.[87] Preoperative imaging predicts non-resectability based on local extension, but is not useful for assessing nodal or peritoneal metastases. The role of laparoscopy and of endoscopic ultrasonography for staging bile duct carcinoma has yet to be defined; however, they are increasingly performed prior to laparotomy.[88]

Biliary Tree Resection and Lymphadenectomy

At the initial phase of exploratory laparotomy, precise assessment of tumour extension often necessitates a biopsy with frozen section of any suspicious lesion or lymph node. Evidence of a multicentric hepatic lesion, distant metastasis, or para-aortic lymph node metastasis precludes resection. Lymphatic spread is common with bile duct and gall bladder carcinoma and often involves pericholedochal lymph nodes. Regional lymph node dissection that includes the hepatoduodenal ligament is part of resection with curative intent.

In addition to complete hepatoduodenal lymphadenectomy with skeletonisation of the portal vein and hepatic artery, the entire portion of the extrahepatic, suprapancreatic bile duct should be removed. Lymphadenectomy of the hepatic hilum without bile duct resection results in incomplete lymph node clearance at best, and may cause stricture or necrosis of the bile duct. Some groups have insisted on using para-aortic lymphadenectomy; however, this procedure is associated with increased morbidity and does not appear to offer any survival benefit. Aortic lymph node samplings can be helpful in the initial phase of surgery to identify advanced cases and avoid proceeding with major hepatobiliary resection in the patient with minimal predicted survival benefit. For complete removal of these nodes, pancreatoduodenectomy in addition to hepatic and biliary resection has been performed by several Japanese groups. However, this procedure cannot be routinely justified, considering the associated high mortality and morbidity in the absence of proven survival benefit.[89,90]

After bile duct resection and skeletonisation of the hepatic artery and portal vein, maintenance of arterial flow is crucial to maintain integrity of the biliaryenteric anastomosis. The hepatic artery must be handled with extreme care to avoid intimal dissection. An accidentally divided hepatic artery must be immediately reconstructed, preferably via microvascular technique.

Biliary Reconstruction

Biliaryenteric continuity is re-established with a hepaticojejunostomy to a Roux-en-Y loop. The Roux-en-Y loop is prepared and brought cephalid, usually in retrocolic fashion. For a very high biliary anastomosis in a deep abdominal cavity, retrogastric placement of the jejunal loop may provide better exposure and angle for manipulation. Mucosa-to-mucosa approximation is mandatory for the hepaticojejunostomy. The authors' preference is to perform the end-to-side anastomosis with a single layer of 5-0 or 6-0 PDS interrupted sutures. Additional layers of suture do not provide extra security. It is preferable to place and tie sutures so that the knots are extraluminal because intraluminal knots can act as niduses for bile stone formation.[91] The use of absorbable monofilament suture also decreases the chance of bile stone formation. Anastomotic stenting with a silastic tube, 5 Fr to 8 Fr in calibre, may ease the biliary reconstruction and facilitate early postoperative patency, particularly with small-calibre ducts. A closed suction drain should be placed adjacent to the anastomosis.

After removal of the tumour, multiple segmental ducts may be exposed. Each orifice should be probed to determine which hepatic segments it drains. Adjacent duct openings may be incorporated to create a situation where there are no more than three separate orifices to be anastomosed to the Roux-en-Y loop. High anastomoses to multiple orifices of bile ducts should not be performed sequentially; rather, the entire posterior row of stitches to all exposed orifices should be placed first, then the jejunal loop brought up, then the posterior row of stitches tied, and then the anterior row completed.

Management of Biliaryenteric Leak

In the first few postoperative days, scant biliary leakage from either the biliaryenteric anastomosis or liver margin may be noted from the drain. This is usually self-limited, provided that hepatic arterial flow is intact and the anastomosis was performed properly. Massive leaks during these few days necessitate expeditious anastomotic revision. Most often, biliary leakage is first noted after the first few postoperative days. Patients present with signs and symptoms of an intra-abdominal abscess. There is predominantly pain and fever, and there may be bilious drainage from the incision site and/or jaundice. Ultrasound or CT of the abdomen localises the biloma. The first priority is to percutaneously drain the collection and start antibiotics. Subsequently, percutaneous transhepatic cholangiography (PTC) delineates the site and extent of the leak. Transhepatic stenting of the biliary tree, and of the anastomosis if possible, diverts the biliary system, decreases pressure in the ducts, and helps to seal the leak. Re-exploration and reanastomosis for biliary leakage is unlikely to be successful in the face of infection, diffuse inflammation or malnutrition, especially after resection of a very high lesion. Most biliaryenteric leaks can be managed indefinitely without surgery by percutaneous drainage of the extrahepatic collection and percutaneous transhepatic decompression of the biliary tree. Although the presence of percutaneous catheters and the requirement that they be changed at least every few months are a serious nuisance for patients, many leaks will eventually resolve after such long-term care. Cholangiograms and hepatobiliary (99m)Tc-iminodiacetic acid (HIDA) scans help to qualify the magnitude of a leak and determine whether it is healing. Those instances where a biliaryenteric anastomotic leak does not resolve may benefit from eventual elective surgical revision, with some type of biliaryenteric anastomosis.

Management of Biliaryenteric Stricture

Strictures may develop after biliaryenteric anastomosis. Most patients become symptomatic months to years after surgery. The usual presentation is right upper quadrant abdominal pain with jaundice. Some patients have cholangitis at initial presentation. Liver function tests show elevated serum bilirubin and alkaline phosphatase levels. Depending on the time of presentation after surgery, patients may present with destruction of liver parenchyma and cirrhosis due to increased pressure in the biliary system. Ultrasound, CT or MRI confirms the presence of a dilated intrahepatic ductal system. PTC helps localise the site of stricture in the biliary tree. Brush samplings at the site of stricture may be taken if recurrent malignancy is a concern. Strictures can be managed by temporary percutaneous transhepatic dilatation and/or stent placement. Fewer than half of patients require lifelong stenting or eventual surgical revision of the hepaticojejunostomy.

COMPLICATIONS OF RADIOFREQUENCY ABLATION FOR HEPATIC LESIONS

Ablation is increasingly used in the management of liver tumours as either palliative or curative treatment for primary, metastatic, or some benign tumours, or as a "bridge" to liver transplantation for patients with unresectable hepatocellular carcinoma. Ablation is used when adequate resection of tumour/s is not possible because of proximity to vascular or biliary structures, multicentricity, or inadequate hepatic functional reserve. Ablation may be performed as RFA, cryoablation, ethanol injection, or hepatic arterial ligation or embolisation. In general, ethanol injection and arterial embolisation are not considered the domain of the surgeon and hepatic arterial ligation is rarely performed today, since embolisation is easily achievable with interventional radiologic techniques. Cryoablation, compared to RFA, is associated with longer Intensive Care Unit and hospital lengths of stay, greater blood loss and higher overall morbidity.[92] Additionally, the performance of cryoablation is considered by many to be more cumbersome, making RFA the preferred ablative technique by many hepatobiliary surgeons. Therefore, this discussion focuses on complications related to RFA.

The passage of radiofrequency current through saline rich tissue causes focal ionic agitation, heat and coagulation necrosis. RFA can be performed laparoscopically, percutaneously, or via laparotomy. Thus, complications from RFA are related to thermal injury and to the particular surgical approach used for the ablation. The percutaneous approach for ablation is the least invasive and may benefit the patient with inadequate hepatic functional reserve, at increased risk for general anaesthesia and laparotomy or laparoscopy. Open or laparoscopic RFA is preferred for peripheral lesions because these approaches make it possible to protect surrounding viscera by separating them from the heated tissue. These approaches are also preferred to percutaneous RFA in the case of large lesions because they allow for inflow occlusion (Pringle manoeuvre) during the ablation, to avoid the heat sink effect of blood flow and thus ensure more complete ablation.[93] Laparoscopic RFA is less invasive than open RFA and therefore preferred to the open technique, provided laparoscopic ultrasonography equipment is available and the surgeon is versatile at performing laparoscopic ultrasonography and RFA needle placement, both of which are somewhat technically challenging.

Table 2. Complications of Hepatic Radiofrequency Ablation (RFA)

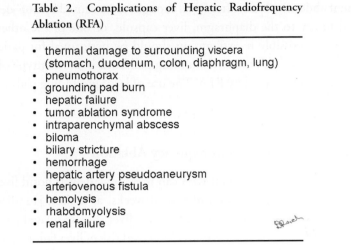

- thermal damage to surrounding viscera (stomach, duodenum, colon, diaphragm, lung)
- pneumothorax
- grounding pad burn
- hepatic failure
- tumor ablation syndrome
- intraparenchymal abscess
- biloma
- biliary stricture
- hemorrhage
- hepatic artery pseudoaneurysm
- arteriovenous fistula
- hemolysis
- rhabdomyolysis
- renal failure

Overall, the reported incidence of complications following RFA is low (2% to 10%).[94–97] and procedure related mortality is rare (<1%).[98] Complications, listed in Table 2, include thermal damage to surrounding viscera, grounding pad burns, hepatic failure, tumour ablation syndrome, intraparenchymal abscess, biloma, biliary stricture, hepatic artery pseudoaneurysm, arteriovenous fistula, haemolysis, rhabdomyolysis, renal failure and haemorrhage.[95,97,99,100] Haemorrhage may be intraperitoneal or subcapsular, but is rare because ablated tissue is not prone to bleeding and the needle track can be heated during removal of the RFA probe.

Thermal Injuries Complicating Radiofrequency Ablation

One of the most dreaded complications after RFA involves thermal damage to surrounding viscera.[97] Injuries are prone to occur if surrounding tissues are not separated from the heated hepatic lesion. Injury to the gall bladder can cause cholecystitis or free bile peritonitis. Cholecystectomy should be performed prophylactically if RFA is to be applied to a lesion within one centimetre of the gall bladder. There have been injuries to the stomach, duodenum and colon, presenting as perforated viscus or as enterocutaneous fistula. Injury to the diaphragm or lung may cause pneumothorax or hydrothorax, necessitating tube thoracostomy and possibly pleurodesis. Some patients complain of persistent abdominal pain after RFA, thought to be caused by non-devastating thermal injury to the diaphragm, liver capsule, or one of the other viscera. CT scan and possibly re-exploration should be performed for patients with severe abdominal symptoms. Grounding pad burn is another type of thermal injury that can be caused by RFA. The use of large grounding pads minimises this risk.[101]

Hepatic Failure after Radiofrequency Ablation

Liver failure that develops after RFA can present acutely as florid liver failure, or insidiously or over a period of several weeks, as ascites, jaundice, failure to thrive, and eventual sepsis. Patients with liver disease related to hepatitis, steatosis, or fibrosis are at significantly increased risk of liver failure, particularly following larger ablations. Nonetheless, the incidence of liver failure after RFA is reportedly low, provided care is taken to leave an adequate volume of perfused, functional parenchyma.[102] Supportive care is often best provided in an Intensive Care Unit. Prophylaxis and treatment of infection is critical as is nutritional support. Liver transplantation should be considered, although many patients are not candidates because of the preablation tumour burden.

Tumour Ablation Syndrome after Radiofrequency Ablation

Following RFA, there is a systemic inflammatory response, also known as tumour ablation syndrome, mediated by inflammatory cytokines and other by-products of cellular destruction released by the necrotic tissue. The severity of this syndrome depends on the amount of tissue ablated. Ablation of larger lesions is often followed by low-grade fever (rarely above 39°C), fatigue, malaise, transient hyperbilirubinemia, and an elevated white blood cell count. Extensive ablation can cause high-grade fever, nausea, vomiting, lethargy and a clinical picture indistinguishable from frank sepsis. The syndrome typically resolves within 10 days but has lasted for up to three weeks after extensive ablations. Clinical management of patients with tumour ablation syndrome involves differentiation from a true infection by means of serial cultures. In the absence of infection, symptomatic care with antipyretics and adequate hydration usually suffices. Treatment with IV broad-spectrum antibiotics may be necessary.[97]

Intraparenchymal Abscess and Other Collections

RFA of hepatic lesions may cause intraparenchymal abscess. In this setting it can be difficult to quickly diagnose a liver abscess because symptoms overlap those of the tumour ablation syndrome, and CT scan or abdominal ultrasound frequently reveal gas at the ablation site, even in the absence of infection. Thus, a high index of suspicion is critical. If the patient appears toxic with haemodynamic compromise, blood cultures should be taken and IV broad-spectrum antibiotics administered, preferably within an Intensive Care Unit. Percutaneous drainage may be required for diagnostic purposes and certainly for treatment of an abscess.

Heat-related injury to the biliary system can lead to biloma, biliary fistula, or biliary stenosis. Biloma is managed by percutaneous drainage. Fistulae are rare and usually self-limited. Biliary stenosis should be managed by endoscopic stenting for distal stenoses and/or percutaneous drainage for more proximal strictures, as well as antibiotic coverage for cholangitis.

CONCLUSION

The field of hepatobiliary surgery has flourished over the past century, since Cantlie first described the right and left lobes of the liver.[103] Continued progress in this field will be fueled by the increasing demand for hepatobiliary surgical therapies. This rising demand is in part due to the hepatitis B and C epidemics and the resultant increase in hepatocellular carcinoma, the rise in metastatic liver disease attributable to the increasing age of the population, the improved screening and earlier diagnosis of surgically treatable disease, and the improved access to care at major liver centres. The increased volume of hepatobiliary surgical work will be performed in an environment where there is a focus on resource utilisation, healthcare cost containment, and quality improvement, all of which will drive a continued decrease in the morbidity and complications related to these high risk procedures. In addition, new developments will lead to improved outcomes. For example, it is a matter of time until there are cytoprotective agents effective at reducing the impact of the ischaemia reperfusion injury involved with certain procedures, and hepatocyte growth factors that will facilitate regeneration after aggressive resections. Outcomes of surgery for malignant disease will be improved as better multimodality adjuvant and neoadjuvant chemo/radiation and bio-logic therapies become available. Another breakthrough will be the widespread use of laparoscopic approaches for hepatobiliary surgery. As the laparoscopic approaches emerge, there will be a learning curve, a rise in certain compli-cations, followed by the development of strategies and equipment to ensure safety. Hepatobiliary surgery has emerged a successful and critically important clinical endeavour and there is still fertile opportunity for this field to continue to mature. Additional refinement of current clinical practice and new devel-opments such as those alluded to above will ensure a continued decrease in the complications related to hepatobiliary surgery, even as there is an increase in both the types of cases and the total volume of surgery performed.

REFERENCES

1. Dimick JB, Cowan JA, Jr, Knol JA, Upchurch GR, Jr. (2003) Hepatic resection in the United States: indications, outcomes, and hospital procedural volumes from a nationally representative database. *Arch Surg* **138**: 185–191.
2. Cunningham JD, Fong Y, Shriver C, *et al.* (1994) One hundred consecutive hepatic resections. Blood loss, transfusion, and operative technique. *Arch Surg* **129**: 1050–1056.
3. Fan ST, Lo CM, Liu CL, *et al.* (1999) Hepatectomy for hepatocellular carcinoma: toward zero hospital deaths. *Ann Surg* **229**: 322–330.
4. Franco D, Smadja C, Meakins JL, *et al.* (1989) Improved early results of elective hepatic resection for liver tumours. One hundred consecutive hepatectomies in cirrhotic and noncirrhotic patients. *Arch Surg* **124**: 1033–1037.
5. Imamura H, Seyama Y, Kokudo N, *et al.* (2003) One thousand fifty-six hepate-ctomies without mortality in eight years. *Arch Surg* **138**: 1198–1206.
6. Jarnagin WR, Gonen M, Fong Y, *et al.* (2002) Improvement in perioperative outcome after hepatic resection: analysis of 1,803 consecutive cases over the past decade. *Ann Surg* **236**: 397–406.
7. Tjandra JJ, Fan ST, Wong J. (1991) Peri-operative mortality in hepatic resection. *Aust N Z J Surg* **61**: 201–206.
8. Belghiti J, Hiramatsu K, Benoist S, *et al.* (2000) Seven hundred forty-seven hepatectomies in the 1990s: an update to evaluate the actual risk of liver resection. *J Am Coll Surg* **191**: 38–46.
9. Belghiti J, Di Carlo I, Sauvanet A, *et al.* (1994) A ten-year experience with hepatic resection in 338 patients: evolutions in indications and of operative mortality. *Eur J Surg* **160**: 277–282.

10. Bismuth H. (1982) Surgical anatomy and anatomical surgery of the liver. *World J Surg* **6**: 3–9.
11. Couinaud C. (1999) Liver anatomy: portal (and suprahepatic) or biliary segmentation. *Dig Surg* **16**: 459–467.
12. Makuuchi M, Hasegawa H, Yamazaki S, *et al.* (1987) The use of operative ultrasound as an aid to liver resection in patients with hepatocellular carcinoma. *World J Surg* **11**: 615–621.
13. Chouillard E, Cherqui D, Tayar C, *et al.* (2003) Anatomical bi- and trisegmentectomies as alternatives to extensive liver resections. *Ann Surg* **238**: 29–34.
14. Makuuchi M, Hasegawa H, Yamazaki S. (1985) Ultrasonically guided subsegmentectomy. *Surg Gynaecol Obstet* **161**: 346–350.
15. Takasaki K, Kobayashi S, Tanaka S, *et al.* (1990) Highly anatomically systematised hepatic resection with Glissonean sheath code transection at the hepatic hilus. *Int Surg* **75**: 73–77.
16. Tsugita M, Takasaki K, Ohtsubo T, *et al.* (1995) Right side hepatic resection under right thoracoabdominal incision with special reference to a highly anatomical systematised method. *Int Surg* **80**: 242–246.
17. Pringle JH. (1908) Notes on the arrest of hepatic haemorrhage due to trauma. *Ann Surg* **48**: 541.
18. Chiappa A, Makuuchi M, Zbar AP, *et al.* (2001) Comparison of continuous versus intermittent hepatic pedicle clamping in an experimental model. *Hepatogastroenterology* **48**: 1416–1420.
19. Clavien PA, Yadav S, Sindram D, Bentley RC. (2000) Protective effects of ischaemic preconditioning for liver resection performed under inflow occlusion in humans. *Ann Surg* **232**: 155–162.
20. Rudiger HA, Kang KJ, Sindram D, *et al.* (2002) Comparison of ischaemic preconditioning and intermittent and continuous inflow occlusion in the murine liver. *Ann Surg* **235**: 400–407.
21. Takayama T, Makuuchi M, Inoue K, *et al.* (1998) Selective and unselective clamping in cirrhotic liver. *Hepatogastroenterology* **45**: 376–380.
22. Smyrniotis V, Kostopanagiotou G, Lolis E, *et al.* (2003) Effects of hepatovenous back flow on ischaemic-reperfusion injuries in liver resections with the Pringle manoeuvre. *J Am Coll Surg* **197**: 949–954.
23. Man K, Fan ST, Ng IO, *et al.* (1997) Prospective evaluation of the Pringle manoeuvre in hepatectomy for liver tumours by a randomised study. *Ann Surg* **226**: 704–711.
24. Emre S, Schwartz ME, Katz E, Miller CM. (1993) Liver resection under total vascular isolation. Variations on a theme. *Ann Surg* **217**: 15–19.

25. Delva E, Barberousse JP, Nordlinger B, *et al.* (1984) Haemodynamic and bio-chemical monitoring during major liver resection with the use of hepatic vascular exclusion. *Surgery* **95**: 309–318.

26. Belghiti J, Noun R, Zante E, *et al.* (1996) Portal triad clamping or hepatic vascular exclusion for major liver resection. A controlled study. *Ann Surg* **224**: 155–161.

27. Grazi GL, Mazziotti A, Jovine E, *et al.* (1997) Total vascular exclusion of the liver during hepatic surgery. Selective use, extensive use, or abuse? *Arch Surg* **132**: 1104–1109.

28. Torzilli G, Makuuchi M, Midorikawa Y, *et al.* (2001) Liver resection without total vascular exclusion: hazardous or beneficial? An analysis of our experience. *Ann Surg* **233**: 167–175.

29. Cherqui D, Malassagne B, Colau PI, *et al.* (1999) Hepatic vascular exclusion with preservation of the caval flow for liver resections. *Ann Surg* **230**: 24–30.

30. Pachter HL, Spencer FC, Hofstetter SR, Coppa GF. (1983) Experience with the finger fracture technique to achieve intra-hepatic haemostasis in 75 patients with severe injuries of the liver. *Ann Surg* **197**: 771–778.

31. Fan ST, Lai EC, Lo CM, *et al.* (1996) Hepatectomy with an ultrasonic dissector for hepatocellular carcinoma. *Br J Surg* **83**: 117–120.

32. Yamamoto Y, Ikai I, Kume M, *et al.* (1999) New simple technique for hepatic parenchymal resection using a Cavitron Ultrasonic Surgical Aspirator and bipolar cautery equipped with a channel for water dripping. *World J Surg* **23**: 1032–1037.

33. Baer HU, Stain SC, Guastella T, *et al.* (1993) Hepatic resection using a water jet dissector. *HPB Surg* **6**: 189–196.

34. Rau HG, Schardey HM, Buttler E, *et al.* (1995) A comparison of different techniques for liver resection: blunt dissection, ultrasonic aspirator and jet-cutter. *Eur J Surg Oncol* **21**: 183–187.

35. Starzl TE, Bell RH, Beart RW, Putnam CW. (1975) Hepatic trisegmentectomy and other liver resections. *Surg Gynaecol Obstet* **141**: 429–437.

36. Schwartz SI. (1984) Right hepatic lobectomy. *Am J Surg* **148**: 668–673.

37. Lorat-Jacob JL, Robert HG. (1952) Well defined technique for right hepatec-tomy. *Presse Med* **60**: 549–551.

38. Makuuchi M, Yamamoto J, Takayama T, *et al.* (1991) Extrahepatic division of the right hepatic vein in hepatectomy. *Hepatogastroenterology* **38**: 176–179.

39. Smyrniotis V, Kostopanagiotou G, Theodoraki K, *et al.* (2004) The role of central venous pressure and type of vascular control in blood loss during major liver resections. *Am J Surg* **187**: 398–402.

40. Melendez JA, Arslan V, Fischer ME, *et al.* (1998) Perioperative outcomes of major hepatic resections under low central venous pressure anaesthesia: blood

loss, blood transfusion, and the risk of postoperative renal dysfunction. *J Am Coll Surg* **187**: 620–625.

41. Moulton CA, Chui AK, Mann D, *et al.* (2001) Does patient position during liver surgery influence the risk of venous air embolism? *Am J Surg* **181**: 366–367.

42. Liu CL, Fan ST, Lo CM, *et al.* (2002) Intraoperative iatrogenic rupture of hepatocellular carcinoma. *World J Surg* **26**: 348–352.

43. Azoulay D, Marin-Hargreaves G, Castaing D, *et al.* (2001) The anterior approach: the right way for right massive hepatectomy. *J Am Coll Surg* **192**: 412–417.

44. Liu CL, Fan ST, Lo CM, *et al.* (2000) Anterior approach for major right hepatic resection for large hepatocellular carcinoma. *Ann Surg* **232**: 25–31.

45. Noun R, Elias D, Balladur P, *et al.* (1996) Fibrin glue effectiveness and tolerance after elective liver resection: a randomised trial. *Hepatogastroenterology* **43**: 221–224.

46. Schwartz M, Madariaga J, Hirose R, *et al.* (2004) Comparison of a new fibrin sealant with standard topical haemostatic agents. *Arch Surg* **139**: 1148–1154.

47. Okuno A, Miyazaki M, Ito H, *et al.* (2001) Nonsurgical management of ruptured pseudo-aneurysm in patients with hepatobiliary pancreatic diseases. *Am J Gastroenterol* **96**: 1067–1071.

48. Miyamoto N, Kodama Y, Endo H, *et al.* (2003) Hepatic artery embolisation for postoperative haemorrhage in upper abdominal surgery. *Abdom Imaging* **28**: 347–353.

49. Tessier DJ, Fowl RJ, Stone WM, *et al.* (2003) Iatrogenic hepatic artery pseudo-aneurysms: an uncommon complication after hepatic, biliary and pancreatic procedures. *Ann Vasc Surg* **17**: 663–669.

50. Ijichi M, Takayama T, Toyoda H, *et al.* (2000) Randomised trial of the usefulness of a bile leakage test during hepatic resection. *Arch Surg* **135**: 1395–1400.

51. Belghiti J, Kabbej M, Sauvanet A, *et al.* (1993) Drainage after elective hepatic resection. A randomised trial. *Ann Surg* **218**: 748–753.

52. Burt BM, Brown K, Jarnagin W, *et al.* (2002) An audit of results of a no-drainage practice policy after hepatectomy. *Am J Surg* **184**: 441–445.

53. Liu CL, Fan ST, Lo CM, *et al.* (2004) Abdominal drainage after hepatic resection is contraindicated in patients with chronic liver diseases. *Ann Surg* **239**: 194–201.

54. Bhattacharjya S, Puleston J, Davidson BR, Dooley JS. (2003) Outcome of early endoscopic biliary drainage in the management of bile leaks after hepatic resection. *Gastrointest Endosc* **57**: 526–530.

55. Reed DN, Jr., Vitale GC, Wrightson WR, *et al.* (2003) Decreasing mortality of bile leaks after elective hepatic surgery. *Am J Surg* **185**: 316–318.

56. Heinemann A, Wischhusen F, Puschel K, Rogiers X. (1999) Standard liver volume in the Caucasian population. *Liver Transpl Surg* 5: 366–368.

57. Urata K, Kawasaki S, Matsunami H, *et al.* (1995) Calculation of child and adult standard liver volume for liver transplantation. *Hepatology* 21: 1317–1321.

58. Abdalla EK, Denys A, Chevalier P, *et al.* (2004) Total and segmental liver volume variations: implications for liver surgery. *Surgery* 135: 404–410.

59. Kubota K, Makuuchi M, Kusaka K, *et al.* (1997) Measurement of liver volume and hepatic functional reserve as a guide to decision-making in resectional surgery for hepatic tumours. *Hepatology* 26: 1176–1181.

60. Hemming AW, Scudamore CH, Shackleton CR, *et al.* (1992) Indocyanine green clearance as a predictor of successful hepatic resection in cirrhotic patients. *Am J Surg* 163: 515–518.

61. Lau H, Man K, Fan ST, *et al.* (1997) Evaluation of preoperative hepatic function in patients with hepatocellular carcinoma undergoing hepatectomy. *Br J Surg* 84: 1255–1259.

62. Matsumata T, Kanematsu T, Yoshida Y, *et al.* (1987) The indocyanine green test enables the prediction of postoperative complications after hepatic resection. *World J Surg* 11: 678–681.

63. Okamoto E, Kyo A, Yamanaka N, *et al.* (1984) Prediction of the safe limits of hepatectomy by combined volumetric and functional measurements in patients with impaired hepatic function. *Surgery* 95: 586–592.

64. Miyagawa S, Makuuchi M, Kawasaki S, Kakazu T. (1995) Criteria for safe hepatic resection. *Am J Surg* 169: 589–594.

65. Regimbeau JM, Kianmanesh R, Farges O, *et al.* (2002) Extent of liver resection influences the outcome in patients with cirrhosis and small hepatocellular carcinoma. *Surgery* 131: 311–317.

66. Poon RT, Fan ST, Ng IO, Wong J. (2000) Significance of resection margin in hepatectomy for hepatocellular carcinoma: a critical reappraisal. *Ann Surg* 231: 544–551.

67. Azoulay D, Raccuia JS, Castaing D, Bismuth H. (1995) Right portal vein embolisation in preparation for major hepatic resection. *J Am Coll Surg* 181: 266–269.

68. Kawasaki S, Makuuchi M, Kakazu T, *et al.* (1994) Resection for multiple metastatic liver tumours after portal embolisation. *Surgery* 115: 674–677.

69. Makuuchi M, Thai BL, Takayasu K, *et al.* (1990) Preoperative portal embolisation to increase the safety of major hepatectomy for hilar bile duct carcinoma: a preliminary report. *Surgery* 107: 521–527.

70. Nagino M, Nimura Y, Kamiya J, *et al.* (1995) Right or left trisegment portal vein embolisation before hepatic trisegmentectomy for hilar bile duct carcinoma. *Surgery* 117: 677–681.

71. Abdalla EK, Barnett CC, Doherty D, *et al.* (2002) Extended hepatectomy in patients with hepatobiliary malignancies with and without preoperative portal vein embolisation. *Arch Surg* **137**: 675–680.

72. Azoulay D, Castaing D, Krissat J, *et al.* (2000) Percutaneous portal vein embolisation increases the feasibility and safety of major liver resection for hepatocellular carcinoma in injured liver. *Ann Surg* **232**: 665–672.

73. Azoulay D, Castaing D, Smail A, *et al.* (2000) Resection of nonresectable liver metastases from colorectal cancer after percutaneous portal vein embolisation. *Ann Surg* **231**: 480–486.

74. Sugawara Y, Yamamoto J, Higashi H, *et al.* (2002) Preoperative portal embolisation in patients with hepatocellular carcinoma. *World J Surg* **26**: 105–110.

75. Farges O, Belghiti J, Kianmanesh R, *et al.* (2003) Portal vein embolisation before right hepatectomy: prospective clinical trial. *Ann Surg* **237**: 208–217.

76. Yigitler C, Farges O, Kianmanesh R, *et al.* (2003) The small remnant liver after major liver resection: how common and how relevant? *Liver Transpl* **9**: S18–S25.

77. Bruix J, Castells A, Bosch J, *et al.* (1996) Surgical resection of hepatocellular carcinoma in cirrhotic patients: prognostic value of preoperative portal pressure. *Gastroenterology* **111**: 1018–1022.

78. Tsao JI, Nimura Y, Kamiya J, *et al.* (2000) Management of hilar cholangiocarcinoma: comparison of an American and a Japanese experience. *Ann Surg* **232**: 166–174.

79. Sewnath ME, Birjmohun RS, Rauws EA, *et al.* (2001) The effect of preoperative biliary drainage on postoperative complications after pancreaticoduodenectomy. *J Am Coll Surg* **192**: 726–734.

80. Sewnath ME, Karsten TM, Prins MH, *et al.* (2002) A meta-analysis on the efficacy of preoperative biliary drainage for tumours causing obstructive jaundice. *Ann Surg* **236**: 17–27.

81. Mann DV, Lam WW, Magnus HN, *et al.* (2002) Biliary drainage for obstructive jaundice enhances hepatic energy status in humans: a 31-phosphorus magnetic resonance spectroscopy study. *Gut* **50**: 118–122.

82. Nakeeb A, Pitt HA. (1995) The role of preoperative biliary decompression in obstructive jaundice. *Hepatogastroenterology* **42**: 332–337.

83. Burke EC, Jarnagin WR, Hochwald SN, *et al.* (1998) Hilar cholangiocarcinoma: patterns of spread, the importance of hepatic resection for curative operation, and a presurgical clinical staging system. *Ann Surg* **228**: 385–394.

84. Schwartz LH, Coakley FV, Sun Y, *et al.* (1998) Neoplastic pancreaticobiliary duct obstruction: evaluation with breath-hold MR cholangiopancreatography. *AJR Am J Roentgenol* **170**: 1491–1495.

85. Hadjis NS, Blumgart LH. (1987) Role of liver atrophy, hepatic resection and hepatocyte hyperplasia in the development of portal hypertension in biliary disease. *Gut* **28**: 1022–1028.

86. Hann LE, Getrajdman GI, Brown KT, *et al.* (1996) Hepatic lobar atrophy: association with ipsilateral portal vein obstruction. *AJR Am J Roentgenol* **167**: 1017–1021.

87. Hadjis NS, Hemingway A, Carr D, Blumgart LH. (1986) Liver lobe disparity consequent upon atrophy. Diagnostic, operative and therapeutic considerations. *J Hepatol* **3**: 285–293.

88. D'Angelica M, Fong Y, Weber S, *et al.* (2003) The role of staging laparoscopy in hepatobiliary malignancy: prospective analysis of 401 cases. *Ann Surg Oncol* **10**: 183–189.

89. Ogura Y, Mizumoto R, Isaji S, *et al.* (1991) Radical operations for carcinoma of the gall bladder: present status in Japan. *World J Surg* **15**: 337–343.

90. D'Angelica M, Martin RC, Jarnagin WR, *et al.* (2004) Major hepatectomy with simultaneous pancreatectomy for advanced hepatobiliary cancer. *J Am Coll Surg* **198**: 570–576.

91. Blumgart LH, Fong Y. (1997) Surgery of the liver and biliary tract, CD-ROM. (Churchill Livingston, New York).

92. Bilchik AJ, Wood TF, Allegra D, *et al.* (2000) Cryosurgical ablation and radiofrequency ablation for unresectable hepatic neoplasms. *Arch Surg* **135**: 657–664.

93. Curley SA, Marra P, Beaty K, *et al.* (2004) Early and late complications after radiofrequency ablation of malignant liver tumours in 608 patients. *Ann Surg* **239**: 450–458.

94. Choi H, Loyer EM, DuBrow RA, Radiofrequency ablation of liver tumours: assessment of therapeutic response and complications. *RadioGraphics* **21**: S41–S54.

95. Iannitti DA, Dupuy DE, Mayo-smith WW, Murphy B. (2002) Hepatic radiofrequency ablation. *Arch Surg* **137**: 422–427.

96. Curley SA, Izzo F, Delrio P, *et al.* (1999) Radiofrequency ablation of unresectable primary and metastatic hepatic malignancies. *Ann Surg* **230**: 1–8.

97. Bleicher RJ, Bilchik AJ. (2004) Complications of hepatic radiofrequency ablation: lessons learned. In: Ellis LM, Curley SA, Tanabe KT (eds.), *Radiofrequency Ablation for Cancer* (Springer Verlag, New York), pp. 121–134.

98. Livraghi T, Goldberg SN, Lazzaroni S, *et al.* (2000) Hepatocellular carcinoma: radiofrequency ablation of medium and large lesions. *Radiology* **214**: 761–768.

99. McGahan JP, Dodd GD III. (2001) Radiofrequency ablation of liver. *AJR Am J Roentgenol* **176**: 3–16.

100. Keltner JR, Donegan E, Hynson JM, Shapiro WA. (2001) Acute renal failure after radiofrequency ablation of metastatic carcinoid tumour. *Anaesth Analg* **93**: 587–9.
101. Ahmed M, Goldberg N. (2004) Principles of radiofrequency ablation. In: Ellis LM, Curley SA, Tanabe KT (eds.), *Radiofrequency Ablation for Cancer* (Springer Verlag, New York), pp. 3–28.
102. Curley SA, Izzo F. (2004) Radiofrequency ablation of hepatocellular carcinoma. In: Ellis LM, Curley SA, Tanabe KT (eds.), *Radiofrequency Ablation for Cancer* (Springer Verlag, New York), pp. 89–106.
103. Cantlie J. (1987) On a new arrangement of the right and left lobes of the liver. *Proc Anat Soc Great Britain Ireland* **32**: 4–9.

Chapter 13

COMPLICATIONS OF PANCREATIC SURGERY

Nicholas Alexakis, Saxon Connor, Paula Ghaneh, Robert Sutton, Jonathan C. Evans and John P. Neoptolemos

INTRODUCTION

Pancreatic disease continues to be challenging. Cancer of the pancreas is still an incurable disease but surgery with adjuvant chemotherapy offers the best opportunity for prolonged survival. Chronic pancreatitis is on the rise and many patients need to be operated upon for complications of the disease. In the 10–20% of patients who develop severe acute pancreatitis, up to 50% will require surgical intervention from which there is a high rate of complications. Twenty years ago, pancreatic resections carried a mortality rate of more than 20%. Since then, there have been many improvements in the technical aspects of surgery and postoperative management, and the mortality rate has reduced to <5% but morbidity remains high at 30–50%. The most common elective pancreas operation is resection of the head of the pancreas with the classic

Kausch-Whipple partial pancreatoduodenectomy (KW-PD) or the pylorus preserving Kausch-Whipple procedure (PP-KW). This chapter will focus on complications of pancreaticoduodenectomy as well as those following pancreatic necrosectomy for acute pancreatitis.

Morbidity and Mortality of the Kausch-Whipple Operation

The current perioperative mortality in high volume specialist centres is 1–3.6%[1-8] (Table 1). The main causes of death are intra-abdominal bleeding, sepsis from leakage of the pancreaticojejunal anastomosis and cardiovascular and pulmonary events. A study from the University of Mainz-Germany with 221 resections found that intraoperative blood loss, preoperative serum bilirubin, diameter of the main pancreatic duct, and occurrence of complications were independent prognostic factors of perioperative mortality.[9]

The significant decline in operative mortality for pancreatic resection has not been mirrored by a decline in postoperative morbidity. Studies report morbidity rates of 38–54% (Table 2).[5-8,10] These variations depend, among

Table 1.   Morbidity and Mortality After Pancreatoduodenectomy

Study	Region	Period	No. of patients	Overall morbidity %	Mortality %
Yeo et al.[7]	Baltimore	1990–1996	650	41	1.4
Bassi et al.[5]	Verona	1997–1999	150	50.6	2
Yeo et al.[4]	Baltimore	1996–2001	294	36	3
Geer et al.*,[2]	New York	1983–1990	146	37	3.4
Delcore et al.*,[1]	Kansas City	1970–1995	100	22	3
Richter et al.*,[3]	Mannheim	1972–1998	194	30	3.1
Balcom et al.[8]	Boston	1990–2000	489	37	1
Sewnath et al.[15]	Amsterdam	1992–1999	290	51.4	1
Bottger et al.*,[9]	Mainz	1985–1997	221	43.5	3.1
Buchler et al.[6]	Bern	1993–1999	216	46.3	2.7
Neoptolemos et al.**	Liverpool	1997–2003	219	47	3.6

*Cancer cases only.
**Unpublished data.

other things, on the underlying pathology and the variable definitions. Most postoperative complications respond to medical treatment and radiological and endoscopic intervention. Complications that require re-operation (2–4% of the cases) are associated with a mortality between 8–67%.[5–7,11,12] Morbidity results from surgical and medical complications which can be divided into major versus minor and early versus late, for didactic reasons.[13]

Effect of Preoperative Biliary Drainage on Postoperative Complications

A study of 300 patients from the MD Anderson Center (USA) found no difference in the incidence of all complications or pancreas-specific complications between stented and non-stented patients.[14] Similar results were also reported by the Amsterdam Medical Centre (Netherlands) in a study of 232 patients.[15] A meta-analysis in 2002 concluded that with the current standards, preoperative biliary drainage has no clear benefit on postoperative morbidity and its use is dependent on logistical factors.[16]

Medical Complications Following Pancreatic Resection

Medical complications include those arising from the cardiovascular system (angina, myocardial infarction, arrhythmias, stroke, deep venous thrombosis and pulmonary embolism), respiratory system (atelectasis, pneumonia, respiratory insufficiency), renal system (acute renal failure) as well as hepatic and metabolic disturbances, urinary tract infection and central line infection. The postoperative medical complication rate varies from 4–19%.[5–7,9]

Surgical Complications Following Pancreatic Resection

Leakage and fistulae of the pancreato-intestinal anastomosis

There is no agreed definition of a pancreatic fistula with over 20 used in the international literature. The Heidelberg and Johns Hopkins groups use a similar definition of pancreatic fistula, which is drainage of more than 30–50 ml of amylase rich fluid (>5000 IU) per day from intra-abdominal drains, on or after the 10th postoperative day.[17,18] The Ulm group define it as an amylase

Table 2. Surgical Complications After Pancreatoduodenectomy

Complication %	Yeo et al.[7] n = 650	Bottger et al.[9] n = 221	Roder et al.[35] n = 85	Balcom et al.[8] n = 489	Sewnath et al.[15] n = 290	Buchler et al.[6] n = 216	Bassi et al.[5] n = 150	Yeo et al.[4] n = 294	Richter et al.[3] n = 194
Pancreatic fistula/leak	14	13.5	17.6	11.5	12.4	1.9	10.7	9.5	3.6
Haemorrhage	5	3.1	2.3	0.2	8.6		2		9.8
Intra-abdominal abscess	5		12.9	1.6	15.5			3.7	3.6
Delayed gastric emptying	19		9.4	12.3	21.4	25	4	11.2	5.7
Intra-abdominal collection		5.4					16.6		
Biliary fistula/leak	3	0.4	1.2	0.8			4	3.4	
Enteric fistula		0.4					7.4		
Pancreatitis	2						5.3		1.5
Cholangitis	5			0.6				1.7	0.5
Wound infection	10	2.2	8.2	5.1	7.6			7.8	8.2
Re-operation	4	8.6		2	14.1	4.1	3.3	4	7.2

rich fluid (three times the serum level) for more than three days postoperatively and with a drainage volume of more than 10 ml per day.[19] Another definition is pancreatic fluid discharge over seven postoperative days with an amylase concentration of more than three times the serum amylase level.[20] Three groups have defined a pancreatic leak (clinical or biochemical) as drainage fluid that is rich in amylase (≥ 2.5 or five times the serum level) or if the leak is radiologically demonstratable.[21–23] A clinically significant leak may be defined as such if there is associated fever $>38°$ C, leukocytosis $>10 \times 10^9/l$, abdominal tenderness, dyspnoea or a need for percutaneous drainage.[22] From these varied definitions it is clear that there is a considerable overlap between the uses of the terms "fistula" and "leak". In our view, these are arbitrary definitions and the terms "fistula", "leak", "leakage" and "anastomotic insufficiency" are interchangeable. The main issue is the impact of the fistula on the clinical course of the patient (delayed hospital discharge, ITU admission, or death versus no clinical impact) and not the comparisons aimed at attempting to define the "best" centres.

The reported incidence of pancreatic fistula or leak ranges from 2–24% with major centres reporting a risk of 11–18%, and usually arising between the third and seventh postoperative days.[4,6–11,24–26] A leak can manifest as a pancreato-cutaneous fistula, a peripancreatic collection or abscess or as delayed gastric emptying. Many leaks are insignificant without clinical symptoms,[11] which may vary from the systemic inflammatory response syndrome to overt sepsis. The mortality from a major pancreatic leak is up to 28% and the cause of death is intra- or retro-peritoneal sepsis and haemorrhage.[9,11,27]

Several studies have reported risk factors such as a soft parenchymal texture of the pancreatic remnant, small main pancreatic duct diameter, ampullary or intrapancreatic bile duct carcinoma, normal preoperative exocrine function and the anastomotic technique itself, for the breakdown of the pancreatic anastomosis; however, other studies have not found any parameter that is predisposed to pancreatic leak.[6,11,27–30] It is not clear which of the different anastomotic techniques produces the optimum results.[31–35] Adherence to a meticulous standardised surgical technique with careful tissue handling and good perioperative management may be more important in reducing the rate of the pancreatic leak.

Reconstruction of the pancreatic-enteric anastomosis

Most specialist units perform a pancreatico-jejunostomy with an end-to-side or side-to-side, duct-to-mucosa technique (with or without an internal or external pancreatic stent). This can be performed with any duct size and pancreatic texture. A randomised trial in 145 patients with benign and malignant peripancreatic disease who also underwent Kausch-Whipple resection compared the use of pancreatojejunostomy (n = 72) with pancreatogastrostomy (n = 73).[18] The incidence of pancreatic anastomotic leak was 11% for the pancreatojejunostomy and 12% for the pancreatogastrostomy, with no perioperative mortality. In a retrospective study with 441 patients from Hanover, Germany, the leakage rates and mortality due to leakage were significantly lower in the pancreatogastrostomy group when compared with the pancreatojejunostomy group.[36]

Role of main pancreatic duct occlusion

A multi-centre randomised trial from France found no benefits in the rate or severity of intra-abdominal complications from pancreatic duct occlusion with fibrin glue after partial pancreatoduodenectomy or left pancreatectomy.[37] A prospective randomised study from Holland found no significant differences in postoperative complications and mortality but rather a significantly higher incidence of diabetes mellitus after duct occlusion.[38]

Management of a pancreatic fistula or leak

The management of a pancreatic fistula depends on the individual patient. In the absence of peritonitis, sepsis or haemorrhage, conservative management (drain *in situ* or percutaneous drain placement to create a controlled fistula using abdominal CT) should be employed. Early recognition and good monitoring is essential. TPN and somatostatin analogues have been shown to achieve closure rates of 70–100% and serve as the standard treatment[39–41] but the true value of octreotide in the treatment of established pancreatic fistulae is not clear with studies showing conflicting data.[42] Laparotomy is indicated if there is a major complication such as haemorrhage that cannot be managed by other means, or if there is a high output fistula with severe sepsis. The recommended procedure is completion pancreatectomy but this carries considerable morbidity and mortality.[11,12] Another operative option is clo-sure of the jejunal and pancreatic stumps and placement of suction-irrigation drains. A study of 29 patients with clinical leakage from the Amsterdam Med-ical Centre (Netherlands) found that patients who underwent completion pancreatectomy (after a mean of five days from the initial operation) had a significantly lower mortality than patients undergoing percutaneous or surgi-cal drainage procedures (0% vs. 38%).[27] These data also correlate with the findings from other major centres.[9,26]

Intra-abdominal abscess

Intra-abdominal abscess following pancreatic resection occurs in 1–12% of the patients.[5–7] The usual cause is anastomotic leak at the pancreatojejunostomy, hepaticojejunostomy, or gastrojejunostomy and often heralds as a right sub-hepatic or left sub-diaphragmatic collection.[43] A contrast-enhanced CT scan is indicated whenever an intra-abdominal collection is suspected. The preferred management of CT-guided percutaneous drainage[44] with appropriate intra-venous antibiotics and if successful, sepsis usually resolves in 24–48 hours. (Image 1)

Haemorrhage

Postoperative haemorrhage occurs in 2–15% of the patients following pan-creatic resection.[6,7,45–48] Reactionary bleeding (within the first 24 h) is usu-ally from the resection bed or bleeding from an anastomosis suture line. An endoscopy must be performed to identify the gastrointestinal suture line bleed-ing and is usually managed conservatively.[43] Selective angiography should be discussed with the interventional radiologists (Image 2) if bleeding persists; if it is not possible or fails, laparotomy is indicated with enterotomies to inspect the anastomoses.[46] Stress ulceration is rare and can usually be managed med-ically and/or endoscopically. Preoperative biliary drainage does not influence the type of bleeding or mortality in jaundiced patients.[45]

Secondary haemorrhage (usually around two weeks following surgery) often has a sinister underlying cause, an anastomotic leak and secondary ero-sion of the retroperitoneal vasculature, with a mortality of 15–58%[27,46,48]; another cause is a pseudo-aneurysm. Bleeding can be from the right and

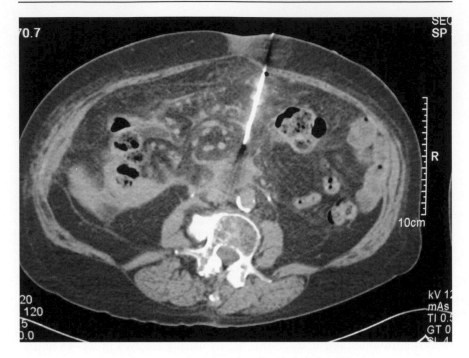

Image 1.   Aspiration-drainage of a postoperative abscess.

common hepatic artery, splenic artery, superior mesenteric artery or the gastro-duodenal artery stump.[47,49] Key investigations include contrast-enhanced CT, endoscopy and selective angiography with selective embolisation if a bleeding point can be identified, with a success rate of 63–79%.[44,48]

Bleeding from the pancreatojejunostomy is particularly problematic with no clear evidence for the optimal re-intervention procedure. The options are a completion total pancreatectomy (but is associated with significant morbidity and mortality), refashioning of the anastomosis after a limited resection of the jejunum and pancreas, or closure of the jejunal stump and drainage of the pancreatic duct and the remaining pancreas.[13,45] Several studies have described that sentinel bleeding indicates local sepsis and possible anastomotic leak.[47–49]

Delayed gastric emptying

There is no uniform definition for delayed gastric emptying. Most definitions include the need for a nasogastric tube more than 7–10 days after the operation

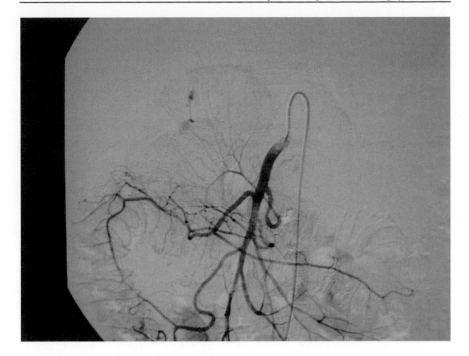

Image 2. Embolisation of a bleeding jejunal Roux loop.

or the inability to tolerate oral intake for more than 7–14 days postoperatively. The incidence of delayed gastric emptying is reported in 4–37% of the patients following resection of the head of the pancreas.[5–7,13] The aetiology of delayed gastric emptying is not entirely clear but includes anastomotic oedema and damage to the fragile vascular supply of the gastroduodenal neuroendocrine axis. Animal studies have also shown that circulating levels of motilin fall following pancreatoduodenectomy.[50]

Yeo *et al.* have shown that delayed gastric emptying can be reduced by up to 37% following pancreatoduodenectomy with intravenous erythromycin, a known motilin agonist.[51] Other supportive measures include the use of metoclopramide and cyclizine. Gastric function normalises at two to four weeks following pancreatoduodenectomy and does not appear to be a significant long-term problem. Although delayed gastric emptying almost invariably resolves with conservative treatment, occasionally operative correction is required. There are studies that suggest that pylorus preservation increases the risk of delayed gastric emptying.[52] There are also many studies indicating that delayed gastric emptying is related to intra-abdominal complications, especially pancreatic leak, and extended radical surgery.[13]

Intra-abdominal fluid collections

The usual definition of an intra-abdominal fluid collection is a collection at least 5 cm in diameter. Their reported incidence is between 6–16%. These are usually harmless and should be drained percutaneously only if they became symptomatic or infected.[5,9]

Enteric and biliary fistula after pancreatoduodenectomy

Enteric and biliary fistulae are uncommon after pancreatoduodenectomy. Biliary fistula, defined as bilirubin-rich drainage fluid lasting for more than five days, occurs in 0.4–4% and indicates leakage from the hepatico-jejunostomy. Most biliary fistulae resolve spontaneously with conservative management or non-operative intervention with percutaneous drainage and transhepatic biliary stenting.[5–9,44,53] Early high output biliary fistulae usually require re-operation. Enteric fistulae occur in 0.4–7.4% and usually indicate a leakage of the gastro-jejunostomy.[5,9] Conservative management including the maintenance of drains, percutaneous drainage, total parenteral or enteral nutrition and the use of octreotide is usually sufficient to heal these fistulae. A reoperation is necessary in case of persistent sepsis.

Other uncommon major complications

Acute cholangitis indicates a partial obstruction due to oedema of the anastomosis or is associated with a local complication. Conservative measures are usually sufficient but a CT scan is mandatory to exclude local complications such as an abscess, bleeding or a pseudo-aneurysm. Acute pancreatitis is rare and usually resolves with conservative management, but bleeding or infection may ensue requiring a completion total pancreatectomy. Small bowel obstruction is also managed conservatively but ischaemia and necrosis may occur. Hepatic portal vein thrombosis is rare but if detected early, percutaneous transhepatic thrombectomy should be performed. Chylous ascites is probably more common than series report and can be troublesome; infection may ensue causing an abscess. External drainage of the ascites is necessary and may need to be supplemented with TPN and octreotide.

*Role of octreotide in decreasing postoperative complications following
pancreatic resection*

The value of octreotide in the prevention and treatment of pancreatic fistulae
and other complications following pancreatoduodenectomy is not yet established. There are five randomised placebo-controlled trials from Europe that
showed it to be beneficial. The group from Ulm[19] randomised 246 patients
undergoing major elective pancreatic surgery of whom 200 underwent resection of the head of the pancreas, 31 underwent left resection, and 15 had other
procedures. The patients were stratified as high risk (peripancreatic tumours
with a soft pancreas) and low risk (chronic pancreatitis with a fibrotic pancreas). The overall complication rate was 32% in the octreotide group versus
55% in the placebo group ($p < 0.005$) and the rate of pancreatic fistula was
18% and 46% respectively. The effect was more prominent in patients with
peripancreatic tumours. The Berne group randomised 247 patients undergoing major resection for chronic pancreatitis.[17] A total of 124 patients underwent resection of the head of the pancreas, 55 had a left resection, 61 had
a pancreatojejunostomy and seven had other procedures. The mortality rates
were similar between the treatment groups. The overall postoperative complication rate in the octreotide group was 16.4% and in the placebo group
29.6% ($p < 0.007$); there was also a significant difference in fistula formation
(10% vs. 22%, $p < 0.05$). Similar findings were reported from two studies in
Italy[54,55] and an institutional study in France.[56]

Three studies were conducted in the USA. The group from Johns
Hopkins studied 211 patients with peripancreatic tumours who had a
pancreatoduodenectomy.[57] The drug was administered within two hours of
surgery and continued for seven days. The pancreatic fistulae rates were 9%
in the control group and 11% in the octreotide group, and the overall complication rates were 34% and 40% respectively. In an open study from the
MD Anderson Cancer Center, Texas, 120 patients who underwent pancreatoduodenectomy for malignancy were randomised to either octreotide or
placebo.[22] The octreotide was administered during or after the operation.
The rate of clinically significant pancreatic leak was 12% in the octreotide
group and 6% in the control group ($p = 0.23$). The perioperative morbidity was 30% and 25% respectively. The third trial from the USA, was a
multi-centre, double-blind, placebo-controlled trial of 275 patients with periampullary neoplasms, of whom 135 received vapreotide and 140 received
the placebo.[10] Pancreatoduodenectomy was performed in 215 patients, distal

pancreatectomy in 52 and central pancreatectomy in eight patients. There was no significant difference in the pancreas-specific complication rates between the two groups (26.4% vs. 30.4% respectively) or the overall complication rate (42% vs. 40% respectively). Marked differences in study design and differences in surgical techniques between institutions may account for the variation in outcomes in the above studies.

Comparison of postoperative complications between standard versus pylorus preserving pancreatoduodenectomy

The lack of standardised descriptions of the Kausch-Whipple (KW) procedure or PP-KW led to inconsistencies in both technique and pathological reporting that have hampered the interpretation of data in reported series. These points were addressed at a pancreatic "workshop" and guidelines on surgery and pathological examination were drawn up and published.[58,59] There are only two prospective randomised trials comparing the two techniques. The first from Taiwan, recruited only a small number of patients (n = 31) and there were no significant differences besides a more frequent delayed gastric emptying in the PP-KW group.[60] The second study from the University of Bern, randomised 77 patients (classic KW = 40, PP-KW = 37) and reported a significantly higher morbidity in the classic KW group.[61] There were no differences in tumour recurrence or long-term survival after a median follow-up of 1.1 years. The advantages of pylorus preservation have not been conclusively established but may include a reduction in post-gastrectomy complications and enterogastric reflux along with improved postoperative nutritional status and weight gain compared to the standard operation.[61–64]

Comparison of postoperative complications between standard and extended resection for pancreas cancer

Two trials have addressed the role of extended lymphadenectomy. A multi-centre, randomised trial from Italy compared conventional pancreatoduodenectomy with and without extended lymph node resection; 40 patients were randomised to conventional resection and 41 were randomised to additional lymphadenectomy and retroperitoneal soft tissue clearance.[65] There were no significant differences regarding perioperative morbidity and mortality. The conventional group had a median survival of 11.2 months with a 3-year survival rate of 10% while the radical group had a median survival of

16.7 months with a 3-year survival rate of 8% (no significant difference). A post-hoc subgroup analysis revealed a significantly longer survival rate in node positive patients after an extended rather than standard lymphadenectomy.

The Johns Hopkins group randomised 56 patients with peripancreatic adenocarcinoma to a standard KW and 58 patients to radical pancreatoduodenectomy. Perioperative morbidity and mortality were not significantly different between the two groups. The one year survival rate was 71% for the standard KW group and 80% for the radical pancreatoduodenectomy group.[66] The updated results in 2002 showed 146 patients in the standard KW arm and 148 in the extended pancreatoduodenectomy group.[4] Perioperative mortality was similar in the two groups but the overall complication rate was significantly higher in the extended pancreatoduodenectomy arm (43% vs. 29%, $p = 0.01$). Radical pancreatoduodenectomy was not associated with a survival benefit (three year survival of 38% vs. 36% respectively). The Johns Hopkins group also studied the quality of life in 105 of these patients at a mean of 2.2 years and the total and subscale scores were comparable between standard and extended resection groups.[67]

Re-admissions after pancreatoduodenectomy

A study from Netherlands with 283 patients, found that 47 (16.6%) patients were readmitted for surgical complications not related to tumour recurrence, mainly for abscesses, fistula and intestinal obstruction.[68] The readmission rate during a 10-year period at Massachusetts General Hospital was 9.6% for dehydration, failure to thrive, wound infection, intra-abdominal abscesses and gastrointestinal bleeding.[8]

Endocrine and exocrine insufficiency after pancreatoduodenectomy

Diabetes mellitus does not usually develop after partial pancreatectomy but the secretory capacity of insulin and glucagon is considerably reduced at three months.[69] Studies in healthy living related pancreatic donors showed deterioration in insulin secretion and glucose tolerance at one year post-resection.[70] Pancreatoduodenectomy may result in steatorrhoea, which in some cases can be profound and difficult to control. The use of high dose pancreatin capsules (Creon) markedly improves symptoms, although they may not entirely normalise stool fat excretion.[71] In patients with chronic pancreatitis, progression of the disease partly accounts for the long-term exocrine and endocrine insufficiency.

Evolution of specialist centres and the volume — mortality effect

The development of high volume specialist centres is probably the main reason for the reduction in perioperative mortality during the last decade. The evidence base around specialist units has grown substantially and now clearly shows a reduced postoperative mortality that is a continuous effect, with no threshold, unaffected by case mix and only a possible single surgeon effect, reduced postoperative morbidity, reduced postoperative length of stay and cost, an increased resection rate, and probable increased long-term survival. Numerous studies from Europe and the USA have demonstrated a clear correlation between caseload and surgical mortality (Table 3).[47,53,72–82] A survey of 2.5 million complex surgical procedures in the USA showed a large inverse relationship between the hospital volume and case mortality rates for pancreatic resection.[83] As a result of these studies the UK National Health Service Executive has instructed regional health providers to concentrate pancreatic surgery into dedicated cancer centres that will serve an adult population of 2–4 million.[84,85] It is expected that health care authorities throughout the western world will adopt this approach.

DIAGNOSIS AND MANAGEMENT OF COMPLICATIONS FOLLOWING PANCREATIC NECROSECTOMY

The indications for surgery for severe acute necrotising pancreatitis have been defined (Table 4).[86,87] Several surgical techniques[88–104] have been described to manage this condition, but are associated with a significant morbidity and mortality. Within the literature mortality is well documented and although isolated series[89,91,96] have reported extremely low mortalities (6–12%) these have not been widely reproduced. In the largest reported series[99] of 340 patients the mortality rate was 39%. The overall morbidity varies between 32–88%.[94,95,103,105,106] Most series (Table 5) include direct complications from the surgical procedure such as bleeding and fistulae but those associated with the disease process or long-term outcome are less commonly reported.

Table 3. Hospital Mortality Following Resection for Pancreatic Cancer: Comparison of High vs. Low Volume Hospitals

Series: author and Ref. no.	Year	Region	Period	No. of institutions	No. of resections	Mortality % (high volume hospitals)	Mortality % (low volume hospitals)
Studies from the USA							
1. Lieberman et al.[72]	1995	New York	1984–1991	184	1972	5.5	11.8–18.9
2. Janes et al.[75]	1996	USA	1983–1990	978	2263	4.2	7.7
3. Gordon et al.[76]	1995	Maryland	1988–1993	39	501	2.2	13–19.1
4. Glasgow et al.[80]	1996	California	1990–1994	298	1705	3.5	6.9–14.1
5. Gordon et al.[79]	1998	Maryland	1984–1995	43	1093	1.8	14.2
6. Begg et al.[78]	1998	USA	1984–1993		742	5.8	12.9
7. Birkmeyer et al.[73]	1999	USA	1992–1995	1246	7229	4.1	12.7–16.1
Studies from Europe							
8. Neoptolemos et al.[77]; Bramhall et al.[81]	1997	UK; West Midlands, UK	1976–1996	21; 28	1026; 421	5.9	8.3–27.6
9. Nordback[74]	2002	Finland	1990–1994	33	350	4	13
10. Gouma et al.[53]	2000	Netherlands	1994–1998		1126	1	16
11. NYCRIS[82]	2000	Yorkshire, UK	1986–1994	17	130	7.8	21

Table 4.   Indications for Surgery in Acute Necrotising Pancreatitis

The presence of infected pancreatic necrosis as demonstrated by CE-CT (extra- intestinal gas) or FNABF culture.

In patients with greater than 50% pancreatic necrosis, irreversible clinical deterioration despite maximum supportive care for at least two weeks from the onset of symptoms or suspicion of infected pancreatic necrosis in the absence of positive CE-CT or FNABF.

In those with extensive (>50%) pancreatic necrosis and a prolonged illness or continuing symptoms (abdominal pain, vomiting and inability to eat) despite resolution of distant organ dysfunction.

CE-CT = Contrast enhanced computed tomography
FNABF = Fine needle aspiration and bacteriological and fungal culture

In the Royal Liverpool University Hospital Regional Pancreas Centre's experience of 80 necrosectomies comprising 40 minimally invasive retroperitoneal pancreatic necrosectomy (MIRP) and 40 open necrosectomies (OPN) between 1997–2003, 76 patients developed a complication due to their disease process or surgery. The complications associated with necrosectomy are shown in Table 6. In the following sections, complications associated with pancreatic necrosectomy and the diagnosis and management strategies involved in successful treatment will be reviewed.

Organ Dysfunction

In the first 14 days of the illness multi-organ dysfunction is a common occurrence in those with severe acute pancreatitis. Following this, the persistence of organ dysfunction is usually due to either extensive or infected pancreatic necrosis. Patients who require surgery for their underlying necrosis are subjected to a further insult that can result in a profound deterioration in their clinical state. The incidence of postoperative organ dysfunction purely due to surgical intervention is not well described as a significant number of patients have pre-existing organ dysfunction. Within the literature, the rates vary between 8–38%.[88,89,91–98,103,105,107] Increasing postoperative organ dysfunction scores have been shown to be associated with an increased mortality[27] indicating the seriousness of this complication.[108] Beattie *et al.* reported a significant deterioration in postoperative organ dysfunction scores following open necrosectomy.[88] Mier *et al.* performed a randomised controlled trial

Table 5. Reported Morbidity Following Pancreatic Necrosectomy

Author (Ref.)	Year	No. of patients	Surgical technique	Post-op. technique	Haemorrhage	Delayed necrosis/collections requiring further intervention	Enteric fistulae	Panc fistulae	Colonic necrosis	Post-op organ dysfunction	Cardio-vascular	Thrombo-embolic	Biliary stricture	Endocrine insufficiency	Exocrine insufficiency	Incisional hernia	Pseudo-cyst	Overall morbidity
Gotzinger[99]	2002	340	TPD+/–R, RD	DC	75/340 (22%)	196/340 (57%)	56/340 (17%)	20/340 (6%)										
Sarr[103]	1991	23	TPD,O,RD	DC	6/23 (26%)	2/23 (4%)	10/23 (43%)	6/23 (26%)	2/23 (9%)	3/23 (13%)		1/23 (4%)		3/23 (13%)	6/23 (26%)		2/23 (9%)	52%
Branum[91]	1998	50	TPD,O,RD	L		6/23 (26%)	16%	32/44 (72%)		22%	1/23 (4%)		1/23 (4%)	7/30 (40%)	7/23 (30%)	2/23 (9%)	6/23 (26%)	
Fugger[97]	1991	102	TPD,O,RD		22/102 (22%)	6/23 (26%)	30/102 (29%)			32/102 (31%)	2/102 (2%)	4/102 (4%)						
Bradley[90]	1993	71	TPD,O, RD	DC,L	5/71 (7%)	3/71(4%)	5/71 (7%)	33/71 (46%)								23/61 (38%)	1/61 (2%)	
Ho[117]	1995	136	TPD+/–O	SD			25/136 (18%)	21/136 (15%)	1/136 (1%)								30/136 (22%)	51%
Tsiotos[104]	1998	75	TPD, RD	SD	13/72 (18%)	9/54 (17%)	19/72 (26%)	14/72 (19%)	2/72 (3%)								1/54 (2%)	
Fernadez-del Castillo[96]	1998	64	TPD	SD	2/64 (3%)	22/64 (31%)	10/64 (16%)	34/64 (53%)		5/64 (8%)	1/64 (2%)	1/64 (2%)		6/64 (9%)	16/64 (25%)			
Gambiez[98]	1998	9	TPD	SD,L	1/9 (11%)	5/9 (56%)				3/9 (33%)				3/6 (50%)		2/6 (33%)	2/6 (33%)	
Ashley[110]	2001	36	TPD	SD,L		12%	9%	9%				1/36 (3%)		15% (includes exocrine insufficiency)				
Beger[89]	1988	74	TPD	L	1/61 (2%)	15/74 (20%)	1/74 (1%)	7/74 (9%)		6/32 (19%)								
Beger[107]	1988	95	TPD	L	1/95 (1%)	24/95 (25%)	1/95 (1%)	10/95 (11%)		16/95 (17%)								
Beger[112]	1999	221	TPD	L	3 (1%)	93 (42%)	9 (4%)	10 (5%)										

Table 5.   (*Continued*)

Author (Ref.)	Year	No. of patients	Surgical technique	Post-op technique	Haemorrhage	Delayed necrosis/collections requiring further intervention	Enteric fistulae	Panc fistulae	Colonic necrosis	Post-op organ dysfunction	Cardiovascular	Thrombo-embolic	Biliary stricture	Endocrine insufficiency	Exocrine insufficiency	Incisional hernia	Pseudocyst	Overall morbidity
Büchler[92]	2000	27	TP;D	L	1/27 (4%)			3/27 (11%)		4/27 (15%)	2/27 (8%)						1/27 (4%)	
Rau[111]	1995	107	TP;D	L	2/107 (2%)	39%	28/107 (26%)											
Beattie[88]	2002	54	TP;D	L	4/54 (7%)	20/54 (37%)	2/54 (4%)			11/54 (20%)	2/54 (4%)			9/31 (29%)	7/31 (23%)		4/31 (13%)	
Hungness[106]	2002	25	TP;D															32%
Castellanos[105]	2002	15	RP;D	L, RP			2/15 (13%)	1/15 (7%)		4/15 (27%)				1/15 (7%)	1/15 (7%)			40%
Faginez[95]	1989	40	RP;D	L,SD	9/40 (23%)		9/40 (23%)	1/40 (3%)	3/40 (8%)	15/40 (38%)		2/40 (5%)		2/40 (5%)		9/40 (45%)		50%
Van Vyve[143]	1992	20	RP;D,O	L	1/20 (5%)	7/20 (35%)	3/20 (15%)		1/20 (5%)					4/16 (25%)				
Lasko[100]	2003	34	PD	L		8/34 (24%)		1/34 (3%)										
Gambiez[98]	1998	20	MIRP	L	3/20 (15%)	4/20 (20%)	2/20 (10%)	2/20 (10%)						3/18 (17%)		2/18 (11%)	2/18 (11%)	
Horvath[116]	2001	6	MIRP	L	0/6 (0%)	4/6 (67%)	1/6 (17%)									1/6 (17%)		
Connor[94]	2003	24	MIRP	L,RP	2/24 (8%)	6/24 (24%)	2/24 (8%)	4/24 (16%)		6/24 (25%)	1/24 (4%)	2/24 (8%)	1/24 (4%)				1/24 (4%)	88%
Carter[93]	2001	10	MIRP	L,RP	1/10 (10%)	1/10 (10%)	1/10 (10%)			2/10 (20%)							2/10 (20%)	

TP = Transperitoneal, D = Debridement, O = Open Wound/Laparostomy, RD = Planned/Demand Repeat Debridement, R = Resection, RP = Retroperitoneal, MIRP = Minimally Invasive Retroperitoneal Necrosectomy, PD = Percutaneous Drainage, DC = Delayed Closure, L = Lavage, SD = Simple Drainage, RP = Repeat Retroperitoneoscopy.

comparing early (48–72 h) versus late surgery (>12 days) in those with severe necrotising pancreatitis.[109] This trial was stopped due to the 3–4 fold increased risk of death in the early surgery group. Within those undergoing early surgery (14 patients), four developed cardiovascular collapse perioperatively.

Although in the last 20 years significant improvement has been made in caring for the critically ill, the only treatment for multi-organ dysfunction remains supportive. Therefore correct timing and the nature of the surgery are crucial in minimising the development of this lethal complication. Carter *et al.* developed a minimally invasive technique to try and reduce the impact of surgery on severely ill patients.[93] The RLUH-Academic Unit adopted this technique as their first choice treatment for patients requiring necrosectomy and recently published their initial results.[94] There was no difference in preoperative prognostic factors or mortality between those undergoing MIRP versus OPN. In the current cohort of 80 patients, 46 did not have organ failure prior to surgery. Of these 46 patients, 12 (OPN–9, MIRP–3) developed postoperative organ failure, 31 (OPN–9, MIRP–22) did not, and in three cases it was unknown ($p = 0.006$, Table 6). These results need to be confirmed by randomised data but it does give some hope that by optimising the type of surgery, the development of postoperative organ failure can reduced.

Bleeding

This is a life threatening complication following pancreatic necrosectomy and can occur perioperatively or at a delayed stage distant to the initial surgical procedure. It can be due to a number of causes and sources. During necrosectomy the involved tissue is friable and surrounds a number of significant vessels. To help minimise torrential intraoperative bleeding a number of points should be adhered to. It is important to proceed with great caution, avoiding sharp dissection and using blunt finger dissection instead, and only removing mature necrotic tissue. It is not imperative to remove every piece of necrotic tissue and anything adherent should be left to demarcate; most authors do not advocate a formal resection of the pancreas.[88–92,96–98,103,104,106,107,110,111] Targeted laparotomies based on up to date contrast-enhanced CT scans should be performed to avoid excessive, unnecessary and potentially dangerous mobilisation (including Kocherisation of the duodenum). At the end of the procedure careful placement of drains (avoiding direct contact with major vessels) will help

Table 6. Post-necrosectomy Complications, Academic
Surgical Unit-RLUH, 1997–2003 (n = 80)

Complication	Number
Postoperative organ failure	12/47
Haemorrhage	8
GI fistula	3
Pancreatic fistula	5
Colonic necrosis	2
Delayed collections	6
Thromboembolic	4
Cardiovascular/respiratory/cerebrovascular	10
Portal/splenic vein complication	7
Biliary stricture	4
Duodenal ulcer/oesophageal stricture	3
Clostridium difficile colitis	4
Miscellaneous	2
Endocrine insufficiency	19
Exocrine insufficiency	14
Pseudocyst formation	5

prevent erosion into them. In the event of uncontrollable bleeding which cannot be rectified with local suture control, abdominal packing can be performed and the patient returned to the operating theatre once they are stabilised. In such a situation, an angiogram may be helpful with a view to embolisation if the source can be ascertained.

Minimally invasive procedures can also result in intraoperative bleeding. In this case it can be due to shear forces from the dilatation of the tract or over-vigorous debridement of the cavity wall while trying to remove the necrosis.[93] The best approach is to proceed to the angiography suite where identification and embolisation of the bleeding source can be performed (Image 3). It is therefore important to have a multi-disciplinary team available while performing these procedures. Proceeding straight to the laparotomy is a formidable task in this situation, as the source will not be readily visible from the peritoneal cavity.

Delayed or secondary haemorrhage can be due to erosion of the drains into major vessels or rupture of the pseudo-aneurysm formed by the disease

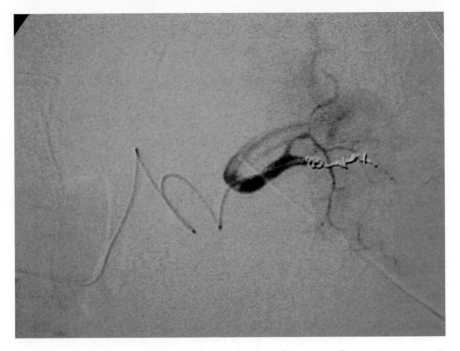

Image 3. Embolisation of bleeding splenic artery after minimally invasive pancreatic necrosectomy.

process. In conjunction with resuscitation, the first investigation will depend on the clinical presentation.

If there is evidence of upper gastrointestinal bleeding, the first investigation should be an upper gastrointestinal endoscopy. If the patient is clinically unstable without evidence of gastrointestinal bleeding or the endoscopy is negative, selective mesenteric angiography in the hope of proceeding to embolisation is the investigation of choice. In the event of portal venous bleeding, embolisation may not be possible and surgical intervention is usually necessary. In those with delayed bleeding it is important to exclude a persistent intra-abdominal sepsis as the underlying precipitant. Reassessment of the disease process with a CT scan is indicated once the patient is stabilised.

In the larger studies the incidence of bleeding ranges between 1–23%.[88,90,95–97,99,104,111,112] Within these studies, various surgical techniques are used. This factor, combined with the heterogeneous nature of necrotising pancreatitis make direct inter-study comparison difficult, but certain observations can be made. The largest series by Gotzinger *et al.* had one of the highest rates of haemorrhage and they are among the few authors who describe formal resection during necrosectomy.[99] Secondly, the major series advocating either laparostomies or repeat laparotomies[97,99,104] have reported rates of haemorrhage between 18–22%, compared to 1–7% for those advocating direct closure with postoperative drainage/lavage.[88,96,111,112] The incidence of postoperative bleeding using an open and minimally invasive retroperitoneal approach is only available from smaller studies but Faginez *et al.*[95] reported an incidence of 23%.

Only a few studies have looked at the effect of postoperative haemorrhage on mortality. Tsiotos *et al.*[104] reported postoperative haemorrhage in 13 (18%) patients. This involved a combination of portal venous and arterial bleeding. Angiography was successful only in one patient. Although there was no direct mortality attributed to haemorrhage, 54% of these patients did not survive and a multivariate analysis revealed that postoperative haemorrhage was an independent prognostic factor. A significant association with gastrointestinal fistula and bleeding (69% of patients who bled developed a fistula) led the authors to conclude that those patients who bleed have a more loco-regionally aggressive form of the disease leading to erosion of adjacent hollow viscera/vessels.

Despite bleeding being a common complication following pancreatic necrosectomy there is relatively little dedicated to its diagnosis and treatment within the literature. Beattie *et al.*[113] describes 10 patients with acute pancreatitis who developed life-threatening bleeding and required an angiography; of these, eight patients had undergone necrosectomy. Three patients suffered from active arterial bleeding, one from venous bleeding secondary to sinustral portal hypertension, one with extensive vasculitis and no bleeding point was found in three. The median time to haemorrhage following surgery was 14 days. Five of the eight patients underwent embolisation with only one case of re-bleeding, and none required open surgery. The mortality in this post-necrosectomy group was 50%.

Local experience (RLUH-Academic Unit) was similar with eight major postoperative bleeds and 50% mortality. Two patients bled from pseudoaneurysms, one of which was successfully embolised; a bleeding point in the other could not be found despite multiple angiograms and the patient eventually underwent a colectomy where a pseudoaneurysm of the transverse colon was found associated with a colo-pancreatic fistula. Both the patients survived. Four patients died after developing delayed bleeding into their pancreatic drains. In three cases, no intervention was undertaken due to co-existing overwhelming multi-organ failure. One patient underwent a laparotomy and although the bleeding from the portal vein (due to erosion of the necrosis into the vein) was staunched, the patient succumbed to ongoing multi-organ failure. Yet another patient developed intraoperative bleeding during the MIRP due to the shearing force of the dilatation, which was successfully embolised; the patient survived.

Fistulae

Fistulae development following necrosectomy can be gastrointestinal or pancreatic in origin.

Gastrointestinal fistulae

The aetiology of gastrointestinal fistulae (Image 4) can be due local erosion by the disease process into adjacent viscera (particularly the transverse and left colon), an iatrogenic cause from surgical intervention, or erosion of drains into adjacent viscera. The necrotising process releases numerous toxic enzymes, which can result in surrounding thrombosis of the mesocolic vessels.[114] This, combined with a low perfusion state due to the systemic inflammatory response associated with pancreatitis can lead to areas of ischaemia within the transverse colon and ultimately fistulation or extensive colonic necrosis.[114,115]

The incidence of fistula ranges from 1–43%[88–91,93–97,99,103–105,107, 110–112,116] The incidence in the major series of laparostomies or repeated laparotomies was between 41–75% while the incidence in studies using a closed approach and postoperative lavage was 15–26% (Table 5). Faginez *et al.* report a series of 40 patients treated with a retroperitoneal approach of whom nine developed a gastrointestinal fistula[95]; eight were colonic in origin and one patient developed a gastric fistula. The authors noted that these were due to repeated surgical procedures and inadequate mobilisation of the left colonic ligaments and all the fistulae occurred early in their experience. Using MIRP, only two (8%) colonic fistulae were seen in 24 patients, of which one was present prior to surgical intervention.[94]

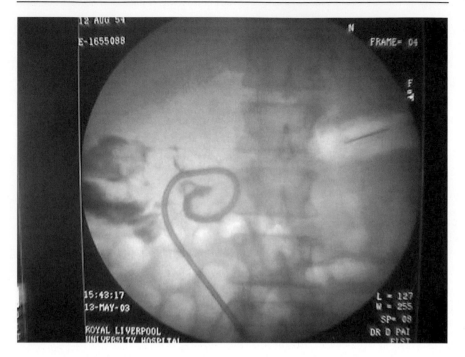

Image 4.   Duodenal fistula after pancreatic necrosectomy.

The clinical diagnosis of gastrointestinal fistulae is made by the persistent abnormal communication between gastrointestinal viscera and cutaneous surface, usually a drainage tract or wound. The patients treated by continuous lavage to the pancreatic bed who develop a fistula may notice profuse watery diarrhoea that ceases with the lavage fluid. Further imaging is required to identify the anatomy and origin of the underlying fistula. This involves proximal or distal (or both) contrast studies depending on the suspicion of fistulograms. Given the association of haemorrhage and gastrointestinal fistula in acute necrotising pancreatitis[104] the development of gastrointestinal bleeding with or without corresponding bleeding from the pancreatic drains should raise the possibility of an underlying fistula.

The usual management guidelines of gastrointestinal fistulae will apply, including protection of the surrounding skin, search for persisting un-drained sepsis and attention to fluid balance and nutrition. The main management issues revolve around the use of enteral nutrition, somatostatin analogues, whether proximal diversion is required and when to perform a definitive surgical procedure. Ho *et al.*[117] reported on 23 (18.4%) patients (with 25 fistulae) from 136 who presented with severe acute pancreatitis and developed gastrointestinal fistulae. The surgical technique for treating the pancreatic necrosis was transperitoneal with simple drainage, and in those with incomplete necrosectomy the abdomen was packed and three gastric fistulae developed along with five duodenal, five jejunal and 12 colonic fistulae. Of these, 39% were reported as present prior to surgical intervention and more likely to have occurred in those with extensive disease: 64% in those with infected necrosis versus 4% in those with sterile necrosis or peripancreatic collections. There was no significant difference in the fistulae rates between those who underwent open packing and those with primary closure of their abdomen. For upper intestinal fistulae the authors recommended a trial of conservative treatment based on a 54% spontaneous resolution rate. The techniques used for surgical intervention included direct repair of gastric fistulae and pyloric exclusion of duodenal fistulae while jejunal fistulae were excised. Colonic fistulae were managed by immediate proximal diversion because spontaneous healing was not reported successfully although no data were provided on the duration of conservative management. The overall mortality rate in this group of patients was 13%, which was not significantly different from those without fistulae in the same study. Similar findings were reported by Tsiotos *et al.*[104] in 19 patients with gastrointestinal fistula. While upper gastrointestinal fistulae healed spontaneously (68%) and did not influence the overall outcome, colonic fistulae were associated with a higher mortality and rarely closed without operative intervention, with six of seven patients requiring intervention.

Although it has been shown that a significant number of the fistulae occur prior to surgery, some are iatrogenic due to repeated trauma associated with ongoing debridement or contact with drains. Bradley, who advocated open management of the abdomen with repeat debridement, reported one of the lowest rates of fistulae post-surgery and describes the use of non-adherent dressings to protect the exposed viscera, which must be carefully removed to avoid unnecessary trauma.[90] Fistulae can also be created by inappropriate decision making with regard to the management of collections in acute pancreatitis.[90,117] Acute fluid collections may be misdiagnosed as "mature pseudocysts" and attempts to perform cyst-enterostomies either percutaneously or operatively result in the conversion of sterile pancreatic necrosis into infected pancreatic necrosis leading to the increased mortality. Although there have been reports of district general hospitals[118] achieving outcomes similar to tertiary referral centres, it is paramount that those involved in the decision making and subsequent management of these patients have a strong interest and clear understanding of the disease process and experience in treating this otherwise fatal disease.

The data regarding the use of somatostatin analogues in the management of gastrointestinal fistulae are contradictory and under-powered. A recent review of the available literature[119] concluded that these analogues may reduce closure time but do not increase the proportion of spontaneous closure. Somatostatin-14 seems to have more potential than octreotide but is difficult to administer and requires a continuous infusion. Further studies are required before definite conclusions can be made.

The use of enteral nutrition in fistulae management is also debatable. Traditionally, TPN has been the standard as it was known to reduce mortality, and increase the rate of spontaneous closure to 60%.[120] In contrast TPN was associated with an increase in systemic morbidity and cost.[121–123] The recent views support the use of enteral feeding in the management of gastrointestinal fistulae as long as the majority of the nutrients are not expelled through the fistula opening.[124] This is often possible by using semi-elemental feeds or feeding distal to the fistula. If the output of the fistula exceeds 10% of the baseline on the commencement of enteral feeding, TPN is recommended.

Pancreatic fistula

The definition used for a pancreatic fistula here is the persistent communication between the pancreatic ductal system and a cutaneous site with the associated discharge of amylase rich fluid. The underlying aetiology is pancreatic duct disruption and may involve the main pancreatic duct or a side branch with a more proximal stricture. In those with severe acute pancreatitis, main pancreatic duct disruption is more likely to have occurred in those requiring surgical intervention.[125,126] Its incidence of following severe acute pancreatitis associated with extensive necrosis is 37–44%.[125,127] Pancreatic duct disruption is also more likely in those who present with pancreatic necrosis and peripancreatic fluid collections.[117,127]

The use of drains post-necrosectomy is universal leading to the possibility of a controlled pancreatic fistula in the event of pancreatic duct disruption.

In fact, one of the goals of the surgery is to minimise the contamination of surrounding spaces and viscera with toxic pancreatic enzymes. It is therefore surprising that there is such a variation in the incidence of pancreatic fistula following necrosectomy (3–72%).[89–92,94–96,98–100,103–105,107,110,112,117] The reasons for this may be multi-factorial but includes heterogeneity between studies with regard to disease severity, the definition of pancreatic fistula, and the duration and volume of fluid. This is highlighted by Branum *et al.*[91] who described 32 of 44 patients being discharged with an elevated amylase in their drain fluid with only one requiring surgery for a non-healing pancreatic cutaneous fistula, eight months post-discharge. An elevated amylase in the cutaneous discharge confirms the diagnosis of pancreatic fistula and when combined with persistent pain suggests a proximal obstruction within the pancreatic duct. With respect to the duration, it is the policy of the RLUH-Regional Pancreas Centre to classify pancreatic fistula in those with a persistent drainage once the drains have been removed.

Radiological imaging is required to determine the nature and cause of the underlying problem. This can be done either by endoscopic retrograde pancreatography (ERCP) or a retrograde fistulogram.[127] Ho *et al.*[117] reported on 21 patients who developed a pancreatic fistula following necrosectomy; six closed spontaneously with a median time of 10 months but two patients developed pseudocysts requiring surgical intervention giving an overall spontaneous resolution rate of 19%. In contrast, several studies[96,104,128] have reported high rates (64–95%) of spontaneous closure. Fielding *et al.*[128] noted that those closing spontaneously (11/15) were low output (<200 ml/day) while the fistulae requiring surgical intervention (4/15) were all high output.

If not adequately managed, uncontrolled pancreatic fistula can quickly result in overwhelming organ failure and death.[129] However, the development of pancreatic fistula has not been associated with an increased mortality.[104] The aim of any fistula management is to achieve closure in the shortest period of time thus limiting the effect on patients' quality of life. The use of TPN and somatostatin analogues are known to speed up closure time by reducing the pancreatic exocrine secretion and are recommended as first line treatment.[130–132] The disadvantages associated with TPN have already been mentioned and unless used properly, somatostatin can result in rebound hypersecretion of pancreatic enzymes between doses.[119] In addition TPN and somatostatin do not seem effective when there is anatomical disruption.[133]

The rate of spontaneous resolution of pancreatic fistula post-necrosectomy is highly variable.[96,104,110,128] It is therefore sensible to try and identify those patients who are likely to require intervention early. The relationship of pancreatic ductal anatomy to the natural history of post-necrosectomy pancreatic fistula has not been extensively studied but certain parallels can be made with patients who develop post-traumatic pancreatic fistula. Wind *et al.*[134] described their experience with 37 patients with pancreatic trauma including 14 with pancreatic fistulae and a pancreatic ductal injury. Seven patients showed a persistent fistula despite conservative treatment, requiring a distal pancreatectomy. In the remaining seven patients whose fistulae healed spontaneously, three developed pseudocysts requiring intervention, one developed recurrent pancreatic pain requiring resection and three patients recovered without further problems. Two of the three that recovered had only a partial injury to the main pancreatic duct. Thus, from the fistulae in 14 patients only one healed spontaneously without further complication. In contrast, four out of 12 patients without main pancreatic duct injury developed pancreatic fistulae; three resolved spontaneously without further complication, while one developed persistent pain requiring surgical intervention.

The available data suggest that those with pancreatic fistulae in the presence of pancreatic ductal disruption are unlikely to heal spontaneously or respond to TPN and somatostatin analogues. However, patients recovering from a necrosectomy are not suitable for immediate further surgery. The optimal treatment for these patients is endoscopic stenting of the pancreatic ductal abnormality.[133] If the problem persists, further surgical intervention can be considered when they have fully recovered and the inflammatory process has long settled (12 months or more). The choice of surgical procedure will be dependant on the location of the ductal disruption; if it is in the body or tail, a distal pancreatectomy can be performed, and a pancreatico-jejunostomy if the disruption is from the head of the pancreas.[128] A flow chart for the management of pancreatic fistulae (Fig. 1) is provided based on the current available evidence.

Pseudocyst

The definition of a pseudocyst is a localised collection of fluid in the region of the pancreas, which is walled off by a membrane of collagen and granulation

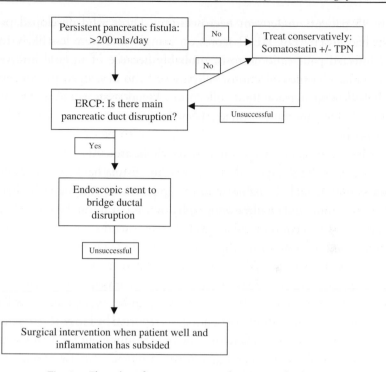

Fig. 1.   Flow chart for management of pancreatic fistulae.

tissue.[135] There may be a communication with the pancreatic ductal system but pus or necrosis is not usually found.[136] This definition has been further subdivided into acute pseudocyst (arising as a consequence of acute pancreatitis, requiring at least four weeks to form and devoid of solid debris) and chronic pseudocyst (arising as a consequence of chronic pancreatitis). The focus of the following section will be on the management of acute pseudocysts.

The incidence following necrosectomy in the major series may be as low as 1–2%[90,104] or as high as 22%.[91,117] The pathogenesis is due to pancreatic parenchymal necrosis involving the ductal system allowing leakage of pancreatic juice.[117,126]

Initially this forms as an acute fluid collection, of which 50–70% will resorb spontaneously but persists in the presence of a major duct disruption or a proximal obstruction. With time these will develop into pancreatic ascites, pseudocyst or pancreatic fistula. Ho *et al.*[117] reported 30/136 (26%) patients who developed pseudocysts following severe acute pancreatitis but only 95 patients underwent necrosectomy. Those who developed pseudocysts had lower APACHE II scores on transfer and were less likely to have had infected pancreatic necrosis, probably because of surgical intervention and drainage of the collections. All patients who developed pseudocysts initially had peripancreatic fluid collections. Pseudocysts can also form following closure of pancreatic fistulae especially if there is a more proximal ductal obstruction.

Clinical suspicion of a pseudocyst should be aroused if there is early satiety or epigastric fullness especially if a pancreatic fistula has recently resolved. A fullness may actually be palpable in the epigastrium. Alternatively there may be no symptoms and an ultrasonography or a CT scan can be the only way to diagnose it. On a contrast-enhanced CT scan, pseudocysts appear as a round or oval fluid collection with either a thin wall (which can be barely perceptible) or a thick wall showing evidence of contrast enhancement.[137] The assessment should include associated local complications. Its subsequent management will depend on a number of factors. A significant number of pseudocysts will resorb spontaneously; in a study of 30 pseudocysts reported by Ho *et al.*, 17% resolved without intervention.[117] Therefore, the only requirement for pseudocysts that are asymptomatic, not enlarging, < 5 cm in diameter and without contrast-enhanced CT evidence of local complications (biliary, duodenal or venous compression) is observation.[137–139]

In patients with pseudocysts that require intervention, the options include endoscopic, percutaneous or surgical approaches. A contrast-enhanced CT scan and high resolution pancreatogram such as magnetic resonance pancreatography, ERCP are required to decide on the best approach.[139] If endoscopic intervention is planned, an endoscopic ultrasound can be a useful adjunct to identify potential complications prior to attempted endoscopic drainage.[139] Sixty-three percent of the pseudocysts will communicate with the main pancreatic duct,[140] implying that trans-papillary drainage by pancreatic stents across strictures can be deployed with excellent results.[133] It is important that the stents are removed six weeks following the resolution of the pseudocyst to avoid chronic ductal changes. If no communication is seen or there is close communication of the pseudocyst with a visceral wall with the absence of intervening vessels (particularly collaterals due to splenic vein thrombosis) trans-mural drainage can be performed. Baron *et al.*[140] reported endoscopic success rates of 74% for acute pseudocysts and 92% for chronic pseudocysts with complication and recurrence rates of 17–19% and 9–12% respectively. Follow up in the form of a contrast-enhanced CT scan is important after 3–6 weeks.

If a percutaneous approach is preferred, the trans-gastric route may be undertaken to minimise the risk of creating an external pancreatic fistula. Success rates for percutaneous drainage of pseudocysts are 76–100%.[138] If there is no communication with the main pancreatic duct, the mean time for resolution is 14–21 days, compared with 5–6 weeks if there is communication.[138] However, surgical intervention by pseudocyst-enterostomy will be required for those with vascular complications to avoid catastrophic bleeding.[139] Although laparoscopic techniques have been described post-pancreatic necrosectomy patients are unlikely to be suitable candidates. In the management of post-pancreatitis pseudocysts, the correct interpretation and decision-making of cystic collections of the contrast-enhanced CT scan is very important. Attempted enteric drainage of acute fluid collections and organised pancreatic necrosis is likely to result in severe retroperitoneal sepsis.

Delayed Necrosis and Distant Collections

One of the most common complications following necrosectomy has been residual necrosis or delayed distant collections. The initial approach of a single laparotomy and simple drainage were associated with high mortality rates due to persistent sepsis and multi-organ failure. The subsequent use of laparostomies, repeat debridement and postoperative lavage of the retroperitoneum have improved the outcome but a high morbidity has remained (Table 2). Retroperitoneal and minimally invasive techniques have also been described in an effort to reduce the associated complications. Unfortunately there have been no randomised controlled trials for surgical technique to confirm the use of one over another and no one technique has achieved the status of "gold standard".

All major series[99,111,112] have a significant incidence of re-intervention (repeat laparotomies or percutaneous intervention) ranging between 39–57%. Bradley[90] who advocated an "open abdomen" technique reported a low re-intervention rate of 4%, yet others using a similar technique have reported re-intervention rates of 26%.[91] Following necrosectomy, patients who develop signs of recurrent or persistent sepsis (including persisting multi-organ failure) should have follow-up contrast-enhanced CT scans to determine if there is residual necrosis or undrained collections.

Those with residual necrosis will require further debridement. The management will depend on the initial surgical technique. However, the clearance of this necrosis is a pre-requisite for long-term survival.[99] Using the minimally invasive technique described earlier, the operating scope is simply reintroduced along the drainage tract and the residual necrosis is removed under direct vision.[94] A targeted laparotomy is required if the residual necrosis was not in communication with the main cavity.

In patients with distant fluid-density collections, radiologically guided percutaneous aspiration can be undertaken; the fluid can be sent for microbiological analysis following which the infected collections can be formally drained. The areas containing heterogeneous solid debris are better approached with a targeted laparotomy to establish adequate drainage. Alternatively a percutaneous approach (using large and multiple catheters) with subsequent lavage may be successful but requires significant and dedicated radiological input including frequent catheter changes.[141]

Disease Related Complications Requiring Surgical Intervention

Colonic necrosis

This severe complication occurs in 1–17% of the patients with pancreatic necrosis.[95,103,104,117,142,143] It is associated with a 53% mortality and is an independent prognostic factor in determining the outcome with a 2.5 fold increased risk of death.[142] The underlying aetiology is due to colonic ischaemia, as discussed above.[114,115] The presentation is variable and can be easily missed; it may present with per rectal bleeding, abdominal pain, and increasing multi-organ failure (advanced septic state) or as peritonitis secondary to perforation. Colonic necrosis can be difficult to diagnose in intensive care patients with co-existing multi-organ failure secondary to the pancreatitis, especially if a retroperitoneal or minimally invasive approach has been used. A high index of suspicion should be maintained in those whose condition is deteriorating despite maximal supportive care. In the largest described series of 17 patients with colonic necrosis treated in a tertiary referral centre,[142] the median time to onset was five days and all occurred in the first three weeks of admission. Fifteen of these cases were associated with infected pancreatic necrosis. The factors associated with an increased risk of colonic necrosis were higher APACHE II scores on admission and alcoholic pancreatitis. The treatment of this rapidly fatal condition requires aggressive colonic resection and defunctioning stoma.[144] Simply defunctioning the colon results in a 100% mortality,[144] and a significant number will die within 24 h from fuliminant septic shock.

Portal-splenic-mesenteric vein thrombosis

Thrombosis of the portal venous system is not a direct complication of necrosectomy but an under-recognised complication that can follow severe acute necrotising pancreatitis. In a case note review of 1,268 patients with inflammatory pancreatic conditions,[145] only four were found to have venous complications, the majority of which were associated with chronic pancreatitis; in a series of 80 patients from the RLUH-Regional Pancreas Centre, there were seven patients with portal-splenic thrombosis. It is an important complication to recognise because patients can be very debilitated[146] and the presence of extensive venous collaterals can make subsequent surgery such as cholecystectomy or pseudocyst-jejunostomy more difficult and hazardous.

Relatively little is known about this complication, its natural history and outcome. Studies examining the causes of extra-hepatic portal hypertension that include pancreatitis as a cause, allow for some extrapolation.[147] The presentation of these patients may be with symptomatic ascites, gastrointestinal bleeding, venous infarction or evidence of hypersplenism. A third of the patients may have a second causative factor such as prothrombotic tendency. The natural history of patients with extra-hepatic portal vein thrombosis is related to co-existing medical conditions and the estimated overall five-year survival is 89%.[147] The risk of oesophageal bleeding is significantly lower when compared with cirrhosis patients[148] with an estimated incidence of 12.5% per 100 patients,[149] and an associated risk of death from haemorrhage at 1–25%.[147,149]

The diagnosis can be made by contrast-enhanced CT scan or duplex ultrasound. Contrast-enhanced CT scan offers the advantage of being able to reconstruct the vascular anatomy to assist in planning for any proposed surgical intervention. Because of the difficulty in treating patients who develop symptoms from portal-mesenteric vein thrombosis, there is some controversy on whether any acute intervention should be undertaken on the diagnosis of this condition. Although a number of interventional radiological techniques are feasible[146,150] they need to be undertaken with a low morbidity in patients who are likely to be severely unwell. Given the association with pro-thrombotic disorders and because recanalisation can occur with anticoagulation, formal anticoagulation is recommended.[151] In the long term, meso-caval shunts offer good relief from debilitating symptoms with minimal long term morbidity.[151]

Biliary Strictures

This relatively uncommon complication can occur following acute pancreatitis.[152] The underlying aetiology is likely to be due to intramural fibrosis from bile duct ischemia or extramural fibrosis of the head of the pancreas as the necrosis resolves. Although uncommon, it is an important complication to recognise as it may arise insidiously and is associated with life threatening side effects such as acute cholangitis and secondary biliary cirrhosis. Its presentation may be with a recurrent episode of jaundice and acute cholangitis or a cholestatic picture of the liver function tests. An abdominal ultrasound will reveal a dilated extra-hepatic biliary tree. Further cholangiography is required, preferably in the form of non-invasive imaging (magnetic resonance cholangiography) if the patient is asymptomatic to avoid the introduction of organisms to an obstructed system. If the patient is jaundiced or presents with acute cholangitis, ERCP following ultrasound is the preferred line investigation to allow at least temporary resolution of the biliary obstruction using plastic stents. The differential includes choledolithasis especially if the initial cause of the pancreatitis was cholelithiasis.

The choice of definitive treatment of the stricture, endoscopically or with surgery (choledo-jejunostomy), is based on the patient's underlying fitness for surgery and associated co-morbidity. In a review of the literature[152] for benign biliary strictures the failure rate for those having endoscopic treatment for chronic pancreatitis was high (90%) versus a 3% failure rate in those undergoing surgery. Given that the strictures are likely to involve the distal third of the bile duct and the proven long-term success and low morbidity of choledocho-jejunostomy this would have to be considered as the current "gold standard".

Miscellaneous Complications

There is a high rate of general complications including cardiovascular, cerebrovascular and respiratory complications. It is important to point out that the incidence of thromboembolic complications within this group of patients is 1–8%[94–97,103,110] with the largest study (of 102 patients) reporting a 4% incidence.[97] Despite the risk of haemorrhage it is important that these patients have an aggressive deep venous thrombosis prophylaxis to minimise the incidence of this life threatening complication.

Long-Term Outcome

Many studies have described the in-hospital outcome following necrosectomy but there are relatively few describing long-term outcomes. In a study by Tsiotos *et al.*[153] 44 patients were studied for a median of 48 months, of whom 22 (50%) maintained normal endocrine and exocrine function. Of the 16 (37%) patients who developed endocrine insufficiency, 12 (75%) required insulin; 11 (69%) were diagnosed prior to discharge (these patients had more extensive necrosis) and the remaining five patients developed diabetes mellitus during follow up (median time to onset was two years, range 1–8 years). With time, the endocrine function tended to deteriorate. Eleven (69%) patients developed exocrine insufficiency (clinical steatorrhoea), which responded to pancreatic enzyme supplementation in 9 (81%). Exocrine insufficiency was present in all patients at the time of discharge (it was also associated with more extensive necrosis) and improved (5/11 resolved with time) or remained stable following discharge. Of the 44 patients in this study, 22 were of working age and 17 were able to return to employment. Poor long-term performance was associated with higher APACHE II scores on admission. Recurrent pancreatitis was uncommon (2/44) but seemed to be related to the underlying cause (alcohol induced).

Incisional hernia can also be a major problem with the incidence (9–45%) depending on the surgical technique used (Table 2). As expected it is more common following techniques using secondary closure. Depending on the size of the defect these can be challenging to repair and require complex techniques in as many as 44% of the cases.[153]

REFERENCES

1. Delcore R, Rodriguez FJ, Forster J, *et al.* (1996) Significance of lymph node metastases in patients with pancreatic cancer undergoing curative resection. *Am J Surg* **172**: 463–468.
2. Geer RJ, Brennan MF. (1993) Prognostic indicators for survival after resection of pancreatic adenocarcinoma. *Am J Surg* **165**: 68–72.
3. Richter A, Niedergethmann M, Sturm J, *et al.* (2003) Long-term results of partial pancreaticoduodenectomy for ductal adenocarcinoma of the pancreatic head: 25-year experience. *World J Surg* **27**: 324–329.
4. Yeo CJ, Cameron JL, Lillemoe KD, *et al.* (2002) Pancreaticoduodenectomy with or without distal gastrectomy and extended retroperitoneal lymphadenectomy for periampullary adenocarcinoma, part 2. *Ann Surg* **236**: 355–368.
5. Bassi C, Falconi M, Salvia R, *et al.* (2001) Management of complications after pancreaticoduodenectomy in a high volume centre: results on 150 consecutive patients. *Dig Surg* **18**: 453–457.
6. Buchler M, Friess H, Wagner M, *et al.* (2000) Pancreatic fistula after pancreatic head resection. *Br J Surg* **87**: 883–889.
7. Yeo C, Cameron J, Sohn T, *et al.* (1997) Six hundred and fifty consecutive pancreaticoduodenectomies in the 1990s. *Ann Surg* **226**: 248–260.
8. Balcom JH, Rattner DW, Warshaw AL, *et al.* (2001) Ten-year experience with 733 pancreatic resections: changing indications, older patients, and decreasing length of hospitalization. *Arch Surg* **136**: 391–398.
9. Bottger T, Junginger T. (1999) Factors influencing morbidity and mortality after pancreaticoduodenectomy: critical analysis of 221 resections. *World J Surg* **23**: 164–172.
10. Sarr MG for the Pancreatic Surgery Group. (2003) The potent somatostatin analogue Vapreotide does not decrease pancreas-specific complications after elective pancreatectomy: a prospective, multicentre, double-blinded, randomized, placebo-controlled trial. *J Am Coll Surg* **196**: 556–565.
11. Cullen J, Sarr M, Ilstrup D. (1994) Pancreatic anastomotic leak after pancreatcoduodenectomy: incidence, significance and management. *Am J Surg* **168**: 295–298.
12. Farley D, Schwall G, Trede M. (1996) Completion pancreatectomy for complications after pancreatoduodenectomy. *Br J Surg* **83**: 176–179.
13. Halloran C, Ghaneh P, Bosonnet L, *et al.* (2002) Complications of pancreatic cancer resection. *Dig Surg* **19**: 138–146.
14. Pisters P, Hudec W, Hess K, *et al.* (2001) Effect of preoperative biliary decompresion on pancreaticoduodenectomy-associated morbidity in 300 consecutive patients. *Ann Surg* **234**: 47–55.

15. Sewnath M, Birjmohun R, Rauws E, *et al.* (2001) The effect of preoperative biliary drainage on post operative complications after pancreaticoduodenectomy. *J Am Coll Surg* **192**: 726–734.

16. Sewnath M, Karsten T, Prins M, *et al.* (2002) A meta-analysis of the efficacy of preoperative biliary drainage for tumors causing obstructive jaundice. *Ann Surg* **236**: 17–27.

17. Friess H, Beger H, Sulkowski U, *et al.* (1995) Randomized controlled multicentre study of the prevention of complications by octreotide in patients undergoing surgery for chronic pancreatitis. *Br J Surg* **82**: 1270–1273.

18. Yeo CJ, Cameron JL, Maher MM, *et al.* (1995) A prospective randomized trial of pancreaticogastrostomy versus pancreaticojejunostomy after pancreaticoduodenectomy. *Ann Surg* **222**: 580–588.

19. Buchler M, Friess H, Klempa I, *et al.* (1992) Role of octreotide in the prevention of postoperative complications following pancreatic resection. *Am J Surg* **163**: 125–130.

20. Suzuki Y, Kuroda Y, Morita A, *et al.* (1995) Fibrin glue sealing for the prevention of pancreatic fistulas following distal pancreatectomy. *Arch Surg* **130**: 952–955.

21. Cunningham J, Weyant M, Levitt M, *et al.* (1998) Complications requiring reoperation following pancreatectomy. *Int J Pancreatol* **24**: 23–29.

22. Lowy A, Lee J, Pisters P, *et al.* (1997) Prospective, randomized trial of octreotide to prevent pancreatic fistula after pancreaticoduodenectomy for malignant disease. *Ann Surg* **226**: 632–641.

23. Mediema B, Sarr M, van Heerden J, *et al.* (1992) Complications following pancreaticoduodenectomy. Current management. *Arch Surg* **127**: 945–950.

24. Bakkevold K, Kambestd B. (1993) Morbidity and mortality after radical and palliative pancreatic cancer surgery. Risk factors influencing the short-term results. *Ann Surg* **217**: 356–368.

25. Conlon K, Labow D, Leung D, *et al.* (2001) Prospective randomized clinical trial of the value of intraperitoneal drainage after pancreatic resection. *Ann Surg* **234**: 487–493.

26. Trede M, Schwall G, Saeger H. (1990) Survival after pancreatoduodenectomiy. 118 consecutive resections without an operative mortality. *Ann Surg* **211**: 447–458.

27. van Berge Henegouwen M, de Witt L, van Guilk T, *et al.* (1997) Incidence, risk factors, and treatment of pancreatic leakage after a pancreatoduodenectomy: drainage versus resection of pancreatic remnant. *J Am Coll Surg* **185**: 18–25.

28. Al Sharaf K, Ihse I, Dawiskiba S, Andren-Sandberg A. (1997) Characteristics of the gland remnant predict complications after subtotal pancreatectomy. *Dig Surg* **14**: 101–106.

60. Lin P, Lin Y. (1999) Prospective randomized comparison between pylorus-preserving and standard pancreatoduodenectomy. *Br J Surg* **86**: 603–607.

61. Seiler C, Wagner M, Sadowski C, *et al.* (2000) Randomized prospective trial of pylorus-preserving vs. classic duodenopancreatectomy (Whipple procedure): initial clinical results. *J Gastrointest Surg* **4**: 443–452.

62. Williamson RCN, Bliouras N, Cooper MJ, *et al.* (1993) Gastric emptying and enterogastric reflux after conservative and conventional pancreatoduodenectomy. *Surgery* **114**: 975–979.

63. Zerbi A, Balzano G, Patuzzo R, *et al.* (1995) Comparison between pylorus-preserving and Whipple pancreatoduodenectomy. *Br J Surg* **82**: 975–979.

64. Mosca F, Giulianotti PC, Balestracci T, *et al.* (1997) Long-term survival in pancreatic cancer: pylorus-preserving versus Whipple pancreatoduodenectomy. *Surgery* **122**: 553–566.

65. Pedrazzoli P, DiCarlo V, Dionigi R, *et al.* (1998) Standard versus extended lymphadenectomy associated with pancreaticoduodenectomy in the surgical treatment of adenocarcinoma of the head of the pancreas. Lymphadenectomy Study Group. *Ann Surg* **228**: 508–517.

66. Yeo CJ, Cameron JL, Sohn TA, *et al.* (1999) Pancreaticoduodenectomy with or without extended retroperitoneal lymphadenectomy for periampullary adenocarcinoma: comparison of morbidity and mortality and short-term outcome. *Ann Surg* **229**: 613–622.

67. Nguyen T, Sohn T, Cameron J, *et al.* (2003) Standard vs. radical pancreaticoduodenectomy for periampullary adenocarcinoma: a prospective randomized trial evaluating quality of life in pancreaticoduodenctomy survivors. *J Gastrointest Surg* **7**: 1–11.

68. van Geenen R, van Guilk T, Busch O, *et al.* (2001) Readmissions after pancreatoduodenectomy. *Br J Surg* **88**: 1467–1471.

69. Ahren B, Andren-Sandberg A. (1993) Capacity to secrete islet hormones after subtotal pancreatectomy for pancreatic cancer. *Eur J Surg* **159**: 223–227.

70. Kendall D, Sutherland D, Najarian J, *et al.* (1990) Effects of hemipancreatectomy on insulin secretion and glucose tolerance in healthy humans. *N Engl J Med* **322**: 898–903.

71. Neoptolemos J, Ghaneh P, Andren-Sandberg A, *et al.* (1999) Treatment of pancreatic exocrien insufficiency after pancreatic resection. *Int J Pancreatol* **25**: 171–180.

72. Lieberman M, Kilburn H, Lindsey M, Brennan M. (1995) Relation of perioperative deaths to hospital volume among patients undergoing pancreatic resection for malignancy. *Ann Surg* **222**: 638–645.

73. Birkmeyer J, Warshaw A, Finlayson S, *et al.* (1999) Relationship between hospital volume and late survival after pancreaticoduodenectomy. *Surgery* **126**: 178–183.

74. Nordbank I, Parviainen M, Raty S, *et al.* (2002) Resection of the head of the pancreas in Finland: effects of hospital and surgeon on short-term and long-term results. *Scand J Gastroenterol* **37**: 1454–1460.

75. Janes R, Niederhuber J, Chmiel J, *et al.* (1996) National patterns of care for pancreatic cancer. *Ann Surg* **223**: 261–272.

76. Gordon T, Burleyson G, Tielsch J. (1995) The effects of regionalization on cost and outcome for one general high risk surgical procedure. *Ann Surg* **221**: 43–49.

77. Neoptolemos JP, Russell RC, Bramhall S, *et al.* (1997) Low mortality following resection for pancreatic and periampullary tumours in 1026 patients: UK survey of specialist pancreatic units. UK pancreatic cancer group. *Br J Surg* **84**: 1370–1376.

78. Begg C, Cramer L, Hoskins W, Brennan M. (1998) Impact of hospital volume on operative mortality for major cancer surgery. *JAMA* **280**: 1747–1751.

79. Gordon T, Browman H, Tielsch J, *et al.* (1998) State-wide regionalization of pancreaticoduodenectomy and its effect on in hospital mortality. *Ann Surg* **228**: 71–78.

80. Glasgow R, Mulvihill S. (1996) Hospital volume influences outcome in patients undergoing pancreatic resection for cancer. *West J Med* **165**: 294–300.

81. Bramhall SR, Allum WH, Jones AG, *et al.* (1995) Treatment and survival in 13,560 patients with pancreatic cancer and incidence of the disease. An epidemiological study. *Br J Surg* **82**: 111–115.

82. Key sites study. Pancreas report. NYCRIS. 2000.

83. Birkmeyer JD, Siewers AE, Finlayson EV, *et al.* (2002) Hospital volume and surgical mortality in the United States. *N Engl J Med* **346**: 1128–1137.

84. NHS Executive. (2001) Guidance on Commissioning Cancer Services. Improving outcomes in upper gastro-intestinal cancers. The Manual. Catalogue Number 23180. Department of Health, London.

85. NHS Executive. (2001) Guidance on Commissioning Cancer Services. Improving outcomes in upper gastro-intestinal cancers. The Evidence. Catalogue Number 23943. Department of Health, London.

86. Toouli J, Brooke-Smith M, Bassi C, *et al.* (2002) Guidelines for management of acute pancreatitis. *J Gastroenterol Hepatol* **17**: S17–S39.

87. Uhl W, Warshaw A, Imrie C, *et al.* (2002) IAP guidelines for the surgical management of acute pancreatitis. *Pancreatology* **2**: 565–573.

88. Beattie G, Mason J, Swan D, *et al.* (2002) Outcome of necrosectomy in acute pancreatitis: the case for continued vigilance. *Scand J Gastroenterol* **37**: 1449–1453.

89. Beger H, Buchler M, Bittner R, *et al.* (1988) Necrosectomy and postoperative local lavage in necrotizing pancreatitis. *Br J Surg* **75**: 207–212.

90. Bradley III E. (1993) A fifteen year experience with open drainage for pancreatic necrosis. *Surg Gynecol Obstet* **177**: 215–222.

91. Branum G, Galloway J, Hirchowitz W, *et al.* (1998) Pancreatic necrosis: results of necrosectomy, packing, and ultimate closure over drains. *Ann Surg* **227**: 870–877.

92. Buchler M, Gloor B, Muller C, *et al.* (2002) Acute necrotising pancreatitis: treatment strategy according to status of infection. *Ann Surg* **232**: 619–626.

93. Carter R, McKay C, Imrie C. (2001) Percutaneous necrosectomy and sinus tract endoscopy in management of infected pancreatic necrosis: an initial experience. *Ann Surg* **232**: 175–180.

94. Connor S, Ghaneh P, Raraty M, *et al.* (2003) Minimally invasive retroperitoneal pancreatic necrosectomy. *Dig Surg* **20**: 270–277.

95. Fagniez P, Rotman N, Kracht M. (1989) Direct retroperitoneal approach to necrosis in severe acute pancreatitis. *Br J Surg* **76**: 264–267.

96. Fernandez-del Castillo C, Rattner D, Makary M, *et al.* (1998) Debridement and closed packing for the treatment of necrotizing pancreatitis. *Ann Surg* **228**: 676–684.

97. Fugger R, Schulz F, Rogy M, *et al.* (1991) Open approach in pancreatic and infected pancreatic necrosis: laparostomies and preplanned revisions. *World J Surg* **15**: 516–520.

98. Gambiez L, Denimal F, Porte H, *et al.* (1998) Retroperitoneal approach and endoscopic management of peripancreatic necrosis collections. *Arch Surg* **133**: 66–72.

99. Gotzinger P, Saunter T, Kriwanek S, *et al.* (2002) Surgical treatment for severe acute pancreatitis: extent and surgical control of necrosis determines outcome. *World J Surg* **26**: 474–478.

100. Lasko D, Habib F, Sleeman D, *et al.* (2003) Percutaneous lavage for infected pancreatic necrosis. *J Gastrointest Surg* **7**: 288–289.

101. Orlando R, Welch J, Akbari C, *et al.* (1993) Techniques and complications of open packing of infected pancreatic necrosis. *Surg Gynecol Obstet* **177**: 65–71.

102. Pamoukian V, Gagner M. (2001) Laparoscopic necrosectomy for acute necrotising pancreatitis. *J Hepatobiliary Pancreat Surg* **8**: 221–223.

103. Sarr M, Nagorney D, Mucha P, *et al.* (1991) Acute necrotizing pancreatitis: management by planned, staged pancreatic necrosectomy/debridement and delayed primary wound closure over drains. *Br J Surg* **78**: 576–581.

104. Tsiotos G, Luque-de Leon E, Soreide J, *et al.* (1998) Management of necrotizing pancreatitis by repeated operative necrosectomy using a zipper technique. *Am J Surg* **175**: 91–98.

105. Castellanos G, Pinero A, Serrano A, *et al.* (2002) Infected pancreatic necrosis. *Arch Surg* **137**: 1060–1063.
106. Hungness E, Robb B, Seeskin C, *et al.* (2002) Early debridement for necrostising pancreatitis: is it worthwhile? *J Am Coll Surg* **194**: 740–745.
107. Beger H, Buchler M, Bittner R, *et al.* (1988) Necrosectomy and post operative local lavage in patients with necrostising pancreatitis: results of a prospective clinical trial. *World J Surg* **12**: 255–262.
108. Connor S, Ghaneh P, Raraty M, *et al.* (2003) Increasing age and APACHE II scores are the main determinants of outcome following pancreatic necrosectomy. *Br J Surg* **90**: 1542–1548.
109. Mier J, Luque-de Leon E, Castillo A, *et al.* (1997) Early vs. late necrosectomy in sever necrotising pancreatitis. *Am J Surg* **173**: 71–75.
110. Ashley S, Perez A, *et al.* (2001) Necrotising Pancreatitis. *Ann Surg* **234**: 572–580.
111. Rau B, Pralle U, Uhl W, *et al.* (1995) Management of sterile necrosis in instances of severe acute pancreatitis. *J Am Coll Surg* **181**: 279–288.
112. Beger H, Isenmann R. (1999) Surgical management of necrotising pancreatitis. *Surg Clin North Am* **79**: 783–800.
113. Beattie G, Hardman J, Redhead D, *et al.* (2003) Evidence for a central role for selective mesenteric angiography in the management of major vascular complications of pancreatitis. *Am J Surg* **185**: 96–102.
114. Gardner A, Gardner G, Feller E. (2003) Severe colonic complications of pancreatic disease. *J Clin Gasterenterol* **37**: 258–262.
115. Hotz H, Foitzik T, Rohweder J, *et al.* (1998) Intestinal microcirculation and gut permeability in acute pancreatitis: early changes and therapeutic implications. *J Gastrointest Surg* **2**: 518–525.
116. Hovarth K, Kao L, Wherry K. (2001) A technique for laparoscopic assisted percutaneous drainage of infected pancreatic necrosis and pancreatic abscess. *Surg Endosc* **15**: 1221–1225.
117. Ho H, Frey C. (1995) Gastrointestinal and pancreatic complications associated with severe pancreatitis. *Arch Surg* **130**: 817–823.
118. Catto J, Alexander D. (2002) Pancreatic debridement in a district general hospital: viable or vulnerable. *Ann R Coll Surg Engl* **84**: 309–313.
119. Hesse U, Ysebaert D, de Hemptinne B. (2002) Role of somatostatin 14 and its analogues in the management of gastrointestinal fistulae: clinical data. *Gut* **49**: 11–20.
120. Rose D, Yarbourgh M, Canizaro P, *et al.* (1986) One hundred and fourteen fistulas of the gastrointestinal tract treated with TPN. *Surg Gynecol Obstet* **163**: 345–350.

121. Abou-Assi S, Craig K, O'Keefe S. (2002) Hypocaloric jejunal feeding is better than total parenteral nutrition in acute pancreatitis: results of a randomised comparative study. *Am J Gastroenterol* **97**: 2255–2262.

122. Abou-Assi S, O'Keefe S. (2002) Nutrition support during acute pancreatitis. *Nutrition* **18**: 938–943.

123. Imrie C, Carter R, McKay C. (2002) Enteral and parenteral nutrition in acute pancreatitis. Best practice and research. *Clin Gastroenterol* **16**: 391–397.

124. Ferreyra M. (2002) Enteral or parenteral nutrition for treatment of post-operative gastrointestinal fistulae: a decision making process. *Nutrition* **18**: 196–197.

125. Neoptolemos J, London N, Carr-Locke D. (1993) Assessment of main pancreatic duct integrity by endoscopic retrograde pancreatography in patients with acute pancreatitis. *Br J Surg* **80**: 94–99.

126. Neoptolemos J. (1993) Endoscopic retrograde cholangio-pancreatography in necrotizing pancreatitis. In: Bradley III E (ed), *Acute Pancreatitis: Diagnosis and Therapy*. (Raven Press, New York), pp. 69–76.

127. Lau S, Simchuk E, Kozarek R, *et al.* (2001) A pancreatic ductal leak should be sought to direct treatment in patients with acute pancreatitis. *Am J Surg* **181**: 411–415.

128. Fielding G, McLatchie G, Wilson C, *et al.* (1989) Acute pancreatitis and pancreatic fistula formation. *Br J Surg* **76**: 126–128.

129. Howard T, Wiebke E, Mogavero G, *et al.* (1995) Classification and treatment of local complications in acute pancreatitis. *Am J Surg* **170**: 44–50.

130. Lansden F, Adams D, Anderson M. (1989) Treatment of external pancreatic fistulae with somatostatin. *Am Surg* **55**: 695–698.

131. Torres A, Landa J, Moreno-Azecita M, *et al.* (1992) Somatostatin in the management of gastrointestinal fistulae. A multicentre trial. *Arch Surg* **127**: 97–99.

132. Tulassay Z, Flautner L, Fehervari I. (1992) Octreotide. *Lancet* **339**: 1428.

133. Kozarek R, Ball T, Patterson D, *et al.* (1991) Endoscopic transpapillary therapy for disrupted pancreatic duct and peri–pancreatic fluid collections. *Gastroenterology* **100**: 1362–1370.

134. Wind P, Tiret E, Cunningham C, *et al.* (1999) Contribution of endoscopic retrograde pancreatography in management of complications following distal pancreatic trauma. *Am Surg* **65**: 777–783.

135. Rosso E, Alexakis N, Ghaneh P, *et al.* (2003) Pancreatic pseudocyst in chronic pancreatitis. Endoscopic and surgical treatment. *Dig Surg* **20**: 397–406.

136. Bradley III E. (1993) A clinically based classification system for acute pancreatitis. *Arch Surg* **128**: 586–590.

137. Balthazar E, Freeny P, van Sonnenburg E. (1994) Imaging and intervention in acute pancreatitis. *Radiology* **193**: 297–306.
138. Lee M, Wittich G, Mueller P. (1998) Percutaneous intervention in acute pancreatitis. *Radiographics* **18**: 711–724.
139. Wilson C. (1997) Management of the later complications of severe acute pancreatitis, pseudocyst, abscess and fistula. *Eur J Gastroenterol Hepatol* **9**: 117–121.
140. Baron T, Harewood G, Morgan D, Yates M. (2002) Outcome differences after endoscopic drainage of pancreatic necrosis, acute pancreatic pseudocysts and chronic pancreatic pseudocysts. *Gastrointest Endosc* **56**: 7–17.
141. Freeny P, Hauptmann E, Althaus S, *et al.* (1998) Percutaneous CT-guided catheter drainage of infected acute necrotising pancreatitis: techniques and results. *Am J Roentgenol* **170**: 969–975.
142. Kriwanek S, Gschwantler M, Beckerhinn P, *et al.* (1999) Complications after surgery for necrotising pancreatitis: risk factors and prognosis. *Eur J Surg* **165**: 952–957.
143. Van Vyve L, Reynaert M, Lengele B, *et al.* (1992) Retroperitoneal laparostomy: a surgical treatment of pancreatic abscess after acute necrotising pancreatitis. *Surgery* **111**: 369–375.
144. Kriwanek S, Armbuster C, Beckerhinn P, *et al.* (1997) Improved results after aggressive treatment of colonic involvement in necrotising pancreatitis. *Hepato-gastroenterology* **44**: 274–278.
145. Nordback I, Sisto T. (1989) Peripancreatic vascular occlusions as a complication of pancreatitis. *Int Surg* **74**: 36–39.
146. Maleux G, Vaninbroukx J, Verslype C, *et al.* (2003) Pancreatitis-induced extrahepatic portal vein stenosis treated by percutaneous transhepatic stent placement: a case report. *Cardiovasc Intervent Radiol* **26**: 395–397.
147. Jannsen H, Wijnhoud A, Haagsma E, *et al.* (2001) Extrahepatic portal vein thrombosis: aetiology and determinants of survival. *Gut* **49**: 720–724.
148. Merkel C, Bolognesi M, Bellon S, *et al.* (1992) Long term follow up study of adult patients with non cirrhotic obstruction of the portal system: comparison with cirrhotic patients. *J Hepatol* **15**: 299–303.
149. Condat B, Pessione F, Denninger M, *et al.* (2000) Recent portal or mesenteric thrombosis: increased recognition and frequent recanalisation on anticoagulant therapy. *Hepatology* **32**: 466–470.
150. Uflacker R. (2003) Applications of percutaneous mechanical thrombectomy in transjugular intrahepatic portosystemic shunt and portal venous thrombosis. *Tech Vasc Intervent Radiol* **6**: 59–69.

151. Wolff M, Hirner A. (2003) Current state of portosystemic shunt surgery. *Langenbeck Arch Surg* **388**: 141–149.
152. Laasch H, Martin D. (2002) Management of benign biliary strictures. *Cardiovasc Intervent Radiol* **25**: 457–466.
153. Tsiotos G, Luque-de Leon E, Sarr M. (1998) Long term outcome of necrotising pancreatitis treated by necrosectomy. *Br J Surg* **85**: 1650–1653.

Chapter 14

COMPLICATIONS OF SPLENECTOMY

Basil Ch. Golematis, Ilias P. Gomatos and
Manousos M. Konstadoulakis

INTRODUCTION

Surgical issues regarding the spleen are multiple and varied. Life-threatening haemorrhage from a lacerated spleen resulting from trauma is a common problem requiring swift surgical intervention. Certain diseases such as idiopathic thrombocytopenic purpura (ITP) and the haemolytic anaemias are often treated by splenectomy when medical management fails. Splenectomy may also be required as an integral part of another operation such as distal pancreatectomy or gastrectomy, whereas the traditional staging workup for Hodgkin's disease has involved removal of the spleen to determine the extent of the disease. The wide range of diseases requiring total or subtotal splenectomy as unique or partial treatment suggests that a multidisciplinary approach has to be established regarding the indications, surgical technique and perioperative care in candidates for splenectomy. This will ensure not only the proper management of the patients undergoing splenectomy, but will also reduce the rate of postoperative complications.

Post-splenectomy complications represent a critical issue in modern surgery, especially after the introduction of minimally invasive laparoscopic techniques. Most of these emerging techniques have been prospectively evaluated based on the incidence and severity of reported complications, shaping evolving guidelines in an evidence-based oriented international surgical community. Furthermore, the current climate of prepaid healthcare with gatekeeper control over hospital costs, progressive reductions in state and federal formulary reimbursement to hospitals and physicians, and the increasing utilisation review by all insurance carriers has raised concern for the frequency of complications that prolong hospital stay.

Post-splenectomy complications can be categorised as non-specific, which potentially develop after any procedure performed in the left upper abdominal quadrant, and as splenectomy-associated complications. The latter group of reported complications associates both with the patients' underlying conditions as well as the intraoperative manipulations. Optimal treatment of these complications requires a high suspicion index for an adverse situation as well as a detailed knowledge of the patients' co-morbidities.

INDICATIONS FOR SPLENECTOMY

An improved understanding of autoimmune anaemia, thrombocytopenia and neutrocytopenia has clarified the role of splenectomy in many haematologic diseases. Since the potential benefit from an operation must always be weighed against the corresponding surgical risk in relation to the patient's underlying conditions, it is obvious that the indications for splenectomy must be well defined. The current indications for splenectomy, either total or partial, are depicted in Table 1.

Splenectomies are commonly performed in order to control diseases such as ITP, hereditary spherocytosis, autoimmune anaemia, a ruptured spleen, thrombotic thrombocytopenic purpura and primary splenic cysts or tumours. Splenectomies are also performed in patients with chronic severe hypersplenism due to hairy cell leukaemia, lymphoproliferative disorders, Felty's syndrome, agnogeneic myeloid metaplasia, thalassaemia major, Gaucher's disease, haemodialysis splenomegaly, splenic vein thrombosis and sickle cell disease. Among these pathologic conditions, traumatic injury, ITP and hypersplenism still remain the most frequent indications for splenectomy.

Table 1. Indications for Splenectomy

Splenectomy always indicated

Primary splenic tumor
Hereditary spherocytosis (congenital haemolytic anaemia)

Splenectomy usually indicated

Primary hypersplenism
Chronic immune thrombocytopenic purpura
Splenic vein thrombosis causing esophageal varices
Splenic abscess

Splenectomy sometimes indicated

Splenic injury
Autoimmune haemolytic disease
Elliptocytosis with haemolysis
Non-spherocytic congenital haemolytic anaemias (pyruvate kinase deficiency)
Haemoglobin H disease
Hodgkin's disease (staging)
Thrombotic thrombocytopenic purpura
Myelofibrosis

Splenectomy rarely indicated

Chronic leukaemia
Splenic lymphoma
Macroglobulinemia
Thalassaemia major
Splenic artery aneurysm
Sickle cell anaemia
Congestive splenomegaly and hypersplenism due to portal hypertension

Splenectomy not indicated

Asymptomatic hypersplenism
Splenomegaly with infection
Splenomegaly associated with elevated IgM
Moderate hereditary haemolytic anaemia
Acute leukaemia
Agranulocytosis

PREOPERATIVE CONSIDERATIONS

Operations for splenic injury or disease should be preceded by specific preoperative preparations. All patients should receive polyvalent polysaccharide pneumonococcal vaccine, polyvalent meningococcal vaccine and Haemophilus influenzae type b conjugate vaccine as early as possible before the operation. Blood and blood products should be sought sufficiently in advance to allow for crossmatching, which may be difficult in patients with acquired haemolytic anaemia, thalassaemia or isoantibodies from previous transfusions. In the presence of haemolytic anaemia, transfusions should not be given before the operation. Platelets should be transfused after splenic artery ligation. The operating room, the blood and blood products should be warmed before use, since patients with chronic lymphocytic leukaemia or lymphoma may have developed cold haemagglutinin disease and thus have an increased risk of haemolysis. In elective splenectomies for massive splenomegaly intestinal preparation is always essential since an enlarged spleen is almost always heavily fixed with the colon with sometimes vascular adhesions. Since these patients develop gastric distention postoperatively, the placement of a nasogastric tube is advisable for all patients undergoing splenectomy.

SURGICAL TECHNIQUE

It has become more than obvious, that the majority of splenectomy-specific complications can be attributed to unfortunate or unstandardised surgical manoeuvers, the extent of which is further reflected by the immediate as well as the long-term postoperative course of the patients involved. Before discussing these complications and their respective management, we consider it essential to provide a detailed update of the existing variations regarding the performance of splenectomy (i.e. total, partial and minimally invasive splenectomy) with respect to common pitfalls and how the surgeon can prevent or escape them in an effective and expeditious manner.

TOTAL SPLENECTOMY (ANTERIOR APPROACH)

Splenectomy can be performed through several standard abdominal incisions. It is rarely necessary to use a thoracoabdominal incision, even to remove massively enlarged spleens. For the anterior approach, which is traditionally applied for a total splenectomy in our Department, the midline incision is preferred, although a left subcostal incision is favoured by some surgeons, especially in children. Palpation is carried out to detect any inflammatory adhesions to the spleen that might cause a capsular tear and troublesome bleeding if not carefully divided. The spleen is mobilised by dividing its posterior ligamentous attachments by electrocauterisation.

First, the spleen is separated from the renal covering with the use of sharp and blunt dissection. The splenocolic and splenorenal ligaments are clamped, divided and safely ligated. The short gastric vessels are clamped, divided and suture-ligated, avoiding injury or ischaemia of the stomach. Then the spleen is mobilised toward the midline before the hilar vessels are secured, a technique applicable for normal-sized, slightly enlarged or ruptured spleens. The spleen, tail and part of the pancreas are elevated, with extra care being paid to the tail of the pancreas. The spleen is now outside the peritoneal cavity and is attached only by the branches of the splenic arteries and veins. Initial ligation of the splenic artery and vein along the upper edge of the pancreas before splenic mobilisation is a very useful technique in patients with massive splenomegaly, because it controls the major portion of the vascular supply, and allows safer mobilisation of the spleen and dissection of its hilar branches. Still, it may predispose to splenic and portal vein thrombosis, encountered in a percentage of patients undergoing splenectomy. Once complete haemostasis has been secured, thorough search for accessory spleens (20% of patients) takes place in all patients undergoing splenectomy for haematologic disease. These spleens vary from a few millimetres to several centimetres in size and may become quite large in myeloproliferative disorders. The accessory spleens most often occur in the hilus, along the splenic vessels, within the attaching ligaments of the spleen, and in the mesentery and omentum. If the spleen is being removed for haematologic reasons, the accessory spleens should be removed as well.

We recommend the use of drains for a few days to reduce the subphrenic accumulation of fluid that occurs in the space previously occupied by the spleen. Closed suction drainage is indicated whenever an injury to the tail of the pancreas occurs as well as for patients where incomplete haemostasis is suspected.

PARTIAL SPLENECTOMY

The major indication for partial splenectomy is trauma to the spleen, not with mentioning its application for non-parasitic splenic cysts, or in patients with Gaucher's disease. Although an effort to save the spleen is of paramount importance, if there is any doubt regarding the safety, therapeutic efficiency and feasibility of partial splenectomy, the entire spleen should be removed. A detailed evaluation of the trauma must be done in order to decide on the most suitable treatment strategy. The alternative procedures include splenorrhaphy; splenorrhaphy with omental fixation; debridement with partial splenectomy and omental fixation; splenic mesh wrap and autotransplantation.

Once the segment chosen for preservation is determined, we begin a systemic stepwise ligation of the arterial and venous branches to the segment to be removed. As the ligation proceeds, evidence of the devascularisation of the spleen becomes increasingly evident as segment after segment undergoes a colour change ranging from dark bluish-purple to dark bluish. Intrasplenic dissection is an integral part of any attempt to perform partial splenectomy. While removing the devascularised segments or part of the ruptured spleen it is essential to avoid cautery and use the scalpel instead. With the scalpel, a superficial anterior incision is made on the viable side of the splenic capsule. By using the scalpel handle, the incision is gradually deepened until the entire spleen has been divided. All vessels are ligated with haemoclips, or with figure-of-eight 4-0 silk, while we always use a haemostatic substance or Argon laser. An alternative technique for treating the raw splenic remnant is the placement of interlocking mattress sutures of 2-0 vicryl or silk, 0.5–1 cm from the divided edge, compressing the splenic parenchyma for haemostasis. These sutures can be tied over pledgets of Gelfoam (absorbable gelatine sponge) or Surgicel (oxidised regenerated cellulose). Nevertheless, with the proper degree of tension on sutures, the application of pledgets of any kind is considered an unnecessary measure. Moreover, a running 2-0 chromic catgut suture is sufficient for a thin exposed splenic area.

In the case of haemorrhage secondary to capsular avulsion or superficial laceration of the spleen a topical haemostatic agent may be applied with satisfactory results, while a partial splenectomy may be handled successfully with stapling devices. For deeply lacerated spleens or whenever a partial splenectomy is performed, an absorbable mesh can be safely applied. A hole is created in the centre of the mesh, through which the injured spleen is passed. Then the spleen is wrapped in the mesh by sewing the opposite edges of the mesh to each other in order to create tamponade. Once again it must be underlined that careful haemostasis is essential for a successful procedure. If blood transfusion becomes necessary during partial splenectomy, then total splenectomy without transfusion is the safer treatment.

LAPAROSCOPIC SPLENECTOMY

Splenectomy has traditionally been transformed through a left subcostal or upper midline incision. Although laparoscopic splenectomy was first described by Cushieri[1] in 1992, it was not often performed until the last five to six years, when the procedure was undertaken in a series of patients large enough to permit objective evaluation of the method and to obtain reliable conclusions.[2,3]

Two alternative positions are used for laparoscopic splenectomy. The modified lithotomy position, where the surgeon stands between the patient's legs with the monitor placed over the patient's left shoulder, and the right lateral position (modified left lateral decubitus position with the iliac crest at table break and kidney rest elevated), which is traditionally used in our Department, where the surgeon stands at the patient's side. The lateral position facilitates posterior dissection of the spleen and of its hilum, while it decreases the amount of splenic retraction required during the operation. The 45-degree modification allows for quick repositioning of the patient and the conversion to open operation if necessary. The position used depends on the indication for the operation and the surgeon's preference.

POST-SPLENECTOMY MORBIDITY AND MORTALITY

Operative mortality for elective splenectomy should be less than 1%, except in patients with myeloproliferative disorders in whom postoperative problems with haemorrhage represent an increased risk. In a recent study splenectomy carried a mortality rate of 0.8%, and a complication rate of 12% in patients operated for haematological disorders.[4] Trauma patients have a variable mortality rate depending on the extent of other injuries. Well-known postoperative complications of splenectomy include left lower lobe atelectasis, wound infection, haemorrhage, subphrenic abscess, acute pancreatitis, (secondary to inadvertent injury to the tail of the pancreas), peripancreatic abscess and pseudocyst, pancreatic fistula formation, gastric fistula/perforation (secondary to

Table 2.   Commonly Observed Complications in Patients Undergoing Splenectomy

Indication	Mortality (%)	Complications (%)		
		Wound Infection	Abdominal Abscess	Wound Dehiscence
Splenic abscess	0		14.3	
Trauma	1.5		2.2	1.1
Iatrogenic injury	10.1	9.4	4.3	0.3

injury/necrosis of the gastric wall during ligation of the short gastric vessels) and portal vein and mesenteric venous thrombosis (Table 2). Late sequelae related to splenectomy are much more common in children, especially those younger than six years of age. Overwhelming post-splenectomy sepsis secondary to encapsulated organisms (pneumococcus, meningococcus, etc.), albeit unusual (<1%), is a well-recognised possibility in children before specific splenic immune function becomes established outside the spleen.

Adequate preoperative evaluation with consequent measures, as well as meticulous surgical manoeuvres can help minimise these complications. Preoperative correction of coagulation defects, excellent visualisation of important structures, careful dissection and rapid control of bleeding can minimise the incidence of intra- and postoperative haemorrhage. Careful dissection, exact application of instruments, staples and clips, and gentle retraction are required to avoid injury to adjacent organs (stomach, colon, or pancreas), which occurs during dissection of splenic attachments, division of splenic vessels or during retraction. Recognised injuries must be repaired immediately.

HAEMORRHAGE

The spleen is a pulpy organ that is easily injured during retraction while the hilar vessels are delicate and can be torn during surgical manipulations. Preoperative correction of coagulation defects, excellent visualisation of important structures, careful dissection and rapid control of bleeding will minimise the incidence of intraoperative and postoperative bleeding. If after splenectomy the patient becomes tachycardiac or hypotensive and has a falling haematocrit, delayed bleeding should be suspected. Most often the safest course for the patient is to evacuate the haematoma and surgically control the source of bleeding. If the patient is bleeding from coagulopathy, the coagulopathy should be controlled before proceeding with the operation.

PROPHYLAXIS AGAINST POST-SPLENECTOMY SEPSIS

Asplenic individuals are at greater risk for developing fulminant bacteremia because of decreased opsonic activity, decreased levels of IgM and decreased clearance of bacteria from the blood after splenectomy. As a rule, children are at greater risk of developing sepsis than adults, and fatal sepsis is more common after splenectomy for haematologic disorders than after trauma.[5] The incidence of post-splenectomy sepsis in asplenic children is 85 times the rate of the normal population and develops in 4.25% of splenectomy patients with a mortality rate exceeding 50%. The risk of sepsis is higher in the first postoperative year, and for adults, each subsequent year carries approximately 1% chance of developing sepsis. As a result of post-splenectomy sepsis syndrome, splenectomy is no longer considered the treatment of choice for splenic injuries. Instead, attempts are made to salvage at least part of the injured spleen. Although the minimal amount of normal functioning spleen needed to protect a patient from post-splenectomy sepsis syndrome has not been established, immunologic protection seems likely if approximately 25% of the spleen remains perfused by either the splenic or the short gastric arteries. Despite the ongoing shift towards splenic salvage procedures, total splenectomy still remains the treatment of choice for a number of diseases. However the prevention of post-splenectomy sepsis is a major issue that will have to be addressed within the next few years. In the meantime, prophylactic protocols have been advocated by the majority of physicians in order to decrease the incidence of this life-threatening complication. Most paediatricians believe that children who have had a splenectomy before the age of five years, should be treated with a daily dose of penicillin until the age of 10 years. The use of prophylactic penicillin is not advocated in children over the age of five years and in adults.

All patients who have undergone a non-elective splenectomy should be immunised with Pneumovax (a non-viable pneumonococcal vaccine containing the more common virulent strains of the pneumonococcus family). Patients for whom an elective splenectomy is planned should also be immunised with Pneumovax, preferably two or more weeks before the operation.[6]

Children under the age of 10 years and all patients who are immunosuppressed or have an associated immunodeficiency should be vaccinated against pneumonococcus, Haemophilus influenza, meningococcus and hepatitis B. Despite the fact that vaccinations and antimicrobial prophylaxis are recommended in these patients, the optimal immunisation schedule for Haemophilus influenzae type b (Hib) vaccine has not been delineated yet. Although the initial vaccination appears to provide immediate and adequate immunity the role of a booster vaccination has to be assessed in the perspective of long-term immunity.[7]

In our department, we do not advocate a post-splenectomy prophylactic antibiotic administration protocol. We only advise our patients to initiate antibiotic treatment for any signs of infection persisting for more than 24 hours, while concomitantly underlining the need to comply with this strategy on a lifelong basis.

POST-SPLENECTOMY ATELECTASIS

Atelectasis is the most common pulmonary complication affecting 25% of patients undergoing abdominal surgery. It is more common in patients who are elderly or overweight, and in those who smoke or have symptoms of respiratory disease. It appears most frequently in the first 48 hours after the operation and is responsible for over 90% of febrile episodes during that period. The pathogenesis of atelectasis involves obstructive and non-obstructive factors including secretions resulting from COPD, intubation and the administration of anaesthetic agents. Small bronchioles (<1 mm) are prone to close when lung volume reaches a critical point. Portions of the lung that are dependent or compressed like during a splenectomy the left lower lobe are the first to experience bronchiole closure, since their regional volume is less than that of non-dependent portions. Post-splenectomy atelectasis is usually manifested by fever, tachypnea and tachycardia. Physical examination may show elevation of the diaphragm, scattered rales and decreased breath sounds, but is often normal. Postoperative atelectasis can be largely prevented by early mobilisation, frequent changes in position, encouragement to cough and the use of incentive spirometer. Preoperative teaching of respiratory exercises and postoperative execution of these exercises prevent atelectasis in patients without pre-existing lung disease.

POSTOPERATIVE INFECTIONS

Once an infection is identified, treatment must be initiated. The single most important aspect of treatment for a surgical infection is drainage of the purulent material. Means of drainage include coughing and suctioning for pneumonia, aspiration of infected sinuses and drainage in the case of an abscess. Many post-splenectomy surgical infections, including postoperative abscesses and wound infections, require adequate incision and drainage. Subphrenic abscess formation is a well-known post-splenectomy complication which may occur as an isolated complication or as a result of injury to an adjacent organ, especially in patients with a massively enlarged spleen. An abdominal CT scan is required, while its treatment includes the administration of antibiotics followed by percutaneous drainage. If patient is not amenable to percutaneous drainage, operative drainage is indicated. Most surgeons do not advocate drainage of the left upper quadrant in patients undergoing splenectomy, but closed suction is mandatory when a large dead space persists. In this respect meticulous haemostasis during the left upper quadrant dissection can help minimise bleeding and the potential for abscess formation.

Any patient with an intermittent spiking temperature is suspected of having a subphrenic abscess. The diagnosis of intraperitoneal abscesses is difficult, resulting in a delay in treatment and poor prognosis. X-ray studies may suggest an abscess in up to one-half of cases. In post-splenectomy subphrenic abscesses the chest X-rays may show pleural effusion, a raised hemidiaphragm, basilar infiltrates or atelectasis. Abnormalities in plain abdominal films include an ileus pattern, soft tissue mass, air fluid levels, free- or mottle-gas pockets, effacement of properitoneal or psoas outlines, and the displacement of viscera. Although many of these findings are vague and non-specific, they may suggest the need for a CT scan. Real-time ultrasonography is sensitive in diagnosing intra-abdominal abscesses in about 80% of cases. CT scan of the abdomen is considered the best diagnostic study with regard to sensitivity (>95%) and specificity. Neither gas shadows nor exposed wounds interfere with CT scanning in postoperative patients, and the procedure is reliable even in areas poorly seen with ultrasonography. Left subphrenic abscesses appear as cystic collections with density measurements ranging between 0 and 15 attenuation units. Resolution can be further increased by the administration of contrast media (e.g. sodium diatrizoate), either intravenously injected, or instilled into hollow viscera adjacent to the abscess. One drawback of CT scan is that diagnosis may be difficult in areas with multiple thick-walled bowel loops, or if a pleural effusion overlies a subphrenic abscess, so that occasionally a very large abscess can be missed. In uncertain cases, CT-guided needle aspiration can distinguish between sterile and infected collections, simultaneously offering an effective resolution of the underlying problem, if followed by percutaneous drainage of the infected site.

Percutaneous drainage is the preferred method for single well-localised, superficial bacterial abscesses that do not have fistulous communications or contain solid debris. Following CT scan or ultrasonographic delineation, a needle is guided into the abscess cavity, infected material is aspirated for culture, and a suitably large drainage catheter is inserted. The success rate of the procedure exceeds 80% in simple abscesses but is often less than 50% in more complex ones.

Open drainage is reserved for abscesses for which percutaneous drainage is inappropriate or unsuccessful. It can be accomplished extraperitonealy by excising the twelfth rib. The infected area must be opened sufficiently to provide free drainage and complete decompression. All loculations must be lysed. All necrotic tissue should be excised, and all infected non-viable tissue debrided, to accelerate healing and reduce the likelihood of a residual infection. Penrose and sump drains are used to allow continued drainage postoperatively, until the infection has resolved.

POST-SPLENECTOMY THROMBOCYTOSIS

Splenectomy is frequently followed by thrombocytosis, which peaks in about seven to 10 days postoperatively, and then returns toward, but rarely, to normal. The number of circulating platelets may exceed 10^6 cells/ml. Thromboembolic complications may be common following splenectomy, but such complications do not correlate with the degree of thrombocytosis. If there are no contraindications, the patient should be mobilised as soon as possible; have their legs elevated while in bed or sitting; wear graduated-pressure compression stockings and receive a platelet function inhibiting drug (e.g. aspirin 300 mg bid with meals, mini-dose heparin 5000 units of heparin subcutaneously every 8 hours, or clopidogrel 75 mg once daily), in order to minimise the risk of deep venous thrombosis and potential thromboembolic events.

DEEP VENOUS THROMBOSIS

Surgery increases the risk of deep venous thrombosis 21-fold. The fact that this disorder is a complication reported in 20% of patients admitted for a general surgical procedure, suggests the need for routine deep venous thrombosis prophylaxis in the surgical patient. The 60% risk of ultimately developing pulmonary thromboembolism among patients with untreated deep venous thrombosis further underlines the essentiality of adopting adequate prophylactic measures. The most commonly used measures are graduated-compression elastic stockings with sequential compression devices and 5000 U of low dose unfractionated heparin given by subcutaneous injection twice daily, or LMWH given at prophylactic dose of 0.5–1 mg/kg subcutaneously daily, which is the current practice in our surgical department. LMWH has been shown to significantly reduce the incidence of postoperative deep venous thromboses and pulmonary embolisms.[8] The platelet count must be monitored in all patients receiving subcutaneous heparin or LMWH, for the early detection of Heparin-Induced Thrombocytopenia (HIT syndrome), which occurs with a peak incidence after 5–10 days of treatment. In cases of suspected post-splenectomy pulmonary thromboembolism as determined by means of spiral CT or magnetic resonance angiography.[9]

The risk of portal vein thrombosis in splenectomy patients is small but important, since this complication may be lethal if not recognised. Symptoms include fever, abdominal pain, diarrhoea and abnormal liver function tests. The primary treatment, similar to any kind of deep venous thrombosis, consists of systemic anticoagulation plus antibiotics. Heparin is initiated immediately and dosed to a goal PTT of 1.5–2 times normal. Warfarin is started after therapeutic heparinisation. Warfarin is continued for 3 to 6 months maintained at a goal INR of 2.0 to 3.0.

PANCREATIC COMPLICATIONS

Since the tail of the pancreas extends toward and frequently into the hilus of the spleen, it can be injured during a splenectomy. Minimal injury to the tail of the pancreas usually requires no care, but a moderately damaged pancreas should be managed with control of bleeding, ligation of exposed ducts and closed drainage. Extensive damage to the tail of the pancreas is usually managed by resection of the pancreatic tail and closed drainage of the area. Unrecognised pancreatic injuries may be followed by pancreatitis, pancreatic pseudocysts or fistulas. We always place a closed suction drainage for at least four days and we give prophylactic somatostatin or its synthetic analogue octreotide, if we suspect pancreatic injury. Furthermore, we carefully examine the removed spleen for pancreatic tissue at the pathology department.

Acute Pancreatitis

In more than two-thirds of patients with post-splenectomy acute pancreatitis, the disease takes a mild course associated with only minimal organ dysfunction. Clinical improvement can be achieved by fluid replacement, pain treatment and nutritional support, while no further complications are observed. Support with TPN is required for approximately 4 to 6 weeks until the inflammatory process in the pancreas subsides and enteric feeding can be resumed. However the initial 72 hours after the onset of symptoms serves as the crossroads after which severe clinical disease develops in as many as 30% of patients with acute pancreatitis. Pancreatic infection rates vary between 40% and 70% in patients not treated with early antibiotics, leading to an incidence of infected necrosis as high as 30%, one week after the onset of symptoms.[10,11] Although the reported rates are not derived from studies focusing specifically on post-splenectomy pancreatitis, they are indicative of the severity of these complications. Prevention of pancreatic infection by means of antibiotics represents a major goal in the treatment of patients with necrotising pancreatitis of all aetiologies. Imipenem alone or ciprofloxacin, ofloxacin, mezlocillin each in combination with metronidazole, have the highest bactericidal activity in cases of pancreatic infection and achieve optimal thaerapeutic levels in pancreatic tissue and necrosis.[12-14] Appropriate antibiotic prophylaxis with one of the suggested regimens should therefore be initiated promptly in order to avoid any of these complications. Thirty to 60% of patients recover from severe post-traumatic pancreatitis without surgical intervention.[15,16] In this context the prevention of pancreatic infection (particularly in the immunocompromised splenectomised patient) is of paramount importance.

Peripancreatic Fluid Collection

Persistent post-splenectomy peripancreatic fluid collections represent a difficult to treat clinical entity. By definition, a pancreatic ductal disruption, caused by intraoperative manoeuvres, is required to allow the peripancreatic fluid collection to develop. Approximately 90% of patients with acute postoperative pancreatitis have a self-limited course of abdominal pain and hyperamylasemia that resolves within one week. When clinical symptoms persist longer than one week, it is likely that many of these patients have a demonstrable pancreatic ductal disruption leading to peripancreatic fluid accumulation plus a variable amount of peripancreatic necrosis. The location of the peripancreatic fluid collection, which can lead to a pseudo-cyst formation, can be determined by dynamic bolus CT imaging. Management of peripancreatic fluid collections can be accomplished by the application of two surgical principles. First, all fluid collections that are symptomatic must be drained by means of endotherapy or surgery and second, if a persistent pancreatic duct fistula is present, downstream obstruction must be recognised and eliminated by means of ERCP. In these cases where the downstream obstruction is a result of oedema, pancreatic ductal stenting aids in healing the fistula without surgery. Occasionally, the disrupted pancreatic ductal system can be bridged by stent placement leading to an optimal resolution of the existing pancreatic fistula. The patient can then develop either a transient leak out of the pancreatic ductal system, or a persistent pancreatic fistula (>50 ml/day of amylase-rich fluid draining from the percutaneous drain). If there is no ductal disruption almost all of these collections heal spontaneously. Follow-up CTs are performed to ensure that fluid collections do not recollect. External drains are removed after catheter drainage has stopped for more than two days and there is no demonstrable cavity or ductal connection by sonogram.

Post-splenectomy Necrotising Pancreatitis

In spite of being very rare, acute post-splenectomy necrotising pancreatitis constitutes a major post-splenectomy complication requiring the timely application of accurate treatment measures. It is currently thought that debridement of dead peripancreatic tissue reduces the mortality rate of acute severe necrotising pancreatitis. Historical controls place the mortality rate at 50% to 80% in the absence of operative treatment and 10%–40% among patients subjected to necrosectomy. Contrast-enhanced CT scans obtained early in the course of the disease are studied for the presence of non-enhancing areas, which indicate the lack of vascular perfusion and reflect the presence of necrotic peripancreatic fat or pancreatic parenchyma. Percutaneous needle aspiration of these areas is used to detect the presence of bacterial colonisation. After the exclusion of infected necrosis through fine-needle aspiration, most patients with proven sterile necrosis should be managed non-surgically. Patients with focal necrosis respond promptly to ICU management. However, patients with extended sterile necrosis (>50% of the pancreas) are candidates for surgical management if they continue to require mechanical ventilation, haemofiltration or haemodialysis.

Pancreatic Fistulas

Pancreatic fistulas occur when the pancreatic duct or one of its branches is disrupted either by direct trauma or as a result of inflammatory disease. They can occasionally complicate unrecognised direct injury to the gland or postoperative pancreatitis. They may communicate externally with the skin or, less frequently, internally with a variety of hollow organs or a body cavity. Complications associated with pancreatic fistulas include fluid and electrolyte losses, bleeding, pulmonary problems, malabsorption, skin breakdown, and autodigestion or the erosion of adjacent viscera. There is a substantial mortality risk of 8% to 10% associated with the development of pancreatic fistula.[17,18] Most deaths are due to intra-abdominal sepsis and haemorrhage. The vast majority of external fistulas occur as complications of elective upper abdominal surgery, including splenectomy, particularly when the latter is performed for trauma. Postoperative fistulas are externalised as a result of either intraoperatively placed drains, spontaneous drainage via the wound, or percutaneous drainage of postoperative fluid collections. They are most often initially noted between postoperative days 3 and 4 and are heralded by an increased surgical drain output of serous to cloudy non-bilious fluid with high amylase content.

External pancreatic fistulas are classified as either high output or low output based on the total daily drainage volume. High output fistulas (>200 ml/day) are more problematic because of their association with pancreatic ductal abnormalities that may preclude closure with conservative therapy. Low output fistulas (<200 ml/day) are more amenable to non-operative management. Pancreatic fistulas that require definitive reoperations are very rare. Irrespective of cause, several important principles are applicable to the treatment of pancreatic fistulas. Unimpeded free drainage of the fistula is essential. Any fistula-associated sepsis must be carefully controlled particularly in the setting of splenectomised patients who are considered immunocompromised. Bowel rest is critical to achieving the reduction of pancreatic exocrine secretion to basal levels that promote fistula closure. Adequate nutritional support with total parenteral nutrition is crucial, as many pancreatic fistulas require prolonged bowel rest. Fluid and electrolyte losses are often substantial in cases of high-output pancreatic fistulas. Excessive losses of bicarbonate lead to a metabolic acidosis that must be corrected. Maintenance of adequate volume status is facilitated by carefully measuring fistula outputs over several days and replacing fluid losses with isotonic crystalloid solutions. Skin breakdown from the exposure to pancreatic digestive enzymes can be avoided if there is effective control of the fistula by means of closed suction drains.

Approximately 80% of external pancreatic fistulas close spontaneously when the principles of conservative management are meticulously followed.[19] The success with internal fistulas has been somewhat less, with spontaneous closure rates in the 40% to 60% range.[20,21] Problems associated with the conservative management of pancreatic fistulas include prolonged hospitalisation and a high cost of care. Since the introduction of clinically efficacious somatostatin analogues, it has become possible to achieve spontaneous closure in a more expedient and cost-effective manner. Octreotide acetate is a long-acting synthetic octapeptide analogue of somatostatin with a half-life of approximately 2 hours.[22] Pharmacologic studies confirm that octreotide dramatically reduces basal and stimulated pancreatic secretion when given in doses as small as 50 μg twice daily.[23] Data obtained from a recent study[24] suggest that pharmacotherapy (either with somatostatin or with octreotide administration) reduces the costs involved in fistula management (by reducing hospitalisation) and also offers increased spontaneous closure rate. Despite the demonstrated superiority of somatostatin versus octreotide, and the lack of difference regarding overall mortality rates, the presented results are considered significant regarding the management of patients with postoperative gastrointestinal and pancreatic fistulas. Currently available information obtained from a recent meta-analysis,[25] indicate a considerable benefit of somatostatin-14 when administered in association with standard conservative treatment in patients with pancreatic fistulas. Nevertheless, these results need to be confirmed in a large prospective controlled study.

Surgery for persistent post-splenectomy pancreatic fistulas is indicated when non-operative management fails. Fistulas arising from the body and tail of the pancreas (susceptible to injury during splenectomy) which are not associated with ductal strictures in the head of the gland are managed by distal pancreatectomy. If a large pseudo-cyst not amenable to resection is present, or if a ductal stricture cannot be encompassed by the resection, then internal drainage of the pseudo-cyst or the actual fistula must be performed. Closed suction drains are routinely placed adjacent to pancreaticojejunostomy or distal pancreatic resection margin to capture any postoperative anastomotic or pancreatic stump leakage.

SPLENOSIS

Precautions must always be taken regarding the manipulation of the spleen in order to avoid capsular disruption which can lead to splenosis and recurrent haematologic disease. In splenosis, multiple small implants of splenic tissue grow in scattered areas on the peritoneal surfaces throughout the abdomen. They arise from the dissemination and autotransplantation of splenic fragments following traumatic rupture of the spleen.[26,27] Although splenic implants or intentional autotransplants are capable of cell culling, their immunologic function appears to be insignificant. Aggressive attempts at surgical excision are not warranted. Splenosis is usually an incidental finding discovered much later during laparotomy for an unrelated problem. However the implants stimulate the formation of adhesions and may be a cause of intestinal obstruction; they must be distinguished from metastatic peritoneal nodules and from accessory spleens.

DISEASE-SPECIFIC COMPLICATIONS

Haematologic Malignancies

Probably the majority of the reported post-splenectomy complications can predominantly be attributed to the patients' underlying conditions and previous medical history. Although splenectomy is routinely performed for haematologic malignancies as a diagnostic and therapeutic tool, its role in this setting of patients remains controversial. A retrospective study performed by Horowitz et al.,[28] analysed the frequency and character of post-splenectomy complications in 135 patients with haematologic malignancies. Reported results indicated splenectomy as a potentially morbid procedure in this setting of patients.

The overall postoperative complication and mortality rates for all patients were 52% and 9%, respectively, while the complication rate was higher for patients whose spleens weighed greater than 2000 g, compared to the rest of the group. Seventy-three percent of the postoperative deaths were due to septic complications, only one of which was caused by an encapsulated organism. Complications occurred in less than 20% of patients with the diagnosis of Hodgkin's disease and hairy cell leukaemia. On the contrary, up to 50% of patients with non-Hodgkin's lymphoma, chronic lymphocytic and chronic lymphogenous leukaemia suffered postoperative complications. These results have been considered significant in shaping the guidelines as to whether a splenectomy should be performed in this group of patients. We believe that surgeons ought to perform a detailed preoperative work-up, follow well-established surgical techniques and closely follow their patients during the immediate and long-term postoperative period to avoid such dismal outcomes.

Sickle Cell Disease

Patients with sickle cell disease also face disease-associated risks following elective splenectomy. Potential complications include sickle cell pain, breathing problems leading to sickle acute chest syndrome, surgical infection, bleeding and difficulty in recovering normal bowel function. Key factors in reducing these risks include the following:

- Scheduling the operation just after one of the patient's regular blood transfusions. This ensures that there are more normal red blood cells in circulation at the time of operation, decreasing the consequences of sickle cell crisis.
- Adequate perioperative administration of intravenous fluids in order to prevent dehydration.
- Appropriate surgical technique in order to minimise postoperative haemorrhage, abdominal injury and septic complications.

COMMENTS ON LAPAROSCOPIC SPLENECTOMY

Laparoscopic splenectomy is as safe as open splenectomy, when performed by experienced laparoscopic surgeons. It has been associated with shortened hospitalisation and decreased time to full recovery, while followed by less severe complications. Although the necessity for intraoperative transfusions is increased compared to the open technique, paying particular attention during the ligation of large splenic vessels and attaining familiarity with the peculiarities of this operation will diminish intraoperative haemorrhagic sequelae. Furthermore, the calculated steep learning curve of the initial 20 cases (as estimated in a paediatric facility)[29] can be easily exceeded in specialised laparoscopic centres, where this procedure is routinely performed.

Despite the fact that the indications of laparoscopic splenectomy are more or less the same as those of open splenectomy, splenic size constitutes an important restraining factor.[3,30,31] Splenic size over 30 cm along the longitudinal axis of the organ has been considered a relative contraindication for the laparoscopic approach.[30–32] Additionally, in a recent study,[33] the incidence of splenectomy-associated complications has been shown to increase in relation to the splenic size, with massive splenomegaly (as defined by a spleen weighing more than 1000 g), leading to a 10% overall complication rate as compared with only a 6.3% complication rate for patients with a spleen weighing less than 1000 g. Nevertheless, other studies[34] suggest that laparoscopic splenectomy can be safely applied in patients with significantly enlarged spleens, especially if a hand-assisted laparoscopic approach is applied.[35]

The reported overall complication rates following laparoscopic splenectomy range from 0% to 24%. These findings are similar to the ones published in the series of open splenectomies.[36–38] However, the primary difference between laparoscopic and open splenectomy resides in the type of complications. Most laparoscopic series reported minor complications such as ileus,[30] seromas of the port sites,[32,39,40] and pleural effusion,[30,39,41] while in more than 450 laparoscopic cases collected, only one series reported more severe complications (i.e. pulmonary embolism, portal vein thrombosis and pancreatic fistula,[42] and one study reported repeat surgery for postoperative bleeding in one patient.[43] On the contrary, in large series of open splenectomy, the prevalence of severe complications was significantly higher. Postoperative subphrenic abscesses requiring repeat surgery were reported in 3% to 5% of cases,[36–38,41] rebleeding requiring exploration occurred in 5% to 7% of cases,[38,44] and pulmonary embolism was found in 2% to 6% of patients.[36,37] Most of these studies are retrospective including patients treated for a variety of different conditions. The inconsistency of the presented results suggests the need for the design and performance of a prospective double-blind randomised study comparing open versus laparoscopic splenectomy with respect to specific postoperative complications as well as their management in patients treated for a specific disease.

In our Department we have recently advocated a treatment protocol involving simultaneous laparoscopic splenectomy and cholecystectomy for patients suffering from β-thalassaemia major.[45] Twenty-eight consecutive β-thalassaemia major patients undergoing elective splenectomy have been randomised for open (n = 14) and laparoscopic splenectomy (n = 14). There has been no operative mortality in our study. Postoperative haemorrhage (observed in three cases) was the major complication observed. Two cases of postoperative bleeding occurred in the laparoscopic group of patients (14.3%), while there was one case of postoperative haemorrhage in the open splenectomy group of patients (7.1%). All bleeding complications were conservatively managed. The two cases of pulmonary atelectasis were equally distributed between the open splenectomy and the laparoscopic group of patients. Although thalassaemia major patients undergoing splenectomy are at increased risk for post-splenectomy sepsis, we did not come across any such event. Despite the fact that the two groups of patients did not differ significantly with respect to postoperative complication rate (14% vs 21%), both the duration of the procedure, as well as the need for blood transfusions, were markedly increased in the laparoscopically-treated group of patients ($p < 0.001$ and $p = 0.018$, respectively). Apart from the shortened hospitalisation period observed in the laparoscopic group of patients (5 days vs 6.5 days, $p = 0.035$), we did not manage to demonstrate either a clear clinical benefit or a decreased overall cost of laparoscopic splenectomy against the conventional open procedure. On the contrary we have come to believe that laparoscopic splenectomy should be regarded with scepticisism before being advocated as the procedure of choice in patients with β-thalassaemia major.

CONCLUSIONS

As our understanding of the role of the spleen in the host immune surveillance system has evolved, the indications for splenectomy have changed. The application of novel treatment strategies for certain haematologic benign and malignant disorders, the development of newer operative techniques for haemostasis and splenic salvage as well as the proliferation of intra-abdominal imaging techniques have markedly changed the way physicians view splenectomy. The development and wide acceptance of minimal invasive techniques in general surgery have further increased the application of laparoscopic splenectomy, which appears to be safe and associated with less pain and more rapid convalescence. Although splenectomy has been considered a routine procedure in large volume centres, occasionally it can prove to be very demanding and associated with severe complications, especially in patients with co-morbidities. Both total and partial splenectomy, either open or laparoscopic, require exact knowledge of the indications, surgical technique and potential pitfalls which are individualised according to the disorder the surgeon is attempting to treat. Overall, surgical experience and technique appear to be the most important factors determining the overall complication rates following electively as well as urgently performed total or partial splenectomy.

REFERENCES

1. Cuschieri A, Shimi S, Banting S, Velpen GV. (1992) Technical aspects of laparoscopic splenectomy. *J R Coll Surg Edinb* **37**: 414–416.
2. Cadiere GB, Verrroken R, Himpens J. (1994) Operative strategy in laparoscopic splenectomy. *J Am Coll Surg* **179**: 668–672.
3. Rege RV, Merriam LT, Joehl RJ. (1996) Laparoscopic splenectomy. *Surg Clin North Am* **76**: 459–469.
4. Baccarani U, Terrosu G, Donini A, *et al.* (1999) Splenectomy in haematology. Current practice and new perspectives. *Haematologica* **84**: 431–436.
5. Golematis B, Tzardis P, Legakis N, Persidou-Golemati P. (1989) Overwhelming postsplenectomy infection in patients with thalassaemia major. *Mt Sinai J Med* **56**: 97–98.
6. Eber SW, Langendorfer CM, Ditzig M, *et al.* (1999) Frequency of very late fatal sepsis after splenectomy for hereditary spherocytosis: impact of insufficient antibody response to pneumococcal infection. *Ann Haematol* **78**: 524–528.
7. Cimaz R, Mensi C, D'Angelo E, *et al.* (2001) Safety and immunogenicity of a conjugate vaccine against Haemophilus influenzae type b in splenectomised and non-splenectomised patients with Cooley anaemia. *J Infect Dis* **183**: 1819–1821.
8. Hirsh J, Bates SM. (2001) Clinical trials that have influenced the treatment of venous thromboembolism: a historical perspective. *Ann Intern Med* **134**: 409–417.
9. Meaney JF, Weg JG, Chenevert TL, *et al.* (1997) Diagnosis of pulmonary embolism with magnetic resonance angiography. *N Engl J Med* **336**: 1422–1427.

10. Banks PA. (1997) Practice guidelines in acute pancreatitis. *Am J Gastroenterol* **92**: 377–386.
11. Beger HG, Bittner R, Block S, Buchler M. (1986) Bacterial contamination of pancreatic necrosis. A prospective clinical study. *Gastroenterology* **91**: 433–438.
12. Banks PA, Gerzof SG, Langevin RE, *et al.* (1995) CT-guided aspiration of suspected pancreatic infection: bacteriology and clinical outcome. *Int J Pancreatol* **18**: 265–270.
13. Gerzof SG, Banks PA, Robbins AH, *et al.* (1987) Early diagnosis of pancreatic infection by computed tomography-guided aspiration. *Gastroenterology* **93**: 1315–1320.
14. Rau B, Pralle U, Mayer JM, Beger HG. (1998). Role of ultrasonographically-guided fine-needle aspiration cytology in the diagnosis of infected pancreatic necrosis. *Br J Surg* **85**: 179–184.
15. Rau B, Pralle U, Uhl W, Schoenberg MH. (1995) Management of sterile necrosis in instances of severe acute pancreatitis. *J Am Coll Surg* **181**: 279–288.
16. Bradley EL III, Allen K. (1991) A prospective longitudinal study of observation versus surgical intervention in the management of necrotising pancreatitis. *Am J Surg* **161**: 19–24.
17. Cullen JJ, Sarr MG, Ilstrup DM. (1994) Pancreatic anastomotic leak after pancreaticoduodenectomy: incidence, significance, and management. *Am J Surg* **168**: 295–298.
18. Edis AJ, Kiernan PD, Taylor WF. (1980) Attempted curative resection of ductal carcinoma of the pancreas: review of Mayo Clinic experience, 1951–1975. *Mayo Clin Proc* **55**: 531–536.
19. Yeo CJ. (1995) Management of complications following pancreaticoduodenectomy. *Surg Clin North Am* **75**: 913–924.
20. Lipsett PA, Cameron JL. (1992) Internal pancreatic fistula. *Am J Surg* **163**: 216–220.
21. Parekh D, Segal I. (1992) Pancreatic ascites and effusion. Risk factors for failure of conservative therapy and the role of octreotide. *Arch Surg* **127**: 707–712.
22. Kuta K, Nuesch E, Rosenthaler J. (1986) Pharmakokinetics of SMS 201–995 in healthy subjects. *Scand J Gastroenterol (Suppl)* **119**: 65–72.
23. Anad BS, Goodgame R, Grahm DY. (1994) Pancreatic secretion in man. Effect of fasting, drugs, pancreatic enzymes and somatostatin. *Am J Gastroenterol* **89**: 267–270.
24. Leandros E, Antonakis PT, Albanopoulos K, *et al.* (2004) Somatostatin versus octreotide in the treatment of patients with gastrointestinal and pancreatic fistulas. *Can J Gastroenterol* **18**: 303–306.

25. Hesse U, Ysebaert D, de Hemptinne B. (2001) Role of somatostatin-14 and its analogues in the management of gastrointestinal fistulae: clinical data. *Gut (Suppl)* **49**: 11–21.

26. Levine JH, Longo WE, Pruitt C, *et al.* (1996) Unresolved issues in laparoscopic splenectomy. *Am J Surg* **172**: 585–589.

27. Holdsworth RJ. (1991) Regeneration of the spleen and splenic autotransplantation. *Br J Surg* **78**: 270–274.

28. Horowitz J, Smith JL, Weber TK, *et al.* (1996) Postoperative complications after splenectomy for haematologic malignancies. *Ann Surg* **223**: 290–296.

29. Cusick RA, Waldhausen JH. (2001) The learning curve associated with paediatric laparoscopic splenectomy. *Am J Surg* **181**: 393–397.

30. Poulin EC, Thibault C, Mamazza J. (1995) Laparoscopic splenectomy. *Surg Endosc* **9**: 172–177.

31. Thibault C, Mamazza J, Letoumau R, Poulin E. (1992) Laparoscopic splenectomy: operative technique and preliminary report. *Surg Laparosc Endosc* **2**: 257–261.

32. Emmermann A, Zornig C, Peiper M, *et al.* (1995) Laparoscopic splenectomy. Technique and results in a series of 27 cases. *Surg Endosc* **9**: 1017–1019.

33. Al-Salem AH. (1999) Is splenectomy for massive splenomegaly safe in children? *Am J Surg* **178**: 42–45.

34. Laopodis V, Kritikos E, Rizzoti L, *et al.* (1998) Laparoscopic splenectomy in b-thalassaemia major patients. Advantages and disadvantages. *Surg Endosc* **12**: 944–947.

35. Kercher KW, Brent D, Matthews BD, *et al.* (2002) Laparoscopic splenectomy for massive splenomegaly. *Am J Surg* **183**: 192–196.

36. Akwari OE, Itani KM, Coleman RE, Rosse WF. (1987) Splenectomy for primary and recurrent immune thrombocytopenic purpura (ITP). Current criteria for patient selection and results. *Ann Surg* **206**: 529–541.

37. Mintz SJ, Petersen SR, Cheson B, *et al.* (1981) Splenectomy for immune thrombocytopenic purpura. *Arch Surg* **116**: 645–650.

38. Musser G, Lazar G, Hocking W, Busuttil RW. (1984) Splenectomy for haematologic disease. The UCLA experience with 306 patients. *Ann Surg* **200**: 40–45.

39. Flowers JL, Lefor AT, Steers J, *et al.* (1996) Laparoscopic splenectomy in patients with haematologic diseases. *Ann Surg* **224**: 19–28.

40. Rhodes M, Rudd M, O'Rourke N, Nathanson L. (1995) Laparoscopic splenectomy and lymph node biopsy for haematologic disorders. *Ann Surg* **222**: 43–46.

41. Park A, Gagner M, Pomp A. (1997) The lateral approach to laparoscopic splenectomy. *Am J Surg* **173**: 126–130.

42. Gigot JF, de Ville de Goyet J, Van Beers BE, *et al.* (1996) Laparoscopic splenectomy in adults and children: experience with 31 patients. *Surgery* **119**: 384–389.

43. Trias M, Targarona EM, Balague C. (1996) Laparoscopic splenectomy: an evolving technique. A comparison between anterior and lateral approaches. *Surg Endosc* **10**: 389–392.

44. Jacobs P, Wood L, Dent DM. (1986) Results of treatment in immune thrombocytopenia. *Q J Med* **58**: 153–165.

45. Konstadoulakis MM, Lagoudianakis E, Antonakis PT, *et al.* (2006) Laparoscopic versus open splenectomy in patients with β-thalassemia major. *J Laparoendosc Adv Surg Tech A* **16**: 5–8.

Chapter 15

COMPLICATIONS OF GROIN HERNIA SURGERY

Enrico Nicolo

INTRODUCTION

Groin hernia repair is a very common surgical procedure, performed today on an outpatient basis in a hospital or surgery centre, electively and with local, spinal or general anaesthesia. Minimal workup is required depending on the age and general condition of the patient. Medical clearance is necessary for patients with chronic heart disease and chronic obstruction pulmonary disease, and other co-morbid conditions as indicated. Anticoagulants such as heparin, coumadin, ASA and plavix should be discontinued a few days prior to surgery, and the coagulation profile should be re-checked just before the surgery.

The operation for groin hernia repair is considered today a satisfactory, safe and simple procedure. The operative technique has become standardised, and the general principles for the management of the sac and repair of the floor are well accepted. The literature today reports a high percentage of cure, negligible mortality, and few complications.

Complications of groin hernia repair are uncommon, rare and possibly avoidable. This chapter will review only those complications related to groin hernia surgery. General and anaesthesia complications are not addressed.

COMPLICATIONS OF HERNIA SURGERY

Injury to Blood Vessels

Bleeding as a result of incomplete haemostasis or injury to blood vessels is the most annoying complications of groin hernia surgery.[1–7] The surgeon should make every effort to maintain a good haemostasis from the beginning and at each operative step of the hernia operation. For example, the fascia should not be incised until all the bleeding points in the superficial layers of skin and sub-cutaneous tissue have been stopped. Bleeding from the superficial branches of the inferior epigastric vessels, external iliac circumflex and external pudendal vessels results in subcutaneous haematoma and/or diffuse ecchymosis. Ecchymosis manifests a few days after the operation in the bluish, green, and then yellow discoloration of the skin, scrotum and foreskin, as a result of blood dissection through the tissue plane. It is harmless, no treatment is necessary, and the patient must be reassured. Wound haematoma appears the day after the operation as a swelling, induration and tenderness, and can be treated conservatively with a heating pad, but it may require evacuation and packing.

The deep epigastric vessels situated in the properitoneal space and running vertically on the medial border of the internal inguinal ring can be accidentally injured during the management of the neck of an indirect sac or during the opening of the transversalis fascia. The deep epigastric vessels when penetrated and transfixed may inadvertently produce an expanding haematoma that may require reoperation, or produce an intraperitoneal bleeding that may require exploratory laparotomy, and in rare occasions thus has been fatal.

When the injury is recognised, the deep epigastric vessels can be ligated free with impunity.

Bleeding from the pampiniform plexus and veins injured during the isolation of an indirect sac from the cord may produce a large, hard, tender haematoma of the scrotum that can extend down to the upper thigh. Aspiration is fruitless. Reabsorption of the haematoma can take considerable time. Elevation of the scrotum with a scrotal support may relieve the discomfort and hasten the reabsorption. The reabsorbed scrotal haematoma can be the cause of a postoperative hydrocele. At times it becomes necessary to make a small incision to evacuate the haematoma, and packing is required to prevent further bleeding.

The iliac and femoral vein and artery may be injured during the placement of deep sutures that are intended to incorporate the anterior femoral sheath, the ileopubic tract or the inguinal ligament. The bleeding is immediate. The needle should be removed and pressure applied. The arterial bleeding responds more rapidly than the venous. In rare occasions the injured vessels require suturing after adequate exposure has been achieved. Delayed complications such as arterial aneurysm and arterio-venous fistula can also be seen.

In the immediate postoperative period we can treat the signs of hypotension and shock that result from intra-abdominal bleeding. Immediate fluid resuscitation and a possible blood transfusion and appropriate workup, including CT scan of the abdomen and pelvis, are part of the initial management. An emergent exploratory laparotomy through an infra-umbilical abdominal midline incision is performed. Usually the bleedings are found to originate from omental or mesenteric vessels, and/or from the inferior deep epigastric vessels. After identification of the offending blood vessel, ligation or suturing is sufficient to stop the bleeding and to stabilise the patient.

Vas Deferens

The vas deferens is recognised by its spaghetti cord-like feel and its special light colour. The vas deferens can be injured especially during hernia repair in children and in recurrences, when it is found strictly adherent to the sac. When accidentally severed, the vas deferens should be re-anastomosed end-to-end with fine interrupted sutures over an intraluminal splint that is removed after the completion of the anastomosis.[2–4]

Obstruction due to fibrosis or kinking can happen when the vas deferens is handled poorly during the operation, when postoperatively it becomes adhered to the posterior wall or to the polypropylene mesh. The obstruction can be complete or partial. When it is partial, it can produce disejaculation,[5] a burning, painful sensation during and after ejaculation. When it is completely obstructed, an interruption in the outflow of sperm will result.

In all of these complications, fertility can be affected and will be dependent upon the function of the opposite testicle and the vas deferens.

Injury to the Nerves

The nerves encountered during inguinal surgery are the ileo-inguinal, ileo-hypogastric, genital femoral and lateral femoral cutaneous nerves, and the femoral nerve.

The anatomy of these nerves must be well kept in mind. Every effort should be made to positively identify the nerves and to preserve their integrity, avoiding trauma, stretching and division, during groin hernia surgery. The ileo-inguinal and the ileo-hypogastric nerves are sensory nerves to the pubis, the back of the penis, and the antero-lateral portion of the scrotum and the upper medial aspect of the thigh. The majority of patients after groin hernia surgery experience anaesthesia and/or pain and paresthesia in the distribution of the ileo-inguinal nerve that is usually transient and subsides without sequelae. In rare occasions however, pain and paresthesia can be severe and at times disabling, and it can persist for a long period of time, months or even years. This is known as "chronic inguinodynia" and is due to the entrapment of the ileo-inguinal nerve, caused by sutures, adhesions, or neuroma.[8,9]

The initial approach to this problem is the ileo-inguinal nerve local block. This may provide substantial or even complete permanent relief from the symptoms. If the local block fails, surgical intervention becomes necessary. Exploration through the same inguinal incision allows the identification of the ileo-inguinal nerve, resection of part of the nerve (neurectomy) including the entrapped segment, and neurolysis or the excision of a neuroma.

The genital branch of the genital femoral nerve is the only motor nerve of the groin and contains motor fibres directed to the cremastatic muscle. Resection of the cremastatic muscles and division of the genital branch eliminate the cremastatic reflex and abolish the suspensory mechanism of the testis. Neuralgia secondary to the entrapment of the genital femoral nerve consists of intermittent or continuous burning pain in the inguinal area radiating to the genitalia and the upper thigh. It is aggravated by walking, stooping or hyper-extension of the hip, and is relieved by recumbency and flexion of the thigh.

If the pain persists after ileo-inguinal nerve surgery and if L1–L2 block results in pain relief, surgical exploration of the genital femoral nerve should be performed. A transverse flank incision lateral to and above the umbilicus is extended to the anterior axillary line, the retroperitoneum is exposed, the ipsilateral psoas and ureter identified. The genital femoral nerve penetrates the psoas as a single trunk along its medial edge. Resection includes the proximal trunk of the genital femoral nerve as well as its bifurcation. Sequelae of the genital femoral neurectomy include hypoesthesia of the scrotum (labium majus), skin over the femoral triangle, and the loss of the cremastatic reflex.

Injury to the femoral nerve is extremely rare. The femoral nerve lies in the lacuna musculorum on the psoas muscle protected by the iliac fascia. The femoral nerve can be injured during pre-peritoneal hernia repair as well as during laparoscopic approach when the prosthesis is sutured or stapled into place. This results in paresis of the extensor muscles of the thigh. Early re-exploration and removal of the offending stitch or staples is the appropriate approach that usually completely relieves the symptoms.

Injury to the Testicular Blood Supply

Ischaemic orchitis, testicular atrophy

The three major arteries and veins of the testicle are: the internal spermatic or testicular artery, which is the main blood supply of the testes and arises from the aorta; the external spermatic artery, which supplies the cremastatic muscles and is a branch of the inferior epigastric vessels; and the deferential artery, which accompanies the vas deferens and is a branch of the superior vesical artery.

A good collateral circulation exists between the branches of the vesical and the prostatic arteries and the testicular and deferential arteries. The scrotal branches of the internal and external pudendal arteries also anastomose the vessels of the spermatic cord. Every effort should be made to prevent injury and preserve intact the vessels of the spermatic cord, the arteries as well as the panpiniform plexus and vein. During primary repair and especially during the repair of recurrent hernia, injury to these vessels can occur followed by two major complications, testicular atrophy and ischaemic orchitis.[1,4,10]

Ischaemic orchitis is mainly due to the interruption of the venous return from the testes as a result of injury to the panpiniform plexus and veins during dissection of the sac from the cord. Thrombosis or ligation is the main cause. Elevation of the testicles and analgesia are usually sufficient. It takes four to eight weeks for the testicles to come back to the normal size or it can progress to testicular atrophy. This can be prevented at times by the trans-scrotal approach in a local anaesthesia incision of the testicular capsule from pole to pole at a point opposite the vessels and epididymis with evacuation of the haematoma.

Atrophy and necrosis of the testicle are rare when the testicular artery alone is ligated because of a good collateral circulation. The artery of the vas deferens usually provides sufficient blood supply to the testicle. When the ligation of the testicular artery is combined with the dissection and mobilisation of the testicle from the scrotum, or during the repair of recurrent inguinal hernia, the necrosis can occur. This manoeuvre (the dissection and mobilisation of the testicle) should be avoided when possible.[1,4,10]

Displacement of the testes up in the scrotum or into the inguinal canal can occur postoperatively. It is a good habit, following the operation and after the dressing has been applied, and the patient is still under anaesthesia, to palpate the testicle and pull it down to the scrotum; this manoeuvre will also straighten up the spermatic cord into the inguinal canal.

Hydrocele and Seroma

Hydrocele and seroma are rare complications of inguinal hernia repair. The implicated etiology is a lymphatic disruption following dissection of the sac from the cord. Usually they resolve in a few days; occasionally needle aspiration is necessary and can be repeated as indicated.[6]

Visceral Complications

Bladder injury

The bladder can be part of the sac as a sliding portion of an indirect inguinal hernia and is almost always present in the sac of an internal oblique hernia. The bladder is recognised by the prevesical fat, and its opening should be prevented. If the bladder is accidentally opened, and recognised by the exposed mucosa, repair should be done with absorbable suture in two layers. A Foley catheter is left in place for five days and removed only after a cystogram is performed and found negative. If the injury is not recognised, and is located in the extraperitoneal portion of the bladder, a urinoma will form. The treatment consists of debridement, closure of the bladder wound, drainage, and a

Foley catheter for three weeks. In rare cases, when the injury is at the intraperitoneal portion of the bladder urinary peritonitis will follow. This will require exploratory laparotomy, closure of the bladder in two layers, irrigation, IV antibiotics and a Foley catheter.

Ureter

The ureter can be injured especially in a large sliding hernia, when the bladder and ureter are down in the sac. The injury to the ureter can be a partial or complete transection or a resection of a segment. The partial or total transection can be sutured over a ureteral catheter; the resection of a segment of the ureter may require a ureteroneocystostomy.

Bowel injury

The large bowel can be injured during ligation of the sac in the sliding hernia when part of the sac is the bowel in incarcerated hernia.

During the repair of an indirect inguinal hernia the ligation of the sac should always be placed only when the sac is open, the content is reduced back into the peritoneal cavity, and the adhesions are lysed. The peritoneum should be sutured, either by transfixion, purse string or in a continuous manner under direct vision and with adequate exposure. This will avoid accidental incorporation into the suture of the small bowel, large bowel and omentum that may bring about possible complications such as abscess, fistula, bowel obstruction and free perforation.

Sliding hernia

A sliding hernia by definition is one in which the viscus itself forms with visceral peritoneum part of the wall of the sac. Bladder, ureter, tubes, ovaries and the uterus can be part of the serosal of the sac. Opening of the sac in a sliding hernia is unnecessary and can be avoided. When the sac has been freed from the structure of the cord, it can be reduced and the floor repaired. When the sac is accidentally opened no attempt should be made to dissect off the organ. The peritoneum and the sac should be closed and reduced, and the hernia repaired.

Laparoscopy

Laparoscopy is a relatively new approach for hernia repair used since the early 1990s. The laparoscopy technique for the repair of inguinal hernia requires general anaesthesia, the use of the mesh all of the time, and violation of the peritoneal cavity in some techniques.

The trans-abdominal peritoneal groin hernia repair consists of an incision of the peritoneum over the defect and the reduction of the sac; the sac can be transected, or left inside. The mesh is placed to cover the defect over the spermatic cord, or it can be split and placed around the cord after its mobilisation. The mesh is fixed in place with staples or tacks to the Cooper ligament inferiorly, and superiorly, above the ileo-pubic tract, to the anterior abdominal wall to either side of the epigastric vessels.

Intraperitoneal onlay mesh repair is still used by few. This approach should be discouraged. Polypropylene mesh should not be left free in direct contact with the peritoneal cavity.

Total or near total extraperitoneal mesh groin hernia repair consists of using the laparoscope and/or the balloon dissector device to create and develop a preperitoneal space. This will allow the management of the sac and the lipoma, and the placement of the mesh in the preperitoneal space, and its fixation in the same fashion to the Cooper ligament and to the anterior abdominal wall.[11-13]

Complications due to the laparoscopic access

Complications due to the laparoscopic access include wound port infection, hernia, subcutaneous emphysema, haemorrhage and visceral perforation.

Wound port infections in hernia are rare and easily treated. Subcutaneous and genital emphysema can appear grotesque, but it is usually well tolerated by the patient, is self-limiting, and rarely requires needle aspiration. The patient needs to be reassured. Bleeding from the abdominal wall vessels caused by trocar insertion is easily controlled by pressure, electrocautery, and occasionally by suturing. Bleeding from major vessels such as the internal or external iliac artery and vein is rare, but serious. Immediate laparotomy will be required to control the bleeding and repair the injury.

Complications specific to the laparoscopic hernia repair

Complications specific to the laparoscopic dissection and repair of groin hernia are bleeding from the preperitoneal space, inferior deep epigastric vessels and iliac vessels, bladder and bowel injuries, and recurrences.

Most of the bleeding from the preperitoneal space is easily controlled with electrocautery. Bleeding from the deep epigastric vessels requires a haemoclip or suturing. Injury to the iliac vessels is very rare, but when it occurs, emergent laparotomy will be life-saving.

Nerve injury

The most common nerve injured during laparoscopic hernia repair is the genital femoral nerve due to its entrapment by staple or tack. This injury can be avoided by the judicious placement of the staples. The ileo-hypogastric, the ileo-inguinal, the laterocutaneous and the femoral nerves can also be injured.

Recurrences

Recurrences after laparoscopic groin hernia repair are between 0.2 and 5%, and they are mostly due to learning curve, mesh size and incomplete fixation.

Most of the recurrences arise during the learning curve, due to the use of a small-size mesh and/or incomplete fixation. The mesh should be large enough to cover the entire myopectineal orifice. The fixation of the mesh must be complete with staples or tacks using a judiciously chosen anatomical site. The use of a larger mesh and a greater number of staples will reduce the incidence of recurrence as demonstrated, but at the same time it will slightly increase the incidence of complications due to mesh and staples.

Visceral injury

The bladder is the most common viscus injury during laparoscopic hernia repair. The small bowel and large bowel as well as the omentum can be occasionally injured.

COMPLICATIONS OF PROSTHETIC HERNIA REPAIR

Prosthetic materials are commonly used today to repair ventral and groin hernias. Polypropylene and PTFE are the most frequent mesh material employed. Prosthetic material is a foreign body and elicits a host tissue reaction.

Complications from the use of prosthetic material for hernia repair are to be considered potentially serious; these include infection, intraperitoneal adhesions with bowel obstruction, erosion with chronic sinus tract formation, and recurrence due to contraction of the prosthesis.

Infection

The use of prosthetic material is associated with a low rate of infection; although it is higher when mesh is not used, it still remains a rare event. The infection is prevented by adequate antisepsis of the surgical site, a shower or bath taken by the patient the night before the operation, shaving of the patient in the operating room, good skin prep, and no breaking of the surgical technique. Prophylactic systemic broad-spectrum antibiotics are given one hour before the operation. The mesh is embedded in betadine solution prior to its use. Good haemostasis and surgical technique are paramount, and fixing of the mesh must avoid redundancy.

When the wound becomes infected after groin hernia repair, the mesh must be removed, debridement of the necrotic tissue performed, and systemic IV antibiotics administered. It is not an easy task to remove the mesh and debride all non-viable tissue. The anatomy is distorted and hidden; the iliac vessel must be carefully identified. The spermatic cord can be affected by the infection, and becomes necrotic jeopardising the viability of the testicle. When debridement of the spermatic cord is completed, orchiectomy may become necessary.

When the mesh becomes infected after an incisional hernia repair, a more conservative approach can be taken.

When the infection is localised, debridement and irrigation are sufficient; and when good granulation tissue appears, the wound can be left to heal by second intention, or skin grafted.

The infection should be treated aggressively when severe, or when accompanied by a chronic sinus tract or enteric fistula. Waiting is not an option.

The management consists of total parenteral nutrition, systemic antibiotics, removal of the mesh, and bowel resection when indicated. The operative field and wound are irrigated with copious saline and an antibiotic solution. The abdomen will be closed with the aid of biological material.[10,14]

There are other rare complications of hernia repair that include osteitis pubis, omental tumour, acute urinary retention, postoperative ileus, postoperative mechanical obstruction and subcutaneous transection of the penis.

CONCLUSION

Knowledge of the anatomy of the groin, accomplished technical skills, the application of well recognised surgical principles, clean anatomical dissection, conservation and respect of nerves and other regional anatomical structures, high ligation of the sac, secure coaptation of tissue, the judicious use of prosthetic material, complete haemostasis, and the gentle handling of the tissues, are of paramount importance in the attainment of success in an operation for groin hernia repair. Success is measured by a low number of recurrences as well as a low incidence of complications.

REFERENCES

1. Fong Y, Wantz GE. (1971) Prevention of ischaemic orchitis during inguinal hernioplasty. *Surg Gynecol Obstet* **50**: 207–212.
2. Sandhu PS, Osborn DE. (1991) Surgical techniques for inguinal surgery and its effect on fertility in the Wistar rat model. *Br J Urol* **68**: 513–517.
3. Shandling B, Janik JS. (1981) The vulnerability of the vas deferens. *J Pediatr Surg* **16**: 461–464.
4. Bendavid R, Andrews DF, Gilbert AI. (1995) Testicular atrophy: incidence and relationship to the type of hernia and to multiple recurrent hernias. *Probl Gen Surg* **12**: 225–227.
5. Bendavid R. (1992) Dysejaculation: an unusual complication of inguinal herniorrhaphy. *Postgrad Gen Surg* **4**: 139–141.
6. Obney N. (1956) Hydroceles of the testicle complicating inguinal hernias. *Can Med Assoc J* **75**: 733.
7. DeBord J. (1994) Vascular complication of hernia surgery. In: Bendavid R (ed), *Prostheses and Abdominal Wall Hernias* (RG Landes Company, Austin), pp. 457–466.

8. Moosman DA, Oelrich TM. (1977) Prevention of accidental trauma to the ilioinguinal nerve during inguinal herniorrhaphy. *Am J Surg* **133**: 146–148.

9. Laha RK, Rao S, Pidgeon CN, *et al.* (1977). Genitofemoral neuralgia. *Surg Neurol* **8**: 280.

10. Wantz GE. (1984) Complications of inguinal hernia repair. *Surg Clin North Am* **64**: 287.

11. Arregui ME, Navrette J, David CJ. (1993) Laparoscopic inguinal herniorrhaphy: techniques and controversies. *Surg Clin North Am* **73**: 513–527.

12. MacFadyen BV, Arregui M, Corbitt J, *et al.* (1993). Complications of laparoscopic herniorrhaphy. *Surg Endosc* **7**(3): 155–158.

13. Phillips EH, Arregui M, Carroll BJ, *et al.* (1995). Incidence of complications following laparoscopic hernioplasty. *Surg Endosc* **9**(1): 16–21.

14. Pollack R, Nyhus LM. (1983) Complications of groin hernia repair. *Surg Clin North Am* **63**: 1362.

Chapter 16

COMPLICATIONS
IN ENDOCRINE SURGERY

Panagiotis B. Kekis, Simon G. T. Smith, John A. Lynn
and William R. Fleming

THYROID AND PARATHYROID SURGERY

Introduction

As with other surgical procedures, thyroidectomy and parathyroidectomy also carry the risk of complications. Surgery of the thyroid and parathyroid glands takes place in an area of complicated anatomy and a thorough knowledge of potential complications is mandatory.[1]

The initial attempts at thyroid surgery by Billroth and Kocher carried very high rates of morbidity and mortality, and was only recommended for life-saving reasons.[2] A thorough understanding of the anatomical and pathological features of the thyroid gland and improvement in surgical technique during the early years of the 20th century has dramatically reduced the incidence of postoperative complications.[3]

The presence of the parathyroid glands and their function went unrecognised for a long time, and their diseases were one of the last to be defined. The glands were identified in humans by Ivar Sandstrom[4] only in the latter part of the 19th century. In the decades that followed, the role of the parathyroids in the regulation of calcium metabolism was recognised, and the place of surgery defined.[5]

Most of the significant contributions to successful thyroid and parathyroid surgery were made in the beginning of the 20th century,[6] and further improvement has led to the recognition of endocrine surgery as a specialty. It is well documented that complication rates in thyroid and parathyroid surgery are lower in expert hands.[7]

In the last decade, minimally invasive techniques have been developed for the surgical treatment of various thyroid and parathyroid disorders,[8–12] but complication rates are similar to standard surgical procedures and will not be discussed separately in this chapter.[13,14]

Nerve Complications

Recurrent laryngeal nerve injury

Recurrent laryngeal nerve injury is a major obstacle in thyroid and parathyroid surgery and the most feared of all potential complications.[15,16] A sound knowledge of the regional anatomy and awareness of the possible course of the nerve is crucial to minimising the risk of damage. The factors that influence its likelihood are the underlying disease (i.e., goitre vs. malignancy), the extent of resection in thyroidectomy or dissection in the case of parathyroidectomy, the experience of the surgeon, anatomical abnormalities, and reoperation (i.e., completion thyroidectomy, persistent hyperparathyroidism).

The paired recurrent laryngeal nerves arise from the vagus, turn back on themselves in the chest and run superiorly into the neck. They supply all the muscles of the larynx, except the cricothyroid, and are sensory to the larynx below the vocal folds. On the right side the nerve hooks around the subclavian artery, while on the left it swings around the ligamentum arteriosum and the arch of the aorta. On both sides the nerve classically ascends in the tracheoesophageal groove but the right nerve courses more obliquely, as it is relatively more lateral in position. The nerves cross the inferior thyroid artery as they ascend superiorly and medially. Their relationship to the branches of the inferior thyroid artery is inconsistent and they may pass deep, superficial, or within the terminal branches of the artery.[17] The most common position of the nerve is deep to the artery (50–80%) and less commonly, within the terminal branches.[18] The surgeon must not only be aware of this, but also remember that this relationship may vary between the two sides of the neck in up to 50% of patients.[19] During ligation of the inferior thyroid artery it is safest to divide the vessel under direct vision on the thyroid capsule to avoid damaging the nerve[20] and devascularising the parathyroid glands.

Finally, the nerves on both sides pass posterior and lateral to the thyroid lobe, beneath the ligament of Berry, a thickened fascia on the trachea just below the cricoid. At this level is the tubercle of Zuckerkandl, a thickening of thyroid tissue that is located at the most posterolateral edge of the thyroid gland. From the surgical point of view it is important to remember that the tubercle is in close anatomic relationship with the recurrent laryngeal nerve and the parathyroid glands.[1,21] Normally, the recurrent laryngeal nerve will course posterior and lateral to the thyroid lobe. However, the tubercle of Zuckerkandl can extend sufficiently posterior to end up behind the nerve.[19]

Before entering the larynx along the posterior aspect of the cricothyroid muscle, the recurrent laryngeal nerve will often break into a number of branches, with all the motor fibres usually in the most medial branch.[19] If this extra-laryngeal branching is not recognised, part of the nerve may be injured.

A difficulty in identifying the recurrent laryngeal nerve during surgery may indicate that the nerve is non-recurrent.[18,22] This variant has a reported incidence of 1% on the right side, but only 0.04% on the left.[18] The presence of non-recurrent laryngeal nerves can be explained by developmental abnormalities of the arterial system. If there is an anomalous origin of the right subclavian artery when the right fourth aortic arch and the proximal right dorsal aorta are obliterated,[18,19] the nerve may be non-recurrent.[23] A left non-recurrent nerve occurs when there is situs inversus, an extremely unusual vascular anomaly.

The nerve may also be totally non-recurrent entering the larynx directly from behind the carotid artery, or very rarely both the recurrent and non-recurrent inferior laryngeal nerves may co-exist.[18,23] The observation of an unusually thin recurrent nerve should alert the surgeon to the possibility of a non-recurrent nerve.[24]

In thyroidectomy, the recurrent laryngeal nerve is at greatest risk during the ligation of the inferior thyroid artery and dissection near the ligament of

Berry.[19] In parathyroid surgery the nerve is at risk during the dissection of the two upper glands. The two upper parathyroids are normally positioned just above or immediately behind the inferior thyroid artery, close to the posterior border of the thyroid and in close relation to the recurrent laryngeal nerve.

The reported incidence of recurrent laryngeal nerve palsy varies considerably (0–17%) for thyroid and parathyroid surgeries.[2] In the hands of an experienced surgeon permanent injury to the recurrent laryngeal nerve should occur in less than 1% of patients, although transient dysfunction may occur more often.[2]

A routine identification of the recurrent laryngeal nerve during thyroidectomy and parathyroidectomy greatly decreases the risk of temporary and permanent nerve injury.[16,25] The authors insist that it is necessary to identify the nerve in all cases and no structure passing medially from the carotid sheath is divided, except the middle thyroid vein, until the nerve is located.[18] The nerve is identified low in the neck and its course followed to the point of entry into the larynx. However, one should be careful not to devascularise the inferior parathyroid glands by dividing the lateral vascular attachments. In identifying the recurrent laryngeal nerves, it is useful to remember that a tiny vessel (vas nervorum) runs parallel to and directly on each nerve. In younger patients the artery is usually readily distinguished from the recurrent laryngeal nerve, but in older patients with arteriosclerosis, the artery appears white and may be mistaken for the nerve.[26] Some surgeons recommend identifying the nerve cephalad to the inferior thyroid artery where it enters the larynx, because its course there is more consistent.[2] Others suggest that palpation against the lateral tracheal wall is a useful technique for identifying the nerve, but the authors have not been impressed with this technique other than as a means to identify the site of the nerve prior to positive visualisation.

Yet another technique to avoid injury is the capsular dissection of the thyroid gland.[18,27] Here, the dissection is maintained on the capsule while keeping the thyroid in tension through medial and anterior traction. The nerve is not routinely identified although it is usually seen at the ligament of Berry.

Retrosternal goitres require special care in the identification of the recurrent laryngeal nerves.[28] In up to 90% of the cases, goitres extending into the thorax lie anterior to the major vessels and recurrent laryngeal nerves,[18] but the remainder descend posteriorly, particularly on the right side of the neck.

Identifying the nerve by a thoracic approach may be limited, and the authors support an initial cervical approach, proceeding to thoracotomy if necessary.

More recently, it has become possible to monitor the recurrent laryngeal nerve by intraoperative nerve stimulation, and is associated with low rates of temporary and permanent nerve paralysis.[29,30] Additionally, knowledge of the status of the nerve following dissection provides the surgeon with important information, should a patient develop stridor postoperatively. This technique may also prove useful during reoperative surgery when the risk of injury is higher because of scarring. Microsurgical techniques have also been reported as being effective in reducing the risk of laryngeal nerve injury.[31]

A routine preoperative laryngoscopy will identify patients with an apparently normal voice but with unrecognised vocal cord dysfunction. However, its necessity may be questioned[32]; most surgeons consider it prudent to perform laryngoscopy when there is a history of voice change or previous neck surgery.[16,33] Routine laryngoscopy at extubation has been found to be unreliable in most studies, and postoperative laryngoscopy should be reserved for patients with symptoms.[34]

Unilateral iatrogenic injury to the nerve is usually manifested by a weak, hoarse and breathy voice. In the postoperative assessment of the larynx, the affected vocal cord tends to lie in a paramedian position. If the nerve has been positively identified over its entire course, the paralysis should be temporary and resolve with time. If the position of the paralysed cord is midline and the "compensation" by the contralateral cord is good, the damage may not be recognised. The symptoms secondary to intubation and oedema of the larynx[35] are similar to those following unilateral injury to the nerve.

The main effect of bilateral nerve injury is on the maintenance of the airway, with the voice often remarkably normal. It produces airway obstruction and respiratory distress, with the vocal cords remaining together in the midline position. Bilateral injury presents with stridor on extubation and the patient must be reintubated or a tracheostomy performed. Furthermore, delayed presentation can also occur due to the splinting effect of the endotracheal tube in the denervated larynx and the abducted position of the vocal cords. These patients are consequently diagnosed late with dyspnoea and stridor, following an increase in the respiratory demand.[19]

Most injuries to the nerves are temporary and only supportive measures may be necessary if there is no acute respiratory distress and the patient's speech is acceptable. Nerve recovery is likely within a few days after surgery, especially if visualised during the operation,[19] but in some cases, is known to take as long as twelve months. Surgical measures may be necessary in patients with a persistently incompetent glottis, resulting in dyspnoea or stridor. In unilateral vocal cord palsy, medialisation of the vocal cord is the goal and can be achieved by injection of materials (Teflon paste, hydrogen gel or silicon), thyroplasty or re-innervation techniques.[18] In bilateral palsy the functional problem to be corrected is the midline position of the vocal cords. Nerve or nerve-muscle transplantation and vocal cord lateralisation procedures have been described.[18,36] However, it must be realised that surgical correction of bilateral abductor palsy cannot result in both normal airway and normal voice.[36] A failed surgery leads to permanent tracheostomy tube with a speaking valve.

superior laryngeal nerve injury

The superior laryngeal nerve arises from the vagus and descends inferiorly, medial to the carotid arteries. It then divides at the level of the hyoid bone to the larger internal and the smaller external laryngeal nerves.[37]

The internal laryngeal nerve is the sensory branch of the superior laryngeal nerve. It penetrates the thyrohyoid membrane and conveys sensory branches from the mucosa of the larynx above the vocal cords and the posterior pharynx. Because of its superior location, the internal branch of the superior laryngeal nerve is rarely subject to injury during thyroidectomy. This nerve is at risk only when an enlarged superior pole of the thyroid gland extends above the upper border of the thyroid cartilage and the surgeon dissects in this area.[38] An injury causes a loss of sensation to the upper half of the larynx and posterior pharynx, resulting in dysphagia, aspiration and consequent pneumonitis.[26]

The external laryngeal nerve provides motor innervation to the cricothyroid muscle and is responsible for tensing the vocal cords when they are approximated; it is also known as the high note nerve or the Amelita Galli-Curci nerve.[19] The injury to this nerve is less well described and overshadowed by the problems associated with damage to the recurrent laryngeal nerve.[39] The loss of innervation of the cricothyroid muscle results in laxity of the vocal cord on the affected side. Unilateral injury will change the timbre of the voice and markedly diminish the capacity to project any volume. Bilateral injury can result in a hoarse, monotonous voice that fatigues easily. An injury to the external branch of the superior laryngeal nerve is underestimated and infrequently reported, because the symptoms are subtle. However, it can be career-threatening for those in professions that require a strong voice, such as singing and teaching.

The terminal part of the external branch of the superior laryngeal nerve runs in close proximity to the superior thyroid artery and is therefore vulnerable when the vessels of the superior pole are ligated. In 20% of the patients, the nerve lies within the thyroid sheath at the level where the superior thyroid artery bifurcates, making it particularly vulnerable during its division.[40] In another 20% the nerve is located within the cricothyroid muscle and therefore unlikely to be injured.[2] In the majority of patients the external laryngeal nerve runs on the surface of the cricothyroid muscle and penetrates the muscle at a low level.[18]

Caudal traction of the upper pole of the thyroid to ligate the branches of the superior thyroid artery may cause transient paresis of the nerve. This can be prevented by providing a gentle traction on the thyroid gland in a caudal and lateral direction and ligating the vessels directly on the capsule of the upper pole individually and low on the thyroid gland. The need for routine identification of this nerve during thyroidectomy is controversial,[3] although the author's opinion is that one should generally try to avoid it rather than identify it.

Miscellaneous nerve injuries

Lymph nodes in the central neck are frequently involved in patients with papillary, medullary and Hürthle cell cancer and a central clearance of para-tracheal lymph nodes between the carotid arteries down to the innominate vessel is necessary.[26,41] In patients with medullary cancer and extensive lym-phadenopathy, a lateral modified neck dissection can be beneficial.[42] The potential complications from this type of dissection include injury to the spinal accessory, phrenic and vagus nerves, the cervical sympathetic trunk and the hypoglossal nerve, all of which may be adherent to or directly invaded by the tumour.

Damage to the cervical sympathetic trunk in a routine thyroidectomy or parathyroidectomy is rare. However, extensive malignancy, retro-oesophageal extension of goitre or anatomical abnormalities can injure this structure.[1] The division of the sympathetic trunk causes Horner's syndrome,[43] but the authors have encountered only two cases in over 8000 thyroidectomies. The dissection of the prespinal surface may damage the sympathetic trunk, such as while mobilising the carotid sheath in parathyroidectomy.

Vascular Complications

Haemorrhage

Thyroid and parathyroid operations should be performed in a blood-free field so that vital structures can be identified. If bleeding occurs, pressure should be applied. The vessel should be clamped only if it can be precisely identified or the recurrent laryngeal nerve has been identified and is not in close proximity to the vessel.[1]

Following thyroidectomy and parathyroidectomy, postoperative bleeding into the deep cervical space can result in a tension haematoma with subsequent laryngeal oedema, tracheal compression and life-threatening respiratory compromise.[3] Massive bleeding is usually arterial in origin and in most cases will occur within four hours of surgery; however, it can also occur any time in the first 24 hours postoperatively. Delayed venous haemorrhage over a few days can also occur, but is usually less serious and its treatment is by aspiration or evacuation of the clot.[18]

Bleeding is the result of inadequately secured vessels. It can be avoided by careful assessment before wound closure, with the patient in a Trendelenberg position and a Valsalva manoeuvre performed, to raise the venous pressure. Substantial blood vessels should be tied with fine ligatures, while small vessels can be managed with diathermy. More recently, haemostatic devices such as the harmonic scalpel and the Ligasure system have been used in thyroid and parathyroid surgeries,[44] but their efficacy over standard techniques is yet to be proved in randomised studies. Haemostatic materials such as methylcellulose can be used to manage bleeding in areas where diathermy or ligation may injure the nervous structures.

Suction drains reduce the consequences of oozing, but fail to help patients with massive haematomas, and may also increase the risk of wound infection.[45] Therefore, most studies suggest that routine drainage is unnecessary following an uncomplicated thyroid or parathyroid surgery.[46] Drainage may be necessary when there is a large dead space, such as after the removal of a large or substernal goitre, or extensive neck dissection for malignant neoplasm.[47] Postoperatively, elevation of the head of the bed and the use of a gentle pressure dressing may be beneficial.

The reported incidence of haematoma following surgery for thyroid and parathyroid disease is low, ranging from 0.7–1.6%.[3,48] If tracheal compression and acute respiratory distress occur from a haematoma in the deep cervical space, the neck incision should be opened and the haematoma evacuated. If respiratory distress is severe, opening of the wound can be performed at the bedside, with haemostasis achieved in the operating theatre. The authors do not favour emergency endotracheal intubation as laryngeal oedema often makes this impossible. Evacuation of the clot at the bedside is much safer and the patient can return immediately to the operating room for exploration of the wound under sterile conditions.[2,3]

Carotid artery and jugular vein injury

The carotid artery and jugular vein are rarely at risk of injury, but may be vulnerable in cases of extensive malignancy or re-exploration. Additionally, unintentional excessive lateral retraction may reduce the carotid artery flow, with subsequent ocular or central nervous damage.[1] This is especially important in older patients where the carotid arteries may be atherosclerotic or stenotic and the blood supply to the brain is already impaired.

Failed Surgery — Metabolic Complications

Thyroid

Postoperative hypocalcaemia — hypoparathyroidism

Hypocalcaemia, either transient or permanent, is the most common surgical complication associated with thyroidectomy,[49] arising from the removal, injury or devascularisation of the parathyroid glands.

The reported incidence of transient hypocalcaemia following thyroid surgery is up to 50%,[2,49–51] while permanent hypocalcaemia has a lower reported incidence ranging between 3–25%.[52–55] The incidence is directly related to the surgeon's experience, the operative technique, the underlying pathology, the extent of the disease and whether or not it is a re-operation procedure.[17,54–58]

A detailed knowledge of the embryology and anatomy of the glands is essential to minimise the risk of damage. Despite care taken to preserve the glands, occasionally a parathyroid within the thyroid parenchyma is inadvertently removed,[59,60] resulting in unexpected hypocalcaemia.[61,62]

Hypocalcaemia is more commonly caused by the devascularisation of the parathyroid glands following ligation of the inferior thyroid artery while identifying the recurrent laryngeal nerve. In 80% of the glands the blood supply is solely derived from the inferior thyroid artery,[2] so that ligation of the branches of the artery close to the thyroid capsule can be protective.[27] The operative field should be kept dry always so that the parathyroids can be identified and their vascular supply preserved.

It has been reported that the incidence of permanent hypoparathyroidism can be diminished substantially by the use of parathyroid autotransplantation.[63,64] If the gland looks partially ischaemic the authors recommend leaving them on their own vascular pedicle, as it has been shown that microcirculation recovers.[65] If there has been complete devascularisation of a parathyroid, part of the gland should be sent for biopsy to confirm its identity and autotransplanted as 1×1 mm pieces into separate pockets in the sternocleidomastoid muscle. After a lobe is removed or especially after a total thyroidectomy, the specimen should be always inspected to be sure that there are no possible parathyroid glands on the thyroid.

Some authors recommend the use of an intraoperative PTH assay in the management of thyroid disease to prevent and treat symptomatic hypocalcaemia, thereby reducing re-admissions following thyroidectomy.[66,67]

The symptoms of hypocalcaemia usually develop 1–5 days postoperatively and include numbness and tingling around the mouth, hands and feet. Chvostek's or Trousseau's signs may be present and progress to tetany. In the asymptomatic patient with low levels of serum calcium, oral supplementation with calcium carbonate should be initiated (2–3 g/day). For mild symptoms, oral supplementation of calcium should be increased combined with a rapid acting Vitamin D analogue (0.5–1 μg/day) and a prolonged hospital stay should be considered. In these instances serum calcium levels should be monitored closely as many cases will resolve spontaneously. Intravenous calcium gluconate is warranted in case of an emergency. Recently some reports have suggested the routine use of oral calcium supplementation, as it appears to prevent symptomatic hypocalcaemia after total thyroidectomy and allows for a safe early discharge.[68,69]

Thyroid storm

Thyroid storm is a rare but serious complication following thyroid surgery in patients with untreated or inadequately treated hyperthyroidism.[70] It is caused by an abnormally high rate of synthesis and release of thyroid hormone. The total thyroid hormone levels do not differ significantly between severe hyperthyroidism and thyroid storm, but the free hormone levels are substantially increased.[70] It can also be triggered by common stressful precipitating factors such as infection and trauma.[71]

The diagnosis is clinical and any delay in the recognition and treatment can be potentially life threatening.[72] The clinical picture is dominated by signs of severe acute hyperthyroidism, such as rapid, high and persistent temperature elevation, tachycardia, altered mental status, delirium, psychosis, nausea, vomiting, abdominal pain and diarrhoea. These signs can be less obvious in the elderly. If left unrecognised and untreated, a thyroid storm can lead to critical failure of a number of organ systems including cardiac, cerebral, hepatic, renal and gastrointestinal.[73]

The goal of treatment is to provide supportive therapy, in an intensive care unit, and inhibit the release and synthesis of thyroid hormone. The supportive measures include fluid and electrolyte balance, sedation, cooling blankets and oxygen supplementation.

The excess thyroid hormone should be counteracted with large doses of an antithyroid drug (Propylthiouracil or Carbimazole) orally or via a nasogastric tube. Propylthiouracil (150–300 mg × 3/day) is preferred because it inhibits the peripheral conversion of T4 to T3 and prevents intraglandular hormone storage. Iodine is also administered to block the release of preformed thyroid hormone from the thyroid gland, given either orally (5 drops × 6/day) or intravenously (0.5 g × 2/day). Glucocorticoid support (Dexamethasone (2 mg/day) or Hydrocortisone Sodium Succinate) given orally or intravenously acts synergistically with propylthiouracil and iodine to prevent the conversion of T4 to T3. Propranolol (40–80 mg × 6/day orally or up to 2 mg IV) and other beta-adrenergic agents are used for symptomatic relief, but care must be exercised in patients with cardiac failure,[74] when diuretics and digoxin may be indicated. Paracetamol should be used for controlling fever as aspirin competes with T3 and T4 for binding to thyroid binding globulin, leading to increased circulating levels of free thyroid hormone.[70,72]

Postoperative hypothyroidism — recurrent hyperthyroidism

Surgery is performed on the thyroid gland to reduce its function (thyrotoxicosis), reduce its volume (non-toxic goitre) or treat malignancy. Surgery must be sufficient for treatment and extensive enough to avoid the need for reoperation, while minimising the risk of injury to the parathyroid glands or recurrent laryngeal nerves. The appropriate extent of surgery for various pathological thyroid conditions remains controversial.[75–77]

Most surgeons regard total thyroidectomy as the preferred treatment for the majority of patients with thyroid cancer, while some feel that hemithyroidectomy is sufficient for those with good-prognosis thyroid cancer.[78–80] Total thyroidectomy is favoured because of the risk of multicentricity of the tumour within the gland, the ability to scan and treat metastases with radioactive iodine, and the ability to follow up with serum thyroglobulin assays.[79,81] There is evidence that a more radical surgery results in a lower local recurrence rate and improved survival, especially with tumours that have a predicted poor prognosis.[79,82] An expert surgeon can safely perform a total thyroidectomy with low morbidity.[49,83] In total thyroidectomy for cancer, hypothyroidism is an inevitable consequence of operation but is not regarded as a complication; it is easily controlled by thyroxine replacement and monitoring.

The surgical treatment of Graves' disease is also controversial, but plays a significant role in patients with failed medical therapy.[76] In some centres, surgery has become the treatment of choice due to the relatively high relapse rate after medical therapy. But it requires striking a balance between the risk of recurrent or persistent hyperthyroidism and postoperative hypothyroidism.

subtotal thyroidectomy has been the traditional operation for a century because of the possibility of avoiding thyroxine therapy, along with an assumed lower risk of complications compared with total thyroidectomy.[84] Unfortunately there is no reliable method to assess the amount of thyroid tissue to be preserved in subtotal thyroidectomy, and the outcome is unpredictable.[84] Thyroid remnants may hypertrophy in the future, causing pressure effects or suspicion of malignancy, especially if the recurrence is nodular. Ectopic thyroid tissue, such as with thyroid rests lying low in the neck or upper mediastinum, may also be left behind in subtotal operations, leading to the recurrence or persistence of symptoms. Similarly, posterior lobes may be missed at subtotal thyroid surgery.

A subtotal thyroidectomy also carries an unavoidable risk of recurrent hyperthyroidism, which may require radioactive iodine treatment or re-operation, with a marked rise in the incidence of complications.[33] The long-term results of subtotal thyroidectomy are not as good as they were previously believed to be, with an increasing incidence of hypothyroidism,[84] which may develop insidiously and remain unrecognised and untreated, increasing in frequency and reaching upto 73% after seven years.[85] The incidence of postoperative hypothyroidism is related to the amount of gland removed, the lymphocytic infiltration of the gland, and maybe even previous iodine intake.[3] The authors believe that if the risks of complications are recognised as equivalent for total and subtotal thyroidectomy, the former procedure offers significant advantages in the surgical management of Graves' disease.

For the treatment of hyperthyroidism in toxic multinodular goitre, surgery is conceived as the last step in a multidisciplinary approach.[86] Some authors believe that surgery is a good alternative to antithyroid agents, which are constraining and often ineffective in the long term, and radioactive iodine which often leads to hypothyroidism.[87] Most surgeons were in favour of bilateral subtotal thyroidectomy or subtotal excision of one lobe and total excision of the other[88,89]; total thyroidectomy is currently favoured, and provides a definitive cure of toxic hyperthyroidism while avoiding the risk of recurrence.[90]

With benign multinodular goitre there is an increasing recognition that total thyroidectomy is appropriate when there is significant nodular disease involving both lobes.[91,92] However, it must be emphasised that protection of the recurrent laryngeal nerve and parathyroid glands is paramount in dealing with benign thyroid disease.[91] subtotal thyroidectomy is not a satisfactory procedure, with a long-term recurrence rate as high as 45% despite the use of thyroxine therapy.[93,94] Total or near-total thyroidectomy in multinodular goitre also eliminates the necessity for early completion thyroidectomy should the final diagnosis be thyroid cancer.[95]

Parathyroid

Persistent or recurrent hyperparathyroidism

In the past, surgery of the parathyroid glands had a notorious reputation, but the outcome has improved substantially during the last 50 years.[96] A better understanding of parathyroid disease, thorough knowledge of the anatomy and embryology, as well as advances in operative technique have led to very high rates of successful surgery.[97]

Normally, there are four parathyroid glands (two pairs) in close association with the thyroid. Each gland measures approximately $6 \times 4 \times 2$ mm and weighs between 30–50 mg. The number and positions of the glands may vary greatly among individuals, with a supernumerary fifth gland occurring in 2–13% of the patients. The supernumerary gland is usually found in the vicinity of the thyrothymic ligament or in the mediastinum. The presence of less than three glands is more unusual, with an incidence of less than 3%.

Embryologically, both glands have an endodermal origin. The superior parathyroid glands originate from the fourth branchial pouch, maintaining a close association with the developing thyroid. They have a short line of embryologic descent and remain close to the lateral lobe of the thyroid, coming to lie at the posterolateral surface of the upper poles of the thyroid. The inferior parathyroid glands originate from the third branchial pouch, follow the descent of the thymus and reach their final location at the posterolateral surface of the lower lobes of the thyroid. These glands have a long line of descent and as a result, their position is much more variable. Migration of the parathyroid glands during foetal development to their final juxtathyroidal location accounts for the complicated surgical approach to these glands.

In most of the cases, the upper glands are located posterior to the middle and upper third of the thyroid lobe and to the recurrent laryngeal nerves, cranially to the inferior thyroid artery. The inferior parathyroid glands are found near the inferior pole of the thyroid in the vicinity of the thyrothymic tract, but their location is more unpredictable. As the thymus migrates inferiorly, these glands can be carried to the superior mediastinum. Ectopic glands may be either within or outside of the thymus, along the line of the oesophagus, or less frequently in the midlower mediastinum, or even the pericardium. In contrast, the inferior parathyroid glands can be left behind, remaining high in the neck, anterior to the carotid bifurcation, in or lateral to the carotid sheath and even more cranially than the upper glands. Occasionally they lie within the thyroid capsule or clefts of thyroid tissue, (intrathyroidal) usually within the lower pole of the thyroid gland.

The variability in the number and location of the parathyroid glands may lead to situations where a patient has four normal glands in the neck and an abnormal fifth located in the mediastinum. Regardless of the inconsistency in their anatomy, there is a symmetrical arrangement between gland positions on either side of the neck in approximately 80% of the cases.

Surgery has an important role in primary, secondary and tertiary hyperparathyroidism,[98,99] and the results are excellent when an experienced endocrine surgeon performs the operation.[100–105]

Surgical failure results in persistent or recurrent hyperparathyroidism.[106–110] Persistent hyperparathyroidism is defined as hypercalcaemia occurring within six months of the initial surgery, while recurrent hyperparathyroidism is defined as hypercalcaemia occurring after a normocalcaemic period of six months. The most common reason for failure of surgery is the surgeon's inexperience, with inadequate exploration of the neck.[106] A detailed understanding of the development of the parathyroid glands, knowledge of their size and weight, and the variety of their position and number is essential.[111]

Surgery is the only curative therapy for primary hyperparathyroidism and should be considered in every patient except those with familial hypocalciuric hypercalcemia. Eighty to eighty-five per cent of the patients with primary hyperparathyroidism have sporadic, benign parathyroid adenomas caused by multi-gland hyperplasia. An experienced endocrine surgeon will cure more than 95% of patients undergoing initial bilateral neck exploration for this type of primary hyperparathyroidism.[104,112–116] Generally, preoperative localisation of the abnormal parathyroid glands is unnecessary for initial bilateral neck exploration.[117] In sporadic cases of primary hyperparathyroidism, a single adenomatous gland is usually found and removed. The golden rule for the endocrine surgeon is to identify all the parathyroid glands in the neck and exclude the possibility of asymmetric hyperplasia.

If bilateral exploration is performed for hyperplasia, all identified glands should be abnormal in size and supernumerary glands and ectopic parathyroid tissue should be excluded. Surgical options include subtotal parathyroidectomy, with removal of three and a half glands, or total parathyroidectomy and autotransplantation of a small remnant into the sternocleidomastoid or the forearm. Autotransplantation can be performed immediately or following cryopreservation[118] but carries a risk of recurrent hyperparathyroidism from the autotransplanted tissue. The most common cause of recurrent or persistent disease is the failure to recognise and remove all abnormal parathyroid tissue, with failed surgery rates ranging 3–8%.[103,115,119–124]

Despite high success rates and low morbidity with bilateral neck exploration for primary hyperparathyroidism, the trend is strongly towards minimally invasive surgery with smaller incisions, minimal exploration, and shorter hospital stay, while maintaining an excellent outcome. Minimally invasive techniques are feasible because of improvements in preoperative localisation by imaging with sestamibi scintigraphy and high-resolution ultrasonography, coupled with intraoperative rapid PTH assay. Minimally invasive parathyroidectomy refers to one of several procedures, including video-assisted endoscopic, radioguided, and unilateral image-guided explorations.[125–132] For a patient to be considered for this approach, the abnormal parathyroid gland must be located preoperatively on imaging studies[127]; patients with known or suspected multi-gland disease or prior neck surgery are generally not suitable for this procedure.

Although most cases are sporadic, up to 10% of the primary hyperparathyroid cases may be hereditary.[133] The hereditary forms often involve an abnormality of multiple parathyroid glands with hyperplasia rather than the single adenomatous parathyroid gland disease that is typically seen in sporadic cases.[134] Therefore, patients with known or suspected hereditary primary hyperparathyroidism should be identified preoperatively as they may require a more aggressive multi-gland resection.[134,135]

The most common form of hereditary primary hyperparathyroidism is Multiple Endocrine Neoplasia syndrome type 1 (MEN 1).[136] Patients with this syndrome present more severe symptoms at a younger age than those with sporadic disease.[137] The management is complex and patients are predisposed to persistent and recurrent disease.[135] Two approaches have been described as the best practice for these patients: subtotal parathyroidectomy and total parathyroidectomy with immediate autotransplantation. Cryopreservation of parathyroid tissue should be performed if possible. The failure to treat these patients can be as high as 40%.[138]

Primary hyperparathyroidism occurs less commonly in patients with MEN 2A and the disease presents in a milder form than in MEN 1.[139] MEN 2A requires resection of only the enlarged glands compared with subtotal resection in patients with other forms of multi-gland disease.[140] The incidence of persistent disease is over 8% and recurrent disease, over 14%.[140]

Nearly all patients with chronic renal failure exhibit some degree of secondary hyperparathyroidism. Despite improvements in the medical management of these patients, therapy often fails and parathyroidectomy becomes necessary to decrease the mass of the hyperplastic parathyroid tissue. The surgical procedure remains controversial; some surgeons prefer subtotal parathyroidectomy, while others prefer total parathyroidectomy with auto-transplantation of a small amount of tissue to the arm, because the transplanted tissue can be removed in the event of recurrent hyperparathyroidism.[117,124,141–148] In patients with renal failure, recurrence rates do not significantly differ with either procedure,[117,124,141–148] with a reported incidence between 5–80%.[113,117,124,141,142,145,146,148–150] Some authors advocate total parathyroidectomy without autotransplantation as a safe procedure with a low rate of recurrent hyperparathyroidism when compared with parathyroidectomy with autotransplantation to the forearm.[147,150] Persistent hyperparathyroidism may occur if there are supernumerary glands or there is a failure to perform total parathyroidectomy.[151–153] Recurrent hyperparathyroidism can be graft dependant and multiple operations to reduce the autograft may be needed.[154–156]

Some patients reveal parathyroid dysfunction after renal transplantation, with a condition known as tertiary hyperparathyroidism.[157] Once the diagnosis is confirmed, a parathyroidectomy is frequently necessary to decrease the mass of the hyperfunctioning parathyroid tissue.[158,159] Four gland parathyroid enlargement (hyperplasia) is often seen, although asymmetric enlargement (adenoma) can occur. Intraoperative findings should dictate surgical strategy, and in case of asymmetric enlargement, only the enlarged parathyroid glands should be resected.[158] Some authors recommend a conservative approach, with surgery reserved for patients with symptomatic disease and patients with asymptomatic persistent hypercalcemia greater than or equal to 3 mmol/l more than one year after transplantation.[159]

Reoperation for persistent or recurrent hyperparathyroidism has been reported to have a very high rate of success in expert hands,[105,109,153,160,161] but is generally associated with a higher incidence of complications. Therefore, it is crucial to refer these patients to a specialised endocrine surgery department.

The approach to the exploration of persistent or recurrent hyperparathyroidism is the same as for an initial exploration. The surgeon must first confirm the diagnosis[162] and all possible details of previous surgery must be obtained. Preoperative localisation is essential as scar tissue and altered anatomy make surgical exploration more demanding. The localisation studies include sestamibi scanning, ultrasound examination, selective venous sampling, MRI, and CT scanning.[161] Sestamibi imaging of the parathyroid gland has the best specificity and sensitivity (90–95% and 80–85%, respectively) but does not replace the need for an experienced endocrine surgeon. Furthermore, intraoperative parathyroid hormone assays and radio-guidance techniques have been used to improve the outcome of reoperation for persistent and recurrent disease.[163–167]

Miscellaneous Complications

Wound healing problem

Thyroid and parathyroid surgery is associated with a very low risk of wound complications and routine antibiotics are not indicated. Some authors have reported an increased incidence of wound infection with drain insertion,[45] but in most studies there has been no difference when a drain is used.[2,57]

Most wound infections in thyroid and parathyroid surgery appear to be endogenous and inflammatory conditions such as an acute pharyngitis must be excluded before surgery.[2] In the past, wound infections were frequently associated with the use of non-absorbable sutures, leading to suture sinuses and frequently re-operation.[48] The administration of antibiotics and opening the wound to drain any pus is usually sufficient treatment.

The cosmetic result in thyroid and parathyroid surgery is of great importance as the wound is central and anterior, and patients see their wounds each time they look in the mirror. However, the cosmetic result needs to be balanced against the need for adequate access so that safe surgery can be undertaken.[1]

A well positioned collar incision approximately 2 cm above the sternal notch and extending laterally to the anterior borders of the sternocleidomastoid gives adequate exposure and excellent cosmetic result.[168] The position and symmetry is very important and the authors recommend marking the line of incision on the skin always prior to surgery. The incision should ideally be placed in one of the natural skin creases of the neck, but not too low as a lower incision is more prone to keloid formation.[2,168] During closure of the wound it is important to appose the strap muscles together in the midline to prevent the skin from tethering to the trachea.[19] Skin closure can be achieved by non-absorbable fine interrupted sutures (nylon 4/0), surgical clips or subcuticular sutures, but the authors recommend the use of fine sutures.

The need for better cosmetic results has provided the impetus for a switch to minimal access thyroid and parathyroid surgery,[8] but a shorter incision length must take into account the specimen volume, patient body mass index, surgeon's experience, and in the case of parathyroidectomy, the extent of the planned exploration.[169]

Inadequate haemostasis during thyroid and parathyroid surgery sometimes leads to superficial haematomas, but bleeding is usually not severe and rarely requires reoperation.[57] Seroma is another rare wound complication after thyroid and parathyroid surgery[170] and its treatment is by aspiration.[2]

Airway compromise and tracheal injury

The preoperative predictive factors for the development of serious postoperative respiratory obstruction are goitre for more than five years, preoperative recurrent laryngeal nerve palsy, significant tracheal narrowing and/or deviation, retrosternal extension, difficult endotracheal intubation and thyroid cancer.[171] If there is any concern about an airway abnormality following thyroidectomy or parathyroidectomy and the patient's condition is stable, fibreoptic endoscopy can be performed.[19] When the patient is unstable endotracheal intubation should be first attempted, in preference to tracheostomy.[172]

Airway obstruction can follow a deep cervical haematoma, causing direct tracheal compression, or more frequently, laryngeal oedema and obstruction. This complication is more likely to occur within four hours of surgery.[18] As previously indicated, the treatment of a haematoma first involves urgent evacuation followed by a return to the theatre for definitive treatment.

Laryngeal oedema can also occur after a difficult and traumatic intubation which may accompany large and cancerous goitres.[173] Steroid therapy can be used in conjunction with prolonged intubation to decrease laryngeal oedema,[19,173] but a tracheostomy may be needed to maintain a secure airway.

Rarely, respiratory obstruction can occur due to bilateral recurrent laryngeal nerve damage after thyroid and parathyroid surgeries. Bilateral injury presents with stridor on extubation, requiring reintubation or tracheostomy, but transient and even permanent palsy of the recurrent laryngeal nerves can result from intubation.[174,175]

The incidence of postoperative respiratory complications after thyroidectomy for large goitres has been reported to be very high.[171,173,176] Besides the aforementioned causes, patients with large goitres may be affected by a condition known as tracheomalacia,[177] resulting in tracheal collapse. It is caused by long standing goitres weakening or destroying the cartilaginous rings of the trachea,[19] so that when the thyroid tissue which has been providing external support to the trachea is removed there is tracheal collapse.[18,19] If the trachea is soft in surgery and tracheomalacia is encountered, elective tracheostomy may be appropriate,[176] but prolonged intubation (ranging from 12–48 hours or more) is usually sufficient.[19,178] Tracheopexy and tracheoplasty are other potential options.[19] In over 27 years of exploring thyroids at the Hammersmith and associated hospitals, the authors have not encountered a tracheal collapse.

An injury to the trachea can occur during mobilisation of the thyroid gland from the trachea, when the gland is very adherent or the trachea is very soft. The authors recently experienced a tracheal injury in a 21-year old female patient with a papillary carcinoma of the thyroid. During antero-lateral traction of the left lobe there was an unnoticed kinking of the soft tracheal rings and the trachea was incised. The incision was sutured with a 2/0 absorbable suture and a graft fashioned from the adjacent muscle. A drain was inserted and left in place for three days, but the postoperative course of the patient was uneventful and emphysema was not noted. A direct injury to the trachea is also possible during thyroidectomy, when there is unnoticed thyroid cancer invasion.[179]

Oesophageal injury

Oesophageal injury is a very rare complication.[180] The oesophagus may be at risk during central neck dissection for thyroid carcinoma, in completion thyroidectomy for recurrent disease, in extensive malignancy, in retro-oesophageal extension of a goitre and during neck exploration for persistent or recurrent hyperparathyroidism.[181] The risk of injury during thyroid surgery may be increased when there is significant displacement of the trachea leaving the anterior esophageal surface exposed.[1]

The clinical presentation is severe pain in the neck and subcutaneous emphysema, and a contrast study will confirm the diagnosis. It is much better to recognise the damage immediately and attempt primary closure; perforations of the cervical oesophagus can be drained without attempting closure. Parenteral nutrition and antibiotic therapy minimise the risk of sepsis,[182] but surgery may still be required.

Thoracic duct damage

Thoracic or right lymphatic duct damage is rare after thyroid surgery and has never been reported after parathyroid surgery.[57] It is more frequently associated with a modified radical neck dissection for carcinoma of the thyroid and often occurs on the left side. A careful intraoperative inspection for a possible chyle fistula is important when thoracic duct damage is suspected.

As a result of the damage a chyle fistula develops, which may impair nutrition, compromise wound healing, and prolong hospitalisation.[183] While further surgery may be required for those with a high fistula output, conservative therapy is usually advocated for others.[184] In most cases, a stepwise conservative approach consisting of dietary modifications and maintaining closed vacuum suction drainage seems sufficient.[185]

Very rarely a chyle fistula may lead to bilateral chylothorax which is potentially lethal,[186,187] but its management by aspiration drainage is usually sufficient to control the consequences.[187]

Mortality

The reported mortality of thyroid and parathyroid surgery is well below 1% in most series,[34,49,57] and many authors have reported no deaths.[3,188–190] However, endocrine surgery is not without life-threatening complications such as respiratory obstruction or thyroid storm,[173,191] and surgeons must be aware of all potential complications for early diagnosis and treatment.[72,192]

REFERENCES

1. Reeve T, Thompson NW. (2000) Complications of thyroid surgery: how to avoid them, how to manage them, and observations on their possible effect on the whole patient. *World J Surg* 24: 971–975.

2. Zarnegar R, Brunaud L, Clark OH. (2003) Prevention, evaluation, and management of complications following thyroidectomy for thyroid carcinoma. *Endocrinol Metab Clin North Am* 32: 483–502.

3. Kahky MP, Weber RS. (1993) Complications of surgery of the thyroid and parathyroid glands. *Surg Clin North Am* 73: 307–321.

4. Eknoyan G. (1995) A history of the parathyroid glands. *Am J Kidney Dis* 26: 801–807.

5. Cope O. (1978) Endocrine surgery. *Surg Clin North Am* 58: 957–966.

6. Cady B, Sedgwick CE. (1980) History of thyroid and parathyroid surgery. *Major Probl Clin Surg* 15: 1–5.

7. Pasieka JL. (2000) The surgeon as a prognostic factor in endocrine surgical diseases. *Surg Oncol Clin North Am* 9: 13–20.

8. Sackett WR, Barraclough BH, Sidhu S, *et al.* (2002) Minimal access thyroid surgery: is it feasible, is it appropriate? *ANZ J Surg* 72: 777–780.

9. Miccoli P. (2002) Minimally invasive surgery for thyroid and parathyroid diseases. *Surg Endosc* 16: 3–6.

10. Miccoli P, Berti P, Materazzi G, Donatini G. (2003) Minimally invasive video assisted parathyroidectomy (MIVAP). *Eur J Surg Oncol* 29: 188–190.

11. Shimizu K, Kitagawa W, Akasu H, *et al.* (2002) Video-assisted minimally invasive endoscopic thyroid surgery using a gasless neck skin lifting method — 153 cases of benign thyroid tumors and applicability for large tumors. *Biomed Pharmacother* 56(Suppl 1): 88s–91s.

12. Maeda S, *et al.* (2002) Video-assisted neck surgery for thyroid and parathyroid diseases. *Biomed Pharmacother* 56(Suppl 1): 92s–95s.

13. McHenry CR. (2002) What's new in general surgery: endocrine surgery. *J Am Coll Surg* 195: 364–371.

14. De Jong SA. (2003) What's new in general surgery: endocrine. *J Am Coll Surg* 197: 436–443.

15. Ahren B, Mansson B. (1992) Recurrent laryngeal nerve palsy after thyroid and parathyroid surgery. Experience from Lund University. *Thyroidology* 4: 87–89.

16. Gavilan J, Gavilan C. (1986) Recurrent laryngeal nerve. Identification during thyroid and parathyroid surgery. *Arch Otolaryngol Head Neck Surg* 112: 1286–1288.

17. Bliss RD, Gauger PG, Delbridge LW. (2000) Surgeon's approach to the thyroid gland: surgical anatomy and the importance of technique. *World J Surg* **24**: 891–897.

18. Studley JGN, Lynn J. (1993) Surgical anatomy of the thyroid gland and the technique of thyroidectomy. In: Lynn J, Bloom SR (eds), *Surgical Endocrinology* (Butterworth-Heinemann, Oxford), pp. 231–239.

19. Prinz RA, Rossi HL, Kim AW. (2002) Difficult problems in thyroid surgery. *Curr Probl Surg* **39**: 5–91.

20. Sturniolo G, *et al.* (1999) The recurrent laryngeal nerve related to thyroid surgery. *Am J Surg* **177**: 485–488.

21. Gauger PG, Delbridge LW, Thompson NW, *et al.* (2001) Incidence and importance of the tubercle of Zuckerkandl in thyroid surgery. *Eur J Surg* **167**: 249–254.

22. Mra Z, Wax MK. (1999) Nonrecurrent laryngeal nerves: anatomic considerations during thyroid and parathyroid surgery. *Am J Otolaryngol* **20**: 91–95.

23. Defechereux T, *et al.* (2000) The inferior non-recurrent laryngeal nerve: a major surgical risk during thyroidectomy. *Acta Chir Belg* **100**: 62–67.

24. Avisse C, *et al.* (1998) Right nonrecurrent inferior laryngeal nerve and arteria lusoria: the diagnostic and therapeutic implications of an anatomic anomaly. Review of 17 cases. *Surg Radiol Anat* **20**: 227–232.

25. Moley JF, Lairmore TC, Doherty GM, *et al.* (1999) Preservation of the recurrent laryngeal nerves in thyroid and parathyroid reoperations. *Surgery* **126**: 673–677.

26. Jossart GH, Clark OH. (1999) Surgical techniques. Thyroid and parathyroid procedures. In: Wilmore DW *et al.* (eds), *Scientific American Surgery* (Scientific American, Inc., New York), pp. 1–30.

27. Delbridge L, Reeve TS, Khadra M, Poole AG. (1992) Total thyroidectomy: the technique of capsular dissection. *Aust N Z J Surg* **62**: 96–99.

28. Sinclair IS. (1994) The risk to the recurrent laryngeal nerves in thyroid and parathyroid surgery. *J R Coll Surg Edinb* **39**: 253–257.

29. Marcus B, *et al.* (2003) Recurrent laryngeal nerve monitoring in thyroid and parathyroid surgery: the University of Michigan experience. *Laryngoscope* **113**: 356–361.

30. Brennan J, Moore EJ, Shuler KJ. (2001) Prospective analysis of the efficacy of continuous intraoperative nerve monitoring during thyroidectomy, parathyroidectomy, and parotidectomy. *Otolaryngol Head Neck Surg* **124**: 537–543.

31. Cavallaro G, Taranto G, Chiofalo MG, Cavallaro E. (1998) Usefulness of microsurgery to isolation of recurrent laryngeal nerve and parathyroid during thyroidectomy operations. *Microsurgery* **18**: 460–461.

32. Green KM, de Carpentier JP. (1999) Are pre-operative vocal fold checks necessary? *J Laryngol Otol* **113**: 642–644.

33. Chao TC, Jeng LB, Lin JD, Chen MF. (1997) Reoperative thyroid surgery. *World J Surg* **21**: 644–647.

34. Fewins J, Simpson CB, Miller FR. (2003) Complications of thyroid and parathyroid surgery. *Otolaryngol Clin North Am* **36**: 189–206, x.

35. Laursen RJ, Larsen KM, Molgaard J, Kolze V. (1998) Unilateral vocal cord paralysis following endotracheal intubation. *Acta Anaesthesiol Scand* **42**: 131–132.

36. Cheesman A, Holden H. (1993) Management of the damaged recurrent laryngeal nerve following thyroid surgery. In: Lynn J, Bloom SR (eds), *Surgical Endocrinology* (Butterworth–Heinemann, Oxford), pp. 324–329.

37. Dozois RR, Beahrs OH. (1977) Surgical anatomy and technique of thyroid and parathyroid surgery. *Surg Clin North Am* **57**: 647–661.

38. Fenton RS. (1983) The surgical complications of thyroidectomy. *J Otolaryngol* **12**: 104–106.

39. Miller FR. (2003) Surgical anatomy of the thyroid and parathyroid glands. *Otolaryngol Clin North Am* **36**: 1–7, vii.

40. Gray SW, Skandalakis JE, Akin JT Jr. (1976) Embryological considerations of thyroid surgery: developmental anatomy of the thyroid, parathyroids and the recurrent laryngeal nerve. *Am Surg* **42**: 621–628.

41. Lennquist S. (1986) Surgical strategy in thyroid carcinoma: a clinical review. *Acta Chir Scand* **152**: 321–338.

42. Cohen MS, Moley JF. (2003) Surgical treatment of medullary thyroid carcinoma. *J Intern Med* **253**: 616–626.

43. Solomon P, Irish J, Gullane P. (1993) Horner's syndrome following a thyroidectomy. *J Otolaryngol* **22**: 454–456.

44. Defechereux T, Rinken F, Maweja S, *et al.* (2003) Evaluation of the ultrasonic dissector in thyroid surgery. A prospective randomised study. *Acta Chir Belg* **103**: 274–277.

45. Tabaqchali MA, Hanson JM, Proud G. (1999) Drains for thyroidectomy/parathyroidectomy: fact or fiction? *Ann R Coll Surg Engl* **81**: 302–305.

46. Kristoffersson A, Sandzen B, Jarhult J. (1986) Drainage in uncomplicated thyroid and parathyroid surgery. *Br J Surg* **73**: 121–122.

47. Wax MK, Valiulis AP, Hurst MK. (1995) Drains in thyroid and parathyroid surgery. Are they necessary? *Arch Otolaryngol Head Neck Surg* **121**: 981–983.

48. Ready AR, Barnes AD. (1994) Complications of thyroidectomy. *Br J Surg* **81**: 1555–1556.

49. Bhattacharyya N, Fried MP. (2002) Assessment of the morbidity and complications of total thyroidectomy. *Arch Otolaryngol Head Neck Surg* **128**: 389–392.

50. Bentrem DJ, Rademaker A, Angelos P. (2001) Evaluation of serum calcium levels in predicting hypoparathyroidism after total/near-total thyroidectomy or parathyroidectomy. *Am Surg* **67**: 249–251.

51. Demeester-Mirkine N, Hooghe L, Van Geertruyden J, *et al.* (1992). Hypocalcemia after thyroidectomy. *Arch Surg* **127**: 854–858.

52. Shaha AR, Burnett C, Jaffe BM. (1991) Parathyroid autotransplantation during thyroid surgery. *J Surg Oncol* **46**: 21–24.

53. Kotan C, *et al.* (2003) Influence of the refinement of surgical technique and surgeon's experience on the rate of complications after total thyroidectomy for benign thyroid disease. *Acta Chir Belg* **103**: 278–281.

54. Abboud B, Sargi Z, Akkam M, Sleilaty F. (2002) Risk factors for postthyroidectomy hypocalcemia. *J Am Coll Surg* **195**: 456–461.

55. Rao RS, Jog VB, Baluja CA, Damle SR. (1990) Risk of hypoparathyroidism after surgery for carcinoma of the thyroid. *Head Neck* **12**: 321–325.

56. Prim MP, de Diego JI, Hardisson D, *et al.* (2001) Factors related to nerve injury and hypocalcemia in thyroid gland surgery. *Otolaryngol Head Neck Surg* **124**: 111–114.

57. Bergamaschi R, Becouarn G, Ronceray J, Arnaud JP. (1998) Morbidity of thyroid surgery. *Am J Surg* **176**: 71–75.

58. McHenry CR, Speroff T, Wentworth D, Murphy T. (1994) Risk factors for postthyroidectomy hypocalcemia. *Surgery* **116**: 641–647.

59. de lC, V *et al.* (1997) Pathologic intrathyroidal parathyroid glands. *Int Surg* **82**: 87–90.

60. Harach HR, Vujanic GM. (1993) Intrathyroidal parathyroid. *Pediatr Pathol* **13**: 71–74.

61. Sasson AR, Pingpank JF Jr, Wetherington RW, *et al.* (2001) Incidental parathyroidectomy during thyroid surgery does not cause transient symptomatic hypocalcemia. *Arch Otolaryngol Head Neck Surg* **127**: 304–308.

62. Lee NJ, Blakey JD, Bhuta S, Calcaterra TC. (1999) Unintentional parathyroidectomy during thyroidectomy. *Laryngoscope* **109**: 1238–1240.

63. Lo CY. (2002) Parathyroid autotransplantation during thyroidectomy. *ANZ J Surg* **72**: 902–907.

64. Lo CY, Lam KY. (1999) Parathyroid autotransplantation during thyroidectomy: is frozen section necessary? *Arch Surg* **134**: 258–260.

65. Ander S, Johansson K, Smeds S. (1997) In situ preservation of the parathyroid glands during operations on the thyroid. *Eur J Surg* **163**: 33–37.

66. Richards ML, Bingener-Casey J, Pierce D, *et al.* (2003) Intraoperative parathyroid hormone assay: an accurate predictor of symptomatic hypocalcemia following thyroidectomy. *Arch Surg* **138**: 632–635.

67. Warren FM, Andersen PE, Wax MK, Cohen JI. (2002) Intraoperative parathyroid hormone levels in thyroid and parathyroid surgery. *Laryngoscope* **112**: 1866–1870.
68. Bellantone R, *et al.* (2002) Is routine supplementation therapy (calcium and vitamin D) useful after total thyroidectomy? *Surgery* **132**: 1109–1112.
69. Moore FD Jr. (1994) Oral calcium supplements to enhance early hospital discharge after bilateral surgical treatment of the thyroid gland or exploration of the parathyroid glands. *J Am Coll Surg* **178**: 11–16.
70. Rennie D. (1997) Thyroid storm. *JAMA* **277**: 1238–1243.
71. Dillmann WH. (1997) Thyroid storm. *Curr Ther Endocrinol Metab* **6**: 81–85.
72. Malchiodi L. (2002) Thyroid storm. *Am J Nurs* **102**: 33–35.
73. Jiang YZ, Hutchinson KA, Bartelloni P, Manthous CA. (2000) Thyroid storm presenting as multiple organ dysfunction syndrome. *Chest* **118**: 877–879.
74. Bewsher PD, Pegg CA, Stewart DJ. (1974) Propranolol in the surgical management of thyrotoxicosis. *Ann Surg* **180**: 787–790.
75. Friedman M, Pacella BL Jr. (1990) Total versus subtotal thyroidectomy. Arguments, approaches, and recommendations. *Otolaryngol Clin North Am* **23**: 413–427.
76. Falk SA. (1990) The management of hyperthyroidism. A surgeon's perspective. *Otolaryngol Clin North Am* **23**: 361–380.
77. Gimm O, Brauckhoff M, Thanh PN. (2002) An update on thyroid surgery. *Eur J Nucl Med Mol Imaging* **29**(Suppl 2): S447–452.
78. Wanebo H, Coburn M, Teates D, Cole B. (1998) Total thyroidectomy does not enhance disease control or survival even in high-risk patients with differentiated thyroid cancer. *Ann Surg* **227**: 912–921.
79. Gough IR, Wilkinson D. (2000) Total thyroidectomy for management of thyroid disease. *World J Surg* **24**: 962–965.
80. Cady B. (1997) Hayes Martin Lecture. Our AMES is true: how an old concept still hits the mark: or, risk group assignment points the arrow to rational therapy selection in differentiated thyroid cancer. *Am J Surg* **174**: 462–468.
81. Clark OH, Levin K, Zeng QH, *et al.* (1988) Thyroid cancer: the case for total thyroidectomy. *Eur J Cancer Clin Oncol* **24**: 305–313.
82. Grant CS, *et al.* (1988) Local recurrence in papillary thyroid carcinoma: is extent of surgical resection important? *Surgery* **104**: 954–962.
83. Delbridge L. (2003) Total thyroidectomy: the evolution of surgical technique. *ANZ J Surg* **73**: 761–768.
84. Barakate MS, *et al.* (2002) Total thyroidectomy is now the preferred option for the surgical management of Graves' disease. *ANZ J Surg* **72**: 321–324.
85. Robert J, *et al.* (2001) Short- and long-term results of total vs subtotal thyroidectomies in the surgical treatment of Graves' disease. *Swiss Surg* **7**: 20–24.

86. Califano G, Abate S, Ferulano GP, Danzi M. (1985) Surgery of toxic goiter: indications and long-term results. *Ital J Surg Sci* **15**: 233–237.

87. Viot A, Babin E, Bequignon A, *et al.* (2003) Surgery for hyperthyroidism on 43 patients. *Rev Laryngol Otol Rhinol (Bord)* **124**: 117–125.

88. Simms JM, Talbot CH. (1983) Surgery for thyrotoxicosis. *Br J Surg* **70**: 581–583.

89. Roka R, Niederle B, Kokoschka R, Fritsch A. (1981) Results following surgical treatment of hyperthyroidism. *Jpn J Surg* **11**: 15–21.

90. Daali M, Tajedine T. (2003) Toxic multinodular goiter. *Ann Endocrinol (Paris)* **64**: 284–288.

91. Reeve TS, Delbridge L, Cohen A, Crummer P. (1987) Total thyroidectomy. The preferred option for multinodular goiter. *Ann Surg* **206**: 782–786.

92. Friguglietti CU, Lin CS, Kulcsar MA. (2003) Total thyroidectomy for benign thyroid disease. *Laryngoscope* **113**: 1820–1826.

93. Rojdmark J, Jarhult J. (1995) High long term recurrence rate after subtotal thyroidectomy for nodular goitre. *Eur J Surg* **161**: 725–727.

94. Marchesi M, Biffoni M, Tartaglia F, *et al.* (1998) Total versus subtotal thyroidectomy in the management of multinodular goiter. *Int Surg* **83**: 202–204.

95. Giles Y, Boztepe H, Terzioglu T, Tezelman S. (2004) The advantage of total thyroidectomy to avoid reoperation for incidental thyroid cancer in multinodular goiter. *Arch Surg* **139**: 179–182.

96. Organ CH Jr. (2000) The history of parathyroid surgery, 1850–1996: the excelsior surgical society 1998 Edward D Churchill lecture. *J Am Coll Surg* **191**: 284–299.

97. Johansson H. (2000) History of endocrinology and Sandstrom's gland. *Lakartidningen* **97**: 4159–4161.

98. Rice DH. (1996) Surgery of the parathyroid glands. *Otolaryngol Clin North Am* **29**: 693–699.

99. Affleck BD, Swartz K, Brennan J. (2003) Surgical considerations and controversies in thyroid and parathyroid surgery. *Otolaryngol Clin North Am* **36**: 159–187, x.

100. Low RA, Katz AD. (1998) Parathyroidectomy via bilateral cervical exploration: a retrospective review of 866 cases. *Head Neck* **20**: 583–587.

101. Piemonte M, Passon P, Palma S. (2002) Selective parathyroidectomy with unilateral cervical exploration for primary hyperparathyroidism. *Acta Otorhinolaryngol Ital* **22**: 289–294.

102. Pino RV, *et al.* (2002) Surgery for secondary and tertiary hyperparathyroidism: 11 years' experience. *Acta Otorrinolaringol Esp* **53**: 418–422.

103. Walgenbach S, Hommel G, Bernhard G, Junginger T. (2000) Surgical therapy of primary hyperparathyroidism. Quality of life after 10 years prospective observation. *Zentralbl Chir* **125**: 666–670.

104. Walgenbach S, Hommel G, Junginger T. (2000) Outcome after surgery for primary hyperparathyroidism: ten-year prospective follow-up study. *World J Surg* **24**: 564–569.

105. Mariette C, *et al.* (1998) Reoperation for persistent or recurrent primary hyperparathyroidism. *Langenbecks Arch Surg* **383**: 174–179.

106. Wells SA Jr, Debenedetti MK, Doherty GM. (2002) Recurrent or persistent hyperparathyroidism. *J Bone Miner Res* **17**(Suppl 2): N158–162.

107. Chou FF, *et al.* (2002) Persistent and recurrent hyperparathyroidism after total parathyroidectomy with autotransplantation. *Ann Surg* **235**: 99–104.

108. Evenepoel P, Kuypers D, Maes B, *et al.* (2001) Persistent hyperparathyroidism after kidney transplantation requiring parathyroidectomy. *Acta Otorhinolaryngol Belg* **55**: 177–186.

109. Shen W, *et al.* (1996) Reoperation for persistent or recurrent primary hyperparathyroidism. *Arch Surg* **131**: 861–867.

110. Penington A, Ihle B, Billson V, Clunie GJ. (1990) Recurrent secondary hyperparathyroidism due to implanted parathyroid tissue: a case report. *Aust N Z J Surg* **60**: 821–823.

111. Hooghe L, Kinnaert P, Van Geertruyden J. (1992) Surgical anatomy of hyperparathyroidism. *Acta Chir Belg* **92**: 1–9.

112. Udelsman R. (2002) Surgery in primary hyperparathyroidism: the patient without previous neck surgery. *J Bone Miner Res* **17**(Suppl 2): N126–132.

113. Olson JA Jr, Leight GS Jr. (2002) Surgical management of secondary hyperparathyroidism. *Adv Ren Replace Ther* **9**: 209–218.

114. Tominaga Y, *et al.* (2001) More than 1,000 cases of total parathyroidectomy with forearm autograft for renal hyperparathyroidism. *Am J Kidney Dis* **38**: S168–S171.

115. Takami H, Ikeda Y, Wada N. (2000) Surgical management of primary hyperparathyroidixsm. *Biomed Pharmacother* **54**(Suppl 1): 17s–20s.

116. Summers GW. (1996) Parathyroid update: a review of 220 cases. *Ear Nose Throat J* **75**: 434–439.

117. Prager G, *et al.* (1999) The value of preoperative localization studies in primary hyperparathyroidism. *Chirurg* **70**: 1082–1088.

118. Ulrich F, *et al.* (2001) Cryopreserved human parathyroid tissue: cell cultures for in vitro testing of function. *Transplant Proc* **33**: 666–667.

119. Kukora JS. (2001) Surgical treatment of primary hyperparathyroidism. *Endocr Pract* **7**: 323–325.

120. Walgenbach S, Junginger T (2001). Results of bilateral surgical technique in primary hyperparathyroidism. *Zentralbl Chir* **126**: 254–260.

121. Arkles LB, Jones T, Hicks RJ, *et al.* (1998) Surgery for primary hyperparathyroidism 1962–1996: indications and outcomes. *Med J Aust* **169**: 118–119.

122. Sakamoto W, Kishimoto T. (1995) Primary hyperparathyroidism — choice of surgical procedures and follow up after surgery. *Nippon Rinsho* **53**: 890–894.

123. Worsey MJ, Carty SE, Watson CG. (1993) Success of unilateral neck exploration for sporadic primary hyperparathyroidism. *Surgery* **114**: 1024–1029.

124. Harding AD, Nichols WK, Mitchell FL. (1990) Total parathyroidectomy and autotransplantation in hyperplasia of the parathyroid gland. *Surg Gynecol Obstet* **171**: 288–290.

125. Lumachi F, Iacobone M, Favia G. (2003) Minimally invasive radioguided parathyroidectomy. *Ann Ital Chir* **74**: 413–416.

126. Lo CY, Chan WF, Luk JM. (2003) Minimally invasive endoscopic-assisted parathyroidectomy for primary hyperparathyroidism. *Surg Endosc* **17**: 1932–1936.

127. Sosa JA, Udelsman R. (2003) Minimally invasive parathyroidectomy. *Surg Oncol* **12**: 125–134.

128. Fahy BN, Bold RJ, Beckett L, Schneider PD. (2002) Modern parathyroid surgery: a cost-benefit analysis of localizing strategies. *Arch Surg* **137**: 917–922.

129. Hallfeldt KK, Trupka A, Gallwas J, Schmidbauer S. (2002) Minimally invasive video-assisted parathyroidectomy and intraoperative parathyroid hormone monitoring. The first 36 cases and some pitfalls. *Surg Endosc* **16**: 1759–1763.

130. Agarwal G, Barraclough BH, Robinson BG, *et al.* (2002) Minimally invasive parathyroidectomy using the 'focused' lateral approach. I. Results of the first 100 consecutive cases. *ANZ J Surg* **72**: 100–104.

131. Sprouse LR, Roe SM, Kaufman HJ, Williams N. (2001) Minimally invasive parathyroidectomy without intraoperative localization. *Am Surg* **67**: 1022–1029.

132. Lowney JK, Weber B, Johnson S, Doherty GM. (2000) Minimal incision parathyroidectomy: cure, cosmesis, and cost. *World J Surg* **24**: 1442–1445.

133. Herfarth KK, Wells SA Jr. (1997) Parathyroid glands and the multiple endocrine neoplasia syndromes and familial hypocalciuric hypercalcemia. *Semin Surg Oncol* **13**: 114–124.

134. O'Riordain DS, *et al.* (1993) Surgical management of primary hyperparathyroidism in multiple endocrine neoplasia types 1 and 2. *Surgery* **114**: 1031–1037.

135. Hubbard JG, Sebag F, Maweja S, Henry JF. (2002) Primary hyperparathyroidism in MEN 1 — how radical should surgery be? *Langenbecks Arch Surg* **386**: 553–557.

136. Katai M, Sakurai A, Ikeo Y, Hashizume K. (2001) Primary hyperparathyroidism in patients with multiple endocrine neoplasia type 1: comparison with sporadic parathyroid adenomas. *Horm Metab Res* **33**: 499–503.

137. Hellman P, *et al.* (1998) Primary and reoperative parathyroid operations in hyperparathyroidism of multiple endocrine neoplasia type 1. *Surgery* **124**: 993–999.

138. Elaraj DM, *et al.* (2003) Results of initial operation for hyperparathyroidism in patients with multiple endocrine neoplasia type 1. *Surgery* **134**: 858–864.

139. Kraimps JL, *et al.* (1996) Primary hyperparathyroidism in multiple endocrine neoplasia type IIa: retrospective French multicentric study. Groupe d'Etude des Tumeurs a Calcitonine (GETC, French Calcitonin Tumors Study Group), French Association of Endocrine Surgeons. *World J Surg* **20**: 808–812.

140. Herfarth KK, Bartsch D, Doherty GM, *et al.* (1996) Surgical management of hyperparathyroidism in patients with multiple endocrine neoplasia type 2A. *Surgery* **120**: 966–973.

141. Decker PA, *et al.* (2001) Subtotal parathyroidectomy in renal failure: still needed after all these years. *World J Surg* **25**: 708–712.

142. Tominaga Y, Johansson H, Takagi H. (1997) Secondary hyperparathyroidism: pathophysiology, histopathology, and medical and surgical management. *Surg Today* **27**: 787–792.

143. Punch JD, Thompson NW, Merion RM. (1995) Subtotal parathyroidectomy in dialysis-dependent and post-renal transplant patients. A 25-year single-center experience. *Arch Surg* **130**: 538–542.

144. Korzets Z, Bernheim J. (1992) Total parathyroidectomy with autotransplantation: revisited. *Nephrol Dial Transplant* **7**: 271.

145. Rothmund M, Wagner PK, Schark C. (1991) Subtotal parathyroidectomy versus total parathyroidectomy and autotransplantation in secondary hyperparathyroidism: a randomized trial. *World J Surg* **15**: 745–750.

146. Fabretti F, Calabrese V, Fornasari V, Poletti I. (1991) Subtotal parathyroidectomy for secondary hyperparathyroidism in chronic renal failure. *J Laryngol Otol* **105**: 562–567.

147. Higgins RM, *et al.* (1991) Total parathyroidectomy alone or with autograft for renal hyperparathyroidism? *Q J Med* **79**: 323–332.

148. Takagi H, *et al.* (1988) Total parathyroidectomy with forearm autograft for secondary hyperparathyroidism in chronic renal failure. *Ann Surg* **208**: 639–644.

149. Garcia-Pallares M, Bernaldez R, Sanchez MC, Gavilan J. (2000) Surgery for secondary hyperparathyroidism in patients undergoing dialysis. *Otolaryngol Head Neck Surg* **122**: 908–910.

150. Ockert S, *et al.* (2002) Total parathyroidectomy without autotransplantation as a standard procedure in the treatment of secondary hyperparathyroidism. *Langenbecks Arch Surg* **387**: 204–209.

151. Amato G, *et al.* (2002) Eight parathyroid glands incidentally discovered during a surgical intervention for secondary hyperparathyroidism: an unusual clinical finding. *J Endocrinol Invest* **25**: 800–803.

152. Aly A, Douglas M. (2003) Embryonic parathyroid rests occur commonly and have implications in the management of secondary hyperparathyroidism. *ANZ J Surg* **73**: 284–288.

153. Alexander PT, *et al.* (1988) Repeat parathyroid operation associated with renal disease. *Am J Surg* **155**: 686–689.

154. Guller U, Schonholzer C, Martinoli S. (2000) Recurrent hyperparathyroidism in kidney failure patients after total parathyroidectomy and autotransplantation. Case report and review of the literature. *Swiss Surg* **6**: 179–181.

155. Niederle B, Roka R, Horandner H. (1988) Recurrent renal hyperparathyroidism: reoperation on the autograft. *Wien Klin Wochenschr* **100**: 369–372.

156. Rothmund M, Wagner PK. (1988) Reoperations in persistent and recurrent secondary hyperparathyroidism. *Wien Klin Wochenschr* **100**: 367–368.

157. Fang JT, Chuang CK, Chu SH, *et al.* (1996) Tertiary hyperparathyroidism after renal transplantation. *Transplant Proc* **28**: 1484–1485.

158. Kilgo MS, Pirsch JD, Warner TF, Starling JR. (1998) Tertiary hyperparathyroidism after renal transplantation: surgical strategy. *Surgery* **124**: 677–683.

159. D'Alessandro AM, *et al.* (1989) Tertiary hyperparathyroidism after renal transplantation: operative indications. *Surgery* **106**: 1049–1055.

160. Hibi Y, *et al.*(2002) Reoperation for renal hyperparathyroidism. *World J Surg* **26**: 1301–1307.

161. Rotstein L, Irish J, Gullane P, *et al.* (1998) Reoperative parathyroidectomy in the era of localization technology. *Head Neck* **20**: 535–539.

162. Henry JF, Denizot A, Audiffret J, France G. (1990) Results of reoperations for persistent or recurrent secondary hyperparathyroidism in hemodialysis patients. *World J Surg* **14**: 303–306.

163. Perrier ND, *et al.* (2000) Intraoperative parathyroid aspiration and parathyroid hormone assay as an alternative to frozen section for tissue identification. *World J Surg* **24**: 1319–1322.

164. Sebag F, *et al.* (2003) Intraoperative parathyroid hormone assay and parathyroid reoperations. *Surgery* **134**: 1049–1055.

165. Sippel RS, Bianco J, Chen H. (2003) Radioguided parathyroidectomy for recurrent hyperparathyroidism caused by forearm graft hyperplasia. *J Bone Miner Res* **18**: 939–942.

166. Takami H, Sasaki Y, Ikeda Y, Tajima G. (2002) Intraoperative quick parathyroid hormone assay in the surgical management of hyperparathyroidism. *Biomed Pharmacother* **56**(Suppl 1): 26s–30s.

167. Hung GU, *et al.* (2000) Recurrent hyperfunctioning parathyroid gland demonstrated on radionuclide imaging and an intraoperative gamma probe. *Clin Nucl Med* **25**: 348–350.

168. Jancewicz S, Sidhu S, Jalaludin B, Campbell P. (2002) Optimal position for a cervical collar incision: a prospective study. *ANZ J Surg* **72**: 15–17.
169. Brunaud L, *et al.* (2003) Incision length for standard thyroidectomy and parathyroidectomy: when is it minimally invasive? *Arch Surg* **138**: 1140–1143.
170. Shaha A, Jaffe BM. (1988) Complications of thyroid surgery performed by residents. *Surgery* **104**: 1109–1114.
171. Abdel Rahim AA, Ahmed ME, Hassan MA. (1999) Respiratory complications after thyroidectomy and the need for tracheostomy in patients with a large goitre. *Br J Surg* **86**: 88–90.
172. Hamilton NT, Christophi C, Swann JB, Robinson GJ. (1987) Endotracheal intubation following thyroidectomy. *Aust N Z J Surg* **57**: 295–298.
173. Lacoste L, *et al.* (1993) Airway complications in thyroid surgery. *Ann Otol Rhinol Laryngol* **102**: 441–446.
174. Ono S, Nishiyama T, Hanaoka K. (2000) Hoarseness after endotracheal intubation caused by submucosal hemorrage of the vocal cord and recurrent nerve palsy. *Masui* **49**: 881–883.
175. Friedrich T, *et al.* (2000) Recurrent laryngeal nerve paralysis as intubation injury? *Chirurg* **71**: 539–544.
176. Ratnarathorn B. (1995) Tracheal collapse after thyroidectomy: case report. *J Med Assoc Thai* **78**: 55–56.
177. Geelhoed GW. (1988) Tracheomalacia from compressing goiter: management after thyroidectomy. *Surgery* **104**: 1100–1108.
178. McHenry CR, Piotrowski JJ. (1994) Thyroidectomy in patients with marked thyroid enlargement: airway management, morbidity, and outcome. *Am Surg* **60**: 586–591.
179. Zannini P, Melloni G. (1996) Surgical management of thyroid cancer invading the trachea. *Chest Surg Clin North Am* **6**: 777–790.
180. Akbulut G, Gunay S, Aren A, Bilge O. (2002) A rare complication after thyroidectomy: esophageal perforation. *Ulus Travma Derg* **8**: 250–252.
181. Cheah WK, *et al.* (2002) Complications of neck dissection for thyroid cancer. *World J Surg* **26**: 1013–1016.
182. Bufkin BL, Miller JI Jr, Mansour KA. (1996) Esophageal perforation: emphasis on management. *Ann Thorac Surg* **61**: 1447–1451.
183. Lucente FE, Diktaban T, Lawson W, Biller HF. (1981) Chyle fistula management. *Otolaryngol Head Neck Surg* **89**: 575–578.
184. al Khayat M, Kenyon GS, Fawcett HV, Powell-Tuck J. (1991) Nutritional support in patients with low volume chylous fistula following radical neck dissection. *J Laryngol Otol* **105**: 1052–1056.

185. de Gier HH, Balm AJ, Bruning PF, *et al.* (1996) Systematic approach to the treatment of chylous leakage after neck dissection. *Head Neck* **18**: 347–351.

186. Eufinger H, Lehmbrock J. (2001) Life threatening and fatal complications of radical neck dissection. *Mund Kiefer Gesichtschir* **5**: 193–197.

187. Jortay A, Bisschop P. (2001) Bilateral chylothorax after left radical neck dissection. *Acta Otorhinolaryngol Belg* **55**: 285–289.

188. Tartaglia F, *et al.* (2003) Complications in total thyroidectomy: our experience and a number of considerations. *Chir Ital* **55**: 499–510.

189. Netterville JL, Aly A, Ossoff RH. (1990) Evaluation and treatment of complications of thyroid and parathyroid surgery. *Otolaryngol Clin North Am* **23**: 529–552.

190. Jacobs JK, Aland JW, Jr, Ballinger JF. (1983) Total thyroidectomy. A review of 213 patients. *Ann Surg* **197**: 542–549.

191. Leow MK, Loh KC. (2002) Fatal thyroid crisis years after two thyroidectomies for graves' disease: is thyroid tissue autotransplantation for post-thyroidectomy hypothyroidism worthwhile? *J Am Coll Surg* **195**: 434–435.

192. Edis AJ. (1979) Prevention and management of complications associated with thyroid and parathyroid surgery. *Surg Clin North Am* **59**: 83–92.

ADRENAL SURGERY

Introduction

Successful adrenal surgery has only become possible in the last 75 years with the unravelling of the complex physiology of the adrenal glands, the development of pharmacological agonists and antagonists to the hormonal functions and the development of cortisone replacement therapy.[1] Sensitive and sophisticated imaging techniques have been developed allowing accurate diagnosis and localisation of tumours.[2]

More recently there has been a change in approach to laparoscopic adrenalectomy, since it was first described in 1992.[3] The small size of the gland, benign nature of most adrenal pathology, and the difficulty in reaching the gland at open operation has led to this change in operative technique.[4,5]

Diagnostic Complications

While it is not within the scope of this chapter to describe the diagnostic pathway for each adrenal condition fully, a few of the pitfalls in diagnosis are worth highlighting.

Cushing's syndrome

Cushing's syndrome (CS) refers to a group of symptoms caused by an excess of circulating glucocorticoids. Although Cushing's disease refers to excess adrenocorticotrophic hormone (ACTH) secretion from the pituitary (approximately 80% of those with CS), the syndrome can also arise from secretion from an adrenocortical adenoma or adenocarcinoma, or from ectopic secretion of ACTH or corticotrophin-releasing hormone (CRH).[6,7] Additionally, the administration of exogenous steroids can produce CS.[8] Hence, the correct establishment of the cause of the symptoms is of absolute necessity in diagnosing CS.[9]

The assessment of steroid use (often without the patient's knowledge in creams, etc.) should be meticulous, as should physical examination, because females with adrenal carcinoma often show virilisation, and males, feminisation.[10] Establishing a diagnosis involves numerous tests but the current investigation algorithm in our unit follows that of Orth.[11]

This approach minimises pitfalls in the diagnosis of CS. However, depression and alcoholism can give rise to pseudo Cushing's, which can be excluded by a low dose dexamethasone suppression test.[9] The differentiation between adrenal or pituitary Cushing's relies on simultaneous measurements of CRH and cortisol during the late afternoon period, and a failure to do this can lead to an inappropriate assumption that the pathology lies within the adrenal glands.[12]

Patients with CS should control their diabetes, and severe cases may require metyrapone, an adrenal-acting inhibitor of cortisol synthesis. Perioperative steroids should be administered and precaution taken to account for the patient's increased risk of infection.[13]

Conn's syndrome

This syndrome caused by hyperaldosteronism is characterised by hypokalaemia, hypertension and alkalosis.[14,15] Some patients feel better by limiting their sodium intake, which helps normalise their potassium, so that hypokalaemia may only be detected if the patient is sodium-loaded 24 hours prior to venesection.[16] When the patient is sodium depleted, plasma renin is low, and subsequent aldosterone measurement should be done only with a normal potassium level as a low level will inhibit aldosterone secretion.[17]

Once hyperaldosteronism is established, CT scanning and venous sampling are performed to differentiate a single adenoma from bilateral zona glomerulosa hyperplasia.[18] Venous sampling is not without complications itself, with possible adrenal haemorrhage and infarction. The consequences of hyperaldosteronism such as hypertension, hypokalaemia and metabolic alkalosis should be pharmacologically controlled preoperatively, frequently utilising spironolactone as first line treatment.[15]

Phaeochromocytoma

The diagnosis in suspected phaeochromocytoma is usually made by measuring plasma and urinary catecholamines, but urinary metabolites may also need to be measured as these can be elevated even in the presence of normal plasma levels.[19] Ten per cent of the cases are multiple, and 10% lie outside the adrenal glands, implying that all patients should undergo MIBG scanning to adequately localise the tumour.[20] Additionally, 10% of cases occur as part of other inherited syndromes, such as MEN 2A and MEN 2B, which when suspected requires appropriate genetic screening.[21] Preoperative control of blood pressure is vital for those with a phaeochromocytoma.[19,22] The authors recommend alpha blockade with phenoxybenzamine, increasing the dosage to a point where the patient has mild postural hypotension. Plasma expansion is vital with alpha blockade, and if tachyarrhythmias occur, beta blockade is added. In cases with severe hypertension, particularly in malignant phaeochromocytomas, alphamethylparatyrosine, a hydroxylase inhibitor, may reduce catecholamine production.[23]

The anaesthetic management of phaeochromocytomas is beyond the scope of this chapter but in summary, continued blood pressure control is sustained with alpha blockade, and arrhythmias are controlled with beta blockade.[24,25] Other drugs including those that induce histamine release (e.g., morphine), drugs that interact with catecholamines, sympathomimetic agents and indirectly-acting sympathomimetic agents should be avoided. A close communication between the surgeon and anaesthetist is vital for phaeochromocytoma, as ligation of the adrenal vein can result in a plummeting of blood pressure, which requires the anaesthetist to be forewarned.[26]

Adrenocortical carcinoma

Forty per cent of adrenocortical carcinomas are functioning lesions and should be included in the investigation of all adrenal tumours, with potential risk of local and metastatic spread.[27]

Incidentaloma

Four per cent of abdominal CT scans find unexpected adrenal masses which must be fully evaluated to assess their nature. The assessment of their size, endocrine function, and tissue composition (assessed by MRI) should be undertaken, and sometimes, a fine needle aspiration is useful.[28] Furthermore, many malignant incidentalomas are metastatic, necessitating a search for the primary site[29]; infections such as tuberculosis can present in this manner.

Operative Complications

Introduction

The operative complications of adrenal surgery are potentially life threatening, as adjacent vasculature and other organs can be easily damaged with subsequent rapid deterioration.[30] Good surgical access is vital to uncomplicated adrenal surgery. The cause, size, side and multiplicity of the pathological lesion, as well as the patient's habitus and the surgeon's preferences determine the route of access.[31] Thoracoabdominal approaches can be used for large lesions, while posterior or modified posterior approaches may be preferred for smaller ones.[29] Multiple lesions usually necessitate a transabdominal approach.

Laparoscopic adrenalectomy

Laparoscopic adrenalectomy has rapidly become the access method of choice, with approximately 60% of surgically treatable adrenal disease approachable this way.[1,32] As the surgical access to the adrenal causes relatively more trauma than the dissection of the gland itself, laparoscopic adrenalectomy is significantly less morbid than open adrenalectomy.[13,33] However, this minimally invasive approach demands advanced laparoscopic skills and experience and may be accompanied by its own specific complications.[34–36] The operation is usually done via the lateral transabdominal approach, with patients in a lateral decubitus position, which may be initially disorientating and a cause of potential complication.[24,37] Established malignancy and frank tumour invasion of adjacent structures are absolute contraindications to laparoscopic adrenalectomy, particularly with the risk of tumour seeding at port sites, and the difficulty of obtaining an adequate resection and node dissection.[38,39]

Traditionally, in adrenal surgery, the patient should be dissected away from the tumour, reducing the risk of tumour fragmentation.[40] Adequate instrumentation is vital to surgical success, with the use of a harmonic scalpel and automated clip applicators allowing uncomplicated laparoscopic or open adrenal surgery.[41]

The overall complication rate of laparoscopic adrenalectomy compares favourably with the open approach, particularly with a decreased likelihood of intraoperative bleeding and postoperative pulmonary complications.[33,42] Brunt reported on a comparison of all published series of open and laparoscopic adrenalectomy and found that while the incidence of bleeding complications was higher for laparoscopic surgery, open adrenalectomy had a significantly higher incidence of associated organ injury, mainly to the spleen, and more wound, pulmonary, cardiac, and infectious complications.[43] The mortality rate was 0.3% for laparoscopic adrenalectomy versus 0.9% after open approaches. Laparoscopic adrenalectomy is now established as the primary method of surgery in many smaller benign lesions that need excision.[44] Many case studies have now been published showing a lower rate of blood loss, transfusion requirement, postoperative analgesia requirement and overall intraoperative complication rate, although the complications themselves are the same as in the open approach.[5,45–47] Its limitations are found when operating on larger and malignant tumours, and the role of laparoscopic adrenalectomy in these situations is as yet unclear.[27,31,38]

Vascular injuries

The adrenal glands are exceedingly vascular structures, being supplied by multiple arterial branches from the inferior phrenic artery, the abdominal aorta and the renal artery.[48] In contrast, the rich venous plexus in each gland tends to drain via a solitary adrenal vein. On the right side this short adrenal vein drains directly into the inferior vena cava, while on the left the adrenal vein drains into the left renal vein.[49] This asymmetric arrangement is important in assessing the risk of haemorrhage from damaged vessels.[50]

Approximately two thirds of the complications associated with this procedure relate to damage to the surrounding vascular structures, particularly by surgeons with little experience.[51] Diffuse circumferential blood supply means that vascular complications can occur at any point around the periphery of the adrenal gland.[49] Vascular injury to the renal and mesenteric vessels should be avoided, and care should be taken when the adrenal mass is very large, as anatomical distortion can result in inadvertent vascular injury.[52]

On the right side, a major pitfall is a tear in the short adrenal vein that drains directly into the IVC on its posterior surface.[4] If a tear does occur, pressure to occlude the IVC should allow placement of a vascular clamp, before either conversion to open operation, or the placement of vascular clips or intracorporeal sutures to oversew the vein stump.[50] Similarly, the drainage branches into the lumbar veins can be easily torn. The low accessory hepatic veins, passing from the caudate lobe to the IVC, can be damaged, and ligation and division early in the dissection avoids inadvertent damage, and allows fuller exposure higher up the IVC. On the left side, Belsey's artery and the left phrenic vein are closely related to the adrenal near the oesophageal hiatus, and should be formally dissected and either preserved or divided electively.[4]

Organ injuries

On both sides, an injury can occur to adjacent organs in the area of dissection; injuries to the spleen, tail of the pancreas, splenic flexure of the colon, stomach and kidney can occur on the left side and patient consent should include details of the potential need for renal, splenic or pancreatic resection.[48,53–55] Right-sided structures at risk include the liver, duodenum, kidney and the hepatic flexure of the colon. Intestinal injuries may not present until several days into the postoperative period when the patient develops peritonitis.[29,55–57]

Dissection high in the abdomen, especially of the right triangular ligament of the liver, may result in diaphragmatic injury with the potential for pneumothorax, and this is particularly common in open posterior approaches which involve removal of the 12th or 11th rib.[55,58–60] Other respiratory complications such as pneumonia and pleural effusion can also arise from surgery very close to the underside of the diaphragm.[1,51,55,61]

Postoperative Endocrine Complications

Postoperative complications arise not only from the surgical insult itself, but also from the inadequate correction of the endocrine deficit created by the operation.[62,63]

Wound infection, dehiscence and delayed healing are more common in Cushing's patients.[6] Secondary hypocorticism is possible and careful attention should be paid to the adequate replacement of cortical function with oral corticosteriods for a prolonged period.[13] These should be weaned slowly, allowing the suppressed contralateral adrenal time to start functioning. Patients with unilateral adrenalectomy should have a short synacthen test in the postoperative period to ensure good contralateral function.[55]

Patients with hyperaldosteronism reveal an unpredictable metabolic response postoperatively, and may become hyper or hypokalaemic, dependant on the function of the contralateral adrenal, and their metabolic imbalance should be closely monitored and corrected.[14,15,30]

The postoperative management of the phaeochromocytoma patient is usually done in the intensive care setting initially, where the blood pressure can be closely monitored.[64] Hypotension due to prolonged alpha blockade should be monitored, and may be prevented if only short acting agents are used perioperatively.[12] Plasma expansion and exogenous alpha agonists can be used to maintain the blood pressure within normal limits.[13]

REFERENCES

1. Staren ED, Prinz RA. (1996) Adrenalectomy in the era of laparoscopy. *Surgery* **120**: 706–709.

2. Sidhu S, *et al.* (2002) Changing pattern of adrenalectomy at a tertiary referral centre 1970–2000. *ANZ J Surg* **72**: 463–466.

3. Gagner M, Lacroix A, Bolte E. (1992) Laparoscopic adrenalectomy in Cushing's syndrome and pheochromocytoma. *N Engl J Med* **327**: 1033.

4. Avisse C, *et al.* (2000) Surgical anatomy and embryology of the adrenal glands. *Surg Clin North Am* **80**: 403–415.

5. Gill IS. (2001) The case for laparoscopic adrenalectomy. *J Urol* **166**: 429–436.

6. Imai T, Kikumori T, Funahashi H, Nakao A. (2000) Surgical management of Cushing's syndrome. *Biomed Pharmacother* **54**(Suppl 1): 140s–145s.

7. Buell JF, Alexander HR, Norton JA, *et al.* (1997) Bilateral adrenalectomy for Cushing's syndrome. Anterior versus posterior surgical approach. *Ann Surg* **225**: 63–68.

8. Beauregard C, Dickstein G, Lacroix A. (2002) Classic and recent etiologies of Cushing's syndrome: diagnosis and therapy. *Treat Endocrinol* **1**: 79–94.

9. Norton JA, Li M, Gillary J, Le HN. (2001) Cushing's syndrome. *Curr Probl Surg* **38**: 488–545.

10. Porpiglia F, *et al.* (2004) Bilateral adrenalectomy for Cushing's syndrome: a comparison between laparoscopy and open surgery. *J Endocrinol Invest* **27**: 654–658.

11. Orth DN. (1995) Cushing's syndrome. *N Engl J Med* **332**: 791–803.

12. Xiao XR, *et al.* (1998) Diagnosis and treatment of adrenal tumours: a review of 35 years' experience. *Br J Urol* **82**: 199–205.

13. Angermeier KW, Montie JE. (1989) Perioperative complications of adrenal surgery. *Urol Clin North Am* **16**: 597–606.

14. Foxius A, *et al.* (1999) Hazards of laparoscopic adrenalectomy for Conn's adenoma. When enthusiasm turns to tragedy. *Surg Endosc* **13**: 715–717.

15. Young WF Jr. (2002) Primary aldosteronism: management issues. *Ann N Y Acad Sci* **970**: 61–76.

16. Miyake, Okuyama A. (2000) Surgical management of primary aldosteronism. *Biomed Pharmacother* **54**(Suppl 1): 146s–149s.

17. Shen WT, *et al.* (1999) Laparoscopic vs open adrenalectomy for the treatment of primary hyperaldosteronism. *Arch Surg* **134**: 628–631.

18. Wu KD, *et al.* (2001) Preoperative diagnosis and localization of aldosterone-producing adenoma by adrenal venous sampling after administration of metoclopramide. *J Formos Med Assoc* **100**: 598–603.
19. Kazaryan AM, Kuznetsov NS, Shulutko AM, *et al.* (2004) Evaluation of endoscopic and traditional open approaches to pheochromocytoma. *Surg Endosc* **18**: 937–941.
20. Miccoli P, Bendinelli C, Materazzi G, *et al.* (1997) Traditional versus laparoscopic surgery in the treatment of pheochromocytoma: a preliminary study. *J Laparoendosc Adv Surg Tech A* **7**: 167–171.
21. Zimmerman P, DaSilva M, Newman T, *et al.* (2004) Simultaneous bilateral laparoscopic adrenalectomy: a surgical option for multiple endocrine neoplasia (MEN 2) patients with bilateral pheochromocytomas. *Surg Endosc* **18**: 870.
22. Maiter D. (2004) Pheochromocytoma: a paradigm for catecholamine-mediated hypertension. *Acta Clin Belg* **59**: 209–219.
23. Kim AW, Quiros RM, Maxhimer JB, *et al.* (2004) Outcome of laparoscopic adrenalectomy for pheochromocytomas vs aldosteronomas. *Arch Surg* **139**: 526–529.
24. Sprung J, *et al.* (2000) Anesthetic aspects of laparoscopic and open adrenalectomy for pheochromocytoma. *Urology* **55**: 339–343.
25. Suzuki K. (2000) Surgical management of pheochromocytoma. *Biomed Pharmacother* **54**(Suppl 1): 150s–156s.
26. Thomson BN, Moulton CA, Davies M, Banting SW. (2004) Laparoscopic adrenalectomy for phaeochromocytoma: with caution. *ANZ J Surg* **74**: 429–433.
27. Saunders BD, Doherty GM. (2004) Laparoscopic adrenalectomy for malignant disease. *Lancet Oncol* **5**: 718–726.
28. Brunt LM, Moley JF. (2001) Adrenal incidentaloma. *World J Surg* **25**: 905–913.
29. Prager G, *et al.* (2002) Surgical strategy in adrenal masses. *Eur J Radiol* **41**: 70–77.
30. Brunt LM, *et al.* (2001) Outcomes analysis in patients undergoing laparoscopic adrenalectomy for hormonally active adrenal tumors. *Surgery* **130**: 629–634.
31. Prager G, *et al.* (2004) Applicability of laparoscopic adrenalectomy in a prospective study in 150 consecutive patients. *Arch Surg* **139**: 46–49.
32. Matsuda T, Murota T, Kawakita M. (2000) Transperitoneal anterior laparoscopic adrenalectomy: the easiest technique. *Biomed Pharmacother* **54**(Suppl 1): 157s–160s.
33. Gonzalez R, *et al.* (2004) Laparoscopic approach reduces likelihood of perioperative complications in patients undergoing adrenalectomy. *Am Surg* **70**: 668–674.
34. Maccabee DL, Jones A, Domreis J, *et al.* (2003) Transition from open to laparoscopic adrenalectomy: the need for advanced training. *Surg Endosc* **17**: 1566–1569.

35. Suzuki K, *et al.* (2001) Comparison of 3 surgical approaches to laparoscopic adrenalectomy: a nonrandomized, background matched analysis. *J Urol* **166**: 437–443.

36. David G, Yoav M, Gross D, Reissman P. (2004) Laparoscopic adrenalectomy: ascending the learning curve. *Surg Endosc* **18**: 771–773.

37. Lal G, Duh QY. (2003) Laparoscopic adrenalectomy — indications and technique. *Surg Oncol* **12**: 105–123.

38. Pisanu A, Cois A, Montisci A, Uccheddu A. (2004) Current indications for laparoscopic adrenalectomy in the era of minimally invasive surgery. *Chir Ital* **56**: 313–320.

39. Guazzoni G, *et al.* (2004) Laparoscopic treatment of adrenal diseases: 10 years on. *BJU Int* **93**: 221–227.

40. Nagesser SK, Kievit J, Hermans J, *et al.* (2000) The surgical approach to the adrenal gland: a comparison of the retroperitoneal and the transabdominal routes in 326 operations on 284 patients. *Jpn J Clin Oncol* **30**: 68–74.

41. Valeri A, *et al.* (2002) The influence of new technologies on laparoscopic adrenalectomy: our personal experience with 91 patients. *Surg Endosc* **16**: 1274–1279.

42. MacGillivray DC, Shichman SJ, Ferrer FA, Malchoff CD. (1996) A comparison of open vs laparoscopic adrenalectomy. *Surg Endosc* **10**: 987–990.

43. Brunt LM. (2002) The positive impact of laparoscopic adrenalectomy on complications of adrenal surgery. *Surg Endosc* **16**: 252–257.

44. Kebebew E, Siperstein AE, Duh QY. (2001) Laparoscopic adrenalectomy: the optimal surgical approach. *J Laparoendosc Adv Surg Tech A* **11**: 409–413.

45. Yokoi S, *et al.* (2002) Comparison of laparoscopic versus open surgery for adrenal tumor. *Hinyokika Kiyo* **48**: 203–206.

46. Schell SR, Talamini MA, Udelsman R. (1999) Laparoscopic adrenalectomy for nonmalignant disease: improved safety, morbidity, and cost-effectiveness. *Surg Endosc* **13**: 30–34.

47. Imai T, Kikumori T, Ohiwa M, *et al.* (1999) A case-controlled study of laparoscopic compared with open lateral adrenalectomy. *Am J Surg* **178**: 50–53.

48. Toniato A, Piotto A, Pagetta C, *et al.* (2001) Technique and results of laparoscopic adrenalectomy. *Langenbecks Arch Surg* **386**: 200–203.

49. Raeburn CD, McIntyre RC Jr. (2000) Laparoscopic approach to adrenal and endocrine pancreatic tumors. *Surg Clin North Am* **80**: 1427–1441.

50. Corcione F, *et al.* (2001) Vena cava injury. A serious complication during laparoscopic right adrenalectomy. *Surg Endosc* **15**: 218.

51. Henry JF, Defechereux T, Raffaelli M, *et al.* (2000) Complications of laparoscopic adrenalectomy: results of 169 consecutive procedures. *World J Surg* **24**: 1342–1346.

52. Terachi T, *et al.* (2000) Complications of laparoscopic and retroperitoneo-scopic adrenalectomies in 370 cases in Japan: a multi-institutional study. *Biomed Pharmacother* 54(Suppl 1): 211s–214s.

53. Suzuki K, *et al.* (1999) Complications of laparoscopic adrenalectomy in 75 patients treated by the same surgeon. *Eur Urol* 36: 40–47.

54. Sung GT, Gill IS. (2000) Laparoscopic adrenalectomy. *Semin Laparosc Surg* 7: 211–222.

55. Jossart GH, Burpee SE, Gagner M. (2000) Surgery of the adrenal glands. *Endocrinol Metab Clin North Am* 29: 57–68, viii.

56. Del Pizzo JJ. (2003) Transabdominal laparoscopic adrenalectomy. *Curr Urol Rep* 4: 81–86.

57. McCallum RW, Connell JM. (2001) Laparoscopic adrenalectomy. *Clin Endocrinol (Oxford)* 55: 435–456.

58. Kalan MM, Tillou G, Kulick A, *et al.* (2004) Performing laparoscopic adrenalec-tomy safely. *Arch Surg* 139: 1243–1247.

59. Assalia A, Gagner M. (2004) Laparoscopic adrenalectomy. *Br J Surg* 91: 1259–1274.

60. Nicolai N. (2003) Laparoscopic adrenalectomy. *Tumori* 89: 556–559.

61. Gagner M. (1996) Laparoscopic adrenalectomy. *Surg Clin North Am* 76: 523–537.

62. Vaughan ED Jr. (2004) Diseases of the adrenal gland. *Med Clin North Am* 88: 443–466.

63. Poulin EC, Schlachta CM, Burpee SE, *et al.* (2003) Laparoscopic adrenalectomy: pathologic features determine outcome. *Can J Surg* 46: 340–344.

64. Gotoh M, Ono Y, Hattori R, *et al.* (2002) Laparoscopic adrenalectomy for pheochromocytoma: morbidity compared with adrenalectomy for tumors of other pathology. *J Endourol* 16: 245–249.

PANCREATIC SURGERY

Introduction

Pancreatic endocrine tumours (PET) represent a rare group of neoplasms that arise from the pancreatic islet cells and account for 1–5% of all pancreatic tumours.[1] Clinically, PET have been classified as nonfunctioning (NF-PET) or functioning (F-PET), depending on the presence or absence of clinical symptoms due to excess hormone secretion.

Distinct F-PET can secrete insulin (**insulinoma**), gastrin (**gastrinoma** or Zollinger-Ellison syndrome), vasoactive intestinal peptide (**VIPoma**), glucagon (), somatostatin (**somatostatinoma**), growth-releasing factor (**GRFoma**), adrenocorticotropin hormone (**ACTHoma**), pancreatic polypeptide (**PPoma**), neurotensin (**neurotensinoma**) and parathyroid hormone releasing peptide (**PTHrPoma**). The presentation of F-PET is usually due to symptoms from the hypersecretion of a particular hormone. However, some tumours may produce a variety of peptides and the clinical presentation may be mixed.

NF-PET may produce hormones but not secrete them, secrete small and non-detectable amounts of hormones, secrete hormone substances that are currently not detectable, or secrete hormones that are biologically inactive and cause no clinical signs. The presentation of NF-PET is usually related to the effect of the tumour mass.

Among F-PET, insulinomas are the most common benign tumours with an estimated annual incidence of five cases per million per year.[2] Gastrinomas are the second most common islet cell secretory tumours, and the most common malignant tumours, with a rising incidence of 1.5 cases per million.[3] VIPomas have a reported incidence around one per 10 million,[4] while glucagonomas have an estimated incidence of one per 20 million.[4] The incidence of somatostatinoma is less than one in 40 million[3] and GRFoma, ACTHoma and PPoma are more rare. The incidence of NF-PET has been rising in recent years and is currently believed to account for 35–50% of all PET.[5,6]

The surgical management of PET depends on the type and location of the tumour, its malignant potential and an assessment of the risks associated with major pancreatic resection compared with medical management. The extent of surgery can vary from enucleation for small benign tumours, to more extensive formal resection of the proximal or distal pancreas in malignant tumours, or in benign tumours close to the pancreatic duct.

In the last decade, there has been widespread adoption of laparoscopic approaches as an alternative to standard open surgical procedures. Laparoscopic management of islet cell tumours, particularly insulinomas, may become the method of choice, being associated with faster postoperative recovery and similar morbidity rates when compared with open surgery.[7] The outcome is encouraging but the number of patients is limited and there has been no randomised controlled study to make safe conclusions.[7,8]

The morbidity and mortality rates of surgical procedures for pancreatic endocrine tumours have decreased substantially due to the better understanding of the biological behaviour of the tumors and the associated clinical syndromes, improvements in preoperative localisation, the introduction of intraoperative ultrasound and advances in perioperative management. Morbidity and mortality are directly related to the degree of surgery[1]; however, some authors have shown that aggressive surgery for advanced neuroendocrine tumours can also be done with acceptable morbidity and low mortality.[9,10] Morbidity tends to be higher if reoperation is required following failure to remove a tumour.[11–13] It is also higher for operations involving the head of the pancreas[14] and without adequate control of hormone secretion preoperatively.[15]

The complications can be divided into pancreatic and non-pancreas related.[11] The major complications are mostly pancreas-related and include pancreatic fistula, pancreatic pseudocyst, abscess formation and pancreatitis. The reported incidence of these pancreatic complications varies between 13–43%.[11,16–22]

Failed Surgery

The inability to localise and perform a complete resection of an endocrine tumour may lead to reoperation and its possible sequelae. The combination of endoscopic ultrasound (EUS) or intraoperative ultrasound (IOUS) and operative palpation has led to an almost 100% success rate at primary operation in experienced hands, but 13% of the patients at referral centres undergo re-exploration.[23]

Failed surgery has been a problem mainly with small and multiple tumours, such as insulinomas and gastrinomas. When operating on PET it is important to have a thorough knowledge of the characteristics of each tumour and tailor the operative procedure accordingly. The exploration must be thorough and meticulous and sites of potential location of the tumour and metastasis must be investigated. The association of MEN 1 must be excluded preoperatively, as these tumours have different characteristics.

Insulinoma

Insulinomas are usually benign (80–90%) and solitary (90%), with a high potential for cure.[2] They can be sporadic or associated with MEN 1. In almost 99% of the cases insulinomas are located within the pancreas, with a relatively even distribution, with up to 80% located in the body and tail.[24] Over 50% are between 1–5 cm in size and 30% are less than 1 cm.[25,26]

In a recent multi-institutional review, the success rate of initial procedures was 94.9%, and 99.5% after reoperation.[21] The reported success rate ranges between 95–100%,[11,21,27,28] and the reasons for failure include missed multiple tumours, MEN 1 syndrome, and diffuse/nodular hyperplasia.[12] Reoperations for persistent hyperinsulinism can be highly successful in experienced hands, but are associated with increased morbidity.[11,13]

Several studies have opposed the need for any preoperative localisation prior to surgical exploration,[29–31] and this is the current recommendation of the British Association of Endocrine Surgeons. This approach is based on the view that most insulinomas are visible and easily palpable, and in combination with IOUS, the success rate can be 100%.[31–33] However, the authors believe that preoperative localisation tests are important because they limit the required mobilisation and exposure of the pancreas, and influence the surgical approach.[34–36]

With the current advances in imaging technology, most insulinomas can be accurately localised in the preoperative setting.[37] Non-invasive studies such as CT and MRI have low sensitivity, but are useful in ruling out metastatic disease.[32,37–40] Invasive studies such as selective angiography (SANG), arterial stimulation venous sampling (ASVS) and EUS have a significantly higher sensitivity.[2,32,37–44]

In addition to accurate preoperative localisation, the exploration of the pancreas must be thorough and meticulous, with adequate exposure, bimanual palpation and suspicious areas sent for frozen section.[45] If the tumour cannot be localised, IOUS can be used, allowing the surgeon to identify the insulinoma in nearly every patient.[46,47] Perioperative monitoring of peripheral glucose can also be used after excision, with rebound hyperglycemia occuring within 30–45 min, but this technique can provide false positive results.[48] Rapid intraoperative insulin radio-immunoassay, similar to quick PTH assay in parathyroid surgery, can be a useful adjunct to ensure complete insulinoma resection and consequently, a successful postoperative outcome.[49,50]

Since the insulinoma may develop throughout the pancreas, the probability of a blind resection being successful is proportional to the amount of pancreas removed.[2] No distal blind resection should be performed in search of occult tumour, because at least 50% of impalpable, and occult insulinomas are located in the proximal pancreas.[11] If the tumour cannot be found, the abdomen should be closed and the patient reinvestigated.

Gastrinoma

It was originally believed that most gastrinomas arose in the pancreas, but now there is evidence that primary duodenal gastrinomas are more common,[51] with the incidence decreasing down the duodenum.[52,53] These are small tumours (microgastrinomas) located in the submucosa, especially occurring in association with MEN 1 syndrome, and are not palpable if they are not invasive. Most gastrinomas (60–90%) are found in the gastrinoma triangle which includes the pancreatic head, uncinate process and duodenum.[54−57] They are usually single in the sporadic group (75% of cases), but often multiple in the MEN 1 patients (25% of cases).[25] Gastrinomas are more frequently ectopic (non-duodenal, non-pancreatic) than insulinomas and can be found in the regional lymph nodes, the proximal mesentery, the omentum, the liver and biliary tree, the stomach and the ovaries.[58,59] The majority of the gastrinomas (60–90%) are malignant with frequent metastases to regional lymph nodes and the liver.[60−62]

The failure to localise a gastrinoma in early studies occurred in 7–48% of the cases,[51] but with the recognition of duodenal gastrinomas and the addition of duodenal exploration and duodenotomy at surgery, success rates are now consistently above 90%.[51,54,63,64] Improvements in preoperative imaging and intraoperative localisation techniques have also increased the surgeon's ability to cure these patients,[65] but early detection remains crucial to allow resection before the tumour has a chance to metastasise. Once the diagnosis of Zollinger-Ellison Syndrome (ZES) has been established, MEN 1 should be excluded and the extent of disease determined to decide whether complete resection, cytoreductive surgery or medical treatment is appropriate.

The preoperative localisation of gastrinomas is less successful than with insulinomas but equally essential, as they can be small and difficult to locate at laparotomy, and occasionally multiple. Primary location and tumour extent can be determined by non-invasive (US, CT, MRI, Somatostatin Receptor Scintigraphy or SRS) and invasive methods (EUS, SANG, ASVS and Transhepatic Venous Sampling or TVS).[66,67] In the presence of metastatic disease, CT and MRI can determine tumour bulk to help decide whether cytoreductive surgery may be beneficial.[68−70] SRS is particularly sensitive in identifying primary tumours and hepatic metastases with a high specificity.[71−74] EUS has the ability to localise pancreatic tumours, but is less sensitive for those located in the duodenum.[75] SANG, ASVS and TVS can be used for localisation if non-invasive methods have failed.[76−79]

There are a number of aids available to assist in the localisation of gastrinomas intraoperatively.[47] Standard palpation allows duodenal tumour detection in approximately 60% of the cases, with IOUS helpful in localising pancreatic gastrinomas, but less sensitive for duodenal tumors.[80] Endoscopic transillumination is more sensitive for duodenal tumours, as it is able to localise more than 80% of the cases and facilitate the planning of the duodenotomy site.[47,81] Duodenotomy increases the success rate up to 97%,[47,56,82] and longitudinal duodenotomy should be mandatory in all patients with MEN 1 and in patients with sporadic ZES when no primary tumour has been identified.[15]

In the past, total gastrectomy or vagotomy was the only effective treatment for acid hypersecretion[60,62,83] but with the advent of proton pump inhibitors, is rarely needed now.[84−88] Some authors propose that parietal cell vagotomy should be routinely performed at laparotomy, because apparently cured patients continue to have mild to moderate acid hypersecretion, requiring daily anti-secretory drugs.[89,90]

Patients with MEN 1 and ZES should undergo parathyroidectomy for hyperplasia[91−93] as fasting gastrin levels and basal acid output have been shown to decrease after parathyroid surgery, and sensitivity to anti-secretory drugs increase, allowing smaller doses to be given.[91–93] The success rate for patients with MEN 1 is low[94] as many have multiple tumours and a high percentage have metastases at the time of surgery.[63,95] Most of these patients have duodenal tumours which is an important factor to remember during surgical intervention.[63,91,95,96] The plasma levels of gastrin can be monitored to assess the response after surgical resection.[97]

Other Pancreatic Endocrine Tumours

A failure to localise other pancreatic endocrine tumours is not usually an issue as they are generally single, large and less frequently extrapancreatic. Most of them have metastasised at the time of diagnosis, but preoperative tests remain important not only for localising the tumours, but also for staging the disease. NF-PET are slow growing tumours, frequently located in the head of the pancreas and often palpable,[4,98] with a rising incidence in recent years.[98–100] Most of them are malignant,[98] but diagnosis is often delayed unless they produce ductal obstruction and jaundice, or symptoms due to metastatic disease.[101] Imaging modalities such as CT and MRI are accurate in localising these tumours.

VIPomas are mostly located in the left area of the pancreas and usually measure over 3 cm in diameter.[102] Tumours in extrapancreatic sites such as the retroperitoneal sympathetic chain and the adrenal medulla can be present in up to 20% of the cases.[103] More than 50% are malignant and the majority have metastasised by the time of diagnosis.[25] They are easily imaged by CT, and SRS can be useful in identifying occult metastatic disease.

Glucagonomas are always located in the pancreas and more frequently in the body and tail,[104] presenting as slow growing tumours, usually larger than 4 cm diameter.[25] The tumours are single, and malignant in more than 70% of the cases,[102] but up to 90% have metastasised by the time of diagnosis, making complete resection rarely possible.[105] CT is the radiological imaging modality of choice.

Somatostatinomas usually develop in the head of the pancreas, but they can also be located in the duodenum in the periampullary region.[106] They are thought to be the slowest growing of all neuroendocrine tumours and are often large.[102] They are malignant at least in 50% of the cases and metastasise to the regional lymph nodes and liver.[107] GRFomas present with acromegaly and can occur in other sites also including lung, adrenal and intestine.[102] Their biological behaviour is benign, and there is a frequent association with MEN 1 syndrome.[108] ACTHomas cause 4–16% of all ectopic CS, and 96% of patients have a malignant tumour.[25] They occur only in the pancreas, tend to grow quickly and almost always metastatic at presentation.[109] Pure PPomas are quite rare,[110] usually located in the body or tail[106] and often multicellular, producing and sometimes secreting more than one hormone or hormone-like substance.[111] The symptoms are non-specific and the tumours may be silent,[106,110,112,113] but are malignant in 20–40% of the patients.[25] Neurotensinoma is a tumour that secretes neurotensin and often other hormones such as VIP and gastrin, but its existence as a separate syndrome is disputed.[112,114] PTHrPoma is often too advanced, with severe life-threatening hypercalcemia.[115]

Pancreas-Related Complications

Pancreas-related complications add considerably to the overall morbidity of pancreatic endocrine tumour resection. Enucleation is preferable to formal resection if the tumour is small, solitary and benign, as it preserves the maximum pancreatic tissue, although distal pancreatectomy may be appropriate for lesions in the tail.[2] Enucleation is particularly suitable for insulinomas, less appropriate for gastrinomas, and rarely for the rest of the pancreatic endocrine tumours. If the tumour is located in the body or tail or is deep in the parenchyma, distal pancreatectomy is an appropriate alternative, while proximal pancreatectomy is rarely needed for benign tumours in the head.

Pancreatic Fistula

Pancreatic fistulae are the most common complication, with an expected incidence of approximately 10%, and may develop after any pancreatic procedure performed for PET.[1,2,11,14,18,21,26,84,116–118] They are more common after enucleation than distal pancreatectomy and this has not changed with the introduction of laparoscopic surgery.[7,18,19,26,36,119] The anatomical relationship of the tumour with the pancreatic duct is an important factor in deciding on enucleation or resection, and IOUS can facilitate this decision. All authors suggest that for tumours deep within the pancreas or in close proximity to the pancreatic duct, resection procedures are preferable.[36,120–125] After enucleation, a close inspection of the pancreatic bed must always be performed to exclude a pancreatic leak, which can be facilitated by the use of intravenous secretin (2 IU/kg body weight).[33,126] If a leak is demonstrated, fibrin glue may be beneficial,[4,126] the defect can be closed with sutures[11] or a roux-en-Y loop can be used to cover the cavity, particularly if it is deep.

Where distal pancreatectomy has been performed, the pancreas can be transected with a stapler or the cut edge of the pancreas oversewn with sutures and the pancreatic duct separately ligated.[127] In recent years ultrasonic dissectors have been used to divide the pancreatic parenchyma in both open and laparoscopic surgery,[127,128] but has not led to a decrease in the fistula rate.[128]

Following all pancreatic procedures, a drain should be left adjacent to the defect to ensure adequate drainage of any pancreatic leak. The perioperative use of somatostatin analogues is controversial[129]; however, it is generally accepted that while somatostatin does not decrease the frequency of the fistulae, it does decrease their output and duration.[4] Fistulae can usually be managed by conservative measures to contain the output, replace fluid and electrolytes, maintain nutrition with TPN and employ somatostatin analogues to decrease the output.[1] Following pancreatoduodenectomy, fistulae tend to discharge mixed enteric content, but can be usually managed by non-operative drainage and anti-secretory therapy.[130] Salvage distal or proximal pancreatectomies have been described for uncontrolled fistulae after enucleation for PET.[18]

Pancreatic Pseudocyst

Ductal disruption during surgery or leakage of pancreatic fluid from small ducts may lead to the formation of a pseudocyst. Its incidence is between 1–6.5%,[2,18,21,26] particularly after enucleation.[18,26] The symptoms are usually related to the compression of an adjacent viscus such as the stomach or duodenum, although a pseudocyst in the head may cause bile duct obstruction and jaundice. Small pseudocysts tend to resolve spontaneously and their treatment should be initially conservative, with close monitoring to detect potential complications such as haemorrhage, rupture or infection.[18] If surgery is indicated the pseudocyst can be resected or drained either externally or internally.

Abscess

Abscess formation may occur after secondary infection of a pancreatic fistula or pseudocyst, presenting with symptoms of sepsis. It can occur with open and laparoscopic surgery for PET as an early or late complication.[116,117,128] Percutaneous drainage under CT guidance may be adequate, but open surgical drainage may be required if symptoms do not resolve.[84,116]

Pancreatitis

The incidence of pancreatitis, occurring particularly after pancreatoduodenectomy, has decreased in recent studies and no longer associated with mortality.[14,21,26,117,131] However, it can be complicated by the formation of pseudocyst or abscess.

Pancreatic Insufficiency

Postoperative pancreatic function is determined by the degree of resection, the presence of underlying pancreatic disease and preoperative pancreatic function. Enucleation is preferred for small, benign tumours as larger resections carry a higher risk of pancreatic insufficiency.[32] Median pancreatectomy has been described as an alternative to distal pancreatectomy for benign and borderline tumours of the pancreatic body in order to decrease the risk of pancreatic insufficiency, but it has a very high pancreatic fistula rate.[132] Pancreatic insufficiency (endocrine, exocrine or both) occurs in up to 17% of the patients after extensive resection of the pancreas for malignant tumours, but may occur even with less extensive surgery.[1,133] Small occult tumours should not undergo unnecessary resection.[39] If a tumour is not detected, the procedure should be terminated and the patient referred to a centre capable of performing advanced preoperative and intraoperative localisation techniques.[39] Blind distal resections are not advised as the likelihood of completion pancreatectomy is high at reoperation.[23] Reoperations can be highly successful in experienced hands but are associated with an increased risk of brittle diabetes that increases mortality.[11,13] In cases of MEN 1 and hyperinsulinism, routine distal pancreatectomy with enucleation of tumours in the head under IOUS guidance is the best way to achieve adequate removal of tumour and minimise the risk of recurrent hypoglycemia, without causing endocrine and exocrine insufficiency.[11]

Bile and Enteric Leak

Although not true pancreatic complications, bile and enteric leaks are directly related to pancreatic surgery. Biliary fistulae are less common than pancreatic fistulae, occurring in up to 9% of the cases, following aggressive surgery and procedures involving the head of the pancreas.[15,133] Their management is conservative unless symptoms of sepsis develop.[14,84]

Enteric leaks have been also reported after operative procedures involving the head of the pancreas,[14,130] particularly the surgical treatment of duodenal gastrinomas. Conservative management may be sufficient if the output is controlled and adequate nutrition is provided to the patient.

Non-pancreas Related Complications

Complications unrelated to pancreatic procedures, such as wound infection, urinary tract infections, cardiopulmonary complications, bleeding, prolonged ileus and deep vein thrombosis, have a reported incidence of approximately 10%.[7,11,84,117,118,130,134]

Cardiopulmonary problems are more common after surgery for PET,[14] particularly in patients with insulinomas who are obese.[26] Patients with glucagonoma have a high risk of deep vein thrombosis, and pulmonary embolism is the most common cause of death.[97,102,135] The incidence of wound infection after laparoscopic surgery seems to be lower than in open surgery, although no randomised trial has been published.[7,36,119,136] The use of perioperative antibiotics is mandatory to decrease the risk of wound infection. Haemorrhage can be either intraoperative,[84,118,130,134] such as in distal pancreatectomy while trying to preserve the spleen, or postoperative, related to bleeding from operation sites or sepsis.[84,117,118,130,134,137,138]

Mortality

Multiple hepatic abscesses, peripancreatic abscesses and uncontrolled fistulae leading to multiple organ failure are the main causes of death.[1,18,84,118,130] Stefanini *et al.* reported an overall mortality rate of 11% in their collective review of insulinomas, with a mortality of 6.7% after the first operation and up to 18% after re-intervention.[26] Acute pancreatitis (37%) was the main cause of death, followed by peritonitis (23%) and pulmonary complications (14%). In a more recent multi-institutional review the operative mortality was significantly lower (2%), possibly because the incidence of pancreatitis has decreased (5.7%) and its management has improved.[21] However, hospital mortality remained almost three times higher at 5.7% following reoperation for failed laparotomy.[21]

The reported mortality for islet cell tumour resections in other studies ranges from 0–16.6%,[1,2,11,14,18,84,116–118,130,134] but mortality in more recent years is extremely uncommon, even after aggressive surgery for metastatic disease.[68,133] This is due to a better understanding of PET accompanied by developments in perioperative management.

REFERENCES

1. Bartsch DK, *et al.* (2000) Management of nonfunctioning islet cell carcinomas. *World J Surg* 24: 1418–1424.
2. Geoghegan JG, *et al.* (1994) Localization and surgical management of insulinoma. *Br J Surg* 81: 1025–1028.
3. Mullan MH, Gauger PG, Thompson NW. (2001) Endocrine tumours of the pancreas: review and recent advances. *ANZ J Surg* 71: 475–482.
4. Proye CA. (1998) Endocrine tumours of the pancreas: an update. *Aust N Z J Surg* 68: 90–100.
5. Gullo L, *et al.* (2003) Nonfunctioning pancreatic endocrine tumors: a multicenter clinical study. *Am J Gastroenterol* 98: 2435–2439.
6. Hochwald SN, Conlon KC, Brennan MF. (2001) Nonfunctional pancreatic islet cell tumors. In: Doherty GM, Skogseid B (eds), *Surgical Endocrinology* (Lippincott Williams & Wilkins, Philadelphia), pp. 361–373.
7. Lo CY, Chan WF, Lo CM, *et al.* (2004) Surgical treatment of pancreatic insulinomas in the era of laparoscopy. *Surg Endosc* 18(2): 297–302.
8. Shimizu S, Tanaka M, Konomi H, *et al.* (2004) Laparoscopic pancreatic surgery: current indications and surgical results. *Surg Endosc* 18(3): 402–406.
9. Norton JA, *et al.* (2003) Morbidity and mortality of aggressive resection in patients with advanced neuroendocrine tumors. *Arch Surg* 138: 859–866.
10. Carty SE, Jensen RT, Norton JA. (1992) Prospective study of aggressive resection of metastatic pancreatic endocrine tumors. *Surgery* 112: 1024–1031.

11. Grant CS. (2001) Insulinoma. In: Doherty GM, Skogseid B (eds), *Surgical Endocrinology* (Lippincott Williams & Wilkins, Philadelphia), pp. 346–360.
12. Simon D, Starke A, Goretzki PE, Roeher HD. (1998) Reoperative surgery for organic hyperinsulinism: indications and operative strategy. *World J Surg* **22**: 666–671.
13. Thompson GB, *et al.* (1993) Reoperative insulinomas, 1927 to 1992: an institutional experience. *Surgery* **114**: 1196–1204.
14. Broughan TA, Leslie JD, Soto JM, Hermann RE. (1986) Pancreatic islet cell tumors. *Surgery* **99**: 671–678.
15. Lowney JK, Doherty GM. (2001) Surgery for endocrine tumors of the pancreas. In: Doherty GM, Skogseid B (eds), *Surgical Endocrinology* (Lippincott Williams & Wilkins, Philadelphia), pp. 381–392.
16. Bieligk S, Jaffe BM. (1995) Islet cell tumors of the pancreas. *Surg Clin North Am* **75**: 1025–1040.
17. Doherty GM, *et al.* (1991) Results of a prospective strategy to diagnose, localize, and resect insulinomas. *Surgery* **110**: 989–996.
18. Lo CY, *et al.* (1997) Pancreatic insulinomas. A 15-year experience. *Arch Surg* **132**: 926–930.
19. Menegaux F, Schmitt G, Mercadier M, Chigot JP. (1993) Pancreatic insulinomas. *Am J Surg* **165**: 243–248.
20. Pasieka JL, McLeod MK, Thompson NW, Burney RE. (1992) Surgical approach to insulinomas. Assessing the need for preoperative localization. *Arch Surg* **127**: 442–447.
21. Rothmund M, *et al.* (1990) Surgery for benign insulinoma: an international review. *World J Surg* **14**: 393–398.
22. van Heerden JA, Edis AJ, Service FJ. (1979) The surgical aspects of insulinomas. *Ann Surg* **189**: 677–682.
23. Richards ML, Gauger PG, Thompson NW, *et al.* (2002) Pitfalls in the surgical treatment of insulinoma. *Surgery* **132**: 1040–1049.
24. Lo CY, *et al.* (2000) Value of intra-arterial calcium stimulated venous sampling for regionalization of pancreatic insulinomas. *Surgery* **128**: 903–909.
25. Aldridge MC, Williamson RCN. (1993) Surgery of endocrine tumours of the pancreas. In: Lynn JA, Bloom SR (eds), *Surgical Endocrinology* (Butterworth-Heinemann, Oxford), pp. 503–520.
26. Stefanini P, Carboni M, Patrassi N, Basoli A. (1974) Beta-islet cell tumors of the pancreas: results of a study on 1,067 cases. *Surgery* **75**: 597–609.
27. Boukhman MP, *et al.* (1998) Insulinoma — experience from 1950 to 1995. *West J Med* **169**: 98–104.

28. Grant CS, van Heerden J, Charboneau JW, *et al.* (1988) Insulinoma. The value of intraoperative ultrasonography. *Arch Surg* **123**: 843–848.

29. Bottger TC, Junginger T. (1993) Is preoperative radiographic localization of islet cell tumors in patients with insulinoma necessary? *World J Surg* **17**: 427–432.

30. Hashimoto LA, Walsh RM. (1999) Preoperative localization of insulinomas is not necessary. *J Am Coll Surg* **189**: 368–373.

31. Huai JC, *et al.* (1998) Localization and surgical treatment of pancreatic insulinomas guided by intraoperative ultrasound. *Am J Surg* **175**: 18–21.

32. Machado MC, *et al.* (2001) Insulinoma: diagnostic strategies and surgical treatment. A 22-year experience. *Hepatogastroenterology* **48**: 854–858.

33. Chapuis Y, Bertrand D. (2002) Laparoscopic enucleation of islet tumors of the pancreas. In: Gagner M, Inabnet WB (eds), *Minimally Invasive Endocrine Surgery* (Lippincott Williams and Wilkins, Philadelphia), pp. 273–281.

34. Patterson EJ, *et al.* (2001) Laparoscopic pancreatic resection: single-institution experience of 19 patients. *J Am Coll Surg* **193**: 281–287.

35. Jaroszewski DE, Schlinkert RT, Thompson GB, Schlinkert DK. (2004) Laparoscopic localization and resection of insulinomas. *Arch Surg* **139**: 270–274.

36. Iihara M, Obara T. (2002) Minimally invasive endocrine surgery: laparoscopic resection of insulinomas. *Biomed Pharmacother* **56**(Suppl 1): 227s–230s.

37. Gramatica L Jr. *et al.* (2002) Videolaparoscopic resection of insulinomas: experience in two institutions. *World J Surg* **26**: 1297–1300.

38. Mabrut JY, *et al.* (2001) Is preoperative localization of insulinomas necessary? *Ann Chir* **126**: 850–856.

39. Hirshberg B, *et al.* (2002) Blind distal pancreatectomy for occult insulinoma, an inadvisable procedure. *J Am Coll Surg* **194**: 761–764.

40. Boukhman MP, *et al.* (1999) Localization of insulinomas. *Arch Surg* **134**: 818–822.

41. Nesje LB, Varhaug JE, Husebye ES, Odegaard S. (2002) Endoscopic ultrasonography for preoperative diagnosis and localization of insulinomas. *Scand J Gastroenterol* **37**: 732–737.

42. Anderson MA, *et al.* (2000) Endoscopic ultrasound is highly accurate and directs management in patients with neuroendocrine tumors of the pancreas. *Am J Gastroenterol* **95**: 2271–2277.

43. O'Shea D, Rohrer-Theurs AW, Lynn JA, *et al.* (1996) Localization of insulinomas by selective intraarterial calcium injection. *J Clin Endocrinol Metab* **81**: 1623–1627.

44. Kuzin NM, *et al.* (1998) Preoperative and intraoperative topographic diagnosis of insulinomas. *World J Surg* **22**: 593–597.

45. Ruckert K, Gunther R. (1982) Is "blind left-pancreatic resection" for insulinoma still indicated? *Chirurg* **53**: 98–102.
46. Cothren CC, Raeburn CD, Chen Y, McIntyre RC Jr. (2003) Insulinoma: identification by EUS and intraoperative US. *Gastrointest Endosc* **58**: 575–576.
47. Norton JA. (1999) Intra-operative procedures to localize endocrine tumours of the pancreas and duodenum. *Ital J Gastroenterol Hepatol* **31**(Suppl 2): S195–197.
48. Tutt GO Jr, Edis AJ, Service FJ, van Heerden JA. (1980) Plasma glucose monitoring during operation for insulinoma: a critical reappraisal. *Surgery* **88**: 351–356.
49. Carneiro DM, Levi JU, Irvin GL, III. (2002) Rapid insulin assay for intraoperative confirmation of complete resection of insulinomas. *Surgery* **132**: 937–942.
50. Proye C, *et al.* (1998) Intraoperative insulin measurement during surgical management of insulinomas. *World J Surg* **22**: 1218–1224.
51. Jensen RT. (2001) Zollinger-Ellison syndrome. In: Doherty GM, Skogseid B (eds), *Surgical Endocrinology* (Lippincott Williams & Wilkins, Philadelphia), pp. 291–343.
52. Thom AK, Norton JA, Axiotis CA, Jensen RT. (1991) Location, incidence, and malignant potential of duodenal gastrinomas. *Surgery* **110**: 1086–1091.
53. Delcore R Jr, Cheung LY, Friesen SR. (1990) Characteristics of duodenal wall gastrinomas. *Am J Surg* **160**: 621–623.
54. Norton JA, Doppman JL, Jensen RT. (1992) Curative resection in Zollinger-Ellison syndrome. Results of a 10-year prospective study. *Ann Surg* **215**: 8–18.
55. Howard TJ, Zinner MJ, Stabile BE, Passaro E Jr. (1990) Gastrinoma excision for cure. A prospective analysis. *Ann Surg* **211**: 9–14.
56. Sugg SL, *et al.* (1993) A prospective study of intraoperative methods to diagnose and resect duodenal gastrinomas. *Ann Surg* **218**: 138–144.
57. Stabile BE, Morrow DJ, Passaro E Jr. (1984) The gastrinoma triangle: operative implications. *Am J Surg* **147**: 25–31.
58. Farley DR, van Heerden JA, Grant CS, Thompson GB. (1994) Extrapancreatic gastrinomas. Surgical experience. *Arch Surg* **129**: 506–511.
59. Wolfe MM, Alexander RW, McGuigan JE. (1982) Extrapancreatic, extraintestinal gastrinoma: effective treatment by surgery. *N Engl J Med* **306**: 1533–1536.
60. Ellison EH, Wilson SD. (1964) The Zollinger-Ellison syndrome: re-appraisal and evaluation of 260 registered cases. *Ann Surg* **160**: 512–530.
61. Creutzfeldt W, Arnold R, Creutzfeldt C, Track NS. (1975) Pathomorphologic, biochemical, and diagnostic aspects of gastrinomas (Zollinger-Ellison syndrome). *Hum Pathol* **6**: 47–76.
62. Fox PS, Hofmann JW, Wilson SD, DeCosse JJ. (1974) Surgical management of the Zollinger-Ellison syndrome. *Surg Clin North Am* **54**: 395–407.

63. Norton JA, *et al.* (1999) Surgery to cure the Zollinger-Ellison syndrome. *N Engl J Med* **341**: 635–644.

64. Jensen RT. (1996) Gastrointestinal endocrine tumours. Gastrinoma. *Baillieres Clin Gastroenterol* **10**: 603–643.

65. Delcore R, Friesen SR. (1994) The place for curative surgical procedures in the treatment of sporadic and familial Zollinger-Ellison syndrome. *Curr Opin Gen Surg* 69–76.

66. Orbuch M, Doppman JL, Jensen RT. (1995) Localization of pancreatic endocrine tumors. *Semin Gastrointest Dis* **6**: 90–101.

67. Rothmund M. (1994) Localization of endocrine pancreatic tumours. *Br J Surg* **81**: 164–166.

68. Norton JA, Warren RS, Kelly MG, *et al.* (2003) Aggressive surgery for metastatic liver neuroendocrine tumors. *Surgery* **134**: 1057–1063.

69. Norton JA, *et al.* (1998) Surgical treatment of localized gastrinoma within the liver: a prospective study. *Surgery* **124**: 1145–1152.

70. Owen NJ, *et al.* (2001) MRI of pancreatic neuroendocrine tumours. *Br J Radiol* **74**: 968–973.

71. Krenning EP, *et al.* (1994) Somatostatin-receptor scintigraphy in gastroenteropancreatic tumors. An overview of European results. *Ann N Y Acad Sci* **733**: 416–424.

72. Alexander HR, *et al.* (1998) Prospective study of somatostatin receptor scintigraphy and its effect on operative outcome in patients with Zollinger-Ellison syndrome. *Ann Surg* **228**: 228–238.

73. Cadiot G, *et al.* (1996) Preoperative detection of duodenal gastrinomas and peripancreatic lymph nodes by somatostatin receptor scintigraphy. Groupe D'etude Du Syndrome De Zollinger-Ellison. *Gastroenterology* **111**: 845–854.

74. Gibril F, *et al.* (1996) Somatostatin receptor scintigraphy: its sensitivity compared with that of other imaging methods in detecting primary and metastatic gastrinomas. A prospective study. *Ann Intern Med* **125**: 26–34.

75. Bhutani MS. (1999) Endoscopic ultrasound in pancreatic diseases. Indications, limitations, and the future. *Gastroenterol Clin North Am* **28**: 747–770, xi.

76. Thom AK, *et al.* (1992) Prospective study of the use of intraarterial secretin injection and portal venous sampling to localize duodenal gastrinomas. *Surgery* **112**: 1002–1008.

77. Imamura M, *et al.* (1987) Usefulness of selective arterial secretin injection test for localization of gastrinoma in the Zollinger-Ellison syndrome. *Ann Surg* **205**: 230–239.

78. Cherner JA, *et al.* (1986) Selective venous sampling for gastrin to localize gastrinomas. A prospective assessment. *Ann Intern Med* **105**: 841–847.

79. Gibril F, *et al.* (1996) Metastatic gastrinomas: localization with selective arterial injection of secretin. *Radiology* **198**: 77–84.
80. Norton JA. (1999) Intraoperative methods to stage and localize pancreatic and duodenal tumors. *Ann Oncol* **10**(Suppl 4): 182–184.
81. Frucht H, *et al.* (1990) Detection of duodenal gastrinomas by operative endoscopic transillumination. A prospective study. *Gastroenterology* **99**: 1622–1627.
82. Jensen RT, Fraker DL. (1994) Zollinger-Ellison syndrome. Advances in treatment of gastric hypersecretion and the gastrinoma. *JAMA* **271**: 1429–1435.
83. Zollinger RM, *et al.* (1980) Primary peptic ulcerations of the jejunum associated with islet cell tumors. Twenty-five-year appraisal. *Ann Surg* **192**: 422–430.
84. Lo CY, *et al.* (1996) Islet cell carcinoma of the pancreas. *World J Surg* **20**: 878–883.
85. Ellison EC. (1995) Forty-year appraisal of gastrinoma. Back to the future. *Ann Surg* **222**: 511–521.
86. Malagelada JR, Edis AJ, Adson MA, *et al.* (1983) Medical and surgical options in the management of patients with gastrinoma. *Gastroenterology* **84**: 1524–1532.
87. Richardson CT, Walsh JH. (1976) The value of a histamine H2-receptor antagonist in the management of patients with the Zollinger-Ellison syndrome. *N Engl J Med* **294**: 133–135.
88. Richardson CT, *et al.* (1979) Effect of vagotomy in Zollinger-Ellison syndrome. *Gastroenterology* **77**: 682–686.
89. Pisegna JR, *et al.* (1992) Effects of curative gastrinoma resection on gastric secretory function and antisecretory drug requirement in the Zollinger-Ellison syndrome. *Gastroenterology* **102**: 767–778.
90. Jensen RT. (1996) Should the 1996 citation for Zollinger-Ellison syndrome read: "Acid-reducing surgery in, aggressive resection out"? *Am J Gastroenterol* **91**: 1067–1070.
91. Jensen RT. (1998) Management of the Zollinger-Ellison syndrome in patients with multiple endocrine neoplasia type 1. *J Intern Med* **243**: 477–488.
92. Norton JA, *et al.* (1987) Effect of parathyroidectomy in patients with hyperparathyroidism, Zollinger-Ellison syndrome, and multiple endocrine neoplasia type I: a prospective study. *Surgery* **102**: 958–966.
93. McCarthy DM, *et al.* (1979) Hyperparathyroidism — a reversible cause of cimetidine-resistant gastric hypersecretion. *Br Med J* **1**: 1765–1766.
94. MacFarlane MP, *et al.* (1995) Prospective study of surgical resection of duodenal and pancreatic gastrinomas in multiple endocrine neoplasia type 1. *Surgery* **118**: 973–979.
95. Thompson NW, Bondeson AG, Bondeson L, Vinik A. (1989) The surgical treatment of gastrinoma in MEN I syndrome patients. *Surgery* **106**: 1081–1085.

96. Thompson NW. (1998) Current concepts in the surgical management of multiple endocrine neoplasia type 1 pancreatic-duodenal disease. Results in the treatment of 40 patients with Zollinger-Ellison syndrome, hypoglycaemia or both. *J Intern Med* **243**: 495–500.

97. Wynick D, Bloom SR. (1993) Diagnosis and Medical Management of Gastoenteropancreatic Tumours. In: Lynn JA, Bloom SR (eds), *Surgical Endocrinology* (Butterworth-Heinemann, Oxford), pp. 487–493.

98. Kent RB, III, van Heerden JA, Weiland LH. (1981) Non-functioning islet cell tumors. *Ann Surg* **193**: 185–190.

99. Kloppel G, Heitz PU. (1988) Pancreatic endocrine tumors. *Pathol Res Pract* **183**: 155–168.

100. Grant CS. (1993) Surgical management of malignant islet cell tumors. *World J Surg* **17**: 498–503.

101. Cheslyn-Curtis S, Sitaram V, Williamson RC. (1993) Management of non-functioning neuroendocrine tumours of the pancreas. *Br J Surg* **80**: 625–627.

102. Doherty GM. (2001) Vipoma, glucagonoma and other rare islet cell tumors. In: Doherty GM, Skogseid B (eds), *Surgical Endocrinology* (Lippincott Williams & Wilkins, Philadelphia), pp. 375–379.

103. Park SK, O'Dorisio MS, O'Dorisio TM. (1996) Vasoactive intestinal polypeptide-secreting tumours: biology and therapy. *Baillieres Clin Gastroenterol* **10**: 673–696.

104. Soga J, Yakuwa Y. (1998) Glucagonomas/diabetico-dermatogenic syndrome (DDS): a statistical evaluation of 407 reported cases. *J Hepatobiliary Pancreat Surg* **5**: 312–319.

105. Zhang M, *et al.* (2004) Clinical experience in diagnosis and treatment of glucagonoma syndrome. *Hepatobiliary Pancreat Dis Int* **3**: 473–475.

106. Howard TJ, *et al.* (1990) Anatomic distribution of pancreatic endocrine tumors. *Am J Surg* **159**: 258–264.

107. Soga J, Yakuwa Y. (1999) Somatostatinoma/inhibitory syndrome: a statistical evaluation of 173 reported cases as compared to other pancreatic endocrinomas. *J Exp Clin Cancer Res* **18**: 13–22.

108. Sano T, Asa SL, Kovacs K. (1988) Growth hormone-releasing hormone-producing tumors: clinical, biochemical, and morphological manifestations. *Endocr Rev* **9**: 357–373.

109. Doppman JL, *et al.* (1994) Adrenocorticotropic hormone-secreting islet cell tumors: are they always malignant? *Radiology* **190**: 59–64.

110. Bellows C, Haque S, Jaffe B. (1998) Pancreatic polypeptide islet cell tumor: case report and review of the literature. *J Gastrointest Surg* **2**: 526–532.

111. Heitz PU, Kasper M, Polak JM, Kloppel G. (1982) Pancreatic endocrine tumors. *Hum Pathol* **13**: 263–271.

112. Shulkes A, Boden R, Cook I, *et al.* (1984) Characterization of a pancreatic tumor containing vasoactive intestinal peptide, neurotensin, and pancreatic polypeptide. *J Clin Endocrinol Metab* **58**: 41–48.

113. Strodel WE, *et al.* (1984) Pancreatic polypeptide-producing tumors. Silent lesions of the pancreas? *Arch Surg* **119**: 508–514.

114. Blackburn AM, Bryant MG, Adrian TE, Bloom SR. (1981) Pancreatic tumours produce neurotensin. *J Clin Endocrinol Metab* **52**: 820–822.

115. Wynick D, *et al.* (1990) Treatment of a malignant pancreatic endocrine tumour secreting parathyroid hormone related protein. *BMJ* **300**: 1314–1315.

116. Grama D, *et al.* (1992) Clinical characteristics, treatment and survival in patients with pancreatic tumors causing hormonal syndromes. *World J Surg* **16**: 632–639.

117. Norton JA, *et al.* (2001) Comparison of surgical results in patients with advanced and limited disease with multiple endocrine neoplasia type 1 and Zollinger-Ellison syndrome. *Ann Surg* **234**: 495–505.

118. Thompson GB, van Heerden JA, Grant CS, *et al.* (1988) Islet cell carcinomas of the pancreas: a twenty-year experience. *Surgery* **104**: 1011–1017.

119. Tagaya N, *et al.* (2003) Laparoscopic resection of the pancreas and review of the literature. *Surg Endosc* **17**: 201–206.

120. Chapuis Y, Bigourdan JM, Massault PP, *et al.* (1998) Videolaparoscopic excision of insulinoma. A study of 5 cases. *Chirurgie* **123**: 461–467.

121. Fabre JM, *et al.* (2002) Is laparoscopic left pancreatic resection justified? *Surg Endosc* **16**: 1358–1361.

122. Vezakis A, Davides D, Larvin M, McMahon MJ. (1999) Laparoscopic surgery combined with preservation of the spleen for distal pancreatic tumors. *Surg Endosc* **13**: 26–29.

123. Machi J. (1999) Intraoperative and laparoscopic ultrasound. *Surg Oncol Clin North Am* **8**: 205–226.

124. Correnti S, Liverani A, Antonini G, *et al.* (1996) Intraoperative ultrasonography for pancreatic insulinomas. *Hepatogastroenterology* **43**: 207–211.

125. Machi J, Oishi AJ, Furumoto NL, Oishi RH. (2004) Intraoperative ultrasound. *Surg Clin North Am* **84**: 1085–1111.

126. Ohwada S, *et al.* (1998) Fibrin glue sandwich prevents pancreatic fistula following distal pancreatectomy. *World J Surg* **22**: 494–498.

127. Suzuki Y, *et al.* (1999) Randomized clinical trial of ultrasonic dissector or conventional division in distal pancreatectomy for non-fibrotic pancreas. *Br J Surg* **86**: 608–611.

128. Ayav A, Bresler L, Brunaud L, Boissel P. (2004) Laparoscopic approach for solitary insulinoma: a multicentre study. *Langenbecks Arch Surg* **390**: 134–140.

129. Gouillat C, Gigot JF. (2001) Pancreatic surgical complications — the case for prophylaxis. *Gut* **48**(Suppl 4): iv32–39.

130. Sarmiento JM, Farnell MB, Que FG, Nagorney DM. (2002) Pancreaticoduodenectomy for islet cell tumors of the head of the pancreas: long-term survival analysis. *World J Surg* **26**: 1267–1271.

131. Chen X, Cai WY, Yang WP, Li HW. (2002) Pancreatic insulinomas: diagnosis and surgical treatment of 74 patients. *Hepatobiliary Pancreat Dis Int* **1**: 458–461.

132. Balzano G, Zerbi A, Veronesi P, *et al.* (2003) Surgical treatment of benign and borderline neoplasms of the pancreatic body. *Dig Surg* **20**: 506–510.

133. Sarmiento JM, *et al.* (2002) Concurrent resections of pancreatic islet cell cancers with synchronous hepatic metastases: outcomes of an aggressive approach. *Surgery* **132**: 976–982.

134. Kaplan EL, *et al.* (1990) Gastrinomas: a 42-year experience. *World J Surg* **14**: 365–375.

135. Stacpoole PW. (1981) The glucagonoma syndrome: clinical features, diagnosis, and treatment. *Endocr Rev* **2**: 347–361.

136. Phan GQ, *et al.* (1998) Surgical experience with pancreatic and peripancreatic neuroendocrine tumors: review of 125 patients. *J Gastrointest Surg* **2**: 472–482.

137. Fernandez-Cruz L, *et al.* (2002) Outcome of laparoscopic pancreatic surgery: endocrine and nonendocrine tumors. *World J Surg* **26**: 1057–1065.

138. Sussman LA, Christie R, Whittle DE. (1996) Laparoscopic excision of distal pancreas including insulinoma. *Aust N Z J Surg* **66**: 414–416.

Chapter 17

SURGICAL COMPLICATIONS IN PAEDIATRIC SURGERY

Muhammad Tariq Dosani, Nadey S. Hakim
and Vassilios E. Papalois

INTRODUCTION

Paediatric surgery combines the technical challenge of performing complex operations in neonate, the appeal of solving a wide array of problems in many anatomic locations and the immense satisfaction of caring for children and offering them a long normal life. The approach to surgical problems in children should consider the long-term effects of the therapy as well as its immediate success rate. The resiliency of children to major surgical stress must always be balanced against their intolerance to inaccurate fluid and medication administration.

During the last 25 years there has been an enormous improvement in the outlook for children who need to undergo surgical procedures. This change in prognosis is the result of a greater understanding of the physiology and an awareness of their special needs. Advances in anaesthesia, surgical procedures and postoperative care have all made it possible to perform complex procedures successfully. The differences between children and adults are most marked immediately after birth, when the infant is adapting to extra-uterine life. However such differences exist throughout childhood and must be understood and acted on if a satisfactory outcome is to be achieved. All staff involved in the care of ill children should have appropriate training and experience. A team approach should include not only nurses and doctors, but pharmacists, laboratory staff, radiographers and social workers. Besides having unique physiological characteristics, children have special psychological needs, which the hospital environment must take into account. The family must be involved in the care of their child; staff must, and therefore be able to, communicate with parents, siblings and others who are close to the patient. The physical environment must provide space for private consultations with parents.

GENERAL CONSIDERATIONS

Differences in topographical anatomy between adults and children are important in surgery. Critically ill children are not "small adults"; unnecessary mistakes in management can occur if the differences are not appreciated. Infants and small children have a wider abdomen, a broad costal margin and a shallow pelvis. The ribs are more horizontal and the respiratory function is much more dependent on diaphragmatic movements. The umbilicus is relatively low lying. Abdominal scars grow with the child, for example a gastrostomy sited in the epigastrium of the newborn infant may migrate and end up as a scar over the costal margin.

Thermoregulation is important in children because of body surface area to weight ratio; therefore children lose heat more quickly. Babies have less subcutaneous fat and immature peripheral vasomotor cortisol mechanism.

Infants undergoing surgery are vulnerable in other ways. Impaired gluconeogenesis renders them more susceptible to hypoglycaemia and blood glucose must be monitored. Newborn infants are at risk of clotting deficiencies and should be given Vitamin K. They are less able to concentrate urine or conserve sodium and have greater obligatory water loss to excrete a given solute load. Immaturity of the immune system increases the risk of infection which can present as poor feeding, vomiting and listlessness. Surgical procedures undertaken in the first few days after birth carry particular risks; the process of adaptation to extra-uterine life must not be adversely affected.

HEAD AND NECK

Surgical lesions of the head and neck are common in children and range from congenital to acquired, from asymptomatic swellings to life-threatening airway obstruction.

Branchial Cleft Remnants

Remnants of embryonic branchial apparatus (cyst, sinuses, fistulae and cartilaginous rest) are common in children. Although congenital by definition, they often go unrecognised. Sinuses, fistulae, and cartilaginous rest are usually apparent at birth and noticed early in life. Cysts are more likely to present later in childhood as neck mass when they fill with secretions. All these lesions are associated with risk of infection and frequently come to clinical attention as an abscess or erythema. Rarely the remnants may harbour malignancy.[1]

With all branchial clefts remnants, the goal of treatment is complete surgical excision. The operation is usually performed at the time of diagnosis provided no active inflammation or infection is present. If there is infection, the operation should be delayed till the inflammation is settled. Formal excision of a branchial cleft lesion attempted in the presence of infection or active inflammation is associated with a higher recurrence rate secondary to incomplete excision and is also associated with an increase likelihood of injury to facial and hypoglossal nerves and other vital structures. Care should be taken during the dissection to avoid injury to facial nerve branches; a nerve stimulator may be helpful.

Thyroglossal Duct Cyst

It is one of the most common midline neck lesions in children. It is present at birth but rarely present clinically in early infancy. It is usually present as a midline cystic neck mass or draining sinus in early childhood. Successful management requires complete removal of the cyst, its entire tract, and the central portion of the hyoid bone. Definitive excision should not be performed in the presence of infection as it increases the risk of incomplete excision and injury to nearby structures. The importance of removing the central portion of the hyoid was described by Sistrunk,[2] along with the possible existence of multiple tracts; therefore it is important to do so as en bloc dissection and removal of a core of tissue to the base of the tongue. This has reduced the recurrence rate to less than 10%.

Lymphangiomas and Cystic Hygroma

Lymphangiomas are masses of disorganised, dilated lymph channels that arise when communications with the internal jugular system fail to develop in a portion of the lymphatic channels. They can vary in size from a few centimetres to huge tumour-like masses extending into the mediastinum. The larger lesions with macrocystic dilated lymphatic channels are often referred to as cystic hygroma. Complete surgical excision is the treatment for lymphatic malformations. Because these lesions are benign, radical extirpation resulting in loss of function or severe deformity is not indicated. One third of these cases require partial excision or staged excision because these are extensive or complex lesions, or as a result of the involvement of vital structures within the lesion. Needle aspiration, radiation treatment, or injection of sclerosants can help in difficult cases but they are associated with significant potential complications.[3]

CHEST

Pectus Excavatum

Pectus excavatum results from the abnormal regulation of growth of the costal cartilages. There is a corresponding posterior curve in the body of the sternum beginning at the maniburum and extending to the xyphoid. It is usually asymmetric with one side more curved than the other. The deformity is usually apparent at birth but may become more prominent with growth and development. Most paediatric surgeons agree that the optimal timing for surgical repair of the pectus excavatum is late childhood and adolescence. It is now recognised that infants and preschool children should not undergo surgical correction because of acquired thoracic dystrophy.[4,5]

Complications generally are limited to wound infections and pneumothorax, which rarely requires tube drainage. Recurrence rates in large series with long-term follow-up range from 5% to 15%[6] and tend to occur in children who have marfanoid habitus. The migration of implanted struts and bars is the cause of most of the serious problems, including cardiac injury.

Pectus Carniatum

This deformity is less common than pectus excavatum and does not cause the same physiologic impairment. However depression deformity of the chest wall may be more troublesome and difficult to hide even when the child is fully clothed. The postoperative course and complications are similar to that of pectus excavatum including pneumothorax, wound infection, recurrence, and postoperative pneumonitis. In the early postoperative period, cardiac pulsation may be particularly visible. With healing, this finding disappears.

Tracheooesophageal Fistula

They are usually described as having five varieties. Oesophageal atresia with proximal pouch and distal fistula is the commonest type accounting for 85% to 95% of cases. Others include oesophageal atresia without fistula, 5% to 7%, tracheooesophageal fistula without atresia, 2% to 6%, oesophageal atresia with proximal tracheooesophageal fistula 1% and oesophageal atresia with proximal and distal traecheooesopahgeal fistula, 1%. Treatment for tracheooesophageal fistula must be initiated as soon as the diagnosis is made to avoid the consequence of an infant's abnormal anatomy. Attempts at feeding are stopped; intravenous fluids and antibiotics started. Endotracheal tube intubation should be avoided unless absolutely necessary because positive pressure ventilation may result in the preferential flow of gases through the fistula. The main aim of surgery is to correct the anatomy with a single operation, avoiding a gastrostomy if possible. High risk infants who cannot safely undergo surgical correction of their oesophageal abnormality may be treated with delayed repair. The presence of major cardiac and chromosomal abnormalities is the most important predictor of survival.[7] Technical problems during the operation occur when the anatomy is misidentified or dissection is carried out improperly, which can result in injury to the vagus nerves, recurrent laryngeal nerve, unplanned pleural entry, or damage to the posterior trachea. Anastomotic leaks occur in about 10% to 20% of cases. Most of these leaks are of little immediate consequence and will heal spontaneously, although this can lead to prolonged hospitalisation and increase the likelihood of stricture. When a leak is detected the retropleural chest tube is left in place and the child is kept nil by mouth with antibiotics. Stricture is very common after repair. This can be due to ischaemia, leakage, gastrooesophageal reflux or excessive tension. Usually the stricture responds well to dilatation. Occasionally a re-operation is required. Gastrooesophageal reflux occurs in most of the infants with oesophageal atresia. Medical treatment can be tried initially, if inadequate, then surgical control of reflux will be required.

Tracheomalacia may occur following an operation. The symptoms are completely relieved by endotracheal intubation. Infants with less severe symptoms may improve over time with tracheal growth. Severe symptoms require a tracheoostomy or tracheal suspension. Recurrent tracheooesophagel fistula may respond to endoscopic dilation or may require an operative division with interposition of pleura, muscle, or pericardium.

Laryngeotracheal Cleft

This is one of the most severe developmental anomalies of the oesophagus and trachea. Associated cardiovascular, gastrointestinal, and genitourinary anomalies are common. A breakdown of the repair and tracheostomy are common after surgery. Oromotor dysfunction and chronic aspiration are long-term problems. Most children require a gastrostomy for feeding. Gastrooesopahgeal reflux is common and may require surgical control.

Congenital Diaphragmatic Hernia

The incidence of congenital diaphragmatic hernia is estimated between 1 in 2000 and 1 in 5000 births, making it one of the most common congenital anomalies.[8] The use of prosthetic material to complete the diaphragmatic closure has gained widespread acceptance. But the major drawback in using a prosthetic patch closure is the risk of infection as well as the risk of dislodgement and subsequent reherniation. The overall survival rate for neonates with congenital diaphragmatic hernia ranges from 39% to 95% with a mean survival rate of 69%.[9] Long-term problems that have been identified with increasing frequency include chronic lung disease, neurological abnormalities with developmental delay, skeletal deformities, and nutritional and growth related problems.

ABDOMEN

Gastroschisis and Omphalocele

Diagnostic ultrasound has led to an increase in the prenatal diagnosis of abdominal wall defects. To prevent injury to the liver, a Caesarean section is preferred for a prenatally diagnosed infant with giant omphalocele. After delivery, the infant should be maintained under an external warmer or a humidified incubator. A nasogastric tube or orogastric sump tube should be inserted early and placed on suction to prevent further intestinal distension. The herniated viscera should be covered with a warm, saline-soaked gauze and covered with a plastic wrap to prevent further contamination. This manoeuvre also helps to prevent hypothermia and volume depletion. Adequate support of the herniated viscera must be provided to prevent intestinal ischaemia. A limiting factor in the primary closure of an abdominal wall defect is the increased intra-abdominal pressure generated by the reduction of the herniated viscera. Increased abdominal pressure can lead to a clinical situation known as the Abdominal Compartment Syndrome, which is characterised by the impaired venous return caused by the compression of the inferior vena cava, mesenteric ischaemia by reduction of splanchanic blood flow and respiratory compromise secondary to impair diaphragmatic excursion. Clinical measurement of intragastric or intravesical pressure less than 200 cm of water, end tidal CO_2 of 50 mm of mercury or less, or a rise in central venous pressure of less than 4 mm of mercury during abdominal wall closure allows for a safe primary abdominal wall closure.[10]

A delay in intestinal function is a common complication following repair in infants with gastrischisis. The use of parenteral nutrition is necessary, as it allows nutritional support. Prolonged TPN can lead to line infection, cholestasis, liver injury, etc. Necrotising entercolitis, a life-threatening inflammatory condition, is another complication that can occur. The use of maternal breast milk may exert a protective effect. Short bowel syndrome and intestinal dysmotility with the inability to tolerate full enteral feeding can evolve in the long run and result in a lifelong dependence on total parenteral nutrition.

Umbilical Hernia

Congenital umbilical hernias are the commonest abdominal wall problems in children. Usually they do not pose any significant problem during childhood. Given the high rate of spontaneous closure and asymptomatic nature, operative repair is not generally performed during the first two years of life. Large defects with significant protrusion may bring the patient with parents desiring repair. An acceptable cosmetic result is almost always achieved and the incidence of infection and recurrence is very low.

Inguinal Hernia

Inguinal hernia is one of the commonest elective procedure in children. It can be direct, indirect or femoral, with the first being the commonest of the three. Congenital inguinal hernias do not resolve spontaneously and are at high risk of incarceration.[11] An operation for indirect inguinal hernia involves high ligation of sac. During dissection all sensory nerves in the inguinal region should be preserved, along with the careful identification and dissection of the vas deferens and testicular blood supply. A major risk of inguinal hernia repair is related to anaesthetic, other risks include wound infection, injury to the vas deferens or testicular vessels, injury or displacement of the testicle, and recurrence.

Hydrocele

Hydrocele is a fluid collection in the tunica vaginalis in the scrotum or the process vaginalis in the inguinal canal and it can be communicating or non-communicating. Communicating hydrocele is treated in a similar manner as indirect inguinal hernia. For non-communicating hydrocele surgery is reserved if it persists after the first year of life. Simple aspiration should be avoided as it is usually ineffective and there is a risk of injury to the bowel.

Intestinal Atresia/Stenosis

This can involve any part of the gastrointestinal tract in any location. Anatomic lesions causing obstruction require operative treatment. The main aim of surgery is to restore continuity of the tract while preserving as much length as possible. It is estimated that 20 cm of the small bowel with an intact ileocecal valve is sufficient for long-term enteral feeding in the neonate.[12] Mortality in these infants is generally related to cardiac anomalies and other congenital defects. Short bowel syndrome usually requires long-term total parenteral nutrition with its risk of liver injury and sepsis. Most of the obstructive duodenal lesion is near the ampulla of Vater, and caution must be exercised to avoid inadvertent injury to the ampulla and pancreas. Late problems that may arise include poor gastric emptying, duodenal dysmotility, and gastrooesophageal reflux.

Meconium Ileus

Meconium ileus occurs in newborn infants with cystic fibrosis resulting in small bowel obstruction. In the majority of infants, operative treatment is not required and non-operative management is effective in 60% to 70% of infants.[13] Initial non-operative treatment consists of performing retrograde irrigation of the terminal ileum with fluids to dissipate the obstructing meconium. Reported complications with this approach include intestinal perforation, mucosal injury and persistent obstruction from meconium concretions. Operative treatment may be necessary in complicated meconium ileus with cyst formation, volvulus, atresia, perforation, or failure to clear the obstruction by enema. Long-term survival following meconium ileus is generally determined by the course of the underlying pulmonary disease.

Malrotation of Gut

The majority of children with malrotation are clinically asymptomatic and are usually found to have malrotation incidentally. Symptoms can occur following a duodenal obstruction from Ladd's band or because of midgut volvulus. The devastating and life-threatening consequences of midgut volvulus are vascular insufficiency and gut ischaemia, and, if untreated, infarction of the bowel supplied by the superior mesenteric artery. Following surgical correction, results are usually very good. Recurrent volvulus or obstruction is unusual if the initial procedure has been technically completed. Adhesions are reported in about 10% of the cases following Ladd's procedure.

Hirchsprung's Disease

Hirchsprung's disease is characterised anatomically by the lack of ganglion cells in the distal intestine. The length of aganglionosis is variable but most commonly involves the distal rectosigmoid colon. Discontinuous aganglionosis has been reported but is distinctively unusual. The major goal of surgery is to provide a resection or bypass of the distal aganglionic rectum with the performance of anastomosis with a normally innervated proximal intestine. Complications resulting from a definitive procedure include anastomotic leakage, stricture, pelvic or rectal muscular cuff abscess, intestinal obstruction, and wound infection. A unique complication following definitive repair is postoperative enterocolitis. Initial treatment for enterocolitis includes resuscitation, broad spectrum antibiotics, cessation of feeding and rectal irrigation. If enterocolitis does not respond to the above, intestinal decompression with an enterostomy is indicated.

Imperforate Anus

Mortality following anorectoplasty is usually related to the presence of associated congenital anomalies. Common complications include leaks, infection and stricture formation. Anorectal strictures are treated by anal dilatation. Recurrent rectourethral fistula or urethral stricture is uncommon. Infants with high lesions are more likely to have difficulty with faecal continence.

Necrotising Enterocolitis

Necrotising enetrocoloitis is characterised by an initial injury of the intestine that may ultimately progress to transmural bowel necrosis. Most infants with necrotising enterocolitis are treated successfully without operative intervention. The overall surgical complication rate is about 30%. Immediate technical complications include leaks, fistula formation, stoma necrosis, bleeding and liver injury during exploration. Late complications include stricture, incisional or parastomal hernia, stomal prolapse, intusseption, wound dehiscence or infection, small bowel obstruction and anastomotic failure. Symptomatic strictures usually require excision and anastomosis but dilatation can be tried.

References

1. Soper RT, Pringle KC. (1986) Cysts and sinuses of the neck. In: Welch KJ, Randolph JG, Ravitch MM, *et al.* (eds), *Paediatric Surgery*, 4th edn (Chicago Year Book), p. 539.
2. Sistrunk WE. (1920) The surgical treatment of cysts of the thyroglossal tract. *Ann Surg* 71: 121–122.
3. Tanaka K, Inomata Y, Utsunomiya H, *et al.* (1990) Sclerosing therapy with bleomycin for lymphangioma in children. *Pediatr Surg Int* 5: 270–273.
4. Haller JA Jr, Colombani PM, Humphries CT, *et al.* (1990) Chest wall constriction after too extensive and too early operation for pectus excavatum. *Ann Thorac Surg* 61: 1618–1625.
5. Weber TR, Kurkchubasche AG. (1998) Operative management of asphyxiating thoracic dystrophy after pectus repair. *J Pediatr Surg* 33: 262–265.
6. Shamberger RC. (1998) Congenital chest wall deformities. In: O'Neill JA Jr, Rowe MI, Grosfeld JL, *et al.* (eds), *Pediatric Surgery*, 5th edn (Mosby, St Louis), pp. 787–817.
7. Choudhary SR, Ashcraft KW, Sharp RJ, *et al.* (1999) Survival of patients with oesophageal atresia: influence of birth weight, cardiac anomaly and late respiratory complications. *J Pediatr Surg* 34: 70–74.
8. Stolar CJH, Dillon PW. (1998) Congenital diaphragmatic hernia and eventration. In: O'Neil JA, Rowe MI, Grosefeld JL, *et al.* (eds), *Pediatric Surgery*, 5th edn (Mosby, St Louis), pp. 819–837.
9. Reickert CA, Hirschl RB, Atkinson JB, *et al.* (1998) Congenital diaphragmatic hernia survival and use of extracorporeal life at selected level III nurseries with multimodality support. *Surgery* 123: 305–310.
10. Puffinbarger NK, Taylor DV, Tuggle DW, *et al.* (1996) End tidal carbon dioxide for monitoring primary closure of gastrschisis. *J Pediatr Surg* 31: 280–282.
11. Rowe MI, Clatworhy HW. (1970) Incarcerated and strangulated hernias in children: a statistical study of high risk factors. *Arch Surg* 101: 136–139.
12. Wilmore DW. (1972) Factors correlating with a successful outcome following extensive intestinal resection in newborn infants. *J Pediatr* 80: 88–95.
13. Oldham KT. (1997) Gastrointestinal disorders. In: Greenfields LJ, Mulholland MW, Oldham KT, *et al.* (eds), *Surgery: Scientific Principles and Practice*, 2nd edn (Lippincott-Raven, Philadelphia), pp. 2034–2078.

Chapter 18

COMPLICATIONS OF UROLOGICAL SURGERY

Tamsin J. Greenwell and Anthony R. Mundy

INTRODUCTION

Urology is a diverse specialty incorporating a wide range of procedures ranging from the simple endoscopic cystoscopy to the major complex cystoprostatectomy with neobladder and supravesical continent catheterisable channel
formation. Recently, laparoscopic versions of minor and major urological procedures have been developed which have made their way into general and
subspecialty urological practice to a variable degree. The complications and
advantages of laparoscopic surgery in general have been dealt with elsewhere
and those specific to the procedure are those of its open counterpart mainly
and therefore, will not be detailed.

COMPLICATIONS OF RADICAL NEPHRECTOMY AND NEPHROURETERECTOMY (Table 1)

radical nephrectomy is the treatment of choice for non-metastatic renal carcinoma and for debulking the metastatic renal cell carcinoma prior to immunotherapy. Nephroureterectomy is the treatment of choice for upper tract transitional cell carcinomas (TCC) that are large or not resectable endo-scopically. radical nephrectomy may be performed via a thoracoabdominal, abdominal or loin approach, while a nephroureterectomy is generally per-formed via a combined loin and abdominal approach.[1-3]

Bleeding from the renal vein and artery, and the adrenal veins may be avoided by double ligating before dividing with 3/0 Vicryl. If the adrenal veins are avulsed from the inferior vena cava (IVC) the bleeding area should be oversewn with 5/0 prolene. If the IVC has been torn and the tear is small, its sides may be grasped with DeBakey forceps and oversewn with 5/0 prolene. In the case of large tears, an assistant should apply occlusive pressure to the IVC with a swab in the region of the tear while access for a Satinsky clamp is obtained above and below the tear. This facilitates cross-clamping the IVC and the tear may then be oversewn with 5/0 prolene.

A lymphocoele is best avoided by careful ligation or diathermy of the lymphatic channels that are encountered especially during hilar dissection.

Hepatic laceration occurs rarely during right-sided procedures following excess hepatic traction. It should be repaired with interrupted hepatic mattress sutures.

Splenic injury occurs in up to 12% of left-sided procedures following traction on the spleen, mainly due to incomplete division of the lienorenal

Table 1. Complications of Radical Nephrectomy and Nephroureterectomy

Complications[1-3]	Incidence (%)
Death	2–5
Significant Bleeding	2–9.5
Lymphocoele	0–2
Hepatic Laceration	0–1.5
Splenic Injury	0–12.4
Pneumonia/Atelectasis	0–3
Colonic Injury	0–0.5

ligament.[1] Minor injuries may be packed with surgical while the more major ones require splenectomy. For immediate control of significant bleeding, the lesser sac can be opened to compress the splenic artery and vein while splenectomy is performed. Post-splenectomy patients require antipneumococcal vaccination and penicillin prophylaxis.[5]

COMPLICATIONS OF ANATROPHIC NEPHROLITHOTOMY AND PERCUTANEOUS NEPHROLITHOTOMY (Table 2)

Anatrophic nephrolithotomy is a rarely performed procedure for large staghorn calculi that has almost completely been superseded by the less invasive percutaneous nephrolithotomy (PCNL). PCNL is currently utilised for the removal of renal or ureteric stones, treatment of pelviureteric junction (PUJ) obstruction, intra-renal and ureteric strictures and upper tract tumour, in particular, TCC.[6–11]

The success rate of anatrophic nephrolithotomy for removal of stones is almost 100% whilst that of PCNL is 70–94%.[7] Atelectasis occurs due to the extreme lateral flexion and Trendelenberg that is required for these procedures, which produces a direct restriction of the chest wall in all directions.[24–26] In the case of anatrophic nephrolithotomy, it can also be due to postoperative wound pain which causes problems with deep breathing and coughing.

Table 2.   Complications of Anatrophic Nephrolithotomy and Percutaneous Nephrolithotomy

Complications[6–23]	PCNL (%)	Anatrophic Nephrolithotomy (%)
Death	0–1.1	0.42
Transfusion	1–34	6.8–10
Atelectasis	3–11	5–37
Pneumothorax	0.1–10.4	3.8–5
PE	0–0.5	0.3–0.9
Others (GI Bleeding, Sepsis)	0–2.8 (bowel injury) 1–29 (infection) 0–3 (sepsis)	16.1
Renal Dysfunction	0–0.2	0–2
Residual Stone	6–30	5–30
Stone Recurrence	10–30	20–30

Pneumothorax is more likely to occur if there has been previous renal surgery or pyelonephritis and/or a 11th or 12th interspace puncture is required. Any small pleural injury during open surgery can be closed with a 4 or 5/0 round bodied Vicryl purse string suture while the lung is hyperinflated. If the injury is large following both open and percutaneous surgery, a chest drain should be inserted for 24–48 hours. A chest X-ray should be obtained and reviewed during the recovery period to confirm the presence of and/or assess the extent of a pneumothorax at the end of all procedures. At PCNL, lung injury should be treated by terminating the procedure and inserting a chest drain; there is known to be an increased risk with upper pole puncture.[17,27]

Significant bleeding occurs in less than 10% of the cases and in open surgery, is best avoided by adhering to the avascular plane and making intrasegmental nephrostomy incisions. The avascular plane may be identified by atraumatically clamping the posterior segment of the renal artery and injecting methylene blue intravenously. If necessary, the main renal artery may be clamped and the kidney cooled to establish control and preserve function. Bleeding during PCNL is best avoided by entry into the apex of the papilla, and the use of a safety wire to allow continual localisation of the tract. Initially, it may be managed with tamponade by the nephrostomy sheath or a ureteric catheter if it is severe. Transfusion is required in up to 34% of PCNL patients.[6,13,17] Secondary bleeding may occur in 0.3–1.5% at around 1–2 weeks postoperatively, often from spontaneous intrapelvic bleeding of inadequately closed intrarenal vessels. In the majority of patients, it settles with conservative treatment. However, if it persists or is severe, superselective arteriographic embolism of the bleeding vessel may be required (0.3–1.0%). In the rare instance that all these measures fail and bleeding is life threatening, open repair may be attempted but nephrectomy is often required (0–1.8%).[13,17,18]

Urinary tract infection (UTI) is a common problem, and up to 28.7% of the patients have a transient increased temperature of about 38.5°C for the first 24 hours postoperatively.[17,19] The best preventive measure is to ensure that preoperative urine is sterile; if a puncture is inadvertently made into infected urine, the procedure should be abandoned and a nephrostomy drain inserted until the urine is sterile. Infection may also be prevented by the use of prophylactic antibiotics, low-pressure irrigation and careful avoidance of venous channels.

Post-procedure renal dysfunction is best prevented at the time of surgery by careful handling of the renal artery following full dissection, the use of atraumatic clamps and avoidance of warm ischaemia (especially for over 30 min),[28–30] and the use of intravenous mannitol following removal of renal arterial clamps.[28–31] Adequate hydration should be ensured after surgery and PCNL.

Stone migration may be avoided at open surgery by looping the ureter distal to the stone, and at PCNL by inflating an endoscopic balloon distal to the stone. The renal pelvis should be open directly onto the stone or in the case of PCNL, the puncture tract made through the tip of the calyces directly onto the stone. A transverse incision away from the pelviureteric junction (PUJ) at open surgery avoids tearing through it. Distal migration may produce obstruction and/or sepsis; and should be managed with either percutaneous nephrostomy or retrograde JJ stent insertion. Extra renal loss of material is not problematic in general and the material can be left *in situ*.[32]

Retained stone fragments are reported in 0–30% and are less common after open procedures. They act as a nidus for further stone formation in 30–70% of the patients,[13,17,20,21,33] and are best avoided by pre- and post-surgical X-ray to localise their presence and ensure removal. Intraoperative ultrasound (US) localisation is used if stones are radioluscent.[34] Intraoperative nephroscopy should be performed at open surgery if there are any localisation difficulties. Residual fragments may be treated by PCNL or extracorporeal shock wave lithotripsy (ESWL).

Decreased renal function follows up to 2%[35] of open or percutaneous nephrolithotomy procedures but is more common following open surgery, with up to 1% of patients requiring eventual nephrectomy for a non-functioning kidney. However, the average renal function is the same pre- and postoperatively with equivalent numbers of patients experiencing a reduction or improvement.[35] Reduction in renal function is best avoided by careful handling of the renal vessels and parenchyma.

Stone recurrence following complete clearance occurs in 20–30% of patients over 6–10 years,[13,17,18,33] and is more common in men than women (10% cf. 40%). Control of UTI reduces recurrence, as does the identification and treatment of any underlying metabolic abnormalities. Hypertension is a rare complication that should be managed with routine anti-hypertensive medication.

Pyelocutaneous fistula may occur consequent to distal ureteric obstruction, UTI and/or intraureteric foreign bodies, and generally resolves spontaneously within 2–3 weeks of surgery. If it does not, antegrade or retrograde insertion of a JJ stent will cure the fistula. Preventive measures include prophylactic placement of a JJ stent.

Urinoma formation occurs rarely, often due to the premature removal of postoperative drains. It may be treated with retrograde insertion of a JJ stent and/or percutaneous or formal drainage.

Liver or spleen injuries should be managed as for those occurring during radical nephrectomy or nephroureterectomy along with an internal drainage of the urinary tract with a JJ stent and urethral catheter, and simultaneous removal of the percutaneous nephrostomy tube to prevent fistula. Both these injuries are rare, with a slightly increased risk in hepatomegaly or splenomegaly.[13,17,18,33]

Another rare complications is colonic injury. Left sided PCNL has an increased risk in patients with a history of constipation, previous abdominal surgery or mobile kidneys. This risk can be reduced by bowel preparation. If the bowel injury is extraperitoneal at PCNL, it may be treated with a JJ stent and urethral catheter insertion along with the simultaneous removal of percutaneous nephrostomy tube under antibiotic cover.[13,17,18,35] If extraperitoneal injury is recognised intraoperatively, management is by withdrawal of the nephrostomy tube into the colon and the insertion of a JJ stent into the ureter. If the injury is intraperitoneal or occurs during open surgery it should be repaired and a defunctioning colostomy formed if required (i.e., gross faecal contamination, poor bowel blood supply, previous radiotherapy).

Duodenal injury is extremely rare but may occur following right-sided procedures. It should be managed conservatively, initially by inserting a nasogastric tube. Open repair may be necessary if conservative management fails.

Splenic injury is extremely rare and requires standard management.[36]

COMPLICATIONS OF OPEN URETERIC SURGERY (Table 3)

Open ureteric surgery is performed to repair any ureteric injury (fistula and/or ligation), stricture and rarely, for removal of stone or tumour.[37–56]

Urine leakage is not uncommon and may be prevented by the insertion of a drain and JJ stent. If the leak persists for over seven days, a ureteric stent should be inserted (if not placed at time of surgery) by either retrograde or antegrade

Table 3.   Complications of Open Ureteric Surgery

Complications	Incidence (%)
Urine Leakage	5–20
Ureteric Stricture	0–1.5
Reduced Renal Function	5–27

route. If this is not possible, a percutaneous nephrostomy should be inserted and the ureteral oedema allowed to settle. A further attempt may be made to insert a JJ stent after 5–7 days. Stent insertion is required to prevent ureteric stricture formation and maintain normal renal function. Suction drainage is best avoided as it may perpetuate the leak.[37–41] Persistent leakage necessitates antegrade imaging to exclude distal ureteric obstruction due to unrecognised stone or distal ureteric abnormality. If conservative management fails, an open repair or nephrectomy may be required. Nephrectomy is indicated in patients with a normally functioning contralateral kidney, especially if they are chronically ill/elderly/debilitated and would benefit from a rapid solution to their ongoing morbidity, or those with vascular grafts, which are at risk of infective complication.

Ureteral stricture occurs in up to 1.5% of the patients following open ureteric surgery. Significant stricture related obstruction may be diagnosed by MAG 3 renogram or Whitaker test. A functionally significant stricture may be treated endourologically by balloon dilation with a 50–76% success rate or by hot or cold knife incision and dilation with 62–100% success.[42–44] Both these techniques may be performed by either ante or retrograde routes. Their advantages include reduced postoperative pain, inpatient stay and convalescence period. However, they have low success rates if the stricture is longer than 1.5–2 cm and/or the affected ureter has poor vascularity secondary to surgery or radiotherapy.[40,42] Open management of a ureteric stricture is indicated following failed endoscopic management, if the stricture is long and/or ischaemic. The type of repair is determined by the location, the stricture, status of the contralateral kidney and the patient, and the surgeon's experience.

1. A psoas hitch ureteric reimplantation is used to repair stricture and other injuries of the lower 1/3 of the ureter. The contralateral superior vesical pedicle is ligated and divided, and the bladder mobilised cephalad and sutured to the

underlying psoas minor tendon prior to reimplantation of the ureter at the most cephalad part of the repositioned bladder. It requires a normal bladder capacity and no history of radiotherapy, bladder outflow obstruction (BOO) or neuropathic bladder. This technique is successful in 98% of patients but carries a small risk of genitofemoral and femoral nerve injury, recurrent ureteric stricture and vesicoureteric reflux.[45]

2. Boari flap +/− psoas hitch procedure can be used to repair ureteric strictures or defects of up to 14 cm of the lower 2/3–1/2 of the ureter. A tubularised anterior bladder wall flap is used to extend the most cephalad part of the bladder prior to ureteric reimplantation. The preoperative requirements are as for a psoas hitch procedure. This technique is successful in 97% but carries a minor risk of reduced renal function, persistent hydronephrosis, reduced bladder capacity, stenosis of the bladder tube and urine leak. The majority of Boari flap reimplants reflux.[46]

3. Transuretero-ureterostomy (TUU) may be used in patients when the bladder is not suitable for primary ureteric reimplantation and, with lower and middle 1/3 ureteric injuries following failure of reimplantation when the pelvis must be avoided (such as after radiotherapy) or when the bladder cannot be mobilised for a psoas hitch or a Boari flap. It is contraindicated in patients with a history of TCC, vesical tuberculosis (TB), pyelonephritis (PN), vesicoureteric reflux or obstruction of the recipient ureter.[47–50] It is successful in 97% and carries a slight risk of recurrent stricture (which puts both kidneys at risk of reduction in function) and of urine leak — both of which may be avoided by stenting until radiological healing has occurred.[51–53]

4. Ileal ureteric replacement is indicated for proximal ureteric injury, extensive ureteric defects and/or following failure of other techniques. The preoperative patient requirements are a serum creatinine level <200 mmol/l with good ipsilateral renal function to avoid progressive renal impairment and normal bladder emptying to avoid BOO secondary to ileal mucus. Ileal ureteric replacement may be performed in conjunction with a vesicopsoas hitch to reduce the length of the ileum required. The success rate is 98% with a minor risk of anastomotic urinary leak, urinary fistula, anastomotic strictures and/or bowel obstruction. Urine leakage is best prevented by the insertion of a percutaneous nephrostomy along with suturing (with dissolvable sutures) a large urinary catheter into the ileum with its tip in the renal pelvis and its opposite

end exiting through the bladder via a suprapubic site for six weeks to allow healing without kinking and free drainage of mucus. All ileal ureteric replacements reflux; however, this does not affect renal function in general.[54] UTI and stone formation can be troublesome in the long term.

5. Anastomotic uretero-ureteric repair may be used for short defects of the upper 2/3 of the ureter in an otherwise healthy ureter. It is successful in 98% with rare complications of recurrent ureteric stricture and fistula.[55]

6. Renal auto transplant is an alternative to ileal ureteric replacement when all other techniques have failed. However, it carries all the risks of a renal transplant including urine leak, bleeding, renal loss and lymphocoele and is rarely successful.[56]

COMPLICATIONS OF URETERO-RENOSCOPY (Table 4)

Uretero-renoscopy (rigid and flexible) is indicated for diagnosis and treatment of urinary tract stones, stricture, obstructed calyceal infundibulum and tumour including TCC.[57–64]

Table 4.   Complications of Uretero-renoscopy

Complications[57–64]	Incidence (%)
Colic Pain	3.5–9
Fever	1.4–6.9
False Passage	0.4–0.9
Minor Bleeding	0–2.1
Prolonged Bleeding	0–1
Extravasation	0.6–1
UTI	1–1.6
Pyelonephritis	0.5
Perforation	0–4.6
Stricture	0.5–1.4
Avulsion	0–0.6
Urinoma	0–0.6
Urosepsis	0–0.3
CVA	0–0.5
DVT	0–0.2

All uretero-renoscopic complications are best prevented by using the smallest diameter scope necessary, prophylactic antibiotics, a safety guide wire at all times to mark the ureteric path, avoiding excess ureteric dilation and postoperative stenting if possible.

The energy sources used to accomplish stone or tumour eradication during uretero-renoscopy contribute to its morbidity. USS results in heat generation and can cause thermal damage. Extrahydraulic lithotripsy (EHL) causes mechanical trauma and results in perforation in 0–19% of the cases (which is generally treated by stenting). Laser causes perforation and/or stricture in 0–6%. The lithoclast is the safest but least efficient in terms of successful stone eradication. When ureteric stricture or avulsion injury occurs it should be managed as detailed previously.[57–64]

COMPLICATIONS OF RADICAL CYSTECTOMY AND RADICAL CYSTOPROSTATECTOMY (Table 5)

For muscle invasive non-metastatic bladder cancer (all types especially TCC), the treatment of choice is radical cystectomy for female patients and radical cystoprostatectomy for males.[65–74]

Table 5.   Complications of Radical Cystectomy and Radical Cystoprostatectomy

Complications	Incidence (%)
Death	1–3
Morbidity	25–41
Transfusion > 10 units	3.4
Rectal Injury	2.2–9.6
Wound Infection	5–10
Sepsis	4.9
Pelvic Abscess	4.7
Pneumonia	1.8
Acute PN	1.8
Cholecystitis	0.3
Erectile Dysfunction (ED)	25–100 depending on nerve sparing or not

Blood loss is expected at cystectomy and a mean of 4.5 units of blood is transfused per patient.[65] In a small percentage, the loss is more extensive and the management involves invasive perioperative monitoring and prompt and appropriate blood and fluid replacement. An elective admission to the intensive care unit (ICU) for postoperative management is routine.

Rectal injury occurs in up to 10%[64,69–71] and is more likely to occur in patients with a history of radiotherapy[70,71] (especially high dose), pelvic surgery, extensive transurethral resection of bladder tumour (TURBT) and inflammatory disease of the rectosigmoid. It is best avoided by carefully mobilising and ensuring that the bowel is fully prepared. If bowel injury is recognised intraoperatively, primary repair should be performed, and this is successful in 89%.[66,67] If in doubt regarding the integrity of the repair, a covering colostomy should be performed; this should also be considered in the elderly if there is significant comorbidity because of poor nutritional status, previous radiotherapy, poor bowel preparation or large injury.

A wound infection requires treatment with appropriate broad-spectrum antibiotics and the release of pus collection. Pelvic abscess may be managed by percutaneous US-guided drain insertion or by open wash out with the insertion of a large calibre drain.

The long-term complications of cystectomy or cystoprostatectomy involve urinary diversion and are discussed in the following section, except ED, which follows conventional management guidelines.

COMPLICATIONS OF URINARY DIVERSION AND URINARY TRACT RECONSTRUCTION

Ileal conduit is the gold standard technique for urinary diversion post-cystectomy or for complicated urinary incontinence. It produces incontinent external urinary drainage. The colon, and in exceptional circumstances the stomach and jejunum can also be used (Table 6).[75–80]

Early complications occur in 26–57%.[75–79] Ileus/intestinal obstruction and small bowel fistula should be managed conservatively in the first instance with intravenous fluid/nutritional replacement. Operative intervention is only required when conservative management fails and/or a non-ileus related small bowel obstruction persists for longer than 48 hours. Operative closure of a small bowel fistula may be required in those patients who fail to settle following

Table 6.   Complications of Ileal Conduit Urinary Diversion

Complications[75–80]	Incidence (%)
Bowel Leak	0–4
Death	0–6
Intestinal Obstruction	0–6.5
Pyelonephritis	0–17
Parastomal Hernia	4.5–31
Stomal Retraction	0–31
Stomal Bleeding	0–7.7
Stomal Stenosis	0–9.5
Incisional Hernia	0–15.4
Stomal Prolapse	0–13
Renal Deterioration	6–25
Renal Improvement	0–37
Ureteroileal Stricture/Obstruction	2–22
Stones	2–8.3

a prolonged (4–6 months) period of conservative management (including total parenteral nutrition if high fistula output). An intraperitoneal bowel anastomotic leak requires immediate reoperative revision. Ureteroileal leakage is generally managed by nephrostomy insertion and antegrade ureteric stent placement, and may be prevented by placing ureteric stents at the time of surgery.

Long-term complications occur in 28–81% of patients, more frequently in females. The rate of long term complications is significantly higher in women with ileal conduit diversion for urinary incontinence, of which 59% require further surgery for stomal complications alone.[78]

Parastomal hernia may be managed conservatively with a truss belt if the patient is unfit for or declines surgery; standard procedure involves open operative repair using a mesh in non-contaminated cases. In difficult recurrent parastomal hernia cases it may be necessary to resite the stoma. Stomal retraction, bleeding and/or stenosis may require revision of stoma. This may be accomplished using the original ileal conduit if it is of sufficient length; an additional segment of ileum is harvested and anastomosed to the original segment if required.[75–80]

Ureteroileal stricture is managed by revision of the anastomosis and renal stones treated according to standard regimes. Metabolic abnormalities do not tend to produce overt clinical problems following conduit formation although there is an increased risk of metabolic abnormalities with increased length of conduit, poor conduit drainage and poor renal function. The type of metabolic abnormality depends on segment of bowel used to form the conduit; ileum and colon produce a hyperchloraemic hypokalaemic metabolic acidosis while the jejunum (used in exceptional circumstances only) produces a hyponatraemic hyperkalaemic hyperchloraemic, metabolic acidosis.[81,82]

Augmentation cystoplasty is used to enlarge and stabilise the bladder in patients with neuropathic hyperreflexia (spinal dysraphism, spinal cord injury, cerebral palsy), idiopathic detrusor instability, congenital anomalies (vesical and cloacal exstrophy, posterior urethral valves, urogenital sinus abnormalities) and following surgery (radical TURBT, partial cystectomy) or infection (TB). The ileum is used in 90% of the cases and colon in the majority of the remainder; the stomach has been used occasionally (Table 7).[81–120]

Table 7.   Complications of Augmentation/Substitution Cystoplasty

Complications[81–120]	Incidence (%)
Bleeding	0.6–6.7
Infection	2.1–9
Fistula	0–29.7
Ileus	0–8.3
Small Bowel Obstruction	1.7–8.7
RTI	0–6
PE/DVT	2.1–7.1
Patch Necrosis	1.1–2.7
Diverticularisation	0–0.5
Death	0–3.2
Metabolic	0–19
Intermittent Self Catheterisation (ISC)	0–100
Reduced Renal Function	0–9
Asymptomatic Bacteriuria	6–100
Symptomatic Bacteriuria	2–28
Stones	0–30
Perforation	0–8.7
Change in Bowel Habit	0–64
Dry	53–100
Dry with Artificial Urinary Sphincter (AUS)	86–100

The early complications of augmentation cystoplasty include cardiovascular, thromboembolic, respiratory and gastrointestinal complications associated with any major abdominal procedure, such as bleeding, wound infection, ileus, DVT/PE, RTI and death. Those specific to the procedure include patch necrosis, bowel anastomotic leak and vesico-cutaneous fistula.

The long-term complications occurring specifically following gastro-cystoplasty include haematuria-dysuria syndrome, peptic ulceration of the bladder,[84] perforation of the gastric segment,[85] and hypergastrinaemia.[86] There are also problems associated with partial gastrectomy, including early satiety and poor feeding, dumping syndrome and exacerbation of pre-existing peptic ulcer disease or gastro-oesophageal reflux.[87]

The metabolic abnormalities are similar to those for ileal conduit diversions. A biochemically detectable acid-base and electrolyte disturbance occurs in virtually all patients but is clinically important in very few.[81,82,88] If symptomatic, treatment with oral bicarbonate supplements is extremely effective.

Renal function deteriorates following bowel augmentation cystoplasty in 15% of patients, with an initial creatinine clearance of at least 15 ml/min,[89,90] compared with 4% of patients with an initial creatinine clearance of at least 40 ml/min.[91] In up to 4% of patients, the renal function improves post-cystoplasty.[89,92]

ISC is required in almost all neuropathic and congenital urinary tract anomaly patients and 15% of idiopathic detrusor overactivity patients following an augmentation cystoplasty.

Diverticularisation may occur if the bladder is inadequately bivalved.[94] It may be managed by CISC in the first instance but if the problem persists, open revision is necessary.[95]

Mucus production can be a problem, especially for those patients requiring CISC.[96] It predisposes to UTI, stone formation, and bladder outlet obstruction and may contribute to bladder perforation.[97] Saline bladder washouts are the best management.[98]

Asymptomatic bacteriuria occurs in the majority of augmentation patients,[100,101] while the incidence of symptomatic UTI is 25%.[102] Increased urinary pH, large post-void residual volumes, the presence of mucus and the need for CISC are predisposing factors. Asymptomatic bacteriuria does not require treatment whereas symptomatic UTI should be treated with a 5–7 day course of appropriate antibiotics.

Stones form in up to 53%[103–105] of cystoplasties. Their formation depends upon the mode of emptying and occur in 2% of patients who void spontaneously per urethra, 10% of the patients requiring CISC per urethra, and 20% of patients with Mitrofanoff-type channels in whom the bladder is emptied by a catheter from above.[106] The risk factors for stone formation are stasis, UTI and intravesical foreign bodies such as staples and mucus.[103,104,107] When stones are detected they must be removed because they represent a nidus for infection and enlarge with time. The majority can be removed endoscopically as long as no fragments are left behind. Large or multiple stones and patients without urethral access require open removal.[104,106]

Spontaneous bladder perforation is a rare but life threatening complication of augmentation with a mortality rate of 23–25%.[108,109] Perforation is a more common occurrence in neuropathy, in the presence of a competent bladder outlet (including an artificial urinary sphincter), in recurrent UTI and in those performing CISC.[108] If the clinical picture reveals bladder rupture, an exploration of the abdomen must be performed urgently, and the defect repaired.[108]

Bowel disturbance has been reported in 30–54% of the patients having augmentation,[109,110] with diarrhoea occurring in up to 25%.[109] Whether this is a consequence of the cystoplasty or an associated disturbance of the bowel function is not clear. Bowel disturbance can be extremely troublesome and is best managed symptomatically with laxatives if constipated, or constipatives if loose.

Incontinence may occur following augmentation cystoplasty, particularly at night and is related to a reduction in urethral closing pressure, relaxation of the pelvic floor muscles, increased urine output and failure of the urethral sphincter to increase in tone in response to contractions from the bowel patch during sleep, because of a loss of sensation.[111–113] In neuropathy or other severe congenital sphincter deficiency, incontinence is best avoided by simultaneous surgical correction. There are a multitude of procedures designed to increase the outlet resistance, and they have been used with some success in combination with augmentation. These include the Young-Dees-Leadbetter bladder neck reconstruction,[114] the Kropp procedure,[115] urethral sling suspension,[116] periurethral injection,[117] bladder neck suspension,[118] and the artificial urinary sphincter.[119,120]

ORTHOTOPIC AND HETEROTOPIC NEOBLADDERS

Orthotopic and heterotopic neobladder formation are performed for bladder replacement, and the primary indications are invasive TCC, aggressive superficial TCC that cannot be controlled by conservative means, pelvic malignancies, congenital and acquired neurological anomalies, congenital urological anomalies and chronic pelvic pain syndromes. The bowel segments used include ileum, ileocaecal, caecum and sigmoid.[121–140]

The complications are essentially those of augmentation cystoplasty with a few additions.

Early complications include cardiovascular, thromboembolic, respiratory and gastrointestinal complications associated with any major abdominal procedure, such as bleeding, wound infection, ileus, DVT/PE, RTI and death, and those related to the formation of the neobladder; uretero-ileal leak, uretero-ileal obstruction, gut leak, and neobladder-cutaneous fistula.[123,124]

The long-term complications may be broadly divided as neobladder-related and general complications. The neobladder-related complications include uretero-ileal complications, metabolic acidosis, UTI, change in bowel function, stone and cancer. The general complications include small bowel obstruction, deterioration in renal function, incisional hernia and abscess. They should be managed as described previously.[121–140]

Changes in the level of consciousness may occur secondary to magnesium deficiency, increased ammonia, enhanced drug reabsorption and failure of drug excretion, especially for those such as theophylline that require renal excretion.[126] Patients require regular review and biochemical assessment to avoid these complications.

Local cancer recurrence occurs in 4–10% of the patients having neobladder formation for malignancy.[128–131] The appearance of a new malignancy is rare and generally arises following a long latent period of 10 or more years after neobladder formation. It may be associated with chronic inflammation, urine stasis and recurrent urinary tract infection.[131–133,140] or related to field change in the colonic mucosa. A high index of suspicion and regular imaging and or cystoscopic review of the neobladder are required to ensure early diagnosis.

Incontinence can be a significant problem after orthotopic neobladder formation, particularly at night and in the elderly patient.[134] Nocturnal enuresis occurs in 15–63%[23,112,113,134,137] while diurnal incontinence occurs in up to 37% of the women and 2–64% of men.[112,113,125,135,136] In patients with orthotopic neobladders, diurnal incontinence may arise from loss of the sacral reflex arc, incomplete neobladder detubularisation and or sphincter damage.[135,136] Timed voiding may help nocturnal enuresis while an artificial urinary sphincter may benefit those with diurnal incontinence.

COMPLICATIONS OF SIMPLE AND RADICAL PROSTATECTOMY (Table 8)

A simple open prostatectomy is performed to remove large (>120 g) obstructive benign prostates, when other problems including bladder stones and diverticulum are present, or when anatomic limitations prevent transurethral resection of prostate (TURP) such as hip or knee contractures or penile prosthesis.[141–148]

In simple open prostatectomy, bleeding may be prevented by the placement of figure of eight stitches at 5 and 7 o'clock that include the bladder mucosa, the bladder neck and the prostatic capsule and by ligation of the dorsal vein before capsulotomy. Packing of the prostatic capsule for at least five minutes following enucleation may also reduce blood loss.[148]

Persistent urinary leak should be treated with urethral dilation and indwelling urethral catheter placement. A pelvic drain should be left *in situ* until after the urethral catheter has been removed.[142]

Table 8.   Complications of Simple and Radical Prostatectomy

Complications	Simple (%)[141–148]	Radical (%)[149–160]
Death	0–5	0–3
Bleeding	0.8–35	0–14
Re-operation for Bleeding	0.8–1.5	0–0.5
Transfusion	1.7–35.5	5–11
Clot Retention	0.8–6.7	0–1.5
Secondary Bleeding	0.45	N/A
Persistent Urinary Leak	1–2	2–5
Bladder Neck Contracture	0.2–6.1	0.2–4
Epididymo-orchitis	2.6	N/A
UTI	13	N/A
DVT/PE	0.3–0.7	0.75
Rectal Injury	0–2.5	<5
Repeat Procedure	2 (at 5 years) 11	0

Urinary incontinence generally settles with time and may be managed with anticholinergic medication if required. Sphincter damage related stress urinary incontinence may respond to pelvic floor exercises but may require the insertion of an artificial urinary sphincter.[142]

Bladder neck contracture may be recurrent and should be treated by bladder neck incision.[147]

Radical perineal or retropubic prostatectomy is used for the curative treatment of prostate cancer. The disadvantage of the perineal route is that a simultaneous pelvic lymph node dissection is not possible unlike in retropubic radical prostatectomy. The perineal route does however allow for more rapid postoperative recovery.[149–159]

Perioperative bleeding from the dorsal venous plexus, the arteries to the prostate and the arteries to the seminal vesicals can be a problem. A pack should be placed and haemostasis achieved with figure of 8 suture(s) for venous bleeding. The arteries should be ligated and divided. Diathermy should be avoided if nerve sparing radical prostatectomy is being attempted.[151]

Delayed bleeding is rare, and generally from the anterior rectal surface or the bladder neck or the bulb of the penis. A careful bladder washout following vesico-urethral anastomosis may detect bleeding areas, which can then be diathermied or ligated. Transfusion is required in fewer than 5% of the cases.[151–154] Rectal injury occurs in less than 1%, generally in the region of the apical dissection or at the base of the prostate. It is due to trauma at the time of taking the superior prostatic plexus, and should be repaired in two layers and the wound washed out copiously and drained. A defunctioning colostomy should be considered but is mandatory only in case of previous radiotherapy.[151–155] Wound infection is rare.

Postoperative loss of the urethral catheter occurs in up to 5%. If it occurs early, a new catheter should be reinserted urethrally, over a guide wire placed via a flexible cystoscope if necessary. If catheter insertion is not possible even with a guide wire, the patient should be re-explored and a new catheter inserted as an open procedure. If the catheter is lost five days or later postoperatively, the patient should have a trial without a catheter, which should only be reinserted if the patient fails to void.[153–156]

Oliguria or anuria may occur following acute tubular necrosis (ATN), displacement or blockage of the urethral catheter or ureteral injury. IV fluids should be administered to ensure adequate hydration and a gentle bladder wash out performed along with catheter re-positioning to ensure free catheter drainage. A cystogram will assess anastomotic integrity and catheter position while an intravenous urogram will assess ureteric injury.[156–158]

Persistent urinary cutaneous fistula may occur following blockage of the urethral catheter or disruption of the vesico-urethral anastomosis. This is best managed by continued urethral catheter drainage if the cystogram indicates an intact anastomosis. Re-exploration is indicated for complete anastomotic disruption.[156–158] The disruption is either physical, related to the passage of the catheter through the anastomosis or tension due to a postoperative bleed or following the removal of an enlarged prostate.

The inability to void following the removal of the catheter occurs in 15% of the cases and is treated by inserting a urethral catheter with a repeat trial of void 48–72 hours later. The failure to void is generally secondary to oedema, a tissue flap or a hypotonic bladder.[146]

Anastomotic stricture occurs in up to 6.7% of the cases and is initially managed by dilatation. If it recurs, stricture incision is required progressing to anastomotic resection with a planned artificial sphincter insertion for subsequent incontinence.[151–158]

Urorectal fistula occurs in up to 2% of the cases and should be managed by continued urinary catheter drainage with delayed repair utilising gracilis flap reconstruction a minimum of three months post-surgery.[151–159]

Erectile dysfunction occurs in almost all male patients. Up to 50% will recover their ability to have satisfactory erections within 12–18 months if they have had a nerve sparing radical prostatectomy and are less than 60 years old.[151–159]

Stress urinary incontinence occurs initially in 50–60% of the male patients but resolves in the majority in 6–8 weeks. However, 2.8–3.1% require long-term pads while 6–12% reported episodes of stress urinary leakage. The risk of post-radical prostatectomy incontinence is greatest for the elderly, the obese, those who have had previous radiotherapy and following non-nerve sparing surgery.[152–159]

COMPLICATIONS OF TRANSURETHRAL RESECTION OF THE PROSTATE (Table 9)

Transurethral resection of the prostate (TURP) remains the gold standard treatment for BOO secondary to BPH. Reduced morbidity has occurred consequent to improvement in surgical technique, perioperative

Table 9.   Complications of Transurethral Resection of the Prostate

Complications	Incidence (%)
Death	0.1–0.37
Bleeding	5–10
Re-operation for Bleeding	0.1
Transfusion	1
Clot Retention	0.37–2
TUR Syndrome	2–10
Secondary Bleeding	3
Persistent Urinary Incontinence	0.5
Persistent Inability to Void	<1
Bladder Neck Contracture	1–5
Urethral Stricture	1–5
UTI	Bacteraemia 25–75; Sepsis15
Retrograde Ejaculation	70–90
Erectile Dysfunction	4–10
Rectal Injury	0–0.37
Repeat Procedure	2% / year (10% at 10 years)

monitoring of fluids and urea and electrolytes, improved anaesthetic care and video-endoscopic equipment. Adverse effects are proportional to the surgeon's experience.[148,161–173]

Perioperative transfusion is required in 1–3% of the cases.[151–161] A return to the theatre for uncontrolled bleeding occurs in <0.5%, and generally requires endoscopic washout and diathermy of bleeding points. Furthermore, 2% of these patients require open washout, enucleation of any remaining prostate, oversewing of the bladder neck and packing of prostatic cavity. This complication may be prevented by perioperatively reducing the pressure of the irrigating fluid, ensuring adequate haemostasis and normal blood pressure to facilitate the identification of all significant bleeding points. The majority of postoperative bleeding can be managed by catheter traction with 25–30 ml of fluid in the catheter balloon and three-way irrigation alone.[148,165,167,169] In general, secondary bleeding occurs 10–14 days postoperatively. It is important to exclude fibrinolysis and primary disseminated intravascular coagulation (DIC) as potential causes especially if the TURP was for prostatic cancer-related BOO. However, the majority of secondary bleeds are related to infection (UTI) or a simple loss of surgical eschar. Secondary bleeding often settles following the insertion of a three-way catheter followed by bladder washout and irrigation to remove any clot.

An inadvertent resection of the intravesical ureteric orifices occurs rarely. If performed using coagulation diathermy, the affected ureter should be stented with a JJ stent for 4–6 weeks. No action is required if performed using cutting diathermy. An IVP is required at six months in all cases to assess upper tract drainage.

Extraperitoneal bladder perforation is an occasional occurrence. If the perforation is small no action is required. However, if it is large, the TURP should be terminated as soon as possible to prevent excess fluid absorption and subsequent TUR syndrome. If the patient has significant retropubic pain, the insertion of a urethral catheter and a suprapubic drain may provide relief.

Intraperitoneal bladder perforation is rare, and if it is large or posterior, open closure and formal assessment for other intra-abdominal injury is required. If the perforation is small, anterior and or lateral it may be managed conservatively with prolonged urethral catheter drainage (21 days).

The TUR syndrome is used to describe a post-TURP symptom complex of any or all of the following: confusion, hypertension, bradycardia, nausea, vomiting, and or visual disturbance related to dilutional hyponatraemia (serum [Na] < 125 mEq). It occurs in varying degrees in 2–10% of TURP patients and is fatal in 0.2–0.8% of cases. It is more common in the elderly, if the resection time is greater than 90 min, if the intraprostatic pressure is greater than 30 mmHg and/or a venous sinus opened or capsular perforation occurred during TURP. It can be treated by lowering the height of the irrigation fluid to less than 60 cm above the patient and completion of the resection as soon as possible. If the patient is relatively well IV furosemide is administered and all irrigation and IV fluids are changed to N saline. If the patient is unwell IV mannitol (2 mg/kg) is administered and the patient transferred to the ICU, where 3% hypertonic saline (250–500 ml over six hours) is administered if the patient is severely unwell.[166,167,173]

UTI and septicaemia are avoided by ensuring that the urine is sterile preoperatively, giving IV antibiotic prophylaxis at the time of TURP and giving IV/im antibiotic prophylaxis prior to the removal of catheter.

Urinary incontinence occurs temporarily in 5% of the patients and generally resolves within 6–12 weeks but sometimes persists for up to 12 months. Permanent urinary incontinence occurs in 0.5% of the patients and may be stress type following perioperative sphincter damage or urge type following new onset or unresolved detrusor overactivity.

The inability to void post-TURP occurs in 6–6.5%.[170,173] There is an increased risk of inability to void if the patient is diabetic or presents with acute retention (10%), acute on chronic retention (38%), chronic retention (44%) and or has a neurogenic bladder dysfunction. Early failure occurs in 0.5–12% of the cases. This resolves in the majority, with persistent failure to void occurring in less than 1%. Persistent obstruction should be excluded by urodynamics and treated with repeat TURP if present. The commonest site for residual tissue is at the apex and in the anterior prostate. There is a repeat TURP rate of 2% per year or 10% at 10 years.[162,163,173]

In the absence of obstruction the patient can be managed by long-term intermittent self-catheterisation or indwelling catheter (urethral or suprapubic).

Urethral stricture occurs in up to 5%[156] of patients post-TURP, most commonly in the membranous, bulbopenile junction and fossa navicularis regions of the urethra secondary to trauma from the resectoscope. Strictures may be prevented by preoperative urethral dilation or urethrotomy (although this is contentious), using the smallest resectoscope possible, generous lubrication of the urethra prior to scope insertion, visual insertion of resectoscope, gentle resection technique, limiting the resection time to less than one hour and the usage of the smallest calibre silastic three-way catheter with the minimal catheter traction time if necessary. Once established, urethral strictures should be treated by dilation, urethrostomy or urethroplasty depending on the position, length and patient wishes.[154,164]

Bladder neck contracture occurs in up to 5%,[162,163] and is more common following TURP of small fibrotic prostates, excess resection and prolonged catheter traction. It is treated by transurethral bladder neck incision in all four quadrants. If this does not open up the bladder neck, a circumferential bladder neck resection is required. The condition has a recurrence rate of 40–50%.[169]

Retrograde ejaculation is almost universal and occurs in 70–90% of the cases. It cannot be prevented or treated and patients must be warned about this preoperatively.[162,163,173]

Following TURP, erectile dysfunction is reported by up to 4%.[162–164] However, it is also reported by about 4% of male patients, undergoing non-urologic surgery postoperatively suggesting that this is an age-related rather than a direct surgical consequence.[161]

COMPLICATIONS OF ARTIFICIAL URINARY SPHINCTER INSERTION (Table 10)

The main indications for the insertion of an artificial urinary sphincter (AUS_ are post-prostatectomy stress incontinence (PPI), sphincter weakness incontinence due to neuropathic dysfunction, intrinsic sphincter deficiency (ISD) and rare congenital causes of incontinence.[174–184]

The mechanical complications are nearly all surgery-related, with physical failure of the device occurring in less than 3%. The majority of mechanical failures are either due to inadequate balloon pressures (33%), blocking of the tubing (16%) or cuff leakage.[174] In patients with inadequate balloon pressure and a bulbar cuff of less than 4.5 cm, changing the balloon to the next highest pressure category balloon is required. For larger cuff sizes, increasing the balloon pressure and reducing the cuff size by 0.5 cm is recommended. These complications occur immediately following a failure to achieve continence upon activation of the device, and the rate reported in all publications is 7.6–12%.[181,182]

Infection may be introduced at the time of implantation via the device or by perforation of the urethra (or vagina or rectum) during surgery. Cuff erosion results from the pressure of the prosthesis on the underlying tissues. Previous irradiation, surgery, trauma, or urethral scarring are associated with an increased risk of erosion. Erosion may occur immediately or at any time after insertion (late erosion).[174,176,183] Treatment is by removal of the device combined with the placement of a urethral silicone catheter for 4–6 weeks until there is radiological evidence of complete healing. The stricture rate after cuff erosion is extremely low.[177]

Table 10.   Complications of Artificial Urinary Sphincter Insertion

Complications	Incidence (%)
Acute Infection/Erosion	2–5
Device Failure	3
Mechanical Failure	7.6–12
Late Erosion	15
Failure to Achieve Continence	16% at 10 years

The reported risk of early infection/erosion is up to 5%, but is higher in neuropathic patients (15%), after failed sling surgery (67%), and following radiotherapy.[170] The incidence of erosion and infection can be minimised by ensuring that the urine is sterile, antibiotic prophylaxis is given, and that surgical technique is meticulous such that neither the urethra nor vagina are perforated during surgery.

Late erosion occurs in up to 15% with a peak incidence at around seven years post-implantation and is probably due to urethral atrophy consequent to cuff pressure.[176,182,183]

Immediate incontinence following implantation is most commonly due to failure to deflate the cuff fully when voiding resulting in incomplete bladder emptying and overflow incontinence. The other causes of early incontinence are predominantly mechanical faults.

Delayed recurrent incontinence may also be secondary to urethral atrophy beneath the cuff.[177,180] This may be corrected by changing the cuff to a smaller size; however, if the original cuff used was the smallest available (4 cm), transcorporal cuff placement[178] or implantation of a second urethral cuff in tandem is required.

COMPLICATIONS OF SUPRAVESICAL CONTINENT CATHETERISABLE CHANNEL FORMATION (MITROFFANOFF OR MONTI CHANNELS) (Table 11)

The formation of a supravesical continent catheterisable channel using the appendix (Mitroffanoff channel) or the reconfigured small bowel (Monti channel) is required in patients with no urethra (following urethrectomy with or without cystectomy for cancer), in those requiring intermittent self-catheterisation to empty their bladder or neobladder for whom urethral CISC is a physical impossibility (quadriplegia, wheelchair bound female spinal dysraphism), or is too painful to perform.[185–198]

Perioperative mortality is currently 0% with higher rates up to 4% reported in the older series.[185–188] Peristomal abscess requires incision and drainage.[189] Small bowel obstruction is managed in the usual way,[186] while ischaemic necrosis of the channel requires re-operation, excision of ischaemic channel and formation of a new channel.[190,191] The higher rates of complication are again reported in the older series,[186] and with the Monti channel.[185,186]

Table 11. Complications of Supravesical Continent
Catheterisable Channel Formation

Complications	Incidence (%)
Mortality	0–4
Peristomal Abscess	0–2.1
Small Bowel Obstruction	4–20
Ischaemic Necrosis of Channel	0–12
Urinary Leakage	0–19
Stomal Stenosis	10–40
Stomal Prolapse	2
Monti Channel Pouch Formation	28
Revision of Channel	16–50
UTI	40
Stones	20–100

Catheterisation difficulties occur in 27% of Mitrofanoff channels and 60% of Monti channels,[185,192] necessitating channel revision in 16–50% of the cases.[185,186,192] This usually follows stomal stenosis, which occurs in 10–40% of the patients,[185,187] and may be prevented by various stomal formation techniques such as the VQ, VQQ or VQZ plasties.[194,195] If it occurs immediately postoperatively, a simple dilation is effective in up to 21% of patients[185,192]; if this fails an excision of the stenotic segment with reformation of the stoma using one of the stomal techniques listed is required. Bladder level stenosis occurs rarely[185]; when it does, an excision of the stenotic segment with revision of the tunnel into bladder/neobladder and lengthening of the channel is necessary.[185,192]

Stomal prolapse occurs in up to 2% of channels,[192] and requires excision of the prolapsed segment and revision of the skin anastomosis. Up to 28% of Monti channels develop catheterisation problems secondary to a pouch-like dilation or diverticulum along the channel, commonly in the area of the anastomosis in double Monti channels.[185] A review of catheterisation technique may be all that is required to correct this. If the problem persists, open resection of any pouch or diverticulum is indicated.[185]

UTI occurs in up to 40% of the cases,[196] and bladder or neobladder stones in 20–100% (the higher rate occurring in those patients with both a Mitrofanoff and an augmentation cystoplasty or neobladder).[186,195,196] Daily bladder/neobladder washouts may prevent stone formation.[196] Once formed, stones under 5 cm may be removed endoscopically either via the native urethra or a percutaneous tract if there is no urethral access, while larger stones require open removal.[191] Open removal may well be the best option as any retained fragments from the minimally invasive techniques will result in stone recurrence.

Persistent postoperative urinary leakage via the channel requires revision of the channel to extend the length of the channel and/or bladder/neobladder tunnel.[186] An extension can be achieved by anastamosing an additional small bowel Monti segment, or in the case of a Mitrofanoff channel by retubularising a segment of the caecum.[197,198] Conversely leakage may occur consequent to channel dilation and lengthening with time — this requires shortening and narrowing of the channel to re-attain continence.

Kinking of the catheterisation channel causing cathetherisation difficulties is most commonly seen in Monti channels, and is due to excessive extravesical length of the channel. A review of the technique may be all that is required to overcome this problem, but if this fails a formal channel revision with reduction in extravesical length is required.[185]

COMPLICATIONS OF FEMALE STRESS URINARY INCONTINENCE SURGERY (Table 12)

Female stress urinary incontinence may be treated by open or laparoscopic retropubic suspension (Burch or VOSURP),[199–202] or by a suburethral slings

Table 12.   Complications of Female Stress Urinary Incontinence Surgery

Complications	Incidence (%)
Bleeding	1–8
GU Injury	1–1.6
RTI	2.1
Wound Infection/Dehiscence	2–5.5
Osteitis Pubis	0.9–3.2
Voiding Dysfunction	2–49
De novo DO	6–25
Prolapse	28
Reduced Quality of Life	25
Sling Erosion	1–23

using autologous, cadaveric (rectus fascia or tensor fascia lata).[203–205] or synthetic material (Transvaginal Tape (TVT or SPARC), Transobturator Tape (TOT).[206–209] All have a similar success rate of 80–90% with the longest available follow up available in the open Burch colposuspension.

Acute complications are similar to those arising from other operative procedures. The risk of bleeding is highest following open colposuspension and lowest following the vaginal sling procedures (TVT/TOT). The risk of genitourinary (GU) tract injury is highest with the vaginal sling procedures (TVT/TOT).[199–209]

Voiding dysfunction occurs following 15% (2–49%) of the procedures, with the open bladder neck slings having a greater degree of dysfunction.[207,210–213] This dysfunction mainly takes the form of frequency, urgency and/or incomplete or slow emptying. The frequency and urgency may follow *de novo* detrusor overactivity (DO), or postoperative outlet obstruction.[210–218] If it relates to *de novo* DO, standard treatment with bladder training, anticholinergic therapy, botulinum toxin injection, neuromodulation or clam augmentation cystoplasty for severe and resistant cases is required.[219–223]

It is best to prevent outlet obstruction with the insertion of a loose sling or by colposuspension. However, if it occurs, CISC will allow bladder emptying without compromising continence. If this is unacceptable, a colposuspension may be taken down whilst open pubovaginal sling procedures require formal urethrolysis and the TVT/TOT procedures require tape division. These revision procedures will restore voiding in up to 80% while continence is maintained in a similar percentage with sling revision but a far lower percentage following colposuspension takedown.[211–218]

A prolapse, especially of the posterior compartment can be a long-term problem in patients having colposuspension procedures, due to support of the anterior compartment by the procedure whilst the posterior compartment is left relatively unsupported. Rectocoele is reported in 22–33%, cystocoele in 2–18%, enterocoele in 3–17% and uterine prolapse following 8–13% of cases of Burch colposuspensions.[214,224–227] Prolapse does not appear to be a problem following sling procedures. It is best avoided by simultaneous repair of any co-existing prolapse at time of colposuspension. If it occurs postoperatively and is symptomatic, formal repair is required with a long-term success reported in 66–100% of the cases.[225–227]

Sling erosion either into the vagina (most commonly) or the urethra may occur in up to 23% of patients with time. It is less common with the current TVT/TOT prolene mesh slings and extremely rare following an autologous sling procedure. Bladder erosion is a very rare complication of the synthetic slings and requires open removal.[206,228] Vaginal or urethral erosion necessitate removal of the sling if possible or, in the case of TVT/TOT, division of the sling with removal of as much as possible and repair of any associated urethrovaginal fistula.[229-231]

COMPLICATIONS OF ENDOSCOPIC AND OPEN MANAGEMENT OF URETHRAL STRICTURE DISEASE (Table 13)

Urethral dilation or optical urethrotomy are the most commonly performed procedures to treat urethral stricture disease. Recurrent or complex strictures are generally treated with urethroplasty, which may involve simple stricture excision and reanastomosis, stricture incision with the placement of a free graft or flap patch or staged free graft or flap replacement of large sections of the urethra.[232-249]

Urethral dilation or urethrotomy have very few complications besides stricture recurrence, which occurs in 50–100% of the patients depending upon the site, length and aetiology of the stricture. Other rare complications include UTI, bleeding and sepsis.

The main complications of urethroplasty in its various forms are stricture recurrence (10–30%), erectile dysfunction (2% or 0–11% depending on type of urethroplasty), post-micturition dribble (occurs in the

Table 13. Complications of Endoscopic and Open Management of Urethral Stricture Disease

Complications of Urethroplasty	Incidence (%)
Stricture Recurrence	10–30
Post Micturition Dribble	70–90
Temporary Erectile Dysfunction	10–30
Permanent Erectile Dysfunction	0–11
Fistulae	0–5

majority of patients), and, fistula formation (following c2% of penile urethroplasties). Stricture recurrence is managed by further urethroplasty or endoscopic treatment followed by weekly ISC. Erectile dysfunction responds to currently available treatment options, especially oral medication. Post-micturition dribble can be simply managed by post-micturition urethral milking to empty the urethra while fistulae require operative repair.[232–249]

REFERENCES

1. Swanson DA, Borges PM. (1983) Complications of transabdominal radical nephrectomy for renal cell carcinoma. *J Urol* **129**: 704.

2. Skinner DG, Colvin RB, Vermillion CD, *et al.* (1971) Diagnosis and management of renal cell carcinoma. A clinical and pathologic study of 309 cases. *Cancer* **28**: 1165.

3. Shuford MD, McDougall EM, Chang SS, *et al.* (2004) Complications of contemporary radical nephrectomy: comparison of open vs. laparoscopic approach. *Urol Oncol* **22**: 121.

4. Roupret M, Hupertan V, Traxer O, Loison G, Chartier-Kastler E, Conort P, Bitker MO, Gattegno B, Richard F, Cussenot O. (2006) Comparison of open nephroureterectomy and ureteroscopic and percutaneous management of upper urinary tract transitional cell carcinoma. *Urology* **67**(6): 1181–1187.

5. Gopal V, Bisno AL. (1977) Fulminant pneumococcal infections in 'normal' asplenic hosts. *Arch Int Med* **137**: 144.

6. Boyce WH. (1983) Surgery of urinary calculi in perspective. *Urol Clin North Am* **10**: 585.

7. Spirnak JP, Renick MI. (1983) Anatrophic nephrolithotomy. *Urol Clin North Am* **10**: 665.

8. White EC, Smith AD. (1984) Percutaneous stone extraction from 200 patients. *J Urol* **132**: 437.

9. Conlin MJ, Bagley DH. (1998) Ureteroscopic endopyelotomy at a single setting. *J Urol* **159**(3): 727.

10. Erdogru T, Kutlu O, Kotsal T, *et al.* (2005) Endoscopic treatment of ureteric strictures: acucise, cold-knife endoureterotomy and wall stents as a salvage approach. *Urol Int* **74**(2): 140.

11. Sonderdahl DW, Fabrizio MD, Rahman NU, *et al.* (2005) Endoscopic treatment of upper tract transitional cell carcinoma. *Urol Oncol* **23**: 114.

12. Pence JR II, Airhart RA, Novicki DE, *et al.* (1982) Pulmonary emboli associated with coagulum pyelolithotomy. *J Urol* **127**: 572.

13. Lang EK. (1987) Percutaneous nephrostolithotomy and lithotripsy: a multiinstitutional survey of complications. *Radiology* **62**: 25.

14. Clayman RV, Suma V, Hunter D, *et al.* (1984) Renal vascular complications associated with percutaneous removal of renal calculi. *J Urol* **132**: 228.

15. Carson CC, Brown MW, Weinerth JL. (1987) Vascular complications of renal surgery. *J Endourol* **1**: 181.

16. Stoller ML, Wolf JS Jr, St Lezin MA. (1994) Estimated blood loss and transfusion rates associated with percutaneous nephrolithotomy. *J Urol* **152**: 1977.

17. Segura JW, Patterson DE, Le Roy AJ, *et al.* (1988) Percutaneous removal of kidney stones: review of 1000 cases. *J Urol* **134**: 1077.

18. Lee WJ, Smith AD, Cubelli V, *et al.* (1986) Percutaneous nephrolithotomy: analysis of 500 consecutive cases. *Urol Radiol* **8**: 61.

19. Nemoy NJ, Stamey TA. (1971) Surgical, bacteriological and biochemical management of infection stones. *JAMA* **215**: 1470.

20. Sleight MW, Wickam JEA. (1977) Long term follow up of 100 cases of renal calculi. *Br J Urol* **49**: 601.

21. Sutherland JW. (1981) Residual post-operative upper urinary tract stones. *J Urol* **126**: 573.

22. Royle G, Smith JC. (1976) Recurrence of infection calculi following postoperative renal irrigation with stone solvent. *Br J Urol* **48**: 531.

23. Li MK, Wong MY, Toh KL, *et al.* (1996) Percutaneous nephrolithotomy — results and clinical experience. *Ann Acad Med S'pore* **25**: 683.

24. Case EW, Stiles JA. (1946) The effect of various surgical positions on vital capacity. *Anaesthesiology* **7**: 29.

25. Jones JR, Jacoby J. (1955) The effect of surgical positions on respirations. *Surg Forum* **5**: 686.

26. Welborn SG. (1978) Anaesthesiologic considerations: urology. In: Martin JT (ed), *Positioning in Anaesthesia and Surgery* (WB Saunders, Philadelphia), p. 170.

27. Korth K. (1984) *Percutaneous Surgery of Kidney Stones: Techniques and Tactics* (Springer, New York).

28. Collins GM, Green RD, Boyer P, *et al.* (1980) Protection of the kidneys from warm ischaemic injury; dosage and timing of mannitol administration. *Transplantation* **29**: 83.

29. Nosowsky EE, Kaufman JJ. (1983). The protective action of mannitol in renal artery occlusion. *J Urol* **89**: 295.

30. McDougal WS. (1988). Renal perfusion-reperfusion injuries. *J Urol* **140**: 1325.

31. Marburger M, Gunther P, Mayer EJ, *et al.* (1976) A simple method for *in situ* preservation of the ischaemic kidney during renal surgery. *Invest Urol* 14: 191.
32. Evans CP, Stoller MC. (1993) The fate of the iatrogenic retroperitoneal stone. *J Urol* 150: 827.
33. Roth RA, Beckmann CF. (1988) Complications of extracorporeal shock wave lithotripsy and percutaneous nephrolithotomy. *Urol Clin North Am* 15: 155.
34. Marshall FF, Smith NA, Murphy JB, *et al.* (1981) A comparison of ultrasonography and radiography in the localisation of renal calculi: experimental and operative experience. *J Urol* 126: 576.
35. Thomas R, Lewis RW, Roberts JA. (1981) The renal scintillation camera study for determination of renal function after anatrophic nephrolithotomy. *J Urol* 125: 287.
36. Kondas J, Szentgyorgy E, Vac ZL, *et al.* (1994) Splenic injury: a rare complication of percutaneous lithotomy. *Int Urol Nephrol* 26: 399.
37. Narasimham DL, Jacobsson B, Nyman U, *et al.* (1990) Primary double pigtail stenting as a treatment of upper tract leaks. *J Urol* 143: 234.
38. Carlton CE, Scott R Jr, Guthrie AG. (1971) The initial management of ureteric injuries: a report of 78 cases. *J Urol* 105: 335.
39. Lang EK. (1984) Antegrade ureteral stenting for dehiscence, strictures and fistulae. *Am J Rientgenol* 143: 795.
40. Chang R, Marshall EF, Mitchell S. (1987) Percutaneous management of benign ureteric strictures and fistulas. *J Urol* 137: 1126.
41. Mailtet PJ, Pelle-Francoz D, Lenche A, *et al.* (1987) Fistula of the upper urinary tract: percutaneous management. *J Urol* 138: 1382.
42. Kramolowsky EV, Tucker RD, Nelson CMU. (1989) Management of benign ureteral strictures; open surgical repair or endoscopic dilation? *J Urol* 141: 285.
43. Goldfischer E, Gerber G. (1997) Endoscopic management of ureteral strictures. *J Urol* 157: 770.
44. Eshgi M. (1989) Endoscopic incision of the urinary tract; part II: endoureterotomy — endoscopic and vascular anatomy of the upper tract. *AUA Update Series* 8: 298.
45. Kowalczyk J, Keating M, Ehrlich R. (1996) Femoral neuropathy after psoas hitch procedure. *Urology* 47: 563.
46. Thompson JM, Ross G Jr. (1974) Long term results of bladder flap repair of ureteral injuries. *J Urol* 111: 483.
47. Hendren WH, Hensle TW. (1980) Transureteroureterostomy: experience with 75 cases. *J Urol* 123: 826.

48. Rushton HG, Parrot TS, Woodard JR. (1987) The expanded role of transureter-oureterostomy in paediatric urology. *J Urol* **138**: 357.

49. Hodges CV, Barry JM, Fuchs EF, *et al.* (1980) Transuretero-ureterostomy: 25 year experience with 100 patients. *J Urol* **123**: 834.

50. Strup S, Sindelar W, Walthe M. (1996) The use of transureteroureterostomy in the management of complex ureteral problems. *J Urol* **155**: 1572.

51. Ehrlich RM, Skinner DG. (1975) Complications of transureteroureterostomy. *J Urol* **113**: 467–473.

52. Sandoz IL, Paull OP, MacFarlane CA. (1977) Complications of transureter-oureterostomy. *J Urol* **117**: 39.

53. Noble J, Lee K, Mundy A. (1997) Transureteroureterostomy: a review of 253 cases. *Br J Urol* **79**: 20.

54. Boxer RJ, Fritzshe P, Skinner DG, *et al.* (1979) Replacement of the ureter by small intestine; clinical application and results of the ileal ureter in 89 patients. *J Urol* **121**: 728.

55. Hussman TK, Kaplan GW, Brock WA, *et al.* (1987) Ipsilateral ureteroureteros-tomy and pyeloureterostomy: a review of 15 years experience with 25 patients. *J Urol* **138**: 1207.

56. Rose MC, Novick AC, Rybila SJ. (1984) Renal autotransplantation in patients with retroperitoneal fibrosis. *Cleve Clin Q* **51**: 357.

57. Grasso M. (1996) Experience with the holmium laser as an endoscopic lithotrite. *Urology* **48**: 199.

58. Razvi HA, Denstedt JD, Chinn SS, *et al.* (1996) Intracorporeal lithotrypsy with the holmium: YAG laser. *J Urol* **156**: 912.

59. Herr HW, Morse MJ. (1988) Endoscopic treatment of upper tract tumours. *Adv Urol* **1**: 101.

60. Grasso M, Lange GS, Loisides P, *et al.* (1995) Endoscopic management of the symptomatic calyceal diverticula calculus. *J Urol* **153**: 1878.

61. Blute ML, Segura JW, Patterson DE. (1988) Ureteroscopy. *J Urol* **139**: 510.

62. Abdel-Razzan OM, Bagley DH. (1992) Clinical experience with flexible ureteropyeloscopy. *J Urol* **148**: 1788.

63. Harrison JW, Serschon PD, Blute ML, *et al.* (1997) Ureteroscopy: current prac-tice and long term complications. *J Urol* **157**: 28.

64. Grasso M, Bagley D. (1998) Small diameter actively deflectable flexible ureteroscopy. *J Urol* **160**: 1648.

65. Johnson DE, Lamy SM. (1977) Staged radical cystectomy and ileal conduit diversion: review of 214 cases. *J Urol* **117**: 171.

66. Freiha FS. (1980) Complications of cystectomy. *J Urol* **123**: 168.

67. Brannan W, Fuselier HA, Ockhsner M, *et al.* (1981) Critical evaluation of 1 stage cystectomy: reducing morbidity and mortality. *J Urol* **125**: 640.

68. Skinner DG, Crawford ED, Kaufman JJ. (1980) Complications of radical cystectomy for carcinoma of the bladder. *J Urol* **123**: 640.

69. Frazier HA, Robertson JE, Paulson DF. (1992) Complications of radical cystectomy and urinary diversion: a retrospective review of 675 cases in two decades. *J Urol* **148**: 1402.

70. Fleichner SM, Spalding JT. (1982) Management of rectal injury after cystectomy. *Urology* **19**: 143.

71. Kozminski M, Konnak JW, Grossman HB. (1989) Management of rectal injury during radical cystectomy. *J Urol* **142**: 1204.

72. Brendler CB, Steinberg GD, Marshall FF, *et al.* (1990) Local recurrence and survival following nerve sparing radical cystoprostatectomy. *J Urol* **144**: 1137.

73. Crawford ED, Skinner DG. (1980) Salvage cystectomy after irradiation failure. *J Urol* **123**: 32.

74. Swanson DA, Von Esschenbach AC, Bracken RB, *et al.* (1981) Salvage cystectomy for bladder cancer. *Cancer* **47**: 2275.

75. Madersbacher S, Schmidt J, Eberle JM, *et al.* (2003) Long term outcome of ileal conduit diversion. *J Urol* **169**: 985.

76. Marshall FF, Leadbetter WF, Dretler SP. (1975) Ileal conduit parastomal repairs. *J Urol* **114**: 40.

77. Klein EA, Montie JE, Montague DK, *et al.* (1989) Stomal complications of intestinal conduit urinary diversion. *Cleve Clin J Med* **56**: 48.

78. Wood DN, Allen SE, Hussain M, *et al.* (2004) Long term stomal complications of ileal conduits in women with complex urinary incontinence. *J Urol* **172**: 2300.

79. Jones MA, Breckman B, Hendry WF. (1980) Life with an ileal conduit: results of questionnaire surveys of patients and urological surgeons. *Br J Urol* **52**: 21.

80. Chadwick DJ, Stower MJ. (1990) Life with urostomy. *Br J Urol* **65**: 189.

81. McDougal WS. (1992) Metabolic complications of urinary intestinal diversion. *J Urol* **147**: 1199.

82. Koch MO, McDougal WS. (1985) The pathophysiology of hyperchloraemic metabolic acidosis after urinary diversion through intestinal segments. *Surgery* **98**: 561.

83. Greenwell TJ, Venn SN, Mundy AR. (2001) Augmentation cystoplasty. *Br J Urol* **88**(6): 511.

84. Atala A, Bauer SB, Hendren WH, *et al.* (1993) The effect of gastric augmentation on bladder function. *J Urol* **149**(5): 1099.

85. Reinberg Y, Manivel JC, Froemming C, *et al.* (1992) Perforation of the gastric segment of an augmented bladder secondary to peptic ulcer disease. *J Urol* **148**(2): 369.

86. Tiffany P, Vaughan ED Jr, Manon D, *et al.* (1986) Hypergastrinaemia following antral gastrocystoplasty. *J Urol* **136**(3): 692.

87. Gold BD, Bhoopalam PS, Reifen RN, *et al.* (1992) Gastrointestinal complications of gastrocystoplasty. *Arch Dis Child* **67**: 1272.

88. Nurse DE, Mundy AR. (1989) Metabolic Complications of cystoplasty. *Br J Urol* **63**(2): 165.

89. Kreder KJ, Webster GD. (1992) Management of the bladder outlet in patients requiring enterocystoplasty. *J Urol* **147**: 38.

90. Fromm D. (1973) Ileal resection or disease and the blind loop syndrome: current concepts and pathophysiology. *Surgery* **73**: 639.

91. Lewis DK, Morgan JR, Weston PMT, *et al.* (1990) The 'clam': indications and complications. *Br J Urol* **65**: 488.

92. Thomalla JV, Mitchell ME, Leapman SB, *et al.* (1989) Renal transplantation into the reconstructed bladder. *J Urol* **141**: 265.

93. Strawbridge LR, Kramer SA, Castillo O, *et al.* (1989) Augmentation cystoplasty and the genitourinary sphincter. *J Urol* **142**(2 Pt 1): 297.

94. Cheng C, Hendry WF, Kirby RS, *et al.* (1991) Detubularisation in cystoplasty: clinical review. *Br J Urol* **67**(3): 303.

95. Elder DD, Stephenson TP. (1980) An assessment of the Frewen regime in the treatment of detrusor dysfunction in females. *Br J Urol* **52**: 467.

96. Hendren WH, Hendren RB. (1990) Bladder augmentation: experience with 129 children and young adults. *J Urol* **144**: 445.

97. Rushton HG, Woodard JR, Parrott TS, *et al.* (1988) Delayed bladder rupture after enterocystoplasty. *J Urol* **140**(2): 344.

98. George VK, Gee JM, Wortley MI, *et al.* (1992) The effect of ranitidine on urine mucus concentration in patients with enterocystoplasty. *Br J Urol* **70**(1): 30.

99. Gillon G, Mundy AR. (1989) The dissolution of urinary mucus after cystoplasty. *Br J Urol* **63**(4): 372.

100. Krieger JN, Stubenbord WT, Vaughan ED Jr. (1980) Transplantation in children with end stage disease of urologic origin. *J Urol* **124**: 508.

101. Kelly JD, Kernohan RM, Keane PF. (1997) Symptomatic outcome following clam ileocystoplasty. *Eur Urol* **32**: 30.

102. Kreder KJ, Webster GD. (1992) Management of the bladder outlet in patients requiring enterocystoplasty. *J Urol* 147(1): 38.
103. Blyth B, Ewalt DH, Duckett JW, *et al.* (1992) Lithogenic properties of entero-cystoplasty. *J Urol* 148(2 Pt 2): 575.
104. Palmer LS, Franco I, Kogan SJ, *et al.* (1993) Urolithiasis in children following augmentation cystoplasty. *J Urol* 150(2 Pt 2): 726.
105. Fontaine E, Bendaya S, Desert JF, *et al.* (1997) Combined modified rectus Fascial sling and augmentation ileocystoplasty for neurogenic incontinence in women. *J Urol* 157(1): 109.
106. Kirby RS, Lloyd-Davies RW. (1985) Adenocarcinoma occurring within a caeco-cystoplasty. *Br J Urol* 57: 357.
107. Nurse DE, McInerney PD, Thomas PJ, *et al.* (1996) Stones in enterocystoplasties. *Br J Urol* 77(5): 684.
108. Ginsberg D, Huffman JL, Lieskovsky G, *et al.* (1991) Urinary tract stones: a complication of the Kock pouch continent urinary diversion. *J Urol* 145(5): 956.
109. Couillard DR, Vapnec JM, Rentzepis MJ, *et al.* (1993) Fatal perforation of an augmentation cystoplasty in an adult. *Urology* 42(5): 31.
110. N'Dow J, Leung HY, Marshall C, *et al.* (1998) Bowel dysfunction after bladder reconstruction. *J Urol* 159(5): 1470.
111. Singh G, Thomas DG. (1997) Bowel problems after enterocystoplasty. *Br J Urol* 79(3): 328.
112. Jakobsen H, Steven K, Stigsby B, *et al.* (1987) Pathogenesis of nocturnal urinary incontinence after ileocaecal bladder replacement: continuous measurement of urethral closure pressure during sleep. *Br J Urol* 59(9): 148.
113. Akerlund S, Berglund B, Kock NG, *et al.* (1989) Voiding pattern, urinary volume, composition and bacterial contamination in patients with urinary diversion via a continent ileal reservoir. *Br J Urol* 63(6): 619.
114. Cher ML, Allen TD. (1993) Continence in the myelodysplastic patient following enterocystoplasty. *J Urol* 149(5): 1103.
115. Salle JL, McLorie GA, Bagli DJ. (1997) Urethral lengthening with anterior bladder wall flap (Pippi Salle procedure): modifications and extended indications of the technique. *J Urol* 158(2): 585.
116. Kropp KA, Angwafo FF. (1986) Urethral lengthening and reimplantation for neurogenic incontinence in children. *J Urol* 135(3): 533.
117. Raz S, Siegel AL, Short JL, *et al.* (1989) Vaginal wall sling. *J Urol* 141(1): 43.
118. Wan J, McGuire EJ, Bloom DA, *et al.* (1992) The treatment of urinary incontinence in children using glutaraldehyde cross-linked collagen. *J Urol* 148(1): 127.

119. Raz S, Ehrlich RM, Zeidman EJ, *et al.* (1988) Surgical treatment of the incontinent female patient with myelomeningocele. *J Urol* **139**(3): 524.
120. Nurse DE, Mundy AR. (1988) One hundred artificial sphincters. *Br J Urol* **61**(4): 318.
121. Lieskovsky G, Boyd SD, Skinner DG. (1987) Management of late complications of the Kock pouch form of urinary diversion. *J Urol* **137**: 1146.
122. Mansson W, Collen S, Sundin T. (1984) Continent caecal reservoir in urinary diversion. *Br J Urol* **56**(4): 359.
123. Mansson W, Davidsson T, Konyves J, *et al.* (2003) Continent urinary tract reconstruction; the Lund experience. *BJU Int* **92**(3): 271.
124. Levy OM, Phillips MH, Algen A, Kivart AM. (1988) Bladder replacement after radical cystectomy using detubularised right colonic segment. *Urology* **32**(6): 492.
125. Kirsch AJ, Olsson CA, Heisle JW. (1996) Pediatric continent reservoirs and colocystoplasty with absorbable staples. *J Urol* **156**(25) Suppl: 611.
126. Elmajnan DA, Stein JP, Esrig D, *et al.* (1996) The Kock ileal neobladder: updates experience in 295 male patients. *J Urol* **156**(3): 920.
127. Fontaine E, Leaver R, Woodhouse CR. (2000) The effect of intestinal urinary reservoirs on renal function: a 10 year follow-up. *BJU Int* **86**: 195.
128. Hautmann RE, Simon J. (1999) Ileal neobladder and local recurrence of bladder cancer; patterns of failure and impact on function in men. *J Urol* **162**: 1963.
129. Ward AM, Olencki T, Peerbook D, Klein EA. (1998) Should continent diversion be performed in patients with locally advanced bladder cancer? *Urology* **51**(2): 232.
130. Tefilli MV, Gheiler EL, Tiguert R, *et al.* (1999) Urinary diversion related outcome in patients with pelvic recurrence after radical cystectomy for bladder cancer. *Urology* **53**: 999.
131. Yossepowitch O, Dalbagni G, Golijanin D, *et al.* (2003) Orthotopic urinary diversion after cystectomy for bladder cancer: implications for cancer control and patterns of disease recurrence. *J Urol* **169**(1): 177.
132. Griffith DP, Musher DM, Itin C. Urease. (1976) The primary cause of infection-induced urinary stones. *Invest Urol* **13**: 346.
133. Hitchcock RJ, Duffy PG, Malone PS. (1994) Ureterocystoplasty: the bladder augmentation of choice. *Br J Urol* **73**: 575.
134. Swami KS, Feneley RC, Hammonds JC, *et al.* (1998) Detrusor myectomy for detrusor overactivity: a minimum 1 year follow up. *Br J Urol* **81**: 68.
135. Fontaine E, Bendaya S, Desert JF, *et al.* (1997) Combined modified rectus fascial sling and augmentation ileocystoplasty for neurogenic incontinence in women. *J Urol* **157**: 109.

136. Beier-Holgersen R, Kirkeby LT, Nordling J. (1994) Clam ileocystoplasty. *Scand J Urol Nephrol* **28**: 55.
137. Bramble FJ. (1990) The clam cystoplasty. *Br J Urol* **66**: 337.
138. Matthews GJ, Churchill BA, McLorie GA, Khoury AE. (1996) Ventriculoperitoneal shunt infection after augmentation cystoplasty. *J Urol* **155**: 686.
139. Shimogaki H, Okada H, Fujisawa M, *et al.* (1999) Longterm experience with orthotopic reconstruction of the lower urinary tract in women. *J Urol* **161**: 573.
140. Iannoni C, Marcheggiano A, Pallone F, *et al.* (1986) Abnormal patterns of colorectal mucin secretion after urinary diversions of different types. *Human Pathol* **17**: 834–840; Rushton HG, Woodard JR, Parrott TS, *et al.* (1988). Delayed bladder rupture after enterocystoplasty. *J Urol* **140**: 344.
141. McConnell J, Barry M, Bruskewitz R. (1994) *Benign Prostatic Hyperplasia: Diagnosis and Treatment*, Clinical Practice Guideline No. 8. US Department of Health and Human Services, Agency for Health Care Policy and Research Publication No. 94–0582, Rockville, MD, USA.
142. Nicoll GS, Riffle GN, Anderson FO. (1978) Suprapubic prostatectomy: the removable purse string: a continuing comparative analysis of 300 consecutive cases. *J Urol* **120**: 702.
143. Nanninga JB, O'Connor VJ. (1972) Suprapubic prostatectomy: a review. *J Urol* **108**: 453.
144. Walsh PC, Oesterling JE. (1990) Improved haemostasis during simple retropubic prostatectomy. *J Urol* **143**: 1203.
145. Meier DE, Tarpley JL, Imediegwu OO, *et al.* (1995) The outcome of suprapubic prostatectomy: a contemporary series in the developed world. *Urology* **46**: 40.
146. Roos NP, Wennberg JE, Matenka DJ, *et al.* (1989) Mortality and reoperation after open and transurethral resection of the prostate for benign prostatic hyperplasia. *N Engl J Med* **320**: 1120.
147. Hannappel J, Krieger S. (1991) Subjective and clinical results after transurethral resection and suprapubic prostatectomy in benign prostatic hypertrophy. *Eur Urol* **20**: 272.
148. Roos NP, Ramsay EW. (1987) A population-based study of prostatectomy: outcomes associated with differing surgical approaches. *J Urol* **137**: 1184.
149. Hautmann RE, Sautre TW, Wenderoth UK. (1994) Radical retropubic prostatectomy: morbidity and urinary continence in 418 consecutive cases. *Urology* **43**(2 Suppl): 47.
150. Harris MJ. (2003) Radical perineal prostatectomy: cost efficient, outcome effective, minimally invasive prostate cancer management. *Eur Urol* **44**(3): 303.

151. Saloman L, Levrel O, de la Taille A, *et al.* (2002) Radical prostatectomy by the retropubic, perineal and laparoscopic approach: 12 years of experience in one center. *Eur Urol* **42**(2): 104.

152. Haab F, Boccon-Gibbod L, Delmas V, *et al.* (1994) Perineal versus retropubic radical prostatectomy for T1, T2 prostate cancer. *Br J Urol* **74**(5): 626.

153. Kerr LA, Zincke H. (1994) Radical retropubic prostatectomy for prostate cancer in the elderly and the young: complications and prognosis. *Eur Urol* **25**(4): 305.

154. Abbas F, Siddiqui K, Biyabani SR, *et al.* (2002) Early surgical results with intent to treat by radical retropubic prostatectomy for clinically localized prostate cancer. *J Pak Med Assoc* **52**(5): 200.

155. Hisasue S, Takahashi A, Kato R, Shimizu T, *et al.* (2004) Early and late complications of radical retropubic prostatectomy: experience in a single institution. *Jpn J Clin Oncol* **34**(5): 274.

156. Martin Marquina Aspiunza A, Zudaire Bergera JJ, Sanchez Zalabardo D, *et al.* (1999) Radical prostatectomy. The surgical complications. *Actas Urol Esp* **23**(1): 5.

157. Maffezzini M, Seveso M, Taverna G, *et al.* (2003) Evaluation of complications and results in a contemporary series of 300 consecutive radical retropubic prostatectomies with the anatomic approach at a single institution. *Urology* **61**(5): 982.

158. Catalona WJ, Carvalhal GF, Mager DE, Smith DF. (1999) Potency, continence and complication rates in 1,870 consecutive radical retropubic prostatectomies. *J Urol* **162**(2): 433.

159. Talcott JA, Rieker P, Propert KJ, *et al.* (1997) Patient-reported impotence and incontinence after nerve-sparing radical prostatectomy. *J Natl Cancer Inst* **89**(15): 1117.

160. Wasson JH, Reda DJ, Bruskewitz RC, *et al.* (1995) A comparison of transurethral surgery with watchful waiting for moderate symptoms of benign prostatic hyperplasia. The Veterans Cooperative Study Group on Transurethral Resection of the Prostate. *N Engl J Med* **332**: 75.

161. Ziada A, Rosenblum M, Crawford ED. (1999) Benign prostatic hyperplasia: an overview. *Urology* **53**: 1.

162. Borboroglu PG, Kane CJ, Ward JF, *et al.* (1999) Immediate and postoperative complications of transurethral prostatectomy in the 1990s. *J Urol* **162**: 1307.

163. Mebust WK, Holtgrewe HL, Cockett AT, *et al.* (1989) Transurethral prostatectomy: immediate and post-operative complications. A co-operative study of 13 institutions evaluating 3885 patients. *J Urol* **741**: 243.

164. Horninger W, Untertechner H, Strasser H, *et al.* (1996) Transurethral prostatectomy: mortality and morbidity. *Prostate* **28**: 195.

165. Brooks MB. (1969) Heparin in the treatment of haemorrhagic diathesis associated with prostate cancer. *J Urol* **106**: 240.

166. Hahn RG. (1991) The transurethral resection syndrome. *Acta Anaesthesiol Scan* **35**: 557.

167. Chambers A. (2002) Transurethral resection syndrome — it does not have to be a mystery. *AORN J* **75**: 156.

168. Henderson DJ, Middleton RG. (1980) Coma from hyponatraemia following transurethral resection of the prostate. *Urology* **15**: 267.

169. Varkarakis J, Bartsch G, Horninger W. (2004) Long-term morbidity and mortality of transurethral prostatectomy: a 10-year follow up. *Prostate* **58**: 248.

170. Reynard JM, Shearer RM. (1999) Failure to void after transurethral resection of the prostate and mode of presentation. *Urology* **53**: 336.

171. Balzarro M, Ficarra A, Bartoloni A, *et al.* (2001) The pathophysiology, diagnosis and therapy of the transurethral resection of the prostate syndrome. *Urol Int* **66**: 121.

172. Madersbacher S, Marberger M. (1999) Is TURP still justified? *Br J Urol* **83**: 227.

173. Emberton M, Neal DE, Black N, *et al.* (1995) The National Prostatectomy Audit: the clinical management of patients during hospital admission. *BJU* **75**: 301.

174. Venn SN, Greenwell TJ, Mundy AR. (2000) The long-term outcome of artificial urinary sphincters. *J Urol* **164**(3): 702.

175. Scott FB, Bradley W, Timm GW. (2002) Treatment of urinary incontinence by an implantable prosthetic urinary sphincter. *J Urol* **167**: 1125.

176. Duncan HJ, McInerney PD, Mundy AR. (1993) Late erosion. A new complication of artificial urinary sphincters. *Br J Urol* **72**: 597.

177. Elliott DS, Barrett DM. (1998) Mayo clinic long-term analysis of the functional durability of the AMS 800 artificial urinary sphincter: a review of 323 cases. *J Urol* **159**(4): 1206.

178. Guralnick ML, Miller E, Toh KL, Webster GD. (2002) Transcorporal artificial urinary sphincter cuff placement in cases requiring revision for erosion and urethral atrophy. *J Urol* **167**: 2075.

179. Furlow WL, Barrett DM. (1985) Recurrent or persistent urinary incontinence in patients with the artificial urinary sphincter: diagnostic considerations and management. *J Urol* **133**(5): 792.

180. Barrett DM, Goldwasser B. (1988) The AUS: current management philosophy. *AUA Update Series* Vol. 5, Lesson 32.

181. Hajivassiloiou CA. (1999) A review of the complications and results of implantation of the AMS artificial urinary sphincter. *Eur Urol* **35**(1): 36.

182. Marks JL, Light JK. (1989) Management of urinary incontinence after prostatectomy with the artificial urinary sphincter. *J Urol* **142**(2 Pt 1): 302.

183. M Hussain, TJ Greenwell, SN Venn, AR Mundy. (2005) The current role of the artificial urinary sphincter in the treatment of urinary incontinence. *J Urol* **174**(2): 418.

184. Litwiller SE, Kim KB, Fone PD, *et al.* (1996) Post-prostatectomy incontinence and the artificial urinary sphincter: a long-term study of patient satisfaction and criteria for success. *J Urol* **156**(6): 1975.

185. Cain MP, Casale AJ, King SJ, Rink RC. (1999) Appendicovesicostomy and newer alternatives for the Mitrofanoff procedure: results in the last 100 patients at Riley Children's Hospital. *J Urol* **162**: 1749.

186. Narayanaswamy B, Wilcox DT, Cuckow PM, *et al.* (2001) The Yang-Monti ileovesicostomy: a problematic channel? *BJU Int* **87**: 861.

187. Duckett JW, Lofti AU. (1993) Appendicovesicostomy (and variations) in bladder reconstruction. *J Urol* **149**: 567.

188. Sumfest JM. Burns MW, Mitchell ME. (1993) The Mitrofanoff principle in urinary reconstruction. *J Urol* **150**: 1875.

189. Castellan MA, Gosalbez R, Labbie A, Monti PR. (1999) Clinical applications of the Monti procedure as a continent catheterizable stoma. *Urology* **54**: 152.

190. Barroso U, Jednak R, Fleming P, *et al.* (2000) Bladder calculi in children who perform clean intermittent catheterisation. *BJU Int* **85**: 879.

191. Suzer O, Vates TS, Freedman AL, *et al.* (1997) Results of the Mitrofanoff procedure in urinary tract reconstruction in children. *Br J Urol* **79**(2): 279.

192. Kajbafzadeh AM, Chubak N. (2001) Simultaneous Malone antegrade continence enema and Mitrofanoff principle using the divided appendix: report of a new technique for prevention of stoma complications. **165**: 2404.

193. Harris CF, Cooper CS, Hutcheson JC, Snyder HM. (2000) Appendicovesicostomy: the Mitrofanoff procedure – a 15-year perspective. *J Urol* **163**(6): 1922.

194. Mor Y, Quinn FM, Carr B, *et al.* (1997) Combined Mitrofanoff and antegrade continence enema procedures for urinary and fecal incontinence. *J Urol* **158**(1): 192.

195. Van Savage JG, Khoury AE, McLorie GA, Churchill BM. (1996) Outcome analysis of Mitrofanoff principle applications using appendix and ureter to umbilical and lower quadrant stomal sites. *J Urol* **156**: 1794.

196. Woodhouse CR, Lennon GN. (2001) Management and aetiology of stones in intestinal urinary reservoirs in adolescents. *Eur Urol* **39**: 253.

197. Sugarman ID, Malone PS, Terry TR, Koyle MA. (1998) Transversely tubularized ileal segments for the Mitrofanoff or Malone antegrade continence enema procedures: the Monti principle. *Br J Urol* **81**: 253.

198. Austin P, Spyropoulos E, Arango H, *et al.* (1997) The failed anti-incontinence mechanism: a flap valve or cecal wrap for surgical reconstruction. *J Urol* 157: 1638.

199. Burch JC. (1961) Urethrovaginal fixation to Cooper's ligament for correction of stress incontinence, cystocele, and prolapse. *J Obstet Gynecol* 81: 281.

200. Marshall FV, Marchetti AA, Krantz KE. (1949) The correction of stress incontinence by simple vesicourethral suspension. *Surg Gynecol Obstet* 88: 509.

201. German KA, Kynaston H, Weight H, Stephenson TP. (1994) A prospective randomized trial comparing a modified needle suspension procedure with the vagina/obturator shelf procedure for genuine stress incontinence. *Br J Urol* 74: 188.

202. Paraiso MR, Falcone T, Walters MD. (1999) Laparoscopic surgery for genuine stress incontinence. *Int Urogynecol* 10: 237.

203. Chaikin DC, Rosenthal J, Blaivas JG. (1998) Pubovaginal fascial sling for all types of stress urinary incontinence: long-term analysis. *J Urol* 160: 1312.

204. Govier FE, Gibbons RP, Correa RJ, *et al.* (1997) Pubovaginal slings using fascia lata for the treatment of intrinsic sphincter deficiency. *J Urol* 157: 117.

205. Amundsen C, Visco AG, Ruiz H, Webster G. (2000) Outcome in 104 pubovaginal slings using freeze-dried allograft fascia lata from a single tissue bank. *Urology* 56: 2.

206. Weinberger MW, Ostergard DR. (1995) Long-term clinical and urodynamic evaluation of the polytetrafluoroethylene suburethral sling for treatment of genuine stress incontinence. *Obstet Gynecol* 86: 92.

207. Morgan JE, Farrow GA, Stewart FE. (1985) The Marlex sling operation for the treatment of recurrent stress urinary incontinence: a 16-year review. *Am J Obstet Gynecol* 151: 224.

208. Ulmsten U, Johnson P, Rezapor M. (1999) A three-year follow up of tension free vaginal tape for surgical treatment of female stress urinary incontinence. *Br J Obstet Gynecol* 106: 345.

209. Hodroff MA, Sutherland SE, Kesha JB, Siegel SW. (2005) Treatment of stress incontinence with the SPARC sling: intraoperative and early complications of 445 patients. *Urology* 66: 760.

210. Ward R, Hilton P. (2002) Prospective multicentre randomised trial of TVT and colposuspension as primary treatment for stress incontinence. *BMJ* 325: 67.

211. Liapis A, Bakas P, Creatas G. (2002) Burch colposuspension and tension-free vaginal tape in the management of stress urinary incontinence. *Eur Urol* 41: 469.

212. Leach GE, Dmochowski RR, Appell RA, *et al.* (1997) Female Stress Urinary Incontinence Clinical Guidelines Panel summary report on surgical management of female stress urinary incontinence. The American Urological Association. *J Urol* **158**: 875.

213. Wiskind AK, Creighton SM, Stanton SL. (1992) The incidence of genital prolapse after the Burch colposuspension. *Am J Obstet Gynecol* **167**: 399.

214. Carr LK, Webster GD. (1997) Voiding dysfunction following incontinence surgery: diagnosis and treatment with retropubic or vaginal urethrolysis. *J Urol* **157**: 821.

215. Nitti VW, Raz S. (1994) Obstruction following anti-incontinence procedures: diagnosis and treatment with transvaginal urethrolysis. *J Urol* **152**: 93.

216. Wang KH, Wang KH, Neimark M, Davila GW. (2002) Voiding dysfunction following TVT procedure. *Int Urogynecol J Pelvic Floor Dysfunct* **13**: 353.

217. Cross CA, Cespedes RD, English RF, McGuire EJ. (1998) Transvaginal urethrolysis for urethral obstruction after anti-incontinence surgery. *J Urol* **159**: 1199.

218. Alcalay M, Monga A, Stanton SL. (1995) Burch colposuspension: a 10–20 year follow up. *Br J Obstet Gynaecol* **102**: 740.

219. Brubaker L, Benson JT, Bent A, *et al.* (1997) Transvaginal electrical stimulation for female urinary incontinence. *Am J Obstet Gynaecol* **177**: 536.

220. Wyndaele JJ, Hoekx L, Vermandel Al. (1997) Bladder biofeedback for the treatment of refractory sensory urgency in adults. *Eur Urol* **32**: 429.

221. Moore KH, Hay DM, Imrie AE, *et al.* (1990) Oxybutynin hydrochloride (3 mg) in the treatment of women with idiopathic detrusor instability. *Br J Urol* **66**: 479.

222. Hasan ST, Robson WA, Pridie AK, Neal DE. (1996) Transcutaneous electrical nerve stimulation and temporary S3 neuromodulation in idiopathic detrusor instability. *J Urol* **155**: 2005.

223. Bosch JL, Groen J. (1995) Sacral (S3) segmental nerve stimulation as a treatment for urge incontinence in patients with detrusor instability: results of chronic electrical stimulation using an implantable neural prosthesis. *J Urol* **154**: 504.

224. Gilja I, Puskar D, Mazuran B, Radej M. (1998) Comparative analysis of bladder neck suspension using Raz, Burch and transvaginal Burch procedures. A 3-year randomized prospective study. *Eur Urol* **33**: 298.

225. Julian TM. (1996) The efficacy of Marlex mesh in the repair of severe, recurrent vaginal prolapse of the anterior midvaginal wall. *Obstet Gynecol* **175**: 1472.

226. Raz S, Nitti VW, Bregg KJ. (1993) Transvaginal repair of enterocele. *J Urol* **149**: 724.

227. Holley RL, Varner RE, Gleason BP, *et al.* (1996) Sexual function after sacrospinous ligament fixation for vaginal vault prolapse. *J Reprod Med* 41: 355.

228. Morgan JL, O'Connell HE, McGuire EJ. (2000) Is intrinsic sphincter deficiency a complication of simple hysterectomy? *Am J Obstet Gynecol* 163: 1645.

229. Blaivas JG, Heritz DM. (1996) Vaginal flap reconstruction of the urethra and vesical neck in women: a report of 49 cases. *J Urol* 155: 1014.

230. Amundsen CL, Flynn BJ, Webster GD. (2003) Urethral erosion after synthetic and nonsynthetic pubovaginal slings: differences in management and continence outcome. *J Urol* 170: 134.

231. Akpinar H, Cetinel B, Demirkesen O, *et al.* (2000) Long-term results of Burch colposuspension. *Int J Urol* 7: 119.

232. Steenkamp JW, Heyns CF, DeKock MS. (1997) Internal urethrotomy versus dilation as treatment of male urethral strictures: a prospective randomised comparison. *J Urol* 157: 98.

233. Mundy AR. (1996) Urethroplasty for posterior urethral strictures. *Br J Urol* 78: 243.

234. Webster GD, Ramon J. (1991) Repair of pelvic fracture posterior urethral defects using an elaborated perineal approach: experience with 74 Cases. *J Urol* 145: 744.

235. Martinez-Pineiro JA, Carcamo P, Garcia Matnes MJ, *et al.* (1997) Excision and anastomotic repair for urethral stricture disease. *Eur Urol* 32: 433.

236. Corriere JN Jr., Rudy DC, Benson GS. (1994) Voiding and erectile dysfunction after delayed 1 stage repair of posterior urethral disruptions in 50 men with fractured pelvis. *J Trauma* 37: 587.

237. Mundy AR. (1996) Urethroplasty for posterior urethral strictures. *Br J Urol* 78: 243.

238. Coursey JW, Morey AF, McAninch JW, *et al.* (2001) Erectile function after anterior urethroplasty. *J Urol* 166: 2273.

239. Mundy AR. (1993) Results and complications of urethroplasty and its future. *Br J Urol* 71: 322.

240. Barbagli G, Selli C, Tosto A, Palminteri E. (1996) Dorsal free graft urethroplasty. *J Urol* 155: 123.

241. Andrich DE, Leach CJ, Mundy AR. (2001) The Barbagli procedure gives the best results for patch urethroplasty of the bulbar urethra. *BJU Int* 88: 385.

242. Bhandari M, Dubey D, Verma BS. (2001) Dorsal or ventral placement of the preputial/penile skin onlay flap for anterior urethral strictures: does it make a difference? *BJU Int* 88: 39.

243. Greenwell TJ, Venn SN, Mundy AR. (1999) Changing practice in anterior urethroplasty. *BJU Int* 83: 631.

244. Venn SN, Mundy AR. (1998) Early experience with the use of buccal mucosa for substitution urethroplasty. *Br J Urol* **81**: 738.

245. Joseph JV, Andrich DE, Leach CJ, Mundy AR. (2002) Urethroplasty for refactory anterior urethral stricture. *J Urol* **167**: 127.

246. Bracka A. (1995) A versatile two stage hypospadias repair. *Br J Plast Surg* **48**: 345.

247. Webster GD, Brown MW, Koefoot RB Jr., Shelnick S. (1984) Suboptimal results in full thickness skin graft urethroplasty using an extrapenile skin donor site. *J Urol* **136**: 1082.

248. Wessells H, McAninch JW. (1996) Use of free grafts in urethral stricture reconstruction. *J Urol* **155**: 1912.

249. Orandi A. (1968) One stage urethroplasty. *Br J Urol* **40**: 717.

Chapter 19

COMPLICATIONS OF GYNAECOLOGICAL SURGERY

Krishen Sieunarine and J. Richard Smith

INTRODUCTION

When asked to write a chapter on surgical complications, one's first instinct is to say "that's something my patients do not experience." Unfortunately all of us who operate have patients with complications occurring because of the surgery. The only surgeon without surgical complications is the "armchair" surgeon who does not do any surgery.

In reality the success of surgery is dependent on thorough preoperative care and assessment, the quality of the surgery, careful asepsis and high quality anaesthesia. Postoperative care can be planned to minimise complications if risk factors such as obesity and smoking are identified preoperatively.

The complications that may occur during any major surgical procedure can be minimised by adequate training and the high level of expertise of the surgeon. However, in any form of major gynaecological surgery, occasional damage to vital internal structures may occur. Early recognition and repair of potential problems, especially during the original operation often makes the difference between complete and rapid recovery and long-term morbidity and further surgery. Seeking appropriate assistance from experienced colleagues or those from another speciality is often invaluable. Intraoperative complications are further minimised by the careful and accurate identification of tissue planes, preferably with sharp dissection and operating under direct vision at all times. Surgery should never be rushed as the outcome is always more important than the operative time. It is good practice to keep the operation under control at all times, such as controlling any bleeding to aid good visibility and to encourage the smooth progress of the procedure.

In general, gynaecologists often benefit from operating on fit and relatively young patients, with the majority of procedures undertaken having a low surgical morbidity. Our goal should be to prevent postoperative complications rather than their diagnosis and treatment. Satisfactory postoperative management is associated with a reduction in morbidity and shorter hospital stay, and hence an increase in patient satisfaction. Playing against the gynaecologist is the narrow field in which we are expected to operate, i.e. the pelvis. This is compounded by the patient's natural desire for small scars. Because their expectations are high there is always enormous disappointment when things go wrong.

Complications that arise during gynaecological surgery may occur during the intraoperative or postoperative period. Intraoperative complications may be further categorised as anaesthetic, surgical and perioperative factors.

INTRAOPERATIVE COMPLICATIONS

Anaesthetic

Surgical

- Ureteric damage
- Bladder damage
- Bowel damage

- Vascular damage and primary haemorrhage
- Uterine perforation and false passage
- Laparoscopic damage/complications

Perioperative factors

- Heat loss
- Circulating blood volume maintenance

Anaesthetic

Intraoperative general anaesthetic complications include laryngospasm, bronchospasm, malignant hyperpyrexia and drug anaphylaxis. Further detailed discussion of the above complications and their management are outside the remit of this chapter.

Ureteric Damage

Ureteric injury occurs in 0.5–2.5% of all major gynaecological procedures. The risk is lower for vaginal versus abdominal hysterectomy and even lower for major laparoscopic surgery.[1] The risk of damage to the ureter can be minimised by recognising when and where they are most at risk and the adoption of a safe surgical technique.

The ureter crosses the pelvic brim in the region of the bifurcation of the common iliac arteries. It usually runs over the external iliac vessels and then down the pelvic sidewall in front of the internal iliac artery and behind the ovary lateral to the ovarian fossae. On reaching the level of the ischial spine, it turns forwards and medially above the pelvic floor and runs lateral to the uterosacral ligaments to pass beneath the uterine arteries, 1–1.5 cm lateral to the cervix and vagina. It then swings medially around the vagina to enter the bladder 2–3 cm below the anterior vaginal fornix.[2]

The ureter is at risk during gynaecological surgery in four regions:

- At the pelvic brim where it can be confused with the infundibulopelvic ligament

- Lateral to the ovarian fossa where it can be adherent to an ovarian mass
- In the ureteric tunnel beneath the uterine artery
- Anterior to the vagina where it runs into the bladder

Locations at which the ureter is at risk	Reason for risk
Pelvic brim	Lies very close to ovarian vessels
Ovarian fossa	May become adherent to an ovarian mass
Ureteric tunnel	Lies immediately inferior to uterine artery
Anterior to vagina at entry into bladder	May not be mobilised during bladder dissection

At the level of the pelvic brim and the ovarian fossa, the ureter can be safely identified by opening the peritoneum of the broad ligament and dissecting the retroperitoneal space. This is achieved by dividing the round ligament and separating the peritoneum superiorly 1.5 cm lateral to the ovarian vessels and inferiorly towards the uterovesical fold. The loose areolar tissue can be bluntly dissected taking care to diathermy any small vessels within the broad ligament. The ureter is seen to lie laterally and can be confirmed by eliciting peristaltic movement along its length by blunt stimulation. The infundibulopelvic ligament can now be safely divided with the ureter under direct vision. This technique is particularly useful when the anatomy of the pelvic sidewall has been distorted.

At the site of the ureteric tunnel, the ureter can be directly palpated within the paracervical tissue between the index finger positioned in the Pouch of Douglas and the thumb placed laterally in front of the uterine pedicle. It feels like a firm cord near the lateral margin of the cervix. Damage to the ureter at this site is avoided by meticulously reflecting the bladder and by not taking too large a pedicle which includes both the uterine artery and the paracervical tissue. Clamping and dividing the uterine artery pedicle at the level of the internal os allows the parametrium to fall laterally taking the ureter with it. The cardinal ligament pedicle is then applied medial to this with the ureter safely out of the way. If the uterine pedicle slips reapplying the clamp can often lead to ureteric damage. After replacing the clamp to arrest any bleeding the ureter should be palpated to ensure it is not included.

The ureter is occasionally damaged in its course across the anterior surface of the vagina during a vaginal hysterectomy, colposuspension or when taking a cuff of vagina. When dissecting the upper vagina it is important to stay in the correct plane close to the vaginal wall. Stitches placed either vaginally or abdominally in this area must be in tissue that has been accurately identified.

In women who require a laparotomy or pelvic surgery in the presence of dense pelvic adhesions (such as those who underwent ovarian conservation following a simple hysterectomy or in those cases of severe endometriosis with alteration of the pelvic sidewall anatomy) cystoscopic placement of a ureteric catheter or stent is a quick, easy and useful procedure that aids identification of the ureters at surgery and reduces the risk of ureteric injury.

Repairing ureteric damage

If a ureter is damaged the presence and condition of the contralateral kidney and ureter should be checked. If the ureter has been crushed or ligated in error and this is recognised during the operation, the ligature can be removed and a stent inserted into the ureter to minimise the risk of stenosis. If the ureter is divided repair will be necessary. Tying off the divided ureter is rarely justifiable.

The following principles should be employed in repairing any ureteric injury:

- Adequate vascular supply
- Adequate surgical exposure
- Gentle tissue handling
- Tension free suturing
- Placing the minimum number of sutures
- Stenting to allow the repair to heal

Repair of the ureter is technically demanding and may lead to long-term complications. It is most appropriately undertaken by an urologist. At the pelvic brim or above an end-to-end anastomosis can be performed. In cases of crush or similar injury the injured ends of the damaged ureter are trimmed, if necessary, to reach viable bleeding tissues. This is generally not necessary for transection injuries. Each end is partially spatulated by making an incision of

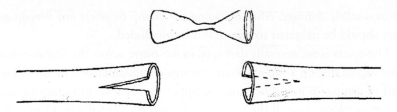

Fig. 1. The injured segment is excised ensuring that the ends to be approximated are well vascularised. Both ends are then spatulated to aid in preventing stenosis at the anastomosis site.

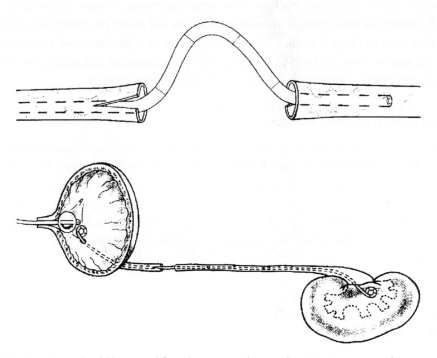

Fig. 2. Repair should be stented for at least two to three weeks. An intravenous pyelogram or pull-back ureterogram is recommended prior to stent removal to ensure patency of ureter.

approximately 3–5 mm longitudinally in each ureter. These incisions should be 180° apart (Fig. 1). The ureter can be stented either by passing a stent through the injured ends towards both the bladder and the renal pelvis or by performing a cystoscopy and passing a stent up through the ureter to the renal pelvis (Fig. 2). Interrupted 4-0 absorbable sutures (polyglycolic acid) are

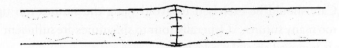

Fig. 3.   Ureteral repair is accomplished with four to six interrupted absorbable sutures.

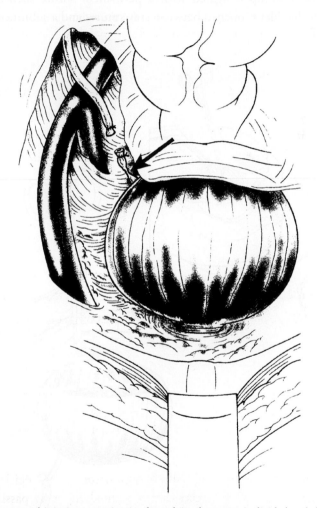

Fig. 4.   For ureteral injuries occurring in the pelvis, the ureter is divided and the distal end permanently ligated with non-absorbable suture.

suitable. Care should be exercised to avoid tying the sutures too tightly or inserting too many sutures.[3] Generally four to six sutures are sufficient (Fig. 3). The stent is removed several weeks later.

For ureteric injuries occurring at the level of the ureteric tunnel or lower the most effective method of repair is to reimplant the ureter into the bladder. The distal stump is ligated with a permanent suture such as 2-0 silk (Fig. 4). The bladder is opened between stay sutures and a submucosal tunnel

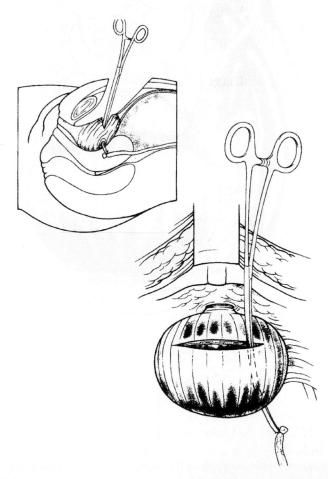

Fig. 5.   Working through an incision in the dome of the bladder, the ureter is brought through the bladder wall at a point that will ensure the most tension-free anastomosis.

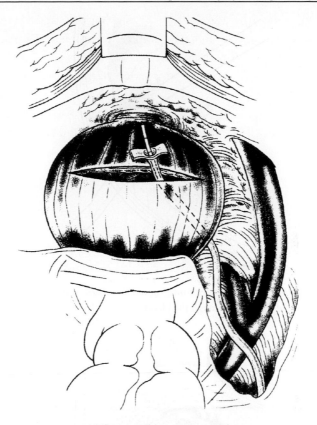

Fig. 6. The ureter is spatulated and stented.

is fashioned along the lateral posterior wall (Fig. 5). The distal end of the ureter is brought through the tunnel and after spatulating the end it is sutured to the bladder mucosa (Fig. 6). The anastomosis is performed using 4-0 absorbable interrupted sutures which include the full thickness of the ureter but only the mucosa and submucosa of the bladder (Fig. 7). A couple of sutures into the serosal surface anchor the ureter to the outer layer of the bladder. Retrograde transurethral filling of the bladder should be performed to ensure a watertight seal. If an indwelling stent is utilised, it may be removed in two weeks if an intravenous pyelogram demonstrates ureteric patency and no leaks.

When damage has occurred higher on the pelvic sidewall, the bladder can be elevated to the cut end of the ureter to allow reimplantation without tension

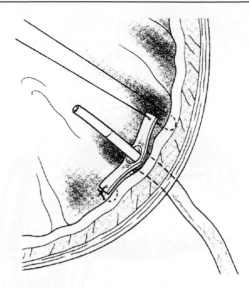

Fig. 7. The anastomosis is created with interrupted absorbable sutures, full thickness through the ureter and partial thickness through the bladder.

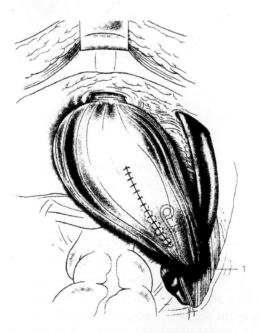

Fig. 8. The cystotomy incision is closed. By making the incision transversely and closing longitudinally, the site of anastomosis can be brought closer to the ureter, thus relieving tension. A psoas hitch can then be performed (1; see text).

using either a psoas hitch or a Boari flap. In the psoas hitch, the appropriate part of the bladder is elevated towards the end of the ureter. To facilitate this, the cystotomy is performed transversely and is closed longitudinally in a perpendicular direction to elongate the bladder and relieve the tension (Fig. 8). Once the ureter is implanted, the bladder is fixed to the psoas muscle to further relieve any tension. This technique allows a ureteric injury at any level in the pelvis up to the pelvic brim to be safely reimplanted. In the Boari flap, a flap of the bladder is elevated, the ureter is reimplanted into this and the flap is closed as a tube (Figs. 9–11). It allows good bladder elevation at the expense of a reduced bladder capacity.

Alternatively a uretero-ureteric anastomosis to the opposite ureter can be performed with the disadvantage that both ureters may be compromised. It may be the only method if bladder access is difficult.

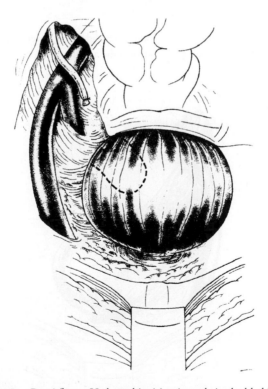

Fig. 9.   Boari flap: a U-shaped incision is made in the bladder.

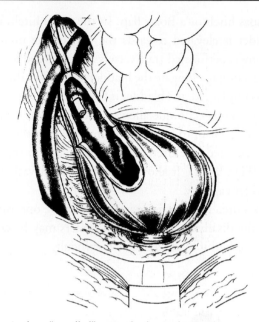

Fig. 10. The flap is then "unrolled" towards the undamaged ureter and the anastomosis performed. Care must be exercised not to perform the anastomosis too close to the cut edge of the bladder.

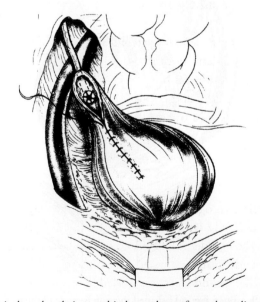

Fig. 11. The flap is then closed. A psoas hitch may be performed to relieve any excess tension.

Bladder Damage

The bladder is an extraperitoneal organ and can rise out of the pelvis up to the level of the umbilicus when full. It is at risk of injury when performing lower abdominal incisions and trocar insertion during laparoscopic surgery, especially after a previous intra-abdominal surgery. Therefore it must always be emptied prior to any pelvic surgery, usually by continuous drainage with an indwelling Foley's catheter to reduce the hazard during the abdominal incision. The peritoneum should be opened superiorly away from the bladder especially during a transverse incision. Blunt dissection with fingers will not necessarily protect the bladder from damage. The technique of tearing the parietal peritoneum open by stretching the wound can lead to damage to the top of the bladder particularly after previous surgery.

An essential part of any hysterectomy is the separation of the bladder from the cervix and upper vagina. After the uterovesical fold of peritoneum is opened, the plane of separation is created by pushing inferiorly with a swab applied firmly to the anterior surface of the cervix above the level of the bladder. This can sometimes lead to very troublesome bleeding points on the back of the bladder which may be difficult to find. The bladder can occasionally be damaged, i.e. a hole made, by this manoeuvre particularly after previous surgery. Alternatively one can use a combination of sharp and blunt dissections.

When performing a vaginal hysterectomy, dissection in the same plane is paramount. If the plane does not develop easily, it is important to use sharp dissection as bluntly pushing on the bladder may tear a hole. A finger over the fundus of the uterus once the pouch of Douglas is opened can define the uterovesical fold of peritoneum and clarify the correct plane for dissection.

Bladder repair

Bladder perforation recognised intraoperatively has an excellent prognosis when managed correctly with a low risk of long-term problems.[4] Should a hole be made in the bladder it is repaired in two layers using 2/0 vicryl interrupted through and through stitches, with the help of stay stitches at either end of the hole. The second layer of absorbable sutures should incorporate the serosa and muscle layers but not the mucosa. The repair should be undertaken without tension to the stitches to achieve an excellent result. Non-absorbable sutures should not be used due to the risk of subsequent stone formation. After repair the bladder is drained with an indwelling catheter for 7–10 days. Alternatively, a suprapubic catheter may be used, it is associated with less urethral irritation and discomfort for the patient.

Bowel Damage

Inadvertent bowel injury occurs in around 0.3% of vaginal and abdominal hysterectomies, and is uncommon in the absence of adhesions or malignant disease.[5] Bowel damage is most likely to occur when dissecting dense intra-abdominal adhesions or opening the peritoneal cavity when intraperitoneal adhesions are present. In addition the rectum lies close to the uterosacral ligaments and posterior wall of the vagina, and may be at risk during extensive pelvic dissection for cervical or vaginal carcinoma.

When performing a laparotomy through a previous scar (especially a midline abdominal scar), the peritoneal cavity should be opened away from the previous closure or otherwise approached with meticulous dissection and attention. Occasionally, when dense intraperitoneal adhesions are encountered, the bowel is so matted together that resection of a small portion may be necessary. Particular care must be exercised in patients who have had radiotherapy, as the bowel is more friable and often densely adherent.

When dividing the uterosacral ligaments close to the pelvic sidewall during a radical hysterectomy, the rectum is at risk of being included in the clamps. When entering the rectovaginal space, it must be adequately opened with complete dissection of the rectum to avoid any direct damage.

Bowel repair

The repair of damaged bowel may involve either the primary closure of a small hole or the excision of a portion of unhealthy bowel and reanastomosis. The small bowel can be anastomosed end-to-end with a single or double layer of sutures. If the bowel lumens are of disparate sizes, an antimesenteric incision parallel to the length of the bowel can be made in the smaller lumen (Cheatle slit) to equalise the lumen sizes (Fig. 12). If two layers are used,

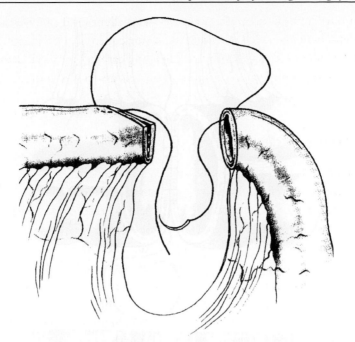

Fig. 12.   End-to-end anastomosis.

the inner layer is a continuous inverted layer of absorbable suture and the outer layer is a series of interrupted inverting silk seromuscular sutures. In a single layer closure, either a continuous inverted or an interrupted inverted single layer technique may be used. Classically, a similar two-layered technique is utilised for colonic anastomoses.[6] A one-layer inverting colonic closure has also been described with satisfactory results[7] (Fig. 13). Many surgeons may also use the endogastrointestinal or thoracoabdominal stapler to achieve bowel anastomosis. Consideration should be given to a defunctioning colostomy proximal to any anastomosis of the large bowel, particularly if the blood supply to the bowel wall is compromised in any way. Adverse factors that benefit from a colostomy are previous radiotherapy, bowel obstruction and gross infection of the operative field, or medical factors such as diabetes, steroid therapy, malignancy and advanced age. The small bowel usually heals without the need for defunctioning. To ensure adequate safety of the repair and medicolegal avoidance, a colorectal surgeon should be involved.

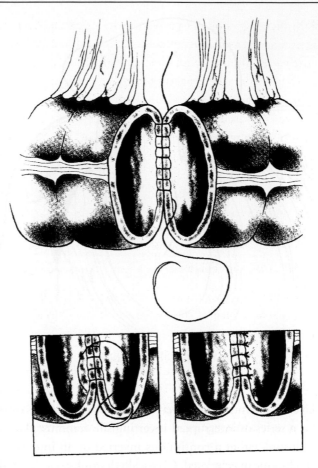

Fig. 13. Single-layer anastomosis, with continuous sutures (inset left) and interrupted sutures (inset right).

Vascular Damage and Primary Haemorrhage

Damage to large vessels is uncommon during routine gynaecological surgery but can occur during radical surgery. Damage to the external or common iliac vessels can result in major compromise to the blood supply to the leg and hence serious morbidity. Usually a vascular surgeon should be involved. The internal iliac vessels may be safely ligated if damage occurs, but bleeding from the thin-walled veins in the pelvic sidewall can be very difficult to control. Initially, bleeding should be controlled by direct pressure either digitally or using a swab. Pressure applied proximally and distally without any dissection can control the bleeding enough to make the defect visible. If the patient's life is at risk, ligation is the available option and is usually well tolerated. During any repair, the vessels should be handled with the utmost care as it is easy to worsen the extent of damage especially during the repair of a vein. In these situations, obtaining help in terms of having both experienced assistants to provide exposure and vascular surgical expertise is of the utmost importance. The technique of ligating the internal iliac artery is often less effective than expected in controlling pelvic haemorrhage because most of such bleeding is often venous in origin. This technique is simple for the experienced surgeon, however, the potential for damaging the underlying vein and compounding the problem should never be underestimated.

Uterine Perforation and False Passage

During dilatation of the cervix, a false passage can result by pushing an instrument through the substance of the cervix rather than along the path of the cervical canal. Instruments may also be inadvertently pushed through the fundus of the uterus into the peritoneal cavity causing a perforation. When learning to dilate the cervix, the technique in inserting the instrument should combine gentle pressure with a sensitivity or feel for the tissues. One should avoid using undue force but rather feel for the path of least resistance. A fine probe will create a false passage more easily and therefore less pressure or force should be applied when in use.

When a false passage has been created, and no damage to any other organ is suspected, and the patient is not pregnant, the situation can be managed conservatively. Any further attempts at dilatation should be resisted. In the pregnant patient significant haemorrhage may occur if there is lateral perforation into the broad ligament and damage to the uterine vessels. Therefore, if vaginal bleeding is persistent and/or the patient's general condition deteriorates, an exploratory laparotomy will be necessary.

The consequences of fundal perforation also depend on whether the patient is pregnant and what instrument has caused the perforation. In a non-pregnant uterus, a dilator through the fundus is very unlikely to cause any problems. Most perforations are often not recognised by the surgeon.[8] The patient can be conservatively managed with regular observation with or without intravenous antibiotics over the next 24 hours and is unlikely to need further intervention. In a pregnant patient, perforation is more likely to cause haemorrhage; however, in general, simple perforations can usually be managed conservatively. One must avoid the repeated reintroducing of instruments into the uterus in an attempt to confirm a perforation as this often worsens the problem. If there is a significant risk of damage to the intra-abdominal organs, e.g. perforation with a connected suction catheter, a laparotomy is indicated because a laparoscopy cannot be relied upon to exclude damage to the bowel.

With a past history of a false passage or perforation any repeat cervical dilation or curettage procedure should be performed either using a small fibre-optic hysteroscope to dilate the cervical canal under vision or with ultrasound guidance to minimise the risk of perforation respectively.

Complications at Laparoscopy

- Bowel damage
- Bladder damage
- Damage to blood vessels
- Diathermy damage

The incidence of complications in laparoscopic surgery is closely related to the experience of the surgeon and the training he or she has received. Most gynaecologists have extensive experience in laparoscopic surgery especially with simple diagnostic procedures. The more advanced operative techniques are performed by those with subspecialty training. The incidence of complications is between 0.6 and 1.0 per 1000 for minor and diagnostic procedures, and between 8.9 and 17.9 per 1000 for advanced procedures.[9,10] The courses available for the various surgical skills further emphasise the principles of laparoscopy and the techniques to reduce operative complications. It is essential that individual surgeons are adequately trained in the procedures they undertake. General complications of laparoscopy are damage to the bowel, bladder, blood vessels, and diathermy damage.

Bowel damage

The incidence of bowel damage during laparoscopic surgery is 0.5%.[1] Blind insertion of the Veress needle and the first trocar may lead to the perforation of intra-abdominal and retroperitoneal structures. The transverse colon is the most common segment perforated during the insertion of the Veress needle or trocar. The bowel is rarely damaged unless it is adherent to the anterior abdominal wall or has reduced mobility by tethering. Patients with a past history of a previous intra-abdominal operation, especially those with longitudinal incisions or past intra-abdominal sepsis, are the high risk group. In these cases, the Veress needle and the initial trocar may be inserted away from the site of the previous incision, e.g. the umbilicus in a previous midline incision, to avoid any underlying adherent bowel. Palmer's point located 3 cm below the left costal margin in the mid-clavicular line is said to be an area where intra-abdominal adhesions are extremely unlikely and is an alternative entry site assuming there is no splenomegaly. Another technique involves entering the abdomen using an open minilaparotomy procedure usually in the intra-umbilical region (Hasson technique) which allows the direct insertion of the laparoscope into the abdominal cavity. The incision can then be sealed around the blunt ended trocar. If there is suspected bowel injury, the safest and recommended practice is to perform a laparotomy to allow careful inspection of the whole bowel and open repair of any damage. It is helpful to leave the offending instrument in place until the abdomen is open because sometimes it can be difficult to find the site of bowel perforation.

Bowel injury should always be suspected after a difficult Veress needle or trocar insertion. Faeces is not always obvious which leads to 60% of small bowel injuries being missed.[11] For litigation, avoidance and risk management consideration, it is essential that a colorectal surgeon be involved in any cases of significant intestinal damage. As laparoscopic perforations are commonly missed, it is sensible to admit any day case patients following a difficult needle or trocar insertion or with a postoperative pyrexia for overnight observation. In addition, some surgeons advocate the use of a temperature chart for 10–14 days postoperatively with advice to the patient to return to hospital if her temperature increases to more than 37.5° C, especially when there is the suspicion of an electrosurgical burn which may take many days to present.

Bladder damage

Laparoscopic surgery carries a lower rate of bladder damage (1%) when compared with open surgery (1–2%),[1] except during colposuspension (4%).[12] Bladder emptying by catheterisation or voiding prior to surgery greatly reduces the risk of injury.[8] Whilst performing a laparoscopic procedure the Veress needle may enter the bladder resulting in a direct leakage of urine from the needle. This does not require further treatment or catheterisation provided it is recognised and the patient voids normally postoperatively.

Laparoscopic trocar insertion into the bladder is rare. The damage can be repaired laparoscopically provided the full extent of the hole can be identified. Mild haematuria is expected and usually clears within 12–24 hours; however, if it persists, a diagnostic cystoscopy is recommended. A six weeks' follow-up appointment should be arranged to ensure there is no persistence of bladder symptoms or other complaints.

Damage to blood vessels

If the Veress needle is inserted via the umbilical incision at an angle of 45°, the direction of the needle thrust must not stray off the midline as this may result in damage to the left or right iliac vessels. For vertical insertion of the Veress needle, as advocated by some, it must be remembered that in a thin patient, the aorta may lie less than 2.5 cm below the skin. Insertion of the first trocar should be angled in such a way that it passes below the sacral promontory and into the free space in the midline of the pelvis. While damage to a major blood vessel may be obvious, the bleeding can sometimes be predominantly retroperitoneal and difficult to see laparoscopically. Therefore, if the patient's blood pressure suddenly drops and the pulse rate rises sufficiently to suggest the possibility of a vascular damage, a laparotomy should be performed immediately.

Lower left or right lateral secondary trocar insertions can result in damage to the inferior epigastric vessels, iliac vessels and bowel. The inferior epigastric vessels can be visualised on the inside of the anterior abdominal wall running just lateral to the obliterated umbilical artery. These vessels cannot reliably be identified by trans-illumination and so the port site should be chosen away from, and usually lateral to, the epigastric vessels. At this site, the external iliac artery and vein are almost directly beneath, and therefore the trocars should be inserted with great care, control and under direct vision.[13] A useful technique is to introduce the tip of the secondary port into the sleeve of the primary trocar with the camera retracted about 3–5 cm up the sleeve. Persistent bleeding from any of the anterior abdominal wall vessels will require suturing which is facilitated by using a J-shaped needle.

Diathermy damage

The problems with laparoscopic use of diathermy usually arise either from the heat generated at the site of tissue destruction or from the current finding an alternative path to earth through an adjacent organ. Tissue coagulated by diathermy becomes very hot and may retain its heat for several minutes. This heat will spread to the underlying structures and adjacent organs and may cause damage. Diathermied tissue must be allowed to cool before coming in contact with adjacent structures. A further problem is the rising impedance in desiccated, diathermied tissue. This may result in the current arcing to a nearby organ that offers a low resistance path to earth. In a similar way, the current may arc to nearby organs if it is activated before the electrode is in contact with the tissue to be treated.

Perioperative Factors

Heat loss can play a significant role in perioperative complications and is often underestimated. This is particularly significant during prolonged operations especially where the bowel is exposed. Measures should be taken to maintain the patient's body temperature and appropriate heating devices should be available in the operating and recovery room.

Maintaining the circulating blood volume during the operation is important. The use of perioperative blood transfusions has been found to be associated with an increased risk of postoperative infections.

POSTOPERATIVE COMPLICATIONS

The majority of potential postoperative complications associated with gynaecological surgery are common to other abdominal surgical procedures and represent the complicated response of the body to the stresses imposed by surgery. There are other complications associated with the specific operation itself.

Postoperative complications can be classified as:

Immediate (within first 6 to 12 hours)

- Haemorrhage — primary/reactionary
- Delayed recovery
- Nausea and vomiting
- Restlessness
- Transfusion reactions
- Pain
- Others — hypoxaemia/cardiac dysrhythmias

Intermediate (from 12 hours up to 5 to 7 days)

- Infection — unexplained
atelectasis
urinary tract infection
wound infection

- Haematomas — subcutaneous/pelvic
- Paralytic ileus
- Surgical damage to the urinary tract
- Surgical damage to the bowel
- Deep vein thrombosis
- Pulmonary embolism
- Urinary retention
- Wound dehiscence

Late (beyond 7 days)

- Wound dehiscence
- Bowel obstruction
- Secondary haemorrhage
- Incisional hernia
- Bladder dysfunction — bladder atony/fistula formation
- Psychosexual disorders

IMMEDIATE

Haemorrhage

Postoperative bleeding is not an uncommon complication seen after major gynaecological procedures. Hysterectomy, for example, is associated with a significant risk of postoperative haemorrhage. This is less with abdominal rather than vaginal procedures. This is thought to be due to better visualisation.

In primary haemorrhage, the bleeding is due to a technical deficiency on the part of the surgeon in that he has failed to control the site of the haemorrhage at the time of the operation. When the haemorrhage is arterial, the most likely cause is a slipped ligature, e.g. from the ovarian pedicle or failure to include an artery in the ligature because it has already retracted by its own elasticity. Venous oozing is a different problem. More often the oozing is indefinable and widespread as when an adherent mass has been freed in severe pelvic inflammatory disease, extensive endometriosis or a malignancy. Immediate firm packing with a warm gauze pack for a few minutes is usually effective in stopping the bleeding or identifying the responsible vessel. Reactionary haemorrhage is really a form of delayed primary haemorrhage when as a result of blood pressure returning to normal or local vasodilatation, a vessel like the uterine or ovarian pedicle, which was improperly secured, starts to bleed.[14] This may occur after a hypotensive shock or a hypotensive anaesthetic. It is also seen where adrenalin has been added to the local anaesthetic and injected to render tissue planes more obvious and to minimise blood loss, e.g. when performing a vaginal hysterectomy.

Evidence of continuing bleeding should be sought by looking at dressings, vaginal loss, any drainage bottles and any apparent abdominal distension or increase in abdominal girth. In cases of excessive postoperative bleeding, clinical monitoring will reveal a tachycardia, pallor and poor perfusion with collapsed veins and cold extremities, hypotension and reduced urine output. Measurement of the difference between the core temperature measured rectally and the peripheral temperature is a very sensitive indicator of peripheral perfusion and hence blood volume and cardiac output. The first priority is to replace the blood volume lost. In the immediate management, crystalloids will maintain the cardiac output and renal function as effectively as colloids although twice the volume is needed. If more than 1000 ml of fluid are required, then a synthetic colloid replacement like gelofusine is recommended until blood becomes available.

When massive blood loss occurs a consumptive coagulopathy may develop as all the coagulation factors are utilised. Therefore, it is important to monitor the coagulation status of the patient throughout any resuscitation, and if an abnormality develops expert advice from a haematologist should be sought. FFP contains all the protein constituents of plasma including the coagulation factors. It is used to replace coagulation factors and should not be used for plasma expansion. Cryoprecipitate contains a high concentration of fibrinogen and may be required in a massive blood transfusion.

One of the most difficult decisions a gynaecologist has to make is deciding when to re-explore a patient who is bleeding postoperatively. The decision should be made by the most experienced person available. The patient should be stabilised by transfusion when possible. If intraperitoneal bleeding is apparent within the first 24 hours after surgery, a single bleeding vessel is usually identified at re-exploration, Beyond this period, at re-exploration, more often a generalised ooze is noticed and adequate haemostasis can be difficult to achieve. In this situation an acceptable alternative management is to transfuse and stabilise the patient, correct any coagulation defect and offer angiographic embolisation if available (see below). If the patient is bleeding vaginally after a hysterectomy, an examination vaginally under anaesthesia usually identifies the source as the vaginal branch of the uterine artery which can be easily sutured vaginally.

At re-laparotomy careful examination of all the pedicles must be performed ensuring that all bleeding points are secured as there can be more than one bleeding site causing the problem. Intra-abdominal bleeding frequently occurs from the ovarian vessels, and the ureter must be clearly identified and dissected because of its close proximity before inserting any securing stitches. Often bleeding in the pelvis is difficult to localise and may be venous rather than arterial as mentioned before. In this instance, large warm pressure packs placed in the pelvis for up to 5 minutes will usually resolve the problem or reduce the general ooze so that the main bleeding points can be observed. If satisfactory haemostasis still cannot be achieved, the omentum can be brought into the pelvis and several large pressure packs placed firmly over it. The abdomen is then loosely closed over the packs with the attached tapes brought through the wound. The packs are then removed under general anaesthesia 24–48 hours later.

Embolisation of actively bleeding blood vessels beyond the first 24–48 hours postoperatively by an interventional radiologist is a highly effective alternative to re-exploratory laparotomy, in the management of postoperative pelvic haemorrhage. Percutaneous angiography is performed using the femoral artery, which can identify the source of the bleeding, and then the pertinent arteries are selectively embolised.[15] It is a reliable and fast method to control postoperative haemorrhage, and avoids what is sometimes a difficult re-laparotomy in a very ill patient.

Delayed Recovery

If anaesthetic recovery is delayed beyond 30 minutes a specific cause should be considered. This may be related to the anaesthetic drugs used. There may be increased sensitivity to the drugs in elderly patients, underweight patients or those with hypothyroidism. Diminished drug metabolism resulting in prolonged action can also be a factor in patients with pre-existing hepatic disorders, hypothyroidism and in the presence of hypothermia. Other causes of delayed recovery include metabolic acidosis, hypoglycaemia, cerebral damage and intravenous infusion of large volumes of cold solutions.[16] The anaesthetist will be primarily involved with diagnosing and treating the patient with these problems.

Nausea and Vomiting

Nausea and vomiting remain common and distressing postoperative symptoms. Nausea is more common after intra-abdominal surgery and is aggravated if pain control is inadequate, although opiate analgesia can itself provoke nausea and vomiting. In the immediate postoperative phase before the patient is fully recovered, there is a risk of aspiration (Mendelson's syndrome or aspiration pneumonitis). Careful attention should be paid to the patient's position in the recovery room. A patient's airway is most easily maintained with the patient in the left lateral "recovery" position.[17] Suction should be immediately available and trolleys capable of rapid tilting are essential. Anti-emetics are most useful but should be reserved for cases when the nausea and vomiting persist or when there is a strong history of postoperative nausea and vomiting. Most anti-emetics can be given intravenously, by deep intramuscular injection or rectally in the early stages.

Restlessness

Restlessness is commonly seen in the immediate postoperative phase and may be caused by a number of factors including reactions to the anaesthetic agents used, pain, anxiety and a full bladder. Patients should respond rapidly to the relief of any of the precipitating factors which are easily detected by a skilled recovery nurse.

Transfusion Reactions

Mild reactions include the appearance of a rash, which may be itchy for the conscious patient, associated with a mild febrile reaction. If it is essential to transfuse blood a mild reaction is not a contraindication to continuing. Antihistamines and paracetamol may offer symptom relief. More severe reactions include a marked febrile reaction which may be associated with rigours, convulsions, bronchospasm and oedema. The transfusion should be stopped immediately and prompt treatment with steroids and adrenaline administered.

Pain

Postoperative pain may be associated with restlessness, hypotension or hypertension. There is a wide range of techniques to ensure effective management of postoperative pain. The most successful approach in the majority of cases is a combination of local anaesthetic around the incision site, the use of non-steroidals either by injection or rectally and opiates which may be administered by a patient-controlled device.[18] The use of epidural analgesia postoperatively may also be very helpful.

Others

Hypoxemia is a common finding for up to five days after major abdominal surgery and is more pronounced at night.[19] Postoperative deaths are more likely to occur at night than during the day and this is associated with the increased hypoxaemia.[20] Should this problem arise prompt assessment is essential using pulse oximetry and a 12 lead ECG to rule out a myocardial infarction.

A wide variety of cardiac dysrhythmias may be seen postoperatively. An ECG is essential to determine the pattern. This may point to an underlying problem such as heart block, supraventricular or ventricular tachycardia or atrial fibrillation. In the immediate postoperative period the anaesthetist will be on hand to direct patient management.[21]

INTERMEDIATE

Infection

Unexplained

Postoperative pyrexia is common after gynaecological surgery but the incidence can be reduced from 20 to 10% with the routine use of prophylactic antibiotics.[22] Almost 40% of women with fever in the first 48 hours postoperatively do not have an identifiable cause[23] and the temperature usually settles without active treatment.

Atelectasis

Pyrexia within the first 48–72 hours is usually caused by pulmonary atelectasis developing during general anaesthesia, which is increased by age, obesity, smoking, poor postoperative analgesia and upper abdominal surgery. Patients may be asymptomatic, but crepitations and reduced air entry will be found on examination. The best treatment is chest physiotherapy, incentive spirometry and adequate analgesia. If atelectasis persists antibiotic therapy may be required.

Urinary tract infection

After 72 hours the most likely cause of a fever is a urinary tract infection, especially if the patient has been catheterised. Often patients are asymptomatic so urine must be sent for microscopy and culture in suspected cases. If the patient is unwell antibiotics may be started empirically. The routine use of prophylactics at the time of surgery does not reduce the incidence of urinary tract infection, but may alter the pattern of bacterial isolates.[24] Urinary tract infections and atelectasis are the commonest causes of postoperative pyrexia.

Wound infection

Wound infections typically present around the 3rd to 5th postoperative day and are usually preceded by induration and erythema around the skin incision with an eventual offensive discharge. If there are signs of a significant collection (e.g. infected haematoma) the wound should be opened in the infected area by removing the sutures. Occasionally, under sterile conditions the wound may need to be probed and any loculations of pus broken down. In the event of wound necrosis, thorough debridement to clean the tissue is essential. The defect should be allowed to heal by secondary intention. Antibiotic therapy is administered if there is significant cellulitis, systemic signs of sepsis or evidence of necrotising infection. Culture swabs should be taken before the commencement of antibiotic therapy. Flucloxacillin or erythromycin is appropriate as empirical treatment while antibiotic sensitivities are awaited.

Necrotising fasciitis is a rare, rapidly progressive and often fatal infection of the superficial fascia and subcutaneous tissues.[25] Diabetic patients are especially vulnerable, but any chronic illness may predispose a patient to this condition. It is seen most often on the vulva or perineum. It is often not related to surgery, but can be seen in the region of a recent surgical wound. There is extensive tissue necrosis and a moderate or severe systemic toxic reaction. Very radical excision is essential with antibiotics and supportive therapy.[26]

Haematomas

Large pelvic or subrectus sheath haematomas may cause a low-grade swinging pyrexia. Transvaginal ultrasound will reveal a pelvic fluid collection after hysterectomy in about one-third of cases, and two-thirds of these develop postoperative pyrexia.[27]

Subcutaneous haematomas are usually self-limiting and will discharge through the wound incision often with symptomatic improvement. Pelvic and subrectus sheath haematomas may need drainage if they fail to resolve spontaneously and continue to cause systemic symptoms. Pelvic haematomas can be drained transvaginally under ultrasound guidance. If the haematoma becomes infected intravenous antibiotics are also indicated. The use of low dose heparin in thromboembolic prophylaxis is associated with a 5–15% increase[28] in the incidence of wound haematomas.

Paralytic Ileus

After manipulation of the small bowel during surgery, normal peristaltic activity usually returns within 16 hours. Failure to do so results in a paralytic ileus. The patient will complain of nausea, abdominal discomfort and distension, and the failure to pass flatus. Vomiting will occur as fluid collects in the stomach and upper gut. On examination the abdomen will be distended and bowel sounds will be absent.

Any abdominal sepsis should be treated and hypokalaemia corrected as both may contribute to an ileus. Management involves the administration of intravenous fluids and bowel decompression by inserting a nasogastric tube and regular aspiration of gastric contents. Most patients will respond to these conservative measures but some may require surgical intervention to rule out a pathological cause.

Surgical Damage to the Urinary Tract

Intraoperative injury to the urinary tract and its management have been previously discussed.

Bladder and ureteric injury

The incidence of bladder injury is typically between 1–2%.[16] Unrecognised bladder perforation can result in postoperative pelvic discomfort or even an intestinal ileus due to peritoneal irritation as urine leaks into the abdominal cavity. In the case of a retroperitoneal perforation, urine can track down the fascial planes into the thighs.

Ureteric injury similarly results in urine leaking into the abdominal cavity and usually presents in the first 24 hours with loin discomfort or an intestinal ileus. It is essential that a urologist be involved in the management of any ureteric injury. This is best practice in risk management and litigation avoidance. Ureteric repair has been previously discussed. Any ureteric stents inserted should be left in place for 2–3 weeks to help maintain free drainage and prevent stricture formation. Long-term follow-up is mandatory to exclude stricture and further ureteric obstruction.

Surgical Damage to the Bowel

Any bowel injury that may have been missed intraoperatively will result in a faecal peritonitis and intestinal ileus. This usually presents in the first 24 hours with abdominal pain, fever, tachycardia, signs of an acute abdomen and vomiting, and abdominal distension due to the intestinal ileus. Management involves stabilisation of the clinical condition followed by an emergency exploratory laparotomy to examine the entire bowel for perforations. Preoperatively, high dose intravenous antibiotics are commenced as soon as possible, the fluid electrolyte balance of the patient maintained by appropriate intravenous fluid replacement and a nasogastric tube passed into the stomach to decompress the bowel and drain the gastric contents. Depending on the size of the defect reanastomosis may be primary with or without excision of the damaged segment of the bowel. Consideration should be given to a defunctioning colostomy proximal to the anastomosis, especially when the sigmoid colon and rectum are involved. The techniques of bowel repair have been discussed previously.

Deep Vein Thrombosis

The development of a deep vein thrombosis (DVT) is a common postoperative event with 30% of patients developing a DVT after moderate and major surgery without adequate prophylaxis. In the past venous thromboembolism (VTE) has accounted for around 20% of perioperative hysterectomy deaths.[29] The level of risk is dependent on various factors including abdomino-pelvic surgery. The degree of risk is highest for surgery associated with malignancy, less in abdominal hysterectomy and lowest for vaginal hysterectomy. Patient related factors that increase the risk of thromboembolism include increasing age, obesity, severe varicose veins, immobility or paralysis, pregnancy or puerperium, previous thromboembolic event and the presence of congenital or acquired thrombophilias. Medical problems such as cardiac failure, recent myocardial infarction, inflammatory bowel disease, nephrotic syndrome, paraproteinaemia polycythemia, infection and malignancy, especially pelvic and abdominal, are all associated with an increased risk.[30] The summation of these factors allows each patient to be assigned a low, moderate or high risk level for developing a DVT.[31] Prophylaxis against thromboembolic disease should be offered to all gynaecology patients undergoing surgery. Low risk patients should be encouraged to mobilise early following the operation and adequate hydration ensured. Those at moderate risk should receive specific prophylaxis with either low dose or low molecular weight subcutaneous heparin and/or graduated compression stockings. Those at high risk should use heparin prophylaxis and be fitted with graduated compression stockings.

The symptoms associated with DVT are pain, swelling and erythema of the affected calf. On examination, there may be a low grade pyrexia, the leg may be warmer and larger in circumference, the peripheral veins distal to the occlusion may be dilated and the calf may be tender to palpation over the site of the thrombosis. Doppler ultrasound of the affected limb is the investigation of choice. Venography is occasionally necessary, but is associated with the risk of embolism. D-dimer levels can be utilised as a screening test for VTE as it has a high negative predictive value. Therefore a low D-dimer level suggests the absence of VTE and further objective tests need not be performed, while an increased level of D-dimer suggests that thrombosis may be present and an objective diagnostic test for DVT and/or pulmonary TE should be performed.[32]

Before anticoagulation treatment is commenced blood should be taken for a full thrombophilia screen, a full blood count and a coagulation screen in addition to D dimer levels. Blood should also be sent for urea, electrolytes and liver function tests to exclude renal or hepatic dysfunction which are precautions for anticoagulation therapy.

Once a DVT is confirmed anticoagulation therapy must be commenced to prevent pulmonary embolism and to restore venous patency. Intravenous unfractionated heparin 2800–40,000 units/24 hours should be administered by continuous infusion for at least 48 hours, following a loading dose of 5000 units.[33] Full anticoagulation with the activated partial thromboplastin time (APTT) at 1.5–2.5 times the control should be achieved within 24 hours with the first APTT level measured six hours after the loading dose. Heparin given subcutaneously 15,000–17,500 units 12-hourly is equally effective. Low molecular weight heparins (LMWHs) given subcutaneously once daily is more effective than the standard unfractionated heparin regimens with lower mortality and fewer haemorrhagic complications in the initial treatment of DVT.[34]

LMWHs are as effective as standard unfractionated heparin for the treatment of pulmonary thromboembolism.[35] It can be given as an outpatient procedure without monitoring coagulation. In the initial management of a DVT the leg should be elevated and a graduated elastic compression stocking applied to reduce oedema. Mobilisation should be encouraged. Conversion to oral anti-coagulation therapy with warfarin should commence after 3–5 days of heparin therapy, and the heparin discontinued once oral anticoagulation is within the therapeutic range. The dosage of warfarin should be adjusted to maintain the international normalised ratio (INR) at between 2.0 and 3.0 and continued for the duration of 3 months. Advice from haematologists should be sought throughout.

In women with factors or a highly suggestive picture of venous throm-boembolism, anticoagulation treatment should be employed until an objective diagnosis is made.

Pulmonary Embolism

The true incidence of pulmonary embolism after surgery is unknown. In patients without prophylactic treatment the incidence of recognised pulmonary embolism is about 4% with about 25–50% of these being fatal.[36] If the clot or embolus is small it passes into the periphery of the lung where it produces a small wedge-shaped infarct. The symptoms and signs in this situation may escape diagnosis or be misdiagnosed as postoperative pneumonitis, chest infection, or even coronary thrombosis. Minor pulmonary embolism is associated with a history of pleuritic chest pain, haemoptysis, a pleural rub and fine crepitations at the base of the lungs. It may present with a dry cough and/or pyrexia. The majority of DVTs which precede pulmonary embolism are not recognised clinically and a high index of suspicion needs to be exercised. At least 50% of the pulmonary tree must be involved to cause any haemody-namic disturbance. In this case of a more massive thrombus the clinical picture is very dramatic. The patient may complain of intense central chest pain and acute dyspnoea, or may have collapsed. This can be associated with cyanosis and tachycardia, and the symptoms and signs of a DVT. The chest X-ray may show the absence of vascular markings over the affected lobe as a result of oligaemia, enlarged pulmonary arteries and an abrupt ending of pulmonary arteries. The ECG may show signs of right-sided ventricular strain with an

S-wave in lead 1, a Q-wave in lead 3 and a T-wave inversion in lead 3 (S_1, Q_3, T_3), and may be helpful in distinguishing the condition from coronary thrombosis. The signs of a pulmonary embolism may include right axis deviation and sometimes right bundle branch block. Arterial blood gas analysis may show a reduced oxygen tension in the presence of a normal carbon dioxide tension. A ventilation/perfusion (V/Q) scan should be requested, which will show an area of hypoperfusion in the presence of normal ventilation thereby confirming the diagnosis. In an emergency a perfusion scan alone can be performed with a ventilation scan being performed only if the perfusion scan is abnormal. If the clinical suspicion and possibility of a pulmonary embolus is high, even if the V/Q scan shows "low" probability and a Doppler ultrasound examination of the legs are negative, consider a spiral computerised tomography (CT) scan, magnetic resonance imaging or pulmonary angiography.[37] Pulmonary angiography requires a degree of expertise that is not always available.

Spiral CT is a new procedure for the diagnosis of pulmonary embolism. Its advantages include rapid results (usually within 30 minutes) and a less invasive method of imaging the lungs. However, CT scans may be less effective in diagnosing blood clots in the smaller peripheral arteries of the lungs. However, a 2001 study concluded that spiral CT provided comparable and in some cases greater sensitivity to that of V/Q scanning.[38] Many physicians now use it as their first choice of imaging investigation.

Blood investigations and the commencement of anticoagulation therapy for the treatment of a pulmonary embolus are described above under the management of a DVT. The involvement of a physician in the management of these patients is recommended. Resuscitation of a patient with a massive pulmonary embolus should ensure that venous return to the heart is maintained to help with right ventricular function. Having stabilised the patient, thrombolysis of the clot may be performed although this is contraindicated within 5 days of surgery. Percutaneous catheter thrombus fragmentation is also another option. Pulmonary embolectomy with cardiac bypass may be life-saving, but is associated with a high mortality.

Urinary Retention

Urinary retention is a commonly observed postoperative complication. It is usually caused by bladder atony due to over distension, or the unwillingness to void due to postoperative discomfort.[26] An alteration in the voiding mechanism, possibly by interference with the parasympathetic detrusor muscle innervation, is seen after a hysterectomy, especially when the cervix is removed. This may lead to long-term voiding dysfunction. Urinary retention is more common after a vaginal hysterectomy, especially if it is performed together with an anterior repair and urethral buttressing. A vaginal hysterectomy leads to urinary retention in 8% of patients compared with 4.8% for abdominal hysterectomy[5] and 0.3% of laparoscopic procedures.[39] If removal of the catheter following re-catheterisation for urinary retention does not lead to a resumption of normal voiding, review by a urologist is advised.

Wound Dehiscence

As well as a late complication, wound dehiscence may occur within the first 7 days postoperatively. Further discussion is covered in the next section.

LATE COMPLICATIONS

Wound Dehiscence

This complication may range from a small skin defect to a burst abdomen. A small dehiscence does not require active management and will heal by secondary intention. Larger skin defects can be closed using sutures or skin tapes under local or general anaesthesia once any infection is treated and the skin edges oppose each other without tension. If the wound is not clean or cannot be closed easily it is better to pack it with gauze soaked in honey or a de-sloughing agent and allow it to heal by secondary intention.

Complete wound dehiscence is rare. It is very unusual after a Pfannensteil incision and can largely be prevented in vertical incisions by mass closure.[40] Contributing factors are wound infection, abdominal distension, postoperative coughing, poor surgical technique, use of incorrect suture material, malnourishment and malignancy. Management involves replacement of the bowel and resuturing the wound. The high mortality (15–24%) associated with this condition is largely due to the co-existing medical problems.[26]

Bowel Obstruction

Bowel obstruction is rare following gynaecological surgery and when it occurs it is usually after the fifth postoperative day. Closure of the pelvic peritoneum does not reduce the incidence of wound infection, postoperative adhesions or bowel obstructions (see Table 1[41]).

In the absence of peritonitis, the initial management should be conservative with nasogastric suction and intravenous fluids. This usually resolves the problem within 48–72 hours. Surgery is usually indicated if there is persistent vomiting or pain, or high volumes of nasogastric aspirate and minimal passage of flatus after 2–3 days of conservative management. If signs of peritonitis develop such as increasing abdominal tenderness, fever and/or tachycardia, immediate surgery or emergency laparotomy is required.

Secondary Haemorrhage

This complication is largely unavoidable and can occur after most gynaecological surgery no matter how satisfactory the initial procedure. For example, a patient who has had a vaginal hysterectomy and pelvic floor repair develops an infection of a small haematoma in the region of the vaginal vault. The suppurative process erodes a vessel at the vault and results in heavy bleeding. A dark red infected discharge usually precedes the actual bleeding which is seldom self-limiting. It usually occurs between days 7–10 postoperatively or sometimes later on. Management should involve more reliance on packing the vagina than direct suturing since most ligatures tend to cut through the area involved causing further bleeding.[14] If an obvious bleeding point is identified, any effort to secure and suture the source should always take into account the proximity of the ureter.

Table 1.   The Effect of Peritoneal Closure on Wound Infection, Adhesion Formation and Bowel Obstruction (% Incidences)

	Peritoneum Closed	Peritoneum Not Closed
Wound infection	3.6	2.4
Adhesions	22.2	15.8
Bowel obstruction	1.6	0

Incisional Hernia

Incisional herniation occurs in 7–8% of patients with midline incisions, with a much lower incidence after lower transverse incisions.[40] Many hernias do not present until at least a year after surgery. Primary closure of the defect may be feasible. The use of synthetic grafts or mesh is helpful in the repair of larger hernias. This should be undertaken by a surgeon who is experienced in hernia repair technique.

Following laparoscopic surgery port site herniae can occur if large 10 mm and 12 mm trocars are used, particularly when they are placed laterally. To obviate the herniation of bowel or omentum through these trocar sites the rectus sheath must also be closed in addition to the skin incision.

Bladder Dysfunction

An atonic bladder with a loss of bladder sensation may occur after a radical or Wertheim's hysterectomy. This usually rectifies itself with time, but some women will need to undertake intermittent self-catheterisation for several months. Bladder and ureteric fistulae may occur in 1–2% of women who had Wertheim's hysterectomies.[42] Conservative management is sometimes successful; however, early surgical repair is usually the patient's preference.

Psychosexual Disorders

A young woman who has had radical gynaecological surgery for a malignant condition with subsequent loss of her fertility will often have her prospects of marriage or her current relationship adversely affected. She can exhibit marked anxiety over her perceived loss of femininity and sexual function. In addition the treatment of gynaecological cancer often produces a premature menopause with its inherent problems. The genital region is psychologically quite unique being both exquisitely sensitive and primal in sexual arousal. A malignancy and surgical treatment in this area is especially disturbing, and different in its emotional impact from cancers and their treatment in other parts of the body.

Specific complications to certain procedures

Burch Colposuspension

In a Burch colposuspension, the most effective surgical procedure for genuine stress incontinence, voiding difficulty has been reported in 10.3% of women. Other complications include *de novo* detrusor overactivity in 17% of women, and genitourinary prolapse such as enterocele and rectocele occurring in 13.6% of women.[43]

SUMMARY

Gynaecological surgery is generally associated with a low morbidity and mortality. Preoperatively all patients should be assessed for risk factors associated with postoperative complications so that steps can be taken to prevent or reduce these complications. Postoperative morbidity and mortality can be reduced by effective postoperative analgesia, good surgical technique, emphasis on sterility, prophylactic antibiotics and thromboembolic prophylaxis. Even with the implementation of all of above the measures, many surgical procedures will inevitably have a small complication rate.

REFERENCES

1. Garry R, Phillips R. (1995) How safe is the laparoscopic approach to hysterectomy. *Gynaecol Endosc* **105**: 77–80.
2. Sinnatamby CS (ed). (2001) *Last's Anatomy Regional and Applied*, 10th edn (Churchill Livingstone, Edinburgh), p. 290.
3. Cosin JA, Fowler JM. (2001) Urologic procedures. In: Smith JR, Del Priore G, *et al.* (eds), *An Atlas of Gynaecologic Oncology*, 1st edn (Martin Dunitz, London). pp. 171–176.
4. Hill DJ. (1997) Complications of hysterectomy. *Baillieres Clin Obstet Gynaecol* **11**: 181–197.
5. Dicker RC, Greenspan JR, Strauss LT, *et al.* (1982) Complications of abdominal and vaginal hysterectomy among women of reproductive age in the United States. The Collaborative Review of sterilisation. *Am J Obstet Gynaecol* **144**: 841–848.
6. Segreti EM, Levenback C. (2001) Bowel surgery. In: Smith JR, Del Priore G, *et al.* (eds), *An Atlas of Gynaecologic Oncology*, 1st edn (Martin Dunitz, London), pp. 157–166.

7. Ceraldi CM, Rypins EB, Monahan M, *et al.* (1993) Comparison of continuous single layer polypropylene anastomosis with double layer and stapled anastomoses in elective colon resections. *Am J Surg* **59**: 168–171.

8. McIndoe GAJ. (1997) Intraoperative complications and their management. In: Shaw RW, Soutter WP, Stanton S (eds), *Gynaecology*, 2nd edn (Churchill Livingstone, Edinburgh), pp. 117–124.

9. Ewen S, Sutton CJD. (1995) Complications of laser laparoscopy: Eleven years experience. *Minim Invasive Ther* **4**: 27–29.

10. Harkki-Siren P, Kurki T. (1997) A natiowide analysis of laparoscopic complications. *Obstet Gynecol* **89**: 108–112.

11. Hill DJ. (1994) Complications of the laparoscopic approach. *Baillieres Clin Obstet Gynaecol* **8**: 865–879.

12. Medical Defence Union. (1998) Annual Report 1998 (Medical Defence Union, London).

13. Ewen S. (1999) Avoiding complications of the laparoscopic approach. *Obstet Gynaecol* **1**: 34–36.

14. Howkins J, Hudson CN. (1983) Postoperative treatment and complications. In: Howkins J, Hudson CN (eds), *Shaw's Textbook of Operative Gynaecology*, 5th edn (Churchill Livingstone, Edinburgh), pp. 69–91.

15. Allison D, Wallace S, Machan LS. (1992) Interventional radiology. In: Grainger RG, Allison DJ (eds), *Diagnostic Radiology*, 2nd edn (Churchill Livingstone, Edinburgh), pp. 2329–2390.

16. Read M, James M. (2002) Immediate postoperative complications following gynaecological surgery. *Obstet Gynaecol* **4**(1): 29–34.

17. Allman K. (2000) Monitoring in the recovery position. In: Wilson I, Walters F (eds), *Update in Anaesthesia,* Issue 11 (NDA Webteam, Oxford), **9**: 1–2.

18. Kehlet H. (1994) Postoperative pain — What is the issue? *Br J Anaesth* **72**: 375–378.

19. Rosenberg J. (1995) Late postoperative hypoxaemia — mechanisms and clinical implications. *Dan Med Bull* **42**: 40–46.

20. Rosenberg J, Pedersen MH, Ramsingh T, Kehlet H. (1992) Circadian variation in unexpected postoperative death. *Br J Surg* **79**: 1300–1302.

21. Mangano DT. (1990) Perioperative cardiac morbidity. *Anesthesiology* **72**: 153–184.

22. Mittendorf R, Aronson MP, Berry RE, *et al.* (1993) Avoiding serious infections associated with abdominal hysterectomy: a meta-analysis of antibiotic prophylaxis. *Am J Obstet Gynecol* **169**: 1119–1124.

23. Hemsell DL, Reisch J, Nobles B, Hemsell PG. (1983) Prevention of major infection after elective abdominal hysterectomy: individual determination required. *Am J Obstet Gynecol* **147**: 520–528.

24. Brown EM, Depares J, Robertson AA, *et al.* (1988) Amoxycillin-clavulanic acid (Augmentin) versus metronidazole as prophylaxis in hysterectomy: a prospective randomised clinical trial. *Br J Obstet Gynaecol* **95**: 286–293.

25. Addison WA, Livengood CH, Hill GB, *et al.* (1984) Necrotising fasciitis of vulvar origin in diabetic patients. *Obstet Gynecol* **63**: 473–479.

26. Tidy J. (1997) Postoperative care. In: Shaw RW, Soutter WP, Stanton S (eds), *Gynaecology*, 2nd edn (Churchill Livingstone, Edinburgh), pp. 125–134.

27. Toglia MR, Pearlman MD. (1994) Pelvic fluid collections following hysterectomy and their relation to febrile morbidity. *Obstet Gynecol* **8**(3): 766–770.

28. Macklon NS, Greer IA. (1997) Thromboprophylaxis in obstetrics and gynaecology. In: RCOG (ed), *PACE Reviews* (RCOG Press, London), **95/10**: 59.

29. Department of Health. Report of the National Confidential Enquiry into Perioperative Deaths 1991/1992 (HMSO, London).

30. Stirrat GM. (1997) Gynaecological surgery. In: Stirrat GM (ed), *Aids to Obstetrics and Gynaecology*, 4th edn (Churchill Livingstone, Edinburgh), pp. 302–305.

31. THRIFT Consensus Group. (1992) Risk of and prophylaxis for venous thromboembolism in hospital patients. *BMJ* **305**: 567–574.

32. Greer IA, Thomson AJ. Thromboembolic disease in pregnancy and the puerperium: acute management. RCOG Guideline 2001, No. 28, RCOG guidelines and audit committee.

33. Hirsh J. (1991) Heparin. *N Engl J Med* **324**: 1565–1574.

34. Gould MK, Dembitzer AD, Doyle RL, *et al.* (1999) Low molecular weight heparins compared with unfractionated heparin for treatment of acute deep vein thrombosis — a meta-analysis of randomised controlled trials. *Ann Intern Med* **130**: 800–809.

35. Simmoneau G, Sors H, Charbonnier B, *et al.* (1997) A comparison of low-molecular weight heparin with unfractionated heparin for unfractionated heparin for acute pulmonary embolism. *N Engl J Med* **337**: 663–669.

36. Kakkar VV, Howe CT, Flanc C, Clarke MB. (1969) Natural history of postoperative deep vein thrombosis. *Lancet* **2**: 230–232.

37. Thomson AJ, Greer IA. (2000) Non-haemorrhagic obstetric shock. *Best Pract Res Clin Obste Gynaecol* **14**: 19–41.

38. Cueto SM, *et al.* (2001) Computed tomography scan versus ventilation-perfusion lung scan in the detection of pulmonary embolism. *J Emerg Med* **21**(2): 155–164.

39. Smith ARB. (2000) Postoperative complications following minimal access surgery. *Baillieres Best Pract Res Clin Obstet Gynaecol* **14**: 123–132.
40. Bucknall TE, Cox PJ, Ellis H. (1982) Burst abdomen and incisional hernia: a prospective study of 1129 major laparotomies. *BMJ* **284**: 931–933.
41. Tulandi T, Hum HS, Gelfand MM. (1988) Closure of laparotomy incisions with or without peritoneal suturing and second look laparoscopy. *Am J Obstet Gynecol* **158**: 536.
42. Anderson MC, Coulter CAE, Mason WP, Soutter WP. (1997) Malignant disease of the cervix. In: Shaw RW, Soutter WP, Stanton S (eds), *Gynaecology*, 2nd edn (Churchill Livingstone, Edinburgh), pp. 549–550.
43. Adams EJ, Barrington JW, Brown K, Smith ARB. Surgical treatment of urodynamic incontinence. RCOG Guideline 2003, No **35**, RCOG guidelines and audit committee.

Chapter 20

COMPLICATIONS OF NEUROSURGERY

Wolff M. Kirsch and Lloyd Dayes

A medical complication is defined as "a disease or adventitious circumstance or condition co-existent with, and modifying, a primary disease".[1] Neurosurgical intervention (neurosurgery) can be considered an adventitious circumstance and the delivery of neurosurgery potentially damaging. This chapter is designed with the purpose of advising the reader on how to avoid, recognise and treat neurosurgical complications. The material for the chapter is based on the clinical experience of two academic neurosurgeons who still maintain clinical appointments and teaching roles in a neurosurgical environment. Each surgeon has had clinical experiences that extend over five decades. This combined experience has been distilled with the following aphorism in mind — "good judgment comes from experience, and experience ... well, that comes from poor judgment".[2]

The guiding principle for avoiding neurosurgical complications is a critical and well considered determination of whether surgical intervention is or is not the appropriate remedy for the disorder. The rationale for the decision to operate on a neurological disorder is formed from the history, physical and neurologic examination, laboratory and radiological evidence plus a recall for previous results which at times can be selective. Even Harvey Cushing had concerns regarding the surgeon's ability to recollect his bad results even with respect to a "golf score". His trusted associate, Louise Eisenhardt, kept track of his operative results.[3] The measured decision of when, or who, should operate is a critical step in avoiding complications. The clinical situations focused on are three common disorders for which neurosurgical intervention may or may not be indicated: low back pain and sciatica, head injury, and pituitary tumours. Though an exhaustive discussion of conceivable neurosurgical complications is beyond the scope of this chapter, a tabular formulation of disorders, interventions, and complications is provided.

AVOIDING, RECOGNISING AND TREATING COMPLICATIONS RELATED TO LUMBAR SPINE SURGERY

The major reasons for complications associated with lumbar intervertebral disc surgery can be cogently summarised: operating on the wrong patient, operating at the wrong level, and operating on the wrong side. Critical reviews of the so-called "failed-back" syndrome after lumbar spine surgery prove that the patient selection plays a very important role in the surgical success rate.[4,5] A history of previous spinal surgery also complicates recovery after secondary or tertiary surgery.[6] Evaluation of a patient with low back or radiating lower extremity pain begins with a detailed and careful history. History taking is directed with the recognition that a number of common medical disorders, e.g. diabetic neuropathy, can imitate the sciatic pain associated with a herniated lumbar disc. Apophyseal joint, gynaecological and urological disorders including prostatitis, result in low back and radiating leg pain. The evaluation should include questioning for significant symptoms such as fever, weight loss, and persistent focal back pain despite rest. The initial evaluation must include a consideration of other conceivable causes for the patient's complaints of back and leg pain. These processes include a wide variety of diseases that the authors have noted in individuals with acute low back pain, sciatica, and the inevitable suggestive but not conclusive radiographic findings for herniated lumbar disc. Osteosarcoma of the iliac crest, distended seminal vesicles, Paget's disease, ankylosing spondylitis, Richter's syndrome, the enteropathic arthritis of ulcerative colitis and Crohn's disease, rheumatoid arthritis, granulomatous disease and neoplasms have presented with low back pain and sciatic pain. Neoplasms, both benign and malignant, including plasmacytomas, osteosarcomas, multiple myeloma and chondrosarcoma, can masquerade as herniated lumbar discs. Retroperitoneal and pelvic disorders, e.g. endometriosis, result in menses-associated leg pain with extension to the lumbosacral plexus. Retroperitoneal inflammatory disease can present with low back pain. Identification of these disorders is accomplished only by detailed history taking — recognising the non-focal nature of the back pain as well as signs of gut dysfunction and peritoneal irritation. Considering causes for low back pain and sciatica other than the common herniated lumbar disc avoids the complication of unindicated surgery, the risks of a lumbar disc exploration, and the identification at times of other treatable disorders.

Usually a clear and somewhat stereotyped history for the herniation of a low lumbar disc at the L4–5, L5–S1 interspace can be obtained from the patient. Backache, either acute or gradual with radiation over the anterolateral aspect of the thigh as referred pain from the stretched or torn annulus fibrosis, is a frequent complaint. There may or may not be a history of trauma or injury. Symptomatology is a function of lumbar spinal canal dimensions and the position of the disc herniation. A narrow lumbar spinal canal and large midline herniated disc result in complaints of back pain and vague leg pain that alternate in intensity from side to side. A large free fragment of the disc can result in a cauda equina syndrome with paraplegia and bowel-bladder incontinence. Recognition of the syndrome is essential since urgent neurosurgical intervention is indicated for this disorder.

A patient with acute sciatica can trace a dermatonal distribution of pain according to the nerve root affected. An L4–5 disc protrusion most usually impinges the L5 nerve root. Pain radiates from the posterior hip to the posterolateral thigh and calf with a sensory disturbance involving the medial toes (great and first two toes). The great toe extensor is weak with the patient standing. An L5–S1 disc herniation catches the S1 nerve root most frequently and pain radiates along the hip, posterior thigh and calf with extension to the lateral toes. The Achilles tendon jerk is reduced. Though less frequent in occurrence, an L3–4 disc herniation is potentially more threatening since the spinal canal narrows, the cauda equina is thicker, and the disc protrusion may be large and midline. The L4 radiculopathy associated with a lateral L3–4 disc herniation is associated with groin discomfort and pain along the anterior thigh. The important feature to remember about the history is that a number of other disorders besides a herniated disc can imitate this symptomatology and a differential diagnosis should always be considered. Though the neurological examination is important for localisation at the level of the disc rupture and defining nerve root irritation and injury, neurological sign variability is notorious. At times textbook findings are only found in textbooks. Examination should include circumferential measurements of the thigh and calf with particular attention to atrophy of the calf musculature. Evidence for the latter finding is readily apparent with the patient standing on tiptoe. Motor function testing is readily appreciated by both static and dynamic testing and minimal weakness of dorsi- and plantar flexion enhanced by asking the patient to walk on heel and toes. Assessment of "mechanical" back pain is readily accomplished by having the patient remove his shoes and socks while sitting. Individuals with a clear-cut herniated lumbar disc will have great difficulty with this manoeuvre. Quadriceps function is assessed by having a patient step up and down on a chair. Though foot or toe extensor weakness is most commonly noted with L5 radiculopathy, the disturbance also occurs with an L4 lesion. Plantar flexion weakness and plantar atrophy is associated with S1 radiculopathy. Reduction in the patellar reflex denotes an L3–4 motor disturbance, and reduction in the Achilles reflex an S1 root disturbance. The well recognised variability of signs associated with a lumbar disc protrusion and disc herniations are associated with free fragment disc migration and the involvement of more than one root. The correlation of disturbances noted by history and neurological examination is tied together for a diagnosis and therapeutic recommendation by laboratory and imaging studies. The importance of imaging studies, even plain X-ray films, cannot be overstated in the avoiding of surgical complications. Disorders such as spondylolisthesis, fractures, primary and secondary tumours of bone, infectious disorders, congenital malformations, inflammatory arthritis can be diagnosed from plain X-rays of the spine. Spine radiography allows determination of the number of lumbar vertebra, a critical fact to ascertain to avoid operating at the wrong lumbar interspace. Transitional development is common in the lumbar spine with lumbarisation of the first sacral segment or sacralisation of the fifth lumbar segment. X-rays can demonstrate a spina bifida or other anomalies. Plain spine films of patients who have had previous lumbar spine surgery determine the extent of bone removal, a particularly important landmark in the event of re-exploration.

In the authors' opinions the optimal imaging technique subsequent to plain X-rays for the accurate diagnosis of lumbar spinal disorders is magnetic resonance imaging (MRI). This technology has displaced myelography to enable an accurate diagnosis of herniated discs, as well as the exclusion of other disorders such as tumours or infection. The complete MRI examination includes both T1 and T2 weighted images. Gadolinium enhancement may be used to help differentiate scar from disc protrusion in patients who have had previous surgery. Though the MRI is an extremely sensitive test, at times interpretation can be ambiguous, since images usually overstate the extent of disc protrusion. The test is so sensitive that virtually every MRI on an adult, and particularly the elderly adult, will reveal abnormalities at both the discs and joints. MRI is not helpful in the event of a far laterally placed disc herniation. In the event that the MRI results are ambiguous or non-diagnostic and do not correlate with history and physical examination, the next step in the evaluation is CT myelography. Computerised tomography (CT) myelography can be a valuable diagnostic aid particularly for evaluating lumbar canal stenosis at multiple levels. This study provides information necessary to decide on the spinal segmental level necessitating surgical decompression. With experience comes the appreciation of the pitfalls of the MRI test in terms of either over-stating or the lack of reading of a laterally situated herniated disc. CT (computed tomography) is valuable for diagnosing lateral herniations that can be missed during routine myelography or are not obvious on MRI. No one imaging test is perfect for all situations, and the CT scan has a number of disadvantages. CT focuses on axial scans of the spine and sagittal reconstructions are necessary in order not to miss an intraspinal tumour or a large central disc herniation. CT does not differentiate scar from recurrent herniated disc.

Once all the evidence has been assembled, a decision as to how to manage the patient with low back pain and sciatica is in order. Complications of operative treatment for herniated lumbar disc are significant. These relate to patient positioning, patient preparation, and patient selection. The generally accepted indications for operative interventions are: a large midline disc fragment or protrusion resulting in compression of the cauda equina; nerve root compression with significant motor weakness; sciatica not responsive to weeks of conservative non-operative management; and long-standing recurrent events of back pain and sciatica that seriously preclude walking or normal activity. Some indications qualify as an emergency, e.g. pressure on the cauda equina mandates an urgent need for decompression. Serious complications ensue if intervention is delayed. A patient with severe pain and with a large free fragment may require intervention without evidence of a motor, sensory, or reflex deficit.

Operative complications associated with lumbar spine surgery begin with patient positioning. Air embolism can occur if the patient is "jack-knifed" on the operating table with lumbosacral spine elevated significantly above the level of the heart. Improper positioning and abdominal compression can cause congestion of Batson's epidural venous plexus resulting in significant venous bleeding during surgery. Lack of protection of the ulnar and femoral nerves can result in compression palsies. Legs should be wrapped to prevent venous thrombosis. These perioperative complications can be avoided by the surgeon's presence in the operating room during anaesthetic induction and positioning.

Intraoperative lumbar spine discectomy complications are numerous and severe: trauma to nerve roots and their dural envelope by retraction, cutting and cauterising instruments, injury to adjacent structures in the retroperitoneal space to include the iliac veins and aorta, wound contamination and production of lumbar spine mechanical instability due to excessive bone and joint removal. Direct injury to neural elements is inherent in any operative procedure that has a "blind component". Bone removal is a chancy procedure since the inferior lip of the Kerrison rongeur cannot be visualised as it is inserted. If the nerve root is displaced upward by a protruded disc there is real risk of root injury during bone removal and the opening of the ligamentum flavum. Complications are avoided by optical magnification (loupes or microscope) and rongeuring with "crisp" punches rather than wrenching and tearing. In the opinion of one author (W.M.K.), use of the high-speed power drill for bone removal is hazardous. Power drill dural tears and root avulsions are responsible for a number of significant cauda equina injuries and medical litigation cases. Any surgeon who uses a power drill should have proof of certification of training with the instrument. Reoperation for disc herniation and root compression is particularly hazardous and often complicated by dural tears, CSF extravasation, and root injury. The detection of a dural tear mandates closure or a postoperative pseudo-meningocele or CSF fistula with the risk of meningitis. Closing dura by suturing is risky, cumbersome, and at times impossible. The use of non-penetrating arcuate-legged clip (the VCS clip) manufactured by the LeMaitre surgical instrument organisation has proven very useful for dural closure.[7] VCS clips provide a convenient and easy repair of the dural sleeve without any risk of damage to the underlying nerve root.

Achieving haemostasis can be a major problem in the constricted, poorly illuminated space that comprises the arena for lumbar intervertebral disc surgery. Anatomical confines raise the possibility of thermal injury to nerve roots secondary to the coagulation of epidural vessels, though risk is minimised by the use of fine-tipped bipolar coagulation and irrigation. Free disc fragments may be difficult to identify in the limited exposure; they may erode through dura or float loose from the interspace to cause problems after the procedure. Lumbar intervertebral disc removal can be complicated by injury to the aorta, vena cava, or iliac vessels without the surgeon recognising that the anterior annulus has been violated with the disc rongeur. This dreaded complication must be recognised promptly. If the surgeon irrigates the interspace and fluid does not return through the posterior annular opening the suspicion of an anterior breach and potential vascular injury must be raised. A precipitous drop in systemic blood pressure is the only sign of this serious complication. Once this complication is identified prompt and unequivocal action is warranted. The back wound is covered, the patient turned supine and an exploratory laparotomy initiated. A vascular surgeon should be summoned to assist with the treatment of the vascular injury. Delayed recognition of an injury in the form of arteriovenous fistulas or abdominal intestinal injury has been reported. These major complications can be minimised by obtaining good exposure of the annulus, disc protrusion and root, magnification and particular care using the intervertebral disc rongeur. The interspace should be entered with the rongeur jaws open to minimise the risk of penetrating the annulus. The surgeon should always be sure that the scraping curette is against bone with scraping movement of the curette always toward rather than away from the operator. The surgeon must be alert in the immediate postoperative period to recognise symptoms suggesting an intra-abdominal injury.

Other late complications of lumbar disc surgery are wound infections, postoperative discitis, severe postoperative back pain secondary to soft tissue and paraspinal muscle injury, adhesive arachnoiditis, and intestinal ileus. Late failures of the operative treatment constitute the so-called "failed back syndrome".[4] Sufficient case experience has proven that a very important cause for "failed back" is the inappropriate identification of surgical indications and poor patient selection.[4] Other causes include operations at the wrong disc level or side and not removing free disc fragments because of inadequate exposure. These complications can be reduced by both pre- and intra-operative radiological examinations, identifying transitional vertebra or conjoined nerve roots, and if there is any doubt at surgery cross-checking the explored disc level by intraoperative radiography.

There is no real difference between the partial lumbar "hemilaminectomy" and so-called "microdiscectomy". A successful operation for a herniated intervertebral disc requires appropriate patient selection, precise localisation with preoperative X-rays, and in the event of any surgical doubts, an intraoperative X-ray to secure the correct level. Any uncertainty about exploration of the proper level or unexplained findings demand an intraoperative radiograph. Constant vigilance is necessary even in the presence of an intraoperative radiograph. The surgeon can inadvertently extend the dissection superiorly, and identify a higher level to result in exploration and removal of the wrong disc.

A very important consideration for successful lumbar disc surgery is adequate exposure of the dural sac, diseased disc space, and nerve root. Without this exposure one cannot localise the disc fragment in an unusual site resulting in an incomplete removal or conceivably injury to a nerve root. Opening and resections of the ligamentum flava must be done, with great care, using a cotton pledget inserted through the opening to push away the extradural fat and dura. In the event of an anomalous or conjoined nerve root the relationship of the nerve root to the disc will complicate exposure.

"Failure" of a lumbar disc operation requires the surgeon to review all of the original indications for surgery, question whether the original diagnosis was correct, whether another disease process is responsible, and repetition of the preoperative studies. Patients with the "failed back" syndrome who have failed with previous laminectomy and surgery are a particularly difficult population to treat. The differential diagnosis include recurrent disc herniation, a retained disc fragment, persistent, recurrent or delayed lateral stenosis, intraspinal or foraminal ganglionic cyst arising from an injured facet joint or a persistent and delayed central spinal stenosis with fibrosis and excessive scar tissue.

The determination of the cause of postoperative pain represents difficult differential diagnoses. A very difficult clinical problem is the differentiation between the pain caused by scarring or fibrosis about a nerve root injury and nerve compressive pain secondary to a bony or cartilage mass. Postoperative epidural fibrosis is a very common finding on MRI and is not an indication for surgery. Repeat surgery for a recurrent disc herniation or retained disc fragment, postoperative intraspinal ganglionic cyst, recurrent persistent lateral stenosis, and spinal stenosis is a demanding procedure with greater risk of surgical neural injury and tearing of the dural sac. Re-explorations are technically difficult procedures and the operating microscope is an essential component of instrumentation for the operative procedure to avoid further nerve root injury and to attain maximal visualisation. The use of magnification reduces the incidence of root injuries. These operations are formidable and particularly great care must be taken if there is a pseudo-meningocele which increases the risk of nerve root or cauda equina injury. In a series reported by one of the authors (W.M.K.) a successful outcome can be anticipated in only one-quarter (26%) of the patients undergoing reoperation for "failed lumbar disc surgery".[6] Success occurred only in those patients with large recurrent herniated disc fragments. Third and fourth lumbar spinal explorative procedures carry an even greater risk of failure and a high risk of permanent neural injury. Complications ensuing after a repeat laminectomy are more likely to occur because of the technical difficulties of working on scar tissue. Complications include nerve root and root sleeve damage, pseudo-meningocele, CSF leak, arachnoiditis, and postoperative instability related to additional facet complex damage.

Lumbar spinal instability resulting from excessive bone facet joint removal elicits the possibility of fusion and stabilisation by instrumentation. Lumbar spinal instrumentation procedures, with particular application to pedicle screw fixation of the spine, generate a new set of complication issues.[8] Spinal instrumentation is a technically demanding procedure and should be performed only by experienced and qualified surgeons who are aware of the significant pitfalls. These pitfalls and liabilities are most apt to occur in elderly patients treated with multi-level lumbar decompressions and arthrodesis. Elderly patients are at increased risk for surgical complications because of the magnitude of the procedure, the trauma of a prolonged operation, and the blood loss associated with this procedure. Despite these caveats, the incidence of spinal fusion surgery is rapidly increasing throughout the world. There were 150,000 spinal fusion operations performed in 1993 in the United States and over 300,000 in the year 2001.[8] The rationale for a spinal fusion is the construction of an arthrodesis to prevent movement in otherwise painful joints. The procedure performed alone or in conjunction with diskectomy and laminectomy has a remarkable geographic diversity and distribution in the United States. Much of the increase of spinal stabilisation and spinal fusion has been in older patients in association with laminectomy for spinal stenosis. There have been increasing and widening indications for spinal fusion surgery and the case is to be built for restraint in applying this procedure because of the complications associated with it.[9]

In contrast to the straightforward lumbar partial hemilaminectomy and discectomy, the lumbar spinal instrumentation requires bone decortication, the placement of implants, an extensive dissection, and longer operative time. The incidence of complications associated with this procedure include: instrument failure occuring in 7% of cases, complications related to bone donor sites such as the iliac crest including infection or chronic pain in about 11% of the cases, neural injuries in approximately 3% of cases, pulmonary embolus in 2%, and infections in about 3%. Failure to achieve a solid fusion occurs in about 15% of cases.[10] There are other complications reported with fusion surgery including blindness as a rare result of ischaemic injury with intravascular volume shifts and patient positioning during surgery.

Surgical restraint in the application of this instrumentation has been encouraged because of the high incidence of complications. These risks include the utilisation of pedicle screw fixation in reconstructive surgery of the cervical spine, another technically demanding procedure associated with a high complication rate.[11] In one series of pedicle screws fixation to achieve lumbar and lumbosacral fusion complications of varying severity were noted in 54% of the patients. Deep infections were found in 4.7%. There were no permanent neurological complications related to the instrumentation but one serious neurological sequela was a paraplegia that appeared to be unrelated to screw placement. Screw misplacement occurs in approximately 6.5% of cases and breakage in 12.4% of patients resulting in a loss of correction. Fortunately most of the complications are not severe and infections can be dealt with by treatment with antibiotics.[12,13]

AVOIDING, RECOGNISING AND TREATING COMPLICATIONS RELATED TO CRANIAL TRAUMA

Current management of the head injured patient by the neurosurgeon is compromised because of aggressive pre-hospital and emergency room care now being practiced in most settings. Critically ill trauma patients, most with multiple injuries are intubated, sedated, and pharmacologically paralysed before a neurosurgeon has had a chance for an evaluation. Thus, to avoid complications it becomes essential that the neurosurgeon has a close relationship and open communication with the trauma or emergency physicians to ascertain the patient's initial clinical neurological status. Appropriate and urgent neurosurgical management decisions are based again on a "blinded" and handicapped clinical situation. Most severe head injuries are intubated, paralysed and anaesthetised before the neurosurgeon arrives on the scene. Thus CT scan of the head and clearance of the cervical spine for fracture-dislocation is an imperative that must be urgently acted upon. The head CT takes priority over diagnostic peritoneal lavages or other investigative studies if the patient is otherwise haemodynamically stable and does not have the indicators for an intra-abdominal or thoracic injury. Exceptional reliance is placed on repeated head computed tomography in the face of a coagulopathy.

The spectrum of head injury severity and the extent of associated injuries play an important role in the initial treatment of the head injured patient. A very important determinant for neurosurgical intervention is the patient's initial level of consciousness when first evaluated. In order to standardise communication between care-givers the Glasgow Coma scale was introduced to grade motor, verbal and eye opening responses.[14] A patient who is fully oriented, following commands and moving all extremities with spontaneous eye opening scores a 15. A score of less than 15 indicates a reduced level of consciousness. The head injury severity on the Glasgow Coma scale would rank 13–15 as a mild injury, 9–12 would be a moderate injury, and anywhere from 3–8 is a very severe injury. Complications associated with evaluating cases with these various degrees of severity in terms of interventions and treatment have been identified.

Establishing an effective airway can be associated with significant complications in managing a head injury patient. The vast majority of head injury patients with a Glasgow Coma scale of 8 or less require intubation and assisted ventilation. Since the cervical spine may be potentially unstable, and as a consequence extension of the neck may lead to new neurological deficits, cervical spine radiography is necessary to avoid further complication. A nasotracheal intubation may lead to complications in patients with skull base fractures. The complication rate of tracheostomy in an emergency setting can be as high as one-third of all cases.

In the moderately or severely injured patient with a Glasgow Coma scale of 13 or less, multiple repeated examinations are necessary and should focus on the level of consciousness, the papillary light reflexes, extraocular eye movements, and lower brain stem reflexes, as well as a motor examination. The true level of a deteriorating level of consciousness, pupillary dilatation, and associated hemiparesis is very suggestive of a hemispheric mass lesion with a transtentorial herniation. These signs can also be seen in patients with diffuse brain injuries. A radiological evaluation with computed tomography is always necessary in the acutely head injured patient. This test determines whether neurosurgical intervention may be required. If there is a suspicion of intracranial hypertension, another neurosurgical intervention is intracranial pressure monitoring. Monitoring of intracranial pressure provides a sensitive way to determine if herniation is going to develop. The general rule of thumb has been that patients with a Glasgow Coma scale of 8 or less should have intracranial pressure monitoring, and that it should be considered with scores of 9–13 in the presence of intracranial haematomas or mass effect.

There are neurosurgical complications associated with the placement of a ventriculostomy. These include injury to the brain, associated haemorrhage, as well as the incidence of infection. Ventriculostomy complications occur in 1–2% of cases.[15] Complications can be caused by co-existent conditions (e.g. haemorrhagic diathesis) as well as difficulty in the placement of the ventricular catheter. Intracranial infection subsequent to ventricular catheterisation appears to be dependent on a function of the time that the catheter remains in place. Though one out of every 10 ventricular catheters will become infected the incidence is related to the duration of placement. If the catheter is removed within five days a 6% infection rate can be expected whereas approximately 18% will have an infection if it remains in longer. Other factors which reduce the risk of infection are prophylactic antibiotics and minimal manipulation and irrigation of the catheter system.[16] Other types of ICP monitors include the fibreoptic intracranial pressure monitor and these are placed between dura and bone.

Other complications occurring in the head-injured patient include post-traumatic seizures, delayed haematoma, subdural empyema, meningitis, brain abscess, electrolyte disturbances, and pneumonia. Complications are associated with both intubation and tracheostomy. It does appear however that if early extubation is not possible because of neurological or pulmonary disturbances, the placement of a traceheostomy tube should be considered. The instance of complications with regard to tracheostomies has been well described, but tracheostomy facilitates the pulmonary toilet as well as more rapid weaning from the ventilator.[17] Thromboembolic events also complicate the management of head injuries and a high degree of suspicion for deep vein thrombosis and pulmonary embolus must be maintained; also prophylaxis with severe head injury because of recurrent gastrointestinal bleeding.

Controversy still exists regarding the indications for the evacuation of intracerebral haematomas and haemorrhagic contusions, and whether their removal actually improves the control of elevated intracranial pressure and improves outcome. Studies suggest that despite the removal of haematomas and contusions there is an aggravation of intracranial hypertension. Thus, the recommendation is for an initial conservative course in most cases, resorting only to surgery if medical management of intracranial hypertension fails.[18] Other opinions maintain that the surgical removal of larger intracerebral haematomas (>2 cm diameter) and cerebral contusions provides early control of intracranial pressure and helps prevent a cascade of secondary deleterious events.[19]

There is agreement that a decision to remove an intracerebral haematoma or contusion should be based on several key parameters: the size of the lesion, its depth and exact location from the cortical surface, the presence of associated lesions, and the patient's neurological status and intracranial pressure.[19] Cerebral contusions and haematomas over 2 cm in diameter are generally removed if there is significant mass effect, although a conservative approach is warranted if important cortical areas such as dominant temporal lobe central sulcus are involved.

A major complication of trephination for the removal of subdural haematoma is repeated bleeding into the subdural space or subdural pneumocephalus. This is a well recognised complication. Walter Dandy claimed that one could determine the quality of the housestaff based on their ability to detect these lesions after the drainage of a subdural haematoma.[20] One must be continually on the alert after the evacuation of a subdural haematoma for haemorrhage recurrence.

AVOIDING, RECOGNISING AND TREATING COMPLICATIONS RELATED TO TRANSSPHENOIDAL PITUITARY SURGERY

Over the past several decades transsphenoidal surgery has evolved as the treatment of choice for the resection of pituitary tumours and other lesions that involve the sella turcica. Pituitary surgery has actually extended over the past century with original approaches being transfacial and transnasal. For example, Cushing did 200 of his 300 pituitary procedures transsphenoidally, but abandoned the approach after catastrophic experiences with intrasellar intracarotid artery aneurysms and suprasellar meningiomas. Inadequate visualisation, misleading diagnostic studies, and the risk of meningitis shifted pituitary surgery approaches from transnasal to transfrontal. Advances in instrumentation and the introduction of adjuvant medications such as corticosteroids and antibiotics popularised the transfrontal operation approximately five decades ago. Subsequently, the advent of the operating microscope and the intraoperative radiological image intensification allowed the transsphenoidal technique to gain wide acceptance. The transsphenoidal approach is now the principal procedure used by most surgeons. As with other procedures that have gained wide acceptance such as the partial lumbar hemilaminectomy for herniated disc, there are definite and serious complications associated with the procedure. Though the mortality rate for transsphenoidal surgery is low, between 0 and 1%, there can be significant complications associated with what could be at times a treacherous procedure.

The key to avoiding complications with the procedure is again appropriate patient selection for the procedure. For example, prolactinomas are pituitary tumours that secrete high levels of prolactin into the bloodstream, and yet at times can be difficult to diagnose despite an available blood test. The pituicytes of the adenohypophysis are geared to manufacture and secrete prolactin unless a restraint in the form of prolactin inhibitory factor is delivered via the pituitary stalk from the hypothalamus. Therefore, lesions that involve the pituitary stalk as well as suprasellar non-functional pituitary tumours can interfere with inhibitory factor transport and result in an elevated serum prolactin. A variety of drugs (phenothiazines, antihypertensives, antidepressants) and medical disorders (hypothyroidism, renal failure) can be associated with an elevated serum prolactin. Values of serum prolactin above 100 nanograms/ml are suggestive of a prolactin-secreting tumour. The values for conditions mimicking prolactinoma are usually in 30–50 nanograms/ml range. Correct diagnosis is an important consideration, since the prolactinoma is a pituitary neoplasm that is very sensitive to medical therapy. Medical rather than surgical therapy is the procedure of first choice for treating a prolactinoma, not transsphenoidal surgery. This caveat must be respected to avoid complications. Treatment consists of oral bromocriptine, a derivative of ergotamine. Bromocriptine administration results in a rapid and significant reduction in tumour size and cessation of the symptoms associated with hyperprolactinemia. Galactorrhoea stops, menses resume in the female and fertility is restored. Bromocriptine is a well tolerated drug and though the tumour is never "cured" lifelong maintenance with the drug avoids a major surgical procedure. The only reservation noted with prolonged medical therapy is a significant lower cure rate if the patient elects later to have a transsphenoidal procedure. The reason for the lower cure rate is claimed to be due to the pituitary fibrosis secondary to bromocriptine-treatment.[21]

An excellent and comprehensive review of the complications associated with transsphenoidal pituitary surgery has been compiled by Ciric.[22] This monograph reviews the subject of complications in a national survey done in the United States and includes his own extensive personal experience. Ciric analysed the complications based on the surgeons' experience with the procedure and organised the problems systematically. For example, he has organised the complications associated with transsphenoidal pituitary surgery as related to: improper indications for surgery; intercurrent medical conditions; anaesthesia; variants of anatomy surrounding the approach and pituitary gland; endocrine systems involved; and surgical technique.

Avoiding complications with transsphenoidal pituitary surgery requires both diagnostic and technical acumen. As noted above, a prolatinoma mandates medical not surgical therapy as the initial step in therapy. Other pituitary tumours bear careful observation and a conservative approach unless visual fields are threatened. The transsphenoidal approach is indicated for small pituitary tumours (microadenomas <0.5 cm O.D.) with symmetrical suprasellar extension and pituitary tumours extending into sphenoid sinus and clivus. Staged transsphenoidal removals are recommended for suprasellar extensions greater than 30 mm. Contraindications to transsphenoidal pituitary surgery are: sphenoid sinusitis, anomalies of optic nerve anatomy, dumbbell-shaped suprasellar adenomas with small introitus at the diaphragm sellae, anomalous or diseased carotid arteries constituting an obstruction to anterior sellar approach, and the superior caval syndrome with venous congestion. Extension of the pituitary adenoma into the cavernous sinus is not a contraindication unless the tumour is centred laterally to the carotid artery. Any suspected vascular anomaly in the region of the sphenoid sinus or sella such as an aneurysmally dilated carotid artery is an important contraindication to this approach.

Ciric noted in his survey that anaesthetic complications associated with transsphenoidal surgery are relatively rare. The transsphenoidal procedure is essentially extracranial if the arachnoid membrane is not penetrated or torn. Transsphenoidal surgery is safe in the elderly so long as medical conditions associated with the cardiac, pulmonary or other metabolic disorders are well handled. The large tongue in an acromegalic patient may offer difficulties for the passage of an endotracheal tube, and metabolic disorders associated with Cushing's disease and acromegaly demand attention and correction. The elevated serum potassium of Cushing's disease constitutes a cardiac risk. The cardiomyopathy of acromegaly should be treated with somatostatins to avoid cardiac complications. Acromegalic patients with large tongues should remain intubated until fully awake. Prevention of deep vein thrombosis and pulmonary emboli with standard prophylaxis is a critical part of the anaesthetic care to avoid complications. There are nasal cosmetic complications resulting from the inappropriate resection and removal of the cartilaginous nasal septum. "Saddle nose" can be avoided by preserving cartilaginous septum and reflecting the inferior incised structure as a single mucoperichondrial flap. The post-operation numbness of the anterior maxillary teeth is usually temporary. Care in reflecting the nasal mucosa will avoid the complication of a nasal septum perforation. The submucosal injection of local anaesthetic elevates the nasal mucosa, an essential technical manoeuvre, in order to reflect the mucosa on both sides. Septal perforations result from creating confluent bimucosal tears.

A dreaded complication of transsphenoidal surgery is injury to the internal carotid artery about the carotid canals and cavernous sinus. Documentation of the position of the carotid canals prior to surgery defines important preoperative landmarks. There must be intraoperative radiological confirmation of an absolute midline approach to the sella. Ciric found that the incidence of carotid injury is 0.4% for most experienced surgeons (over 500 cases) to

1.0% for least experienced surgeons (less than 200 cases). The preoperative assessment establishes both the carotid positions and intracarotid space to work with to enter the anterior sellar wall. Serious complications ensue if the carotids are not accounted for. One very experienced transsphenoidal surgeon recounted in a personal communication how he mistook the tortuous right internal carotid artery for the left, attempted to push it to the left and in the process tore the artery. Carotid arteries as an anomaly can be located within the sella and the working space between the two arteries be as little as 4 mm.[23] A T1 weighted carotid MR angiogram can delineate the anatomic relationships of both carotid arteries to the sella. Any evidence of a carotid abnormality by magnetic resonance angiography should be confirmed by digital subtraction angiography. The complication of tearing the carotid artery during a transsphenoidal pituitary operation is treated emergently by packing. The procedure is discontinued and with the packs in place angiography performed. If angiography is negative, packing should be removed in the angiogram suite and angiography repeated. Intraoperative endovascular occlusion of the carotid artery may be necessary to control bleeding. Other options include endovascular occlusion and trapping for false aneurysm and carotid cavernous fistulas. The resection of pituitary tumours that invade the mesial compartments of the cavernous sinus may result in injury to the sixth cranial nerve. The incidence of this complication was found by Ciric to be between 0.4% for the most experienced surgeons and 1.9% for the least experienced.[22]

Pituitary tumours arise outside the arachnoidal membrane and in this respect are comparable to acoustic neurinomas. As pituitary tumours grow into the suprasellar space they gradually stretch the dural ring and displace the arachnoid membrane. Consequently, pituitary tumours can be considered as extra-arachnoidal masses just as an acoustic tumour grows in an extra-arachnoidal plane. This anatomical fact makes preservation of the arachnoidal membrane an important objective in order to reduce and avoid associated complications. Anomalies of the arachnoid membrane may make an arachnoidal breech inevitable if the membrane is low-lying and extends around the anterior sella. The surgeon will have no choice in this circumstance but to enter the subarachnoid space before dealing with the tumour. In the usual case, the arachnoid membrane will start to drop into the sella as the tumour is removed. Care must be exercised to avoid tearing of the membrane — the consequence being a higher risk for cerebrospinal fluid rhinorrhoea. The incidence of CSF rhinorrhoea subsequent to transsphenoidal surgery ranges from 1.5% for the "most experienced surgeons" to 4.2% for the "least experienced" according to Ciric.[22] Literature reports of CSF rhinorrhoea subsequent to transsphenoidal pituitary surgery range from 1 to 4%.[22] Another risk of opening of the arachnoid membrane is meningitis. Though the reported incidence of meningitis is 0.2%, it is potentially deadly. Another risk associated with the arachnoid tear is tension pneumocephalus. This is a very serious and potentially deadly complication. Ciric's method for sealing a tear in the arachnoid membrane employs covering the tear with autologous fascia, fat and autologous fibrin glue. A small cartilaginous graft is deployed to keep material in place. A persistent CSF fistula is treated by spinal drainage and re-exploration or packing if necessary. Other consequences of penetration of the arachnoid membrane are severe: injury to the hypothalamus, optic nerves and chiasm, and related vessels. Hypothalamic injuries after an arachnoid tear are purported to be the principal cause of operative deaths. Visual loss is another complication of penetration to the arachnoid membrane. The incidence of acute perioperative visual loss is 0.4% for the "most experienced" and 2.4% for the "least experienced" surgeons. Mechanisms for visual loss are related to either direct trauma or vascular compromise by optic nerve and chiasm displacement. Injuries to optic nerve chiasm and hypothalamus are more frequent in patients undergoing transsphenoidal surgery for recurrent pituitary tumours. The reason may be the tearing of surgically induced adhesions of the residual tumour to the optic apparatus and hypothalamus. As a consequence, Ciric does not recommend a transsphenoidal approach for patients with recurrent pituitary tumours previously operated on transcranially. Delayed visual loss can occur as a consequence of optic nerve and chiasm prolapse into an empty sella. Chiasmapexy is rarely necessary but has been used to maintain the proper positioning of the optic chiasm. Manipulations of the suprasellar tumour can be complicated by subarachnoid haemorrhage from an aneurysm, bilateral frontal epidural haematomas as well as temporal lobe epilepsy.

The most frequent endocrine complications associated with transsphenoidal surgery are diabetes insipidus and anterior pituitary insufficiency. The incidence of these endocrine disturbance ranges between 1 and 10% although one series reported an incidence as high as 27%.[24] Temporary post-transsphenoidal diabetes insipidus has been reported to occur in 10 to 60% of cases. Permanent diabetes insipidus occurs with an incidence ranging between

0.5 and 15%. A delayed but enhanced secretion of antidiuretic hormone can complicate the postoperative course. This phenomenon usually occurs a week after surgery and is probably related to necrosis of the posterior lobe resulting in a sudden release of the antidiuretic hormone.

These studies of complications make it clear that results are a function of the previous experience of the surgeon. The established mortality rate of 0.9%, and the incidence of complications of a serious nature, e.g. carotid artery injury 1.1%, central nervous system injury 1.3%, loss of vision 1.8%, CSF fistula 4%, meningitis 1.5%, nasal septum perforation 6.7%, indicate the potentially hazardous features of the procedure.

CONCLUSIONS

Complications in neurosurgical practice are always disappointing, and their treatment most challenging. At times they can be anticipated, at other times they are unexpected; they may be easily correctible or they may be devastating to the point of being lethal. With this in mind the surgeon is obliged to think ahead of the possibilities and make every effort to stay clear of anything that would invite the introduction of such events.

This starts with the doctor's very first examination of the patient and taking a detailed history. A thorough detailed examination of the patient is a compulsory requirement and this includes not only the nervous system but all body systems since the latter may profoundly impact the future care of the patient. Often the condition of other body systems will determine if modifications of care are warranted. With this in mind, personal interaction between patient and surgeon is a prerequisite prior to any surgical intervention. Much of this interaction involvas history taking followed by a thorough detailed examination of the patient, although the urgency of neurosurgical intervention, as in some neurosurgical emergencies, will modify the details somewhat. The more complex the neurosurgical issue the more detailed the examination including laboratory investigation.

Neurosurgeons and most physicians for that matter are "poor writers", and details may be overlooked on a chart with sloppy writing. Typewritten materials today supercede handwriting, but often handwritten notes are still adopted for charting. The interaction of the surgeon with the patient and family is a critical relationship. Not only are the patient and his family or other responsible person comforted and reassured by the physician/surgeon explaining about the disease process, its ramifications and possible untoward results or complications of surgery, such interaction also reduces the stress and fear which undoubtedly accompany the very thought of the surgical knife. An informed consent is of paramount importance and requires this type of interaction.

The standard preliminaries include the detailed, complete medical record and laboratory tests. In many instances prophylactic antibiotics will be indicated. The operative site is examined to certify that no untoward findings in the area of operation will be a surprise. The operations most frequently performed carry with them the ongoing organisation of the operative instruments and procedure; the not so common procedures should have, as a part of the preparation, a list of any unusual equipment or personnel needed. Radiological studies and laboratory test results, including the availability of blood for transfusion if necessary, are part of the attempt to reduce the chances of complications. Intraoperative medications including antibiotics, steroids and cardiac medications should receive due attention. Communication with the anaesthesiologist, the surgical assistants and the operating room staff is of paramount importance — particularly in the unusual or complicated cases.

All preoperative evaluations of patients should include cardiac evaluation, particularly those with known cardiac disease. When less than appropriate measures are exercised, to do surgery without such evaluation, one may be obliged to treat any inadvertent cardiac dysrhythmias secondary to medication, abnormal oxygen tension, or administered drugs given by the anaesthesiologist. The position of the patient could easily determine the treatment and outcome; compare the technical difficulties associated with the supine to the face down position with the sitting position and the associated secondary possibilities of embolisation. Without question continuous cardiac monitoring is always a recommended adjunct to the care of the patient undergoing any technical neurosurgical procedure. "Heartbreak" for the healthcare givers comes when there is a cardiac arrest with its attendant "silent panic" and the surgeon, anaesthesiologist, nurses and all present in the operating theatre at the time of occurrence.

Though cataloging of all neurosurgical complications is clearly an impossible task for this chapter, an attempt to tabulate certain problems has been

Table 1. Neurosurgical Pitfalls: Warnings for the Unwary

Disorder	Procedure	Complications	
Meningiomas of the free tentorial edge[26]	Craniotomy in the semi-sitting position	Keratitis, blindness, secondary V nerve injury	
		Sigmoid sinus resection with only one sinus on the tumour side	
		Acute subdural haematoma	2.9%
		An additional unrecognised spinal tumour	2.0%
Occipital falcine meningioma[27]	Craniotomy in the prone position	Bilateral frontal epidural haematomas	3.5%
All neurosurgical procedures at a university teaching hospital between 1977 to 2001[28]	All neurosurgical procedures — cranial, spinal, peripheral nerve	Wound haematomas	
		CSF leaks	
		Wound infections	
Spontaneous subarachnoid haemorrhage[29]	Craniotomy, aneurysm, clipping	Anxiety — significant in 40% of survivors	
Arterio-venous malformation of brain[30]	Craniotomy, resection of arteriovenous malformation	Death	2%
		Permanent neurological deficit	12%
		Delayed postoperative haemorrhage 4.4 to 1% with aggressive perioperative BP control	
Temporal lobe epilepsy[31]	Selective amygdalo-hippocampectomy	Seizure-free 85%, loss in verbal learning, memory	10%
Cerebral arterial aneurysm[32]	Intravascular coil embolisation	Makes clipping and exposure of aneurysm in neck difficult, visualisation of neck obliteration, incomplete	
Penetrating brain wounds (Vietnam War)[33]	Field debridement	Retained foreign bodies	17%
		Positive brain microbial cultures	8%
		Superficial scalp infections	6%
		CSF leaks	3%
		Death	4.5%

Table 1.   (*Continued*)

Disorder	Procedure	Complications
Movement disorders[34]	Deep brain stimulation	Lead dysfunction, fracture, slipping — 5.3%
Instability of the spinal column (thoracic, thoracolumbar spine)[35]	Transthoracic approach to spine with video–endoscopic guidance, instrumentation	Temporary intercostal neuralgia — 12.9% Pulmonary insufficiency — 2.3% Thoracic duct injury } Abdominal wall lesions — 4.7%
Dural defect[36]	Synthetic dural graft (polyester urethane) versus pericranial graft	Deep wound infection Synthetic graft = 15% Pericranial = 6% P = 0.006 CSF leaks Synthetic graft = 13% Pericranial = 1.6% P < 0.05
Adult hydrocephalus; "Normal pressure hydrocephalus"[37]	Ventriculo-peritoneal CSF shunt	30% chance of a significant problem related to the shunt; subdural haematoma, obstruction, infection, overdrainage
Movement disorders, Parkinson's disease, tremor[38]	"Gamma knife" radiosurgery Stereotactic RF pallidotomy and thalamotomy	Transient side effects — 18% Long-term complications — 9.2% (fatigue, sleepiness, memory loss, depression, aphasia, scotoma, facial and leg paresis, delayed stroke)
Apparently "minor head injury"[39]	Observation	Required a major neurosurgical procedure — 3%
Low grade isthmic spondylolisthesis[40]	Stabilisation of spine; posterior lumbar interbody or posterolateral	Exquisite narrowing of the exiting foramen producing nerve root compression, non-fusion
Severe osteoporosis[41]	Reinforcing degenerated bone	Adjunct stabiliser advances fracture of osteoporotic bone
Multiple prior cervical spine surgeries[41]	Multiple cervical corpectomies, titanium cages, anterior plating	Often the anchoring site is sparse and one has to go multiple levels above or below the defective area

made in Table 1. This guideline is for the unwary and will serve to advise the patient, the family and the surgeon of the risks that may be encountered.

REFERENCES

1. Webster's New International Dictionary (1934), 2nd edn Unabridged (G and C Merriam Co., Publisher, Springfield, MA).
2. Quotation of Cousin Woodman, see Famous Quotations Network.www
3. Davey LM. (1994) Louise Eisenhardt, MD: first editor of the Journal of Neurosurgery (1944–1965). *J Neurosurg* **80**(2): 342–346.
4. Sypert GW, Arpin-Sypert EJ. (1996) Evaluation and management of the failed back syndrome. In: Youmans JR (ed), *Neurological Surgery: A Comprehensive Reference Guide to the Diagnosis and Management of Neurosurgical Problems*, 4th edn (WB Saunders, Philadelphia), pp. 2432–2448.
5. White L, Doak G. (1999) Outcomes analysis can provide new directions for the management of patients undergoing lumbar spine surgery. *Can J Anaesth* **46**(1): 3–6.
6. Law JD, Lehman RAW, Kirsch WM. (1978) Reoperation after lumbar intervertebral disc surgery. *J Neurosurg* **48**: 259–263.
7. Marks P, Koskuba D. (2000) Use of a non-penetrating staple device for spinal dural closure. *Br J Neurosurg* **14**(5): 468.
8. Deyo RA, Nachemson A, Mirza SK. (2004) Spinal-fusion surgery — the case for restraint. *N Engl J Med* **350**(7): 722–726.
9. Lipson SJ. (2004) Spinal-fusion surgery — advances and concerns. *N Engl J Med* **350**(7): 643–644.
10. Jutte PC, Castelain RM. (2002) Complications of pedicle screws in lumbar and lumbosacral fusions in 105 consecutive primary operations. *Eur Spine J* **11**(6): 594–598.
11. Abumi K, Shono Y, Ito M, Taneichi H, Kotani Y, Kaneda K. (2002) Complications of pedicle screw fixation in reconstructive surgery of the cervical spine. *Spine* **25**(8): 962–969.
12. Katonis P, Christoforakis J, Kontakis G, *et al.* (2003) Complications and problems related to pedicle screw fixation of the spine. *Clin Orthop* **411**: 86–94.
13. Carreon LY, Puno RM, Dimar JR II, *et al.* (2003) Perioperative complications of posterior lumbar decompression and arthrodesis in older adults. *J Bone Joint Surg Am* **85-A**(11): 2089–2092.
14. Teasdale G, Jennett B. (1974) Assessment of coma and impaired consciousness: a practical scale. *Lancet* **2**: 82–84.

15. Narayan RK, Kishore PR, Becker DP, *et al.* (1982) Intracranial pressure: to monitor or not to monitor? A review of our experience with severe head injury. *J Neurosurg* **56**: 650–659.

16. Winfield JA, Rosenthal P, Kanter RK, Casella G. (1993) Duration of intracranial pressure monitoring does not predict daily risk of infectious complications. *Neurosurgery* **56**: 424–431.

17. Gallagher JT. (1992) Endotracheal intubation. *Crit Care Clin* **8**: 665–676.

18. Miller JD, Butterworth JF, Gudeman SK, *et al.* (1981) Further experience in the management of severe head injury. *J Neurosurg* **54**: 289–299.

19. Bullock R, Golek J, Blake G. (1989) Traumatic intracerebral haematoma — which patients should undergo surgical evacuation? CT scan features and ICP monitoring as a basis for decision making. *Surg Neurol* **32**(3): 181–187.

20. *Selected Writings of Walter E Dandy.* (1957) Compiled by Charles E Troland and Frank J Otanesek (Charles C Thomas Publishing).

21. Landolt AM, Osterwalder V. (1984) Perivascular fibrosis in prolactinomas: is it increased by bromocriptine? *J Clin Endocrinol Metab* **58**(6): 1179–1183.

22. Ciric I, Ragin A, Baumgartner C, Pierce D. (1997) Complications of transsphenoidal surgery: results of a national survey, review of the literature, and personal experience. *Neurosurgery* **40**(2): 225–236.

23. Lee KJ. (1978) The sublabial transseptal transsphenoidal approach to the hypophysis. *Laryngoscope* **88**: 1–65.

24. Riche H, Jaboulay JM, Chiara Y, Peloux A. (1992) Postoperative complications of transsphenoidal surgery. *Minerva Anaestesiol* **58**: 71–72.

25. Barker FG II, Klibanski A, Swearingen B. (2003) Transsphenoidal surgery for pituitary tumours in the United States, 1996–2000: mortality, morbidity, and the effects of hospital and surgeon volume. *J Clin Endocrinol Metab* **88**(10): 4709–4719.

26. Firsching R, Synowitz HJ, Grimm C. (2003) Pitfalls in surgery of meningeomas of the free tentorial edge. *Zentralbl Neurochir* **64**(4): 151–158.

27. Chandra PS, Jaiswal A, Mahapatra AK (2002). Bifrontal epidural haematomas following surgery for occipital falcine meningioma: an unusual complication of surgery in the prone position. *J Clin Neurosci* **9**(5): 82–84.

28. Smith SF, Simpson JM, Sekhon LH. (2004) A quarter of a century of neurosurgery: the value of a relational database to document trends in neurosurgical practice of a tertiary referral hospital. *J Clin Neurosci* **11**(1): 31–36.

29. Morris PG, Wilson JT, Dunn L. (2004) Anxiety and depression after spontaneous subarachnoid hemorrhage. *Neurosurgery* **54**(1): 52–54.

30. Morgan MK, Winder M, Little NS, *et al.* (2003) Delayed haemorrhage following resection of an arteriovenous malformation in the brain. *J Neurosurg* **99**(6): 967–971.
31. Helmstaedter C, Van Roost D, Clusmann H, *et al.* (2004) Collateral brain damage, a potential source of cognitive impairment after selective surgery for control of mesial temporal lobe epilepsy. *J Neurol Neurosurg Psychiatry* **75**(2): 323–326.
32. Veznedaroglu E, Benitez RP, Rosenwasser RH. (2004) Surgically treated aneurysms previously coiled: lessons learned. *Neurosurgery* **54**(2): 303–305.
33. Hagan RE. (1971) Early complications following penetrating wounds of the brain. *J Neurosurg* **34**(2 Pt 1): 132–141.
34. Yianni J, Nandi D, Shad A, *et al.* (2004). Increased risk of lead fracture and migration in dystonia compared with other movement disorders following deep brain stimulation. *J Clin Neurosci* **11**(3): 243–245.
35. Borm W, Hubner F, Haffke T, *et al.* (2004) Approach-related complications of transthoracic spinal reconstruction procedures. *Zentralbl Neurochir* **65**(1): 1–6.
36. Malliti M, Page P, Gury C, *et al.* (2004) Comparison of deep wound infection rates using a synthetic dural substitute (neuro-patch) or pericranium graft for dural closure: clinical review of one year. *Neurosurgery* **54**(3): 599–603.
37. Puca A, Anile C, Maira G, Rossi G. (1991) Cerebrospinal fluid shunting for hydrocephalus in the adult: factors related to shunt revision. *Neurosurgery* **29**(6): 822–826.
38. Okun MS, Stover NP, Subramanian T, *et al.* (2001) Complications of gamma knife surgery for Parkinson is disease. *Arch Neurol* **58**(12): 1995–2002.
39. Dacey RG Jr, Alves WM, Rimel RW, *et al.* (1986) Neurosurgical complications after an apparently minor head injury. Assessment of risk in a series of 610 patients. *J Neurosurg* **65**(2): 203–210.
40. Madan S, Boeree NR. (2002) Outcome of posterior lumbar interbody fusion versus posterolateral fusion for spondylolytic spondylolisthesis. *Spine* **27**(14): 1536–1542.
41. Hee HT, Majd ME, Holt RT, *et al.* (2003) Complications of multilevel cervical corpectomies and reconstruction with titanium cages and anterior plating. *J Spinal Disord Tech* **16**(1): 1–8.

Chapter 21

COMPLICATIONS IN ORTHOPAEDIC SURGERY

Wael Dandachli and Justin P. Cobb

INTRODUCTION

Orthopaedics constitutes a vast surgical field. With an ageing population and the associated increase in the prevalence of degenerative joint disease, more and more orthopaedic procedures are being performed especially in the field of joint replacement. Joint arthroplasties have offered a dramatic improvement in the quality of life of millions of patients.

Risks are inherent in every surgical procedure, and orthopaedic procedures are no exception. However, during the 20th century, there has been a significant reduction in the number of complications owing to improved sterile techniques, prophylactic antibiotic use, early postoperative mobilisation of the patient, prophylactic anticoagulation methods, and enhanced implant designs.

In this chapter, we will describe the most common complications in orthopaedic surgery with focus on their diagnosis and treatment. Although acute blood loss is a commonly encountered problem, it has not been included in this chapter as it is not specific to orthopaedic surgery.

DEEP INFECTION

A. Pathology

Despite elective orthopaedic procedures being considered "clean" as well as the advances in surgical technique and perioperative care, deep infection remains a significant cause of morbidity and failure. Although the reported rate of deep periprosthetic infection after total hip arthroplasty is around 0.3–2%, some studies have reported rates as high as 8.4–9.7%.[1,2]

Various organisms have been implicated in deep periprosthetic sepsis. The most prevalent of these are gram-positive cocci, with *Staphylococcus aureus* accounting for 50–65% of the infections and *Staphylococcus epidermidis* for 25–30%. Other bacteria, fungi and mycobacteria account for 10–15% of deep infections.

Schmalzried *et al.* described four modes by which infections can get established.[3] These are namely, contamination at the time of operation; haematogenous spread; recurrence of sepsis in a previously infected site; and contiguous spread from a local source. Once at the surgical site, micro-organisms take advantage of the presence of any foreign material, i.e. prosthetic implants, making them less accessible to the host's immune system.

There have been several methods of classifying periprosthetic infections. The original classification was that of Coventry, who described three stages by which infection clinically presents: stage I: acute postoperative infections; Stage II: delayed infections occurring six months to two years postoperatively; and Stage III: late haematogenous infections.[4] Recently, this system has been expanded to take into consideration current treatment guidelines. The modified classification consists of four categories: (1) positive intraoperative culture; (2) early postoperative infection; (3) acute haematogenous infection; and (4) late chronic infection (Table 1).

There are several factors that increase the risk of infection after surgery. General factors include a history of diabetes mellitus, rheumatoid arthritis, chronic renal impairment, malnutrition, malignancy, systemic steroid intake, or any other conditions associated with immunosuppression. On the other hand, procedures which are prolonged, those which involve an open skin lesion

Table 1.   Classification of Deep Periprosthetic Infection[5]

Classification Variables	Type 1	Type 2	Type 3	Type 4
Timing	Positive intra-operative culture	Early postoperative infection	Acute haematogenous infection	Late chronic infection
Definition	Two or more positive cultures after surgery	Infection occurs within first month after surgery	Haematogenous seeding of a well-functioning arthroplasty	Chronic infection present for more than 1 month
Treatment	Antibiotics	Attempt at debridement with prosthesis salvage	Attempt at debridement with prosthesis salvage	Prosthesis removal

on the affected extremity, and those done on a site that had been operated on previously are all associated with a higher risk of infection.[5]

B. Diagnosis

The diagnosis of deep infection should start with a detailed history. Pain is the most common presenting symptom. This may be associated with a history of fever or wound discharge. There may be a history of remote or recent infection causing bacteraemia. The presence of any risk factor which may increase the likelihood of infection should be investigated. Unless the operation site is deep seated as in the case of hip arthroplasty, signs of infection may be seen. These include swelling, erythema, and tenderness, with or without a draining sinus.

Laboratory tests are helpful in diagnosing deep infection. The white cell count (WCC) with differential, erythrocyte sedimentation rate (ESR), and serum C-reactive protein (CRP) are most widely used. Studies looking at the reliability of these tests showed a respective sensitivity and specificity of 36–89% and 85–99% for the WCC; 79–82% and 78–85% for the ESR; and 96% and 92% for the CRP. The high sensitivity of serum CRP stems from the fact that it returns to normal more quickly than the ESR following surgery. Consequently, a persistently raised serum CRP is more accurate in identifying deep infection.[6–8]

Plain radiography is another simple and useful investigative tool. Signs of deep infection include radiolucent lines, focal osteolysis, and especially periosteal bone formation. The absence of these findings, however, does not rule out the presence of infection.

Another modality that may prove valuable in the diagnosis is nuclear medicine. This includes Technetium (^{99}Tc) bone scans and Gallium (^{67}Ga)-labelled and Indium (^{111}In)-labelled white cell scans. A significant problem with the ^{99}Tc bone scans is that these scans may be abnormal for as long as one year after surgery, and cannot be used to differentiate septic from aseptic implant loosening. Most studies involving the other two tests have yielded disappointing results in terms of sensitivity and specificity, and hence, most centres have abandoned them.[9,10] Technetium-labelled mono-clonal antibody-labelled granulocyte scans have recently been investigated. Although the results are promising, the technique is still not in routine clinical use.

Finally, magnetic resonance imaging has been studied as a diagnostic tool, but more experience is needed before it is widely used.

C. Treatment

The treatment options available for deep infection take into account the main therapeutic goals, these being eradication of infection, alleviation of pain, and restoration of function. It is important to note that the general principles of treatment are thorough surgical debridement, with or without exchange of the prosthesis, combined with the use of antibiotics. Using antibiotics alone should be reserved only for patients who are too frail or too ill to withstand a further surgical procedure. At the same time, the microorganism should be of low virulence and susceptible to an antibiotic which will be tolerated by the patient. The limited data available in the literature shows successful retention of the prosthesis in only 31% of infected total hip arthroplasties treated with antibiotic suppression alone.[11]

Open surgical debridement remains the mainstay of deep infection eradi-cation. It involves excision of all infected and necrotic tissues, sending of tissue specimens for microbiological and histological examination, and thorough irrigation of the wound. In the case of an endoprosthesis, the options then are either retention or removal of the prosthesis. Attempted salvage of the prosthesis should be done only if certain conditions are met. These are namely, short duration of symptoms, susceptibility of the microorganisms to antibiotics that are tolerable by the patient, and absence of prosthetic loosening.[12–14] A relative contraindication to prosthesis retention is the presence of multiple joint replacements or prosthetic heart valves due to the risk of infection in these other prosthetic devices.[15]

If a decision has been made to remove an infected endoprosthesis, thorough surgical debridement should include removal of all foreign material including cement, metalwork, and suture material. The available options then are either revision surgery with implantation of another prosthesis or amputation. In the case of an infected joint replacement, arthrodesis and excision arthroplasty are other options (Fig. 1). It is worthwhile noting that re-implantation of another prosthesis may be done either as a single-stage (direct exchange) or two-stage procedure. Nowadays, most surgeons opt for the latter, as it allows observation of the patient's response to treatment and assessment for possible recurrence of infection. There have been no studies looking at the length of time that should elapse between stages, but six weeks seem to be the most accepted figure. In the interim period, and especially in the treatment of infected joint replacements, surgeons have been using antibiotic-loaded cement spacers such as Prostalac. These act as a local antibiotic delivery system and help in maintaining limb length and anatomical relationships.

VENOUS THROMBOEMBOLISM

A. Pathology

Venous thromboembolism, a term which encompasses deep vein thrombosis (DVT) and pulmonary embolism (PE), is a common and potentially fatal condition. Patients undergoing major orthopaedic surgery, particularly hip or knee arthroplasty, are considered to be at the greatest risk since the surgical trauma involved markedly activates the coagulation cascade. Indeed, without prophylaxis, DVT, detectable by venography, occurs in as many as 84% of patients undergoing total knee arthroplasty and 57% of those undergoing

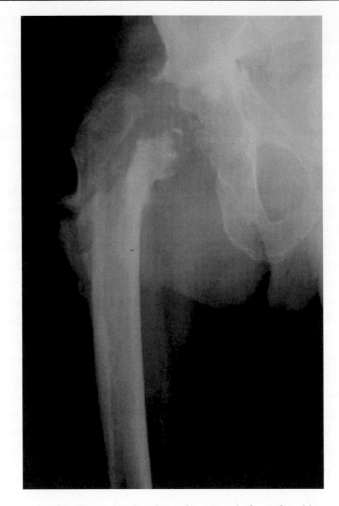

Fig. 1.   Resection (Girdlestone) arthroplasty after removal of an infected hip prosthesis.[5]

total hip arthroplasty.[16] Moreover, proximal DVT, which is more likely to lead to potentially fatal pulmonary embolism than is distal DVT, occurs in up to 70% and 36% of those having total knee and total hip arthroplasty, respectively.[16]

Deep vein thrombosis can be the consequence of one or more of three pathological states which constitute Virchow's triad. These are vascular

Table 2.   Patient-Specific Risk Factors Influencing the Perioperative Risk of Thrombosis[17]

Clinical Risk Factors	Drugs	Inherited Thrombophilia	Acquired Thrombophilia
History of thromboembolism	Oral contraceptives	Activated protein C resistance (FV Leiden mutation)	Antiphospholipid antibody syndrome
Malignancy	Hormone replacement therapy	Prothrombin gene mutation G20210A	Sustained elevated FVIII levels
Age >40 yr		Antithrombin deficiency	
Obesity		Protein C deficiency	
Varicose veins		Protein S deficiency	
Prolonged immobilisation		Hyper-homocysteinaemia	
Dehydration			
Heart failure			
Nephrotic syndrome			
Stroke			
Myeloproliferative syndrome			
Behçet's disease			
Pregnancy, puerperium			

endothelial damage, venous stasis, and hypercoagulability of blood. When any of these processes occurs, a procoagulant state arises.

There are numerous risk factors that increase the likelihood of a patient developing DVT postoperatively. Some of these factors are patient-related, while others are specific to the procedure. Table 2 lists patient-specific factors with varying contribution to the overall risk. Moreover, in order to simplify risk assessment, models have been created to help surgeons make a decision regarding whether prophylaxis is needed or not. One such risk assessment model (RAM) is the one used by the American College of Chest Physicians (Table 3).

Table 3.   Risk Assessment Model (RAM) from the American College of Chest Physicians[18]

Low Risk	Moderate Risk	High Risk	Very High Risk
Uncomplicated minor surgery in patients < 40 yr with no clinical risk factors	Major and minor surgery in patients 40–60 yr with no clinical risk factors	Major surgery in patients >40 yr who have additional risk factors	Major surgery in patients >40 yr plus previous venous thromboembolic or malignant disease or hypercoagulable state
	Major surgery in patients <40 yr with no additional risk factors		Elective major orthopaedic surgery or hip fracture or stroke or spinal cord injury or multiple trauma
	Minor surgery in patients with risk factors		

B. Diagnosis

1. Deep vein thrombosis

The diagnosis of DVT starts with a good history taking. Risk factors predisposing to thromboembolism should be sought. Commonly, the patient presents with pain, erythema, tenderness, and swelling of the affected limb. In a lower limb with DVT, the affected leg is usually swollen with the circumference of the calf larger than that of the unaffected side.

The differential diagnosis of DVT should include ruptured Baker's cyst and infective cellulitis. The former commonly appears in the context of osteoarthritis and rheumatoid arthritis. Infective cellulitis, on the other hand, usually presents with clearly demarcated areas of erythema. Breaks in the skin and coexistent fungal infection are additional clues to cellulitis.

B-mode duplex ultrasonography remains the non-invasive investigation of choice for the diagnosis of suspected DVT. It is highly sensitive in detecting proximal DVT but less so for isolated calf DVT. Moreover, it has been shown to be highly technician-dependent with an accuracy varying from 0% to 90%.[19]

Another modality that may be helpful in diagnosing DVT, especially in pregnant women and suspected recurrent DVT, is impedance plethysmography. Compared with untrasonography, this test is slightly less specific and sensitive and is not as popular, as it needs purpose-built equipment.

Contrast venography remains the definitive investigation for DVT. Although it is an invasive technique, it is still used when a definitive answer is needed. Newer, less invasive imaging techniques are being developed. Tools such as magnetic resonance venography and computerised tomography could possibly detect pelvic vein thromboses, but further testing is needed to establish their role in the diagnosis of DVT.

Finally, certain blood tests are sometimes used to aid in the diagnosis of thromboembolism. One such test, the plasma fibrin D-dimer, showed a sensitivity and specificity of 98% and 39%, respectively, when the concentration was higher than 500 µg/l.[20]

2. Pulmonary embolism

The clinical presentation of patients with pulmonary embolism is usually that of dyspnoea, with or without haemoptysis and pleuritic chest pain. The patient may, however, present with collapse and shock in the absence of other causes. A history of suspected DVT along with risk factors for thromboembolism will make the diagnosis of PE more likely. In many cases the accurate diagnosis of PE remains difficult, with studies showing the confirmation of a clinical suspicion in only 5% to 20% of cases.[21]

Ventilation-perfusion scanning is widely used to confirm the diagnosis of PE (Fig. 2). However, it was shown that although a high-probability scan may indicate PE, only a minority of patients with emboli have high-probability scans.[21] Moreover, fat embolism, now a recognised common problem after hip and knee arthroplasty, may result in false-positive scans, leading to inappropriate treatment.

The gold standard investigative tool for pulmonary embolism remains pulmonary angiography. It is, however, invasive and associated with 0.5% mortality. Contrast-enhanced spiral computerised tomography is also reliable, but diagnosis is limited to emboli in larger vessels only.[22]

C. Prophylaxis

The prevention of postoperative thromboembolism remains a challenge. When considering prophylaxis against DVT, it is important to weigh the benefits of preventing a potentially fatal PE against the risks of potential bleeding

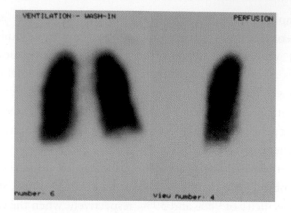

Fig. 2.   Ventilation-perfusion scan showing massive pulmonary thromboembolism, showing a mismatch between (*right*) perfusion and (*left*) ventilation scans.[22]

complications. There are two main types of preventative measures, namely chemoprophylaxis and the use of mechanical aids.

Chemoprophylaxis is done with pharmacological agents such as low-molecular-weight heparin, warfarin, and aspirin, with the former two being more effective in preventing DVT. Although LMW heparin is the most widely used agent in the UK, its administration outside the hospital setting can be difficult. The limitation with warfarin, on the other hand, is the need to have the patient's coagulation monitored regularly. Moreover, warfarin's antithrombotic effect only becomes apparent 3–5 days after the first dose; hence, it has to be used with other agents until its levels are adequate.

Direct thrombin inhibitors, such as hirudin and its recombinant form desirudin, are newer anticoagulants that are licensed for use in patients undergoing orthopaedic surgery. Since they are administered parenterally, they do not offer any practical advantage over LMW heparin. Oral direct thrombin inhibitors, such as ximelagatran and dabigatran, have been developed and are being evaluated.

Although there is consensus among orthopaedic surgeons that some form of chemoprophylaxis should be used in major surgery, there is no such consensus as to which agents are most appropriate, when prophylaxis should start, and for how long it should be continued. In Europe, initiation of prophylaxis has usually been before the operation, whereas in North America, prophylaxis is usually started postoperatively.

Finally, mechanical aids used to prevent DVT include calf and plantar compression devices. They may be useful adjuvants in the prevention of DVT, but they have not been shown to prevent PE.[23]

D. Treatment

The treatment of thromboembolism depends on the site and extent of the thrombus and whether pulmonary embolism has occurred. In general, patients who have a large proximal venous thrombus or pulmonary embolism must be treated. The most widely accepted regimen involves the immediate establishment of a therapeutic level of heparin, followed by three to six months of warfarin treatment. Heparin administration is continued until a therapeutic level of warfarin is achieved. This treatment regimen, however, is associated with a significant risk of bleeding complications. Studies have shown that if therapeutic levels of anticoagulants are achieved in the first week after total hip arthroplasty, there is a 45% chance of significant bleeding.[24] Moreover, achieving therapeutic levels of heparin have been associated with a 10% chance of bleeding and a 1% mortality rate.[25]

The treatment of distal below-knee venous thrombosis is less straightforward. It is not clear whether thrombi below the knee present a significant risk of embolisation. Likewise, it is unclear whether calf thrombi will propagate proximally, and if they do, at what rate. Studies have shown that calf thrombi produce symptomatic emboli in only 0.5% to 1.6% of patients.[26,27]

Lastly, in addition to anticoagulation, the treatment of pulmonary embolism may involve other modalities, including local thrombolysis and embolectomy. They are not commonly performed as they are quite invasive and associated with a significant risk of morbidity and mortality.

JOINT INSTABILITY AND DISLOCATION

A. Introduction

Dislocation is defined as the complete loss of contact between the joint's articular surfaces requiring intervention to relocate the joint. Subluxation, on the other hand, refers to an often transient and incomplete loss of contact that usually reduces spontaneously. As dislocation after total hip arthroplasty represents a good example of this complication, we will discuss its risk factors, diagnosis, and treatment in relation to total hip anthroplasty (THA).

It is well appreciated that dislocation after THA is associated with significant morbidity and even mortality. What are less appreciated are the emotional impact and the financial implications to the patient and society associated with this complication. The incidence of THA dislocation varies greatly in the orthopaedic literature. Traditionally, the risk after primary THA has ranged between 1% and 3%, with a comprehensive review published in 1992 concluding that the long-term dislocation rate averaged 2.25%.[28] It has been suggested that more than half of all dislocations occur within the first three months postoperatively, and that more than three fourths occur within a year.[29]

B. Risk Factors

Several risk factors have been implicated in dislocation after THA. They can be grouped as patient factors and surgical factors. Patient factors include, among others, a history of neuromuscular and cognitive disorders such as cerebral palsy, muscular dystrophy, psychosis, dementia and substance abuse. Such a history was found in 22% of patients who had a single dislocation and 75% of those who had recurrent dislocation.[30] In another study, a comparable increased risk of dislocation (13% versus 3%) was reported in patients with these or similar disorders. Muscle weakness or imbalance and lack of compliance with activity restrictions were considered to be likely explanations.

Age has often been cited as a risk factor for dislocation, with older age groups being at a higher risk.[31,32] The evidence is, however, inconclusive as reports of increased rates in the elderly may be confounded by the increased prevalence of neuromuscular and cognitive problems in that age group. Other patient factors that may increase the rate of dislocation include body habitus (tall, thin patients), prior hip surgery, and a diagnosis of fracture or developmental hip dysplasia.

Among the different surgical factors influencing hip dislocation, the surgical approach is the most controversial. Several studies have shown a higher incidence of dislocation with the posterolateral approach as compared with the anterolateral or transtrochanteric approach.[33–35] In a recent meta-analysis involving 13,203 procedures, the dislocation rate was found to be 3.23% after a posterior approach, whereas it was 2.18% after an anterolateral, 1.27% after a transtrochanteric, and 0.55% after a direct lateral approach.[36]

Regardless of the type of approach, perhaps the most important factor influencing the stability of a prosthetic hip is component orientation. Excessive anteversion or retroversion of the acetabular component, for instance, may lead to anterior or posterior dislocation, respectively. Other surgical factors that may enhance stability include implant variables such as a larger head size, and meticulous capsular and soft tissue repair.

C. Diagnosis

The diagnosis of dislocation after THA is usually straightforward. The patient presents with sudden onset of pain and inability to weight bear on the affected side. A click might also be felt. There may be shortening of the affected limb and a marked reduction in the range of motion. Plain radiography, including an anteroposterior view of the pelvis and a cross-table lateral view of the hip, usually confirms the diagnosis (Fig. 3). Computerised tomography may be a

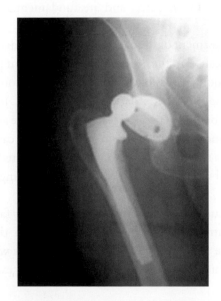

Fig. 3. AP radiograph of a hip showing a dislocated THA.

useful tool to investigate the aetiology of the dislocation and help in planning the management.

D. Prevention and Treatment

Prevention remains the best treatment. Patient education is paramount to the success of a joint replacement, and both the surgeon and the physiotherapist play an important role here.

All efforts at implanting the prosthetic components in the optimum position and orientation should be made. Although implant-specific jigs can be useful and are currently the standard guide to the surgeon, they are inaccurate and depend heavily on the patient's position on the operating table. Recently, computer assistance has been emerging as a helpful tool. This may involve CT-based and CT-free image guidance and navigation, as well as active and semi-active robotics. Outcomes in unicompartmental knee arthroplasty, for instance, have been shown to be significantly better with such accurate systems.[37] Moreover, several reference frames have been introduced that are independent of the patient's position, and hence, elim-inate the errors inherent in alignment jigs. These may involve the pelvis or femur in hip surgery, for instance, and are fundamental in image-guidance systems.[38,39]

After proper assessment of the patient with an acute dislocation, including noting any obvious causes of the dislocation, the treatment priority is to reduce the dislocation as soon as possible. First, closed reduction is attempted after proper muscle relaxation with sedation and analgesia. In some cases, it is necessary to use regional or general anaesthesia to achieve adequate relaxation. Although closed reduction is successful in the majority of cases, open reduction is unavoidable in 3% to 6% of dislocations.[29,30,40] Once reduction is achieved, the patient is treated with either a hip brace or spica casting for approximately six weeks.

In cases of recurrent dislocation, the aetiological factors must be re-evaluated. The treatment options available depend on the aetiology. They include conservative measures, revision surgery, with or without exchanging parts or all of the implant, and, in some failed revisions, excision arthroplasty (Girdlestone).[41]

VASCULAR COMPLICATIONS

A. Introduction

Although arterial injury is an uncommon complication of limb surgery, the sequelae can be disastrous. They include problems with wound healing, infection with or without overwhelming sepsis, and amputation. In a study involving 68 patients who suffered vascular complications after a total hip arthroplasty, the incidence of limb loss was 15%, and the overall mortality rate was 7%.[42] The exact incidence of arterial complications after orthopaedic procedures is difficult to establish. The figures reported in the literature for total knee arthroplasty vary from 0.03% to 0.3%.[43–45]

A history of arterial insufficiency is a very important predisposing factor to arterial complications. This may manifest as intermittent claudication, rest pain, and/or previous arterial ulcers. Absent or asymmetrical pedal pulses are other manifestations that need to be investigated prior to surgery. There may also be evidence of calcification of an artery on a plain radiograph.

Tourniquet use is another risk factor associated with indirect arterial injury. It has been suggested that mechanical pressure from the tourniquet can traumatise atheromatous vessels causing fracture of the plaque, and that lack of blood flow as a result of the tourniquet may cause thrombosis in atherosclerotic vessels.[46] It is therefore prudent to avoid using a tourniquet in patients with severe atherosclerotic disease or prior to bypass surgery.

There are several mechanisms of direct arterial injury. The most frequently encountered mechanism is acute arterial thromboembolism associated with atherosclerotic disease and leading to distal ischaemia. Due to the decreased elasticity of atheromatous vessels manipulation, causing distortion or traction on the vessel, intimal tears or fracture of the plaque can occur, leading to thrombosis, with or without distal embolisation of the thrombus or part of the plaque. Direct laceration of a vessel is another mechanism of arterial injury. It goes without saying that a good understanding of the normal anatomical relationships can limit the extent of these injuries. Other injury mechanisms include formation of arteriovenous fistulae and pseudoaneurysms.

Examples of common arterial injuries encountered in lower limb surgery include the external iliac, the common femoral, the superficial femoral, and the popliteal arteries.

B. Diagnosis

Arterial complications after orthopaedic procedures usually present in the immediate postoperative period. The vascularity of the limb involved should be assessed at the end of the procedure. Pallor, coldness, or absence of pulses that were present preoperatively should alert the surgeon. Once the patient is awake, the symptoms and signs also include pain, parasthesiae, and loss of function. It is worthwhile noting that the neurological assessment of the affected limb may be difficult due to the residual effects of a spinal or epidural anaesthetic. Ankle brachial index measurement may be helpful in establishing the diagnosis. Finally, arteriography should be performed to confirm the diagnosis and aid in planning the treatment.

C. Treatment

Once the diagnosis of an arterial injury is suspected, during or after an orthopaedic procedure, a vascular surgeon should be consulted and an emergency arteriogram should be performed (Fig. 4). Revascularisation is the goal of the treatment, and this can be done by either thrombectomy or bypass surgery. If a distal bypass is required, contralateral saphenous vein grafts are preferred. The prognosis is poor if the diagnosis or treatment is delayed.[48]

NERVE INJURIES

A. Introduction

Perioperative nerve injuries are not rare complications of orthopaedic procedures. The physiological demands and the proximity of many nerves to certain joints predispose these structures to injury during procedures on the joints. Moreover, nerves with a partly superficial course, such as the ulnar nerve near the elbow and the common peroneal nerve near the fibular neck, may be at risk due to the positioning of the patient during surgery.

The reported incidence of nerve injury associated with orthopaedic procedures is quite variable and depends on the procedure and the nerve involved. nerve injuries are also under-recognised and under-reported. The overall incidence of lower extremity nerve injuries after total hip and total knee arthroplasties is about 1% to 2%.[49,50] The nerves most commonly affected in total

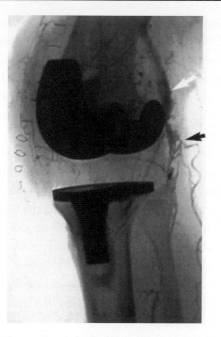

Fig. 4.   An arteriogram in a patient who had a total knee arthroplasty showing a popliteal artery aneurysm (*white arrow*) and occlusion of the popliteal artery (*black arrow*) distal to the aneurysm.[47]

hip arthroplasty are the sciatic nerve (incidence of 0.6% to 3.7%), the femoral nerve (0.04% to 0.4%), and less commonly, the superior gluteal and the obturator nerves.[51,52] The incidence is higher in revision procedures (3% to 8%) and in reconstructions for developmental dysplasia of the hip (5.8%).[52]

As for total knee arthroplasty (TKA), most reports relating to nerve injuries focus on the common peroneal branch of the sciatic nerve. Because of its superficial position at the fibular neck, the common peroneal nerve is vulnerable to injury, with an incidence ranging from 0.3% to 2%.[53] Moreover, it was found that 94% of sciatic nerve injuries involve the peroneal branch, as opposed to only 2% involving the tibial branch.[52] Risk factors for injury include a preoperative flexion contracture, valgus deformity, and prior knee surgery.

The variation in the reported incidence of nerve injuries also applies to shoulder surgery. With procedures for rotator cuff tears and instability, the incidence ranges from 1.1% to 2.6%.[54] On the other hand, studies looking at nerve injuries during total shoulder arthroplasty and hemiarthroplasty found an incidence of 0.9% and 2.8%, respectively.[55] The nerves most commonly affected are the musculocutaneous, axillary, radial, ulnar, and median nerves.

Three types of nerve injuries have been described by Seddon (Fig. 5). Neuropraxia refers to a conduction block in a structurally intact nerve caused by minor trauma. It is usually self-limiting and associated with a complete recovery. Axonotmesis, on the other hand, is a relatively more severe injury and is associated with disruption of the axons. The investing connective tissue remains intact and acts as a guide for axonal regeneration at an approximate rate of 1 mm per day. Finally, a complete disruption of a nerve is called neurotmesis. This is the most severe of injuries and hence carries the worst prognosis. It may lead to unsuccessful attempts at regeneration with associated painful neuromas.

There are several mechanisms by which nerves can be damaged during surgery. These include direct trauma from a scalpel or reamers; constriction by suture or wire; heat from polymerising cement or diathermy; compression from dislocation, a tight dressing, a tourniquet, or a haematoma; and traction from retractors or lengthening.

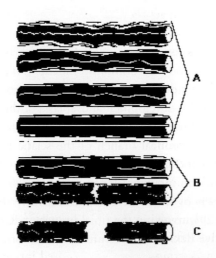

Fig. 5. Spectrum of injury to a nerve as it is stretched. (Only one axon in its connective tissue layers is shown.) A = Neuropraxia, with all the anatomic structures intact. B = Axonotmesis, with disruption of the axons but intact connective tissues. C = Neurotmesis, with complete disruption of all layers.[49]

B. Diagnosis

The diagnosis of neuropathy related to a surgical procedure is often delayed. This is particularly true when epidural anaesthesia has been used. In most cases, the diagnosis is not suspected until the second postoperative day.

The symptoms of neuropathy are usually straightforward. The patient may complain of parasthesiae or numbness, weakness, and pain. Examination will reveal weakness in the muscle group supplied by the injured nerve. In the lower limb, gait may be affected. For instance, injury to the superior gluteal nerve leads to a Trendelenberg gait due to weakness of the hip abductors. It is important to note that neuropathy, in association with diabetes mellitus, for example, may be present preoperatively. Hence, it is essential that a thorough neurological assessment is done prior to surgery.

Electrodiagnostic tests may be helpful in establishing the diagnosis. These include evoked potentials and electromyography. The former tool refers to voltage changes in sensory nerve fibres after stimulation of peripheral nerves. The electrical signal is usually affected by damage or irritation of the nerves. This is manifested by a decrease in the amplitude or an increase in the latency of the evoked potential. Electromyography (EMG) studies, on the other hand, are useful in assessing the integrity of motor nerve fibres. Stimulation of a peripheral nerve leads to an action potential which in turn produces a muscle contraction measured by an EMG response. The use of electrodiagnostic tests intraoperatively remains controversial.

C. Treatment

Like many medical and surgical conditions, the best treatment of iatrogenic nerve injury remains prevention. This is best done by carefully identifying the patients and/or procedures at risk. For instance, in hip surgery, patients with hip dysplasia and those undergoing revision surgeries are clearly at an increased risk. Technical measures to reduce the risk of nerve injury include factors such as wide exposures, meticulous haemostasis, clear understanding of the anatomy, and careful placement of retractors.

In cases where nerve transection is recognised intraoperatively, attempts at immediate repair are warranted. Immediate re-exploration of a nerve is otherwise not usually indicated unless, postoperatively, there is concern about transection or clear evidence of a haematoma. Apart from these relatively uncommon scenarios, treatment of nerve injury is by and large conservative. Any offending agent such as a constrictive dressing should be removed. The joint should be placed in a position of minimum tension on the affected nerve. Physiotherapy and the use of orthoses to prevent contactures are of paramount importance. For instance, the treatment of foot drop associated with sciatic or common peroneal nerve injury should include the use of an ankle-foot orthosis together with stretching exercises to prevent equinus contracture. If there is no recovery of nerve function by three months, neurolysis may be indicated.[50]

PERIPROSTHETIC FRACTURES

A. Introduction

Over the past two or three decades, there has been a significant increase in the number of joint replacements being performed, especially total hip (THA) and total knee (TKA) arthroplasties. With that, there has been an associated rise in the number of periprosthetic fractures. Occurring in close proximity to implanted prostheses either intraoperatively or postoperatively, these fractures present a significant challenge to the orthopaedic surgeon.

The reported incidence of periprosthetic fractures is variable, ranging from 0.3% to 2.5% for supracondylar periprosthetic femoral fractures after TKA, and from 0.6% to 2.4% for postoperative fractures following primary and revision THA, respectively.[56–58] It has been found that fractures related to uncemented prostheses are more common than those related to cemented implants. A large study of intraoperative periprosthetic femoral fractures during primary total hip arthroplasty by Berry showed a prevalence of 5.4% when the femoral component is inserted without cement as opposed to 0.3% when it is inserted with cement. Similarly, for revision procedures, these rates were 21% for the uncemented arthroplasties and 3.6% for the cemented ones.[59]

Several risk factors have been found to be associated with periprosthetic fractures. Patient-related factors include a history of rheumatoid arthritis, neurological disorders, osteoporosis, osteomalacia, Paget's disease, and chronic steroid use. Local factors, on the other hand, include a revision procedure, osteolysis associated with aseptic loosening of the implant, under-reaming of the acetabulum in THA, and anterior cortical notching of the femur in TKA.[60]

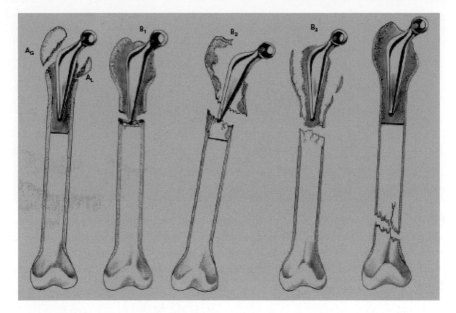

Fig. 6.   The Vancouver classification of periprosthetic femoral fractures. Type A, with fracture at the greater trochanter (A_G) and at the lesser trochanter (A_L). Type B, with fracture around or just below a well-fitted stem (B_1), around or just below a loose stem with adequate bone (B_2), and at or just below a loose stem with poor proximal bone stock (B_3). Type C fracture well below the stem.[62]

Most classification systems for periprosthetic fractures give information about the site of the fracture but do not help in planning the management. One of the classification systems that do provide good assistance in such planning is the Vancouver classification of postoperative femoral fractures after THA[61] (Fig. 6). Another system that may be helpful is the one describing supracondylar periprosthetic fractures following TKA (Fig. 7).

B. Diagnosis

periprosthetic fractures can occur either intraoperatively during reaming or implant impaction, or postoperatively in relation to, most frequently, a minor traumatic episode. When they do occur during the procedure, they can sometimes go undetected, and only when the postoperative radiographs are obtained, that the problem is recognised.

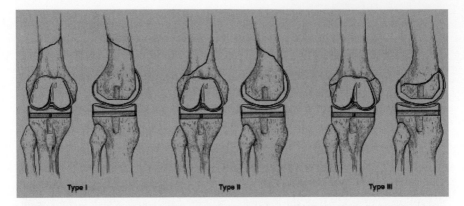

Fig. 7.   Anteroposterior and lateral views of supracondylar periprosthetic femoral fracture classification. Type I: Fracture proximal to femoral knee component. Type II: Fracture originating at the proximal aspect of the femoral knee component and extending proximally. Type III: Any part of the fracture line is distal to the upper edge of the anterior flange of the femoral knee component.[63]

With postoperative fractures, the patient complains of pain. There is localised tenderness and possibly a visible swelling from the fracture haematoma. A deformity might be present, and there is usually a reduction in the range of motion of the nearby joint.

The diagnosis is mostly confirmed with plain radiography. Computerised tomography may be helpful in defining the fracture configuration, revealing the underlying pathology, defining any bone loss, and assisting in planning the management.

C. Treatment

Any management plan for a patient with a periprosthetic fracture must take into account several factors. These include the patient's medical and functional status, fracture site and pattern, integrity of the bone-prosthesis interface, and quality of bone stock. The aims of treatment are early union and mobilisation, restoration and maintenance of pain-free function, a stable implant, and conservation of bone stock.

Historically, the management of periprosthetic fractures involved mostly conservative measures. These included skeletal traction, cast immobilisation, and cast-bracing. However, because of the problems associated with prolonged recumbancy, such as pressure ulcers, thromboembolism, and basal atelectasis and pneumonia, surgical intervention has been more favoured recently. This has also been the case because of advances in instrumentation and implant design, improved experience in revision surgery, as well as unsatisfactory results from non-operative treatment, with high rates of non-union and malalignment.

In broad terms, the surgical options for the treatment of periprosthetic fractures consist of open reduction and internal fixation with plates, screws, and/or wires; indirect reduction and internal fixation with an intramedullary device; and revision arthroplasty. Specific treatment options depend on the site and configuration of the fracture, as well as on the state of the bone-implant interface. For instance, the surgical treatment of a displaced type A_G or A_L periprosthetic femoral fracture (see Fig. 6) is usually with circlage wires supplemented with screws or plates if necessary. For a long oblique or spiral type B1 fracture, the treatment consists of circlage wires or cables with or without a cortical strut graft or a plate. Because the implant is loose in a type B2 fracture, it is necessary to revise the stem with one that bypasses the fracture site (Fig. 8).

In a type B3 fracture, the implant is loose and the bone stock is deficient; therefore, internal fixation is supplemented with two cortical onlay grafts, and a cancellous allograft is used to augment the bone stock further. If this is not feasible, the proximal femur may have to be replaced with a customised prosthesis. Finally, type C fractures are so distal in the femoral shaft that they can be essentially treated without consideration of the proximal prosthesis.[62]

HETEROTOPIC OSSIFICATION

A. Introduction

heterotopic ossification (HO) is a condition characterised by bone formation in soft tissues other than the periosteum. It may be related to a surgical procedure, peripheral nerve injury, spinal cord injury, or fracture or dislocation involving the hip on knee joints. However, in most cases, no precipitating factor can be found. Myositis ossificans is a similar condition to HO, but the fundamental difference is that the former develops after a traumatic muscle injury causing inflammation. In the context of THA and TKA, bone formation related to HO usually occurs around the neck of the femoral component and lateral to

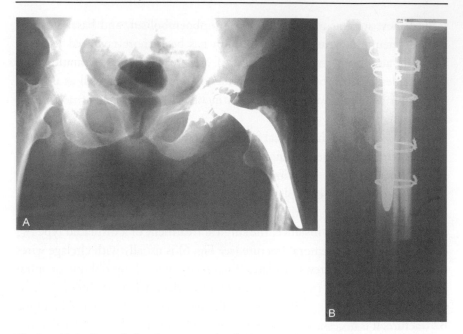

Fig. 8. (A) Radiograph showing an example of a Vancouver Type B2 fracture. (B) The patient was treated with long stem diaphyseal fixation bypass and circlage wires.[64]

the greater trochanter in THA, and on the anterior distal aspect of the femur and within the quadriceps mechanism in TKA.

Although heterotopic ossification following hip or knee arthroplasty is frequently observed radiographically, it has much less clinical significance. However, in a minority of patients, symptoms related to heterotopic ossification are severe enough to warrant surgical intervention. The reported rates of HO after THA range from 2% to 90%, but clinically significant cases account for only 3% to 10% of those with HO.[65,66] In comparison, HO after TKA is relatively rare with rates ranging from 1% to 42%.[67,68] Moreover, less than 1% of patients with HO following TKA are symptomatic.[69]

Several factors have been identified which predispose to the development of heterotopic ossification after THA. Male gender, previous history of HO, post-traumatic arthritis with hypertrophic osteophytosis, bilateral hypertrophic osteoarthritis, ankylosing spondylitis, Paget's disease, and diffuse idiopathic skeletal hyperostosis have all been linked to HO.[70,71] In addition, the type of surgical approach also seems to be of significance. Studies have shown that the anterior and certain lateral approaches are associated with higher rates of HO compared with the transtrochanteric approach. Moreover, the posterior approach was found to be the least associated with the development of HO.[72,73]

As for total knee arthroplasty, the risk factors that are associated with HO include hypertrophic osteoarthritis, high lumbar mineral density, notching of the anterior part of the femur, wide exposure of the distal femur for instrumentation placement, and surgical trauma to the quadriceps mechanism.[67,68,74] It has also been noted that forced manipulation of the knee joint to improve the range of motion may increase the incidence of HO.[74]

B. Diagnosis

Most patients with HO are asymptomatic, and so the diagnosis is only established radiographically more than 3 or 4 weeks postoperatively (Fig. 9). The main clinical presentations related to HO after THA include pain, impingement, instability, decreased range of motion, sciatic nerve irritation, and trochanteric bursitis. In TKA, the rare symptomatic cases may present with pain, decreased range of motion, quadriceps muscle snapping, and patellofemoral instability.

C. Prevention and Treatment

During the preoperative assessment of patients having THA or TKA, it is prudent to identify any risk factor predisposing to the development of HO. If the patient is at a high risk, prophylaxis against HO should be seriously considered. Apart from a careful surgical technique, two main modalities may be used. Low-dose radiation and non-steroidal anti-inflammatories (NSAID) postoperatively have both been shown to be effective prophylactic measures.

There has been no universal agreement as to the duration that NSAIDs should be administered. Studies have shown good efficacy from regimens lasting from 7 days to 6 weeks. The main problems with NSAIDs, though, are their associated complications such as wound problems secondary to bleeding and haematoma formation, and gastrointestinal bleeding. They may also have an adverse effect on bone ingrowth into a porous-coated cementless implant.[76]

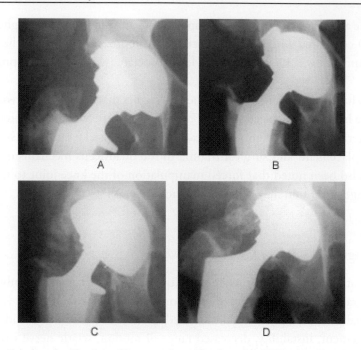

Fig. 9. Brooker classification of heterotopic ossification after THA. (A) Class I: Islands of bone in the soft tissues, (B) Class II: Visible spurs of bone leaving more than 1 cm between opposing bone surfaces, (C) Class III: Visible spurs of bone leaving less than 1 cm between opposing bone surfaces, and (D) Class IV: Apparent ankylosis of the hip.[75]

External beam radiation therapy is also an effective means of preventing HO. The radiation dose is considered safe, but proper shielding is necessary so that the beam targets only the affected area. Single and multi-dose regimens have been suggested, and some authors even advise the use of a preoperative prophylactic dose.[77]

Surgical excision of heterotopic bone is rarely required for patients after THA and TKA. When it is necessary in symptomatic cases, it should be performed after 6 to 12 months postoperatively, when HO is likely to have matured. Isotope bone scans can be helpful in assessing the maturity of the heteroptopic bone and can guide the timing of excision. One other helpful test is the serum alkaline phosphatase, the levels of which generally return to normal as the HO matures. Prophylaxis against HO should be carried out in all patients following excision of the heterotopic bone.

COMPLEX REGIONAL PAIN SYNDROME

A. Introduction

Complex regional pain syndrome (CRPS) is a condition of unknown aetiology characterised by pain disproportionate to the degree of insult, swelling, vasomotor instability, contracture, and osteoporosis. It can be a significantly disabling problem poising a difficult therapeutic challenge. There are numerous synonyms associated with CRPS, including reflex sympathetic dystrophy, Sudeck's dystrophy, causalgia, and algodystrophy. For that reason the International Association for the Study of Pain (IASP) suggested the new term "complex regional pain syndrome".[78,79] Two types of CRPS have been described according to whether or not there is a peripheral nerve injury. In reflex sympathetic dystrophy, or CRPS type 1, there is no nerve injury, whereas in causalgia, or CRPS type 2, there is a definable injury to a peripheral nerve.[79]

CRPS 1 can occur after any type of insult to a limb including surgery, such as arthroscopy and total knee arthroplasty. Although chronic CRPS 1 is uncommon with a prevalence of <2% in retrospective studies, prospective studies have shown the rate of mild CRPS 1 after fractures and surgical trauma to range from 30% to 40%.[80–82] Fortunately, most of these cases resolve within one year, but some features, especially stiffness, may persist.

Any part of the limb can be affected by CRPS, and in some cases, the whole limb may be involved. Sites where CRPS is common include the hand, the foot, the knee, and the shoulder. It rarely affects the elbow, but the hip may be affected in pregnancy.

B. Clinical Features and Diagnosis

The most prominent feature of CRPS is pain which is out of proportion to that anticipated after a similar injury or surgical procedure. The pain is typically not localised to areas supplied by a single peripheral nerve. There is an increased sensitivity to noxious stimuli (hyperalgesia), and even innocuous stimuli, such as a gentle touch, provoke pain (allodynia).

Certain vasomotor symptoms and signs usually accompany the condition. These have been described as occurring in three phases. In phase 1, which occurs within 3 months of the insult, swelling and vasodilatation are dominant leading to warm, pink, and dry skin. In the second phase, the dystrophic phase, vasoconstriction predominates leading to cold, blue, and thin skin with associated stiffness. This phase usually develops between 3 and 12 months after the onset. Finally, phase 3 is the atrophic phase, occurring at least after 12 months. It is characterised by increasing skin, muscle, and soft tissue atrophy, with fibrosis and contracture.

Complex regional pain syndrome is a clinical diagnosis; there is no single diagnostic test. The patient with CRPS is well with no systemic signs. The clinician must have a high index of suspicion, otherwise the diagnosis would be missed. The differential diagnosis should include infection, fracture, cellulitis, inflammatory arthritis, deep vein thrombosis, and malignancy. Laboratory tests such as FBC, ESR, CRP, rheumatoid factor, uric acid, and serum biochemistry are helpful, as they will be normal in CRPS.

Changes on plain radiography normally appear between 2 and 8 weeks after the onset of symptoms. Due to demineralisation, there is visible osteoporosis, which is commonly patchy and affecting mostly the subchondral bone, but demineralisation can also affect the epiphyseal and metaphyseal areas (Fig. 10). Both cortical and cancellous bone may be affected.[84] The "joint space" is preserved, and there is absence of erosions. The radiographs in a minority of cases may be normal. Isotope bone scans are helpful, and although they are not specific, they are quite sensitive. Increased uptake is noted in the affected areas early in the disease process, before any changes occur on plain radiographs.

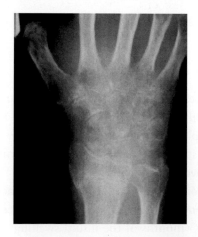

Fig. 10.   Profound osteoporosis in a patient with late severe CRPS type I affecting the hand.[83]

C. Treatment

The management of patients with CRPS is quite complex. Treatment must be started in the early stages, otherwise the outcome is poor. The main treatment objectives are alleviation of pain and preservation of function. A multidisciplinary team approach to management is vital, including the surgeon, pain clinic specialist, physiotherapist, and occupational therapist.

Effective analgesia is essential to the success of treatment. Numerous pharmacological agents have been used. These include non-steroidal anti-inflammatories; anticonvulsants such as gabapentin; α-adrenergic blockers such as prazosin; β-adrenergic blockers such as propranolol; calcium channel blockers such as nifedipine; and membrane stabilising drugs such as mexilitene. The use of corticosteroids has been shown to be helpful in some cases, and results with bisphosphonates have been encouraging. Another option that has been used extensively with good results is intravenous regional sympathetic blockade with agents such as guanethidine. Trancutaneous electrical nerve stimulation (TENS) may also play a role.

Although physiotherapy plays an important role in the management of patients with CRPS, it must be performed gently and with caution. Overly aggressive therapy to try and restore function can have a detrimental effect and increases pain.

The role of surgery in the treatment of CRPS is limited. It may be rarely indicated for the treatment of contractures, in which case, it should be delayed until after the active phase of the disease has passed. Amputation should be avoided if possible as results are poor and unpredictable and CRPS often recurs in the stump.[85]

ACUTE COMPARTMENT SYNDROME

A. Introduction

Compartment syndrome is a condition that was defined by Matsen in 1978 as one "in which increased pressure within a limited space compromises the circulation and function of the tissues within that space".[86] Delays in recognising and treating acute compartment syndrome (ACS) can lead to catastrophic consequences. These range from neurological deficit, muscle necrosis, and ischaemic contracture to infection, acute renal failure, cardiac arrhythmias, amputation and even death.

Although most commonly seen after traumatic injuries to the leg and forearm, compartment syndrome may affect other sites such as the thigh, upper arm, hand, foot, and abdomen. Fractures of the tibial shaft constitute approximately 40% of all cases of ACS, while those of the forearm account for 18%. In 23% of cases, there is only soft tissue injury with no fracture.[86] The incidence of ACS after tibial shaft fractures has been found to range from 1% to 10%.[87–89]

Acute compartment syndrome usually follows a traumatic injury, but it can also be associated with other aetiologies. In the orthopaedic setting, these may include fracture surgery such as intramedullary nailing, ischaemic reperfusion injuries, prolonged limb compression, casts and circular dressings, and pulsatile irrigation.[90] The exact pathophysiology of ACS is still not completely understood, but most hypotheses revolve around the arteriovenous pressure gradient theory. The increase in intracompartmental pressure seen in ACS raises the venous pressure, leading to a drop in the arteriovenous pressure gradient and a resultant reduced local tissue perfusion. Consequent to a drop in venous drainage, the tissue interstitial pressure rises and tissue oedema ensues. With further rises in intracompartmental pressure, the lymphatic system is overwhelmed and eventually collapses.[91,92]

B. Diagnosis

The key to diagnosing acute compartment syndrome is having a high index of suspicion. Often, the clinical signs are subtle. The most important symptom is pain which is usually out of proportion to the injury. Other significant findings include paraesthesia, pain on passive stretching of the affected muscle compartment, and a tense and swollen compartment. Pulselessness, muscle weakness and paralysis are late signs.

Laboratory tests are often unhelpful in the diagnosis of ACS. Highly elevated levels of creatine kinase usually indicate muscle damage, but this test is not useful in the early diagnosis.

In many cases, the clinical findings related to a suspected ACS are inconclusive or difficult to assess objectively. This is certainly the case in patients who are unconscious or uncooperative, as well as in children. When the diagnosis is doubtful, intracompartmental pressure (ICP) monitoring has proven to be an invaluable aide. The concept of ICP monitoring was introduced in the 1970s after Matsen identified a raised ICP in all his cases of ACS, regardless of the aetiology.[93] Several systems for monitoring ICP have since been introduced. The earlier ones were based on needle manometers and required the injection of saline. Their problem was that the column of saline needed to be free of bubbles, and that they could not monitor the ICP continuously. Later devices have been designed to incorporate a transducer-tipped probe, and have proved to be versatile and highly accurate.[94] There has been no consensus on the critical level of the absolute ICP, and hence the concept of the Δp pressure has gained a lot of popularity. It was introduced after the observation that the level of ICP at which ischaemia occurs depends on the perfusion pressure. Numerically Δp is the diastolic pressure minus the intracompartmental pressure. Most studies describe the critical Δp level to be less than or equal to 30 mm Hg. The use of Δp has reduced the number of unnecessary fasciotomies without significant complications.[95]

Other modalities that have been investigated in the diagnosis of ACS include near-infrared spectroscopy (NIRS) and magnetic resonance imaging (MRI). Although both techniques have been found to be useful, both have limitations at present, making them unreliable in diagnosing early compartment syndrome.

C. Treatment

As soon as a diagnosis of ACS is suspected, the management plan should include removal of all circumferential dressings down to skin; achievement of an adequate blood pressure if the patient has been hypotensive; and maintenance of the limb at heart level. Supplemental oxygen can be helpful by maintaining a good level of oxygenation.

If there are clear signs of ACS and/or the Δp is below 30 mm Hg, an emergency fasciotomy to all the relevant compartments should be carried out. The skin incision should be long enough, and the so-called "percutaneous fasciotomies" should be avoided. In the leg, this can be done through a single incision, with or without a fibulectomy, or by a double-incision technique.

REFERENCES

1. Kaltsas DS. (2004) Infection after total hip arthroplasty. *Ann R Coll Surg Engl* **86**: 267–271.
2. Della Valle CJ, Zuckerman JD, Di Cesare PE. (2004) Periprosthetic sepsis. *Clin Orthop Relat Res* **420**: 26–31.
3. Schmalzried TP, Amstutz HC, Au MK, *et al.* (1992) Etiology of deep sepsis in total hip arthroplasty: The significance of hematogenous and recurrent infections. *Clin Orthop Relat Res* **280**: 200–207.
4. Coventry MB. (1975) Treatment of infections occurring in total hip surgery. *Orthop Clin N Am* **6**: 991–1003.
5. Feldman DS, Lonner JH, Desai P, *et al.* (1995) The role of intraoperative frozen sections in revision total joint arthroplasty. *J Bone Joint Surg* **77A**: 1807–1813.
6. Spangehl MJ, Masri BA, O'Connell JX, *et al.* (1999) Prospective analysis of pre-operative and intraoperative investigations for the diagnosis of infection at the sites of two hundred and two revision total hip arthroplasties. *J Bone Joint Surg* **81A**: 672–683.
7. Aalto K, Osterman K, Peltola H, Rasanen J. (1984) Changes in erythrocyte sedimentation rate and C-reactive protein after total hip arthroplasty. *Clin Orthop Relat Res* **184**: 118–120.
8. Charnley J. (1972) Postoperative infection after total hip replacement with special reference to air contamination in the operating room. *Clin Orthop Relat Res* **87**: 167–187.
9. Kramer WJ, Saplys R, Waddell JP, *et al.* (1993) Bone scan, gallium scan, and hip aspiration in the diagnosis of infected total hip arthroplasty. *J Arthroplasty* **8**: 611–616.
10. Merkel KD, Brown MN, Dewanjee MK, *et al.* (1985) Comparison of indium-labelled-leukocyte imaging with sequential technetium-gallium scanning in the diagnosis of low-grade musculoskeletal sepsis: A prospective study. *J Bone Joint Surg* **67A**: 465–476.
11. Hanssen AD, Spangehl MJ. (2004) Treatment of the infected hip replacement. *Clin Orthop Relat Res* **420**: 63–71.
12. Brandt CM, Sistrunk WW, Duffy MC, *et al.* (1997) *Staphylococcus aureus* prosthetic joint infection treated with debridement and prosthesis retention. *Clin Inf Dis* **24**: 914–919.
13. Crockarell JR, Hanssen AD, Osmon DR, *et al.* (1998) Treatment of infections with debridement and retention of the components following hip arthroplasty. *J Bone Joint Surg* **80A**: 1306–1313.
14. Tattevin P, Cremieux AC, Pottier P, *et al.* (1999) *Clin Inf Dis* **29**: 292–295.

15. Murray RP, Bourne MH, Fitzgerald RH Jr. (1991) Metachronous infection in patients who have had more than one total joint arthroplasty. *J Bone Joint Surg* **73A**: 1469–1474.
16. Geerts WH, Heit JA, Clagett GP, *et al.* (2001) Prevention of venous thromboembolism. *Chest* **119**: 132S–175S.
17. Bombeli T, Spahn DR. (2004) Updates in perioperative coagulation: physiology and management of thromboembolism and haemorrhage. *Br J Anaes* **93**: 275–287.
18. Samama CM. (1999) Applying risk assessment models in general surgery: effective risk stratification. *Blood Coagul Fibrinolysis* **10**: S79–S84.
19. Garino JP, Lotke PA, Kitziger KJ, Steinburg ME. (1996) Deep venous thrombosis after total joint arthroplasty: the role of compression ultrasonography and the importance of the experience of the technician. *J Bone Joint Surg* **78A**: 1359–1365.
20. Bounameaux H, Cirafici P, De Moerloose P, *et al.* (1991) Measurement of D-dimer in plasma as diagnostic aid in suspected pulmonary embolism. *Lancet* **337**: 196–200.
21. The PIOPED Investigators. (1990) Value of the ventilation/perfusion scan in acute pulmonary embolism: Results of the prospective investigation of pulmonary embolism diagnosis (PIOPED). *JAMA* **263**: 2753–2759.
22. Turpie AG, Chin BS, Lip GY. (2002) Venous thromboembolism: Pathophysiology, clinical features, and prevention. *Br Med J* **325**: 887–890.
23. Westrich GH, Sculco TP. (1996) Prophylaxis against deep venous thrombosis after total knee arthroplasty: Pneumatic plantar compression and aspirin compared with aspirin alone. *J Bone Joint Surg* **78A**: 826–834.
24. Patterson BM, Marchand R, Ranawat C. (1989) Complications of heparin therapy after total joint arthroplasty. *J Bone Joint Surg* **71A**: 1130–1134.
25. Hull RD, Raskob GE, Rosenbloom D, *et al.* (1990) Heparin for five days as compared with 10 days in the initial treatment of proximal venous thrombosis. *N Engl J Med* **322**: 1260–1264.
26. Lotke PE, Steinberg ME, Ecker ML. (1994) Significance of deep venous thrombosis in the lower extremity after total joint arthroplasty. *Clin Orthop Relat Res* **299**: 25–30.
27. Haas SB, Tribus CB, Insall JN, *et al.* (1992) The significance of calf thrombi after total knee arthroplasty. *J Bone Joint Surg* **74B**: 799–802.
28. Morrey BF. (1992) Instability after total hip arthroplasty. *Orthop Clin Am* **23**: 237–248.
29. Woo RY, Morrey BF. (1982) Dislocations after total hip arthroplasty. *J Bone Joint Surg* **64A**: 1295–1306.

30. Fackler CD, Poss R. (1980) Dislocation in total hip arthroplasties. *Clin Orthop Relat Res* **151**: 169–178.

31. Ekelund A, Rydell N, Nilsson OS. (1992) Total hip arthroplasty in patients 80 years of age and older. *Clin Orthop Relat Res* **281**: 101–106.

32. Morrey BF. (1997) Difficult complications after hip joint replacement. *Clin Orthop Relat Res* **344**: 179–187.

33. Coventry MB. (1985) Late dislocations in patients with Charnley total hip arthroplasty. *J Bone Joint Surg* **67A**: 832–841.

34. Mallory TH, Lombardi AV Jr, Fada RA, *et al.* (1999) Dislocation after total hip arthroplasty using the anterolateral abductor split approach. *Clin Orthop Relat Res* **358**: 166–172.

35. Woo RY, Morrey BF. (1982) Dislocations after total hip arthroplasty. *J Bone Joint Surg* **64A**: 1295–1306.

36. Masonis JL, Bourne RB. (2002) Surgical approach, abductor function, and total hip arthroplasty dislocation. *Clin Orthop Relat Res* **405**: 46–53.

37. Cobb JP, Henckel J, Gomes P, *et al.* (2005) Hands-on robotic unicompartmental knee replacement. A prospective randomised controlled clinical investigation of the Acrobot System. In *Proceedings of the 5th Annual Meeting of Computer Assisted Orthopaedic Surgery International*. Pro Business: Berlin. pp. 65–68 .

38. Dandachli W, Richards R, Harris S, *et al.* (2005) A Practical reference coordinate system for planning hip resurfacing arthroplasty. In *Proceedings of the 5th Annual Meeting of Computer Assisted Orthopaedic Surgery International*. Pro Business: Berlin. pp. 78–80.

39. Dandachli W, Cobb JP, Richards R, *et al.* (2005) The transverse pelvic plane: A new and practical reference frame for hip arthroplasty. To be submitted to the *J Comput Aided Surg.*

40. Joshi A, Lee CM, Markovic L, *et al.* (1998) Prognosis of dislocation after total hip arthroplasty. *J Arthroplasty* **13**: 17–21.

41. Soong M, Rubash HE, Macaulay W. (2004) Dislocation after total hip arthroplasty. *J Am Acad Orthop Surg* **12**: 314–321.

42. Shoenfeld NA, Stuchin SA, Pearl R, *et al.* (1990) The management of vascular injuries associated with total hip arthroplasty. *J Vasc Surg* **11**: 549–555.

43. Choksey A, Noble J, Brown JJ, *et al.* (1998) Angiography in vascular problems with total knee replacement: A report of three cases. *Knee* **5**: 63–67.

44. Calligaro KD, DeLaurentis DA, Booth RE, *et al.* (1994) Acute arterial thrombosis associated with total knee arthroplasty. *J Vasc Surg* **20**: 927–932.

45. Rand JA. (1987) Vascular complications of total knee arthroplasty: report of three cases. *J Arthrosc* **2**: 89–93.

46. Rush JH, Vidovich JD, Johnson MA. (1987) Arterial complications of total knee replacement: the Australian experience. *J Bone Joint Surg* **69B**: 400–401.
47. Smith DE, McGraw RW, Taylor DC, *et al.* (2001) Arterial complications and total knee arthroplasty. *J Am Acad Orthop Surg* **9**: 253–257.
48. Ohira T, Fujimoto T, Taniwaki K. (1997) Acute popliteal artery occlusion after total knee arthroplasty. *Orthop Traumatol Surg* **116**: 429–430.
49. DeHart MM, Riley LH. (1999) Nerve injuries in total hip arthroplasty. *J Am Acad Orthop Surg* **7**: 101–111.
50. Lonner JH, Lotke PA. (1999) Aseptic complications after total knee arthroplasty. *J Am Acad Orthop Surg* **7**: 311–324.
51. Weber ER, Daube JR, Coventry MB. (1976) Peripheral neuropathies associated with total hip arthroplasty. *J Bone Joint Surg* **58A**: 66–69.
52. Schmalzried TP, Amstutz HC, Dorey FJ. (1991) Nerve palsy associated with total hip replacement: Risk factors and prognosis. *J Bone Joint Surg* **73A**: 1074–1080.
53. Idusuyi OB, Morrey BF. (1996) Peroneal nerve palsy after total knee arthroplasty: Assessment of predisposing and prognostic factors. *J Bone Joint Surg* **78A**: 177–184.
54. Mansat P, Cofield RH, Kersten TE, *et al.* (1997) Complications of rotator cuff repair. *Orthop Clin N Am* **28**: 205–213.
55. Lynch NM, Cofield RH, Silbert PL, *et al.* (1996) Neurologic complications after total shoulder arthroplasty. *J Shoulder Elbow Surg* **5**: 53–61.
56. Lewallen DG, Berry DK. (1996) Femoral fractures associated with total hip arthroplasty. In *Reconstructive Surgery of the Joints*, (ed. Morrey BF), pp. 1273–1288. (Churchill-Livingstone, New York.)
57. Figgie MP, Goldberg VM, Figgie HE III, *et al.* (1990) The results of treatment of supracondylar fracture above total knee arthroplasty. *J Arthroplasty* **5**: 267–276.
58. Merkel KD, Johnson EW Jr. (1986) Surpracondylar fracture of the femur after total knee arthroplasty. *J Bone Joint Surg* **68A**: 29–43.
59. Berry DJ. (1999) Epidemiology of periprosthetic fractures after major joint replacement: Hip and Knee. *Orthop Clin N Am* **30**: 183–190.
60. Sharkey PF, Hozack WJ, Callaghan JJ, *et al.* (1999) Acetabular fracture associated with cementless acetabular component insertion: a report of 13 cases. *J Arthroplasty* **14**: 426–431.
61. Duncan CP, Masri BA. (1995) Fractures of the femur after hip replacement. *Instr Course Lect* **44**: 293–304.
62. Learmonth ID. (2004) The management of periprosthetic fractures around the femoral stem. *J Bone Joint Surg* **86A**, 13–19.
63. Su ET, DeWal H, Di Cesare PE. (2004) Periprosthetic femoral fractures above total knee replacements. *J Am Acad Orthop Surg* **12**: 12–20.

64. Masri BA, Meek RM, Duncan CP. (2004). Periprosthetic fractures evaluation and treatment. *Clin Orthop Relat Res* **420**: 80–95.

65. Berry DJ, Garvin KL, Lee SH, *et al.* (1999) Hip and pelvis reconstruction. In: *Orthopaedic Knowledge Update 6: Home Study Syllabus*, (ed. Beaty JH), pp. 455–492. American Academy of Orthopaedic Surgeons: Rosemont, Illinois.

66. Ahrengart L, Lindgren U. (1989) Functional significance of heterotopic bone formation after total hip arthroplasty. *J Arthroplasty* **4**: 125–131.

67. Rader CP, Barthel T, Haase M, *et al.* (1997) Heterotopic ossification after total knee arthroplasty: 54/615 cases after 1–6 years' follow-up. *Acta Orthop Scand* **68**: 46–50.

68. Furia JP, Pellegrini VD Jr. (1995) Heterotopic ossification following primary total knee arthroplasty. *J Arthrosc* **10**: 413–419.

69. Austin KS, Siliski JM. (1995) Symptomatic heterotopic ossification following total knee arthroplasty. *J Arthroplasty* **10**, 695–698.

70. Ritter MA, Vaughan RB. (1977) Ectopic ossification after total hip arthroplasty: Predisposing factors, frequency, and effect on results. *J Bone Joint Surg* **59A**: 345–351.

71. DeLee J, Ferrari A, Charnley J. (1976) Ectopic bone formation following low friction arthroplasty of the hip. *Clin Orthop Relat Res* **121**: 53–59.

72. Pai VS. (1994) Heterotopic ossification in total hip arthroplasty: the influence of the approach. *J Arthroplasty* **9**: 199–202.

73. Horwitz BR, Rockowitz NL, Goll SR, *et al.* (1993) A prospective randomised comparison of two surgical approaches to total hip Arthroplasty. *Clin Orthop Relat Res* **291**: 154–163.

74. Harwin SF, Stein AJ, Stern RE, *et al.* (1993) Heterotopic ossification following primary total knee arthroplasty. *J Arthropsc* **8**: 113–116.

75. Iorio R, Healy WL. (2002) Heterotopic ossification after hip and knee arthroplasty: Risk factors, prevention, and treatment. *J Am Acad Orthop Surg* **10**: 409–416.

76. Vaughan BK. (1995) Other complications of total hip arthroplasty. In *Orthopaedic Knowledge Update: Hip and Knee Reconstruction* (eds. Callaghan JJ, Dennis DA, Paprosky WG, and Rosenberg AG), pp. 163–170. American Academy of Orthopaedic Surgeons.

77. Pellegrini VD Jr, Gregoritch SJ. (1996) Preoperative irradiation for prevention of heterotopic ossification following total hip arthroplasty. *J Bone Joint Surg* **78A**: 870–881.

78. Merskey H, Bogduk N. (1994) *Classification of Chronic Pain: Description of Chronic Pain Syndromes and Definitions of Pain Terms*, 2nd edn. International Association for the Study of Pain Press: Seattle.

79. Stanton-Hicks M, Janig W, Hassenbusch S, *et al.* (1995) Reflex sympathetic dystrophy: changing concepts and taxonomy. *Pain* **63**, 127–133.

80. Bickerstaff DR, Kanis JA. (1994) Algodystrophy: an under-recognized complication of minor trauma. *Br J Rheumatol* **33**: 240–248.

81. Sarangi PP, Ward AJ, Smith EJ, *et al.* (1993) Algodystrophy and osteoporosis after tibial fractures. *J Surg* **75B**: 450–452.

82. Field J and, Atkins RM. (1997) Algodystrophy is an early complication of Colles' fracture: what are the implications? *J Surg* **22B**: 178–182.

83. Atkins RM. (2003) Complex regional pain syndrome. *J Bone Joint Surg* **85B**: 1100–1106.

84. Allum R. (2002) Complications of arthroscopy of the knee. *J Bone Joint Surg* **84B**: 937–945.

85. Dielissen PW, Claassen AT, Veldman PH, *et al.* (1995) Amputation for reflex sympathetic dystrophy. *J Bone Joint Surg* **77B**: 270–273.

86. Matsen F, Winquist R, Krugmire R. (1980) Diagnosis and management of compartmental syndromes. *J Bone Joint Surg* **62A**: 286.

87. McQueen M, Gaston P, Court-Brown C. (2000) Acute compartment syndrome: who's at risk? *J Bone Joint Surg* **82B**: 200–203.

88. Blick SS, Brumback RJ, Poka A, *et al.* (1996) Compartment syndrome in open tibial fractures. *J Bone Joint Surg* **68A**: 1348–1353.

89. Tischenko GJ, Goodman SB. (1990) Compartment syndrome after intramedullary nailing of the tibia. *J Bone Joint Surg* **72A**: 41–44.

90. Kostler W, Strohm PC, Sudkamp NP. (2004) Acute compartment syndrome of the limb. *Injury* **35**: 1221–1227.

91. Vollmar B, Westermann S, Menger MD. (1999) Microvascular response to compartment syndrome-like external pressure elevation: an fluorescence microscopic study in the hamster striated muscle. *J Traumatol* **46**: 91–96.

92. Mars M, Hadley GP. (1998) Raised intracompartmental pressure and compartment syndromes. *Injury* **29**: 403–411.

93. Matsen F. (1975) Compartment syndrome: a unified approach. *Clin Orthop Relat Res* **113**: 8–14.

94. Willy C, Gerngross H, Sterk J. (1999) Measurement of intracompartment pressure with the use of a new electronic transducer-tipped catheter system. *J Bone Joint Surg* **81A**: 158–168.

95. McQueen M, Court-Brown C. (1996) Compartment monitoring in tibial fractures. The pressure threshold for decompressions. *J Bone Joint Surg* **72B**: 99–104.

79. Senton HGS, Ming X, Hanrahan S, et al. (1997) Relic-guided chondrocyte display: changing concepts and discoveries. New 60: 127-133.

80. Buckwalter HG, Kang H. (1999) Articular cartilage: tissue design and chondrocyte matrix interactions. Instr Course Lect 47: 477-486.

81. Saraglia D, Ward A, Smith E, et al. (1998) Bioabsorbable and osteoconductive interbody fixtures. J Surg 73B: 450-454.

82. Vella L, McCahon RM, et al. Shortterm light treatment on chondrocytes of bone tissue vs. osteochondromatosis. J Surg 21B: 453-457.

83. Athanc Phil. (2000) Complex marginal growth and synovitis. J Bone Joint Surg 85B: 1100-1102.

84. Athanc R. (2002) Complications of arthroscopy of the knee. J Bone Joint Surg 84B: 82-85.

85. Dalhoun PW, Gresser AT, Waldman PH, et al. (1995) Amputation for reflex sympathetic dystrophy. J Bone Joint Surg 77B: 270-273.

86. Marson B, Wollmer R, Augustin R, et al. (2001) Diagnosis and management of compartment syndromes. J Bone Joint Surg 82A: 864-866.

87. McGinnem K, Clancy F, Salter Evans A. (2002) Acute compartment syndrome below the elbow. J Bone Joint Surg 82B: 200-204.

88. Platt SC, Brundidge PJ, Dahan J, et al. (2003) Complications from fractures of the tibial diaphysis. J Bone Joint Surg 82B: 1504-1509.

89. Garabedo LG, Souchanc SK. (1996) Compartment syndromes after limb occlusion following tibial fracture. J Bone Joint Surg 73A: 184-195.

90. Laubers M, Steger P, Newton MH. (2001) Acute compartment syndrome of the hand. J Bone Joint Surg 85A: 182-189.

91. Nelson HB, Symmonds S, Sander AG. (1996) Microvascular suture fixation patterns and disorder. Vascular plantar disorders on fluorescent microscope study in the human vitreous. J Anaesth J Aust 47: 89-99.

92. Nell NH, Hall JP, et al. (1990) Bone remodelling in tibial pseudarthrosis. J Anat pseudarthrosis J Surg 29: 101-103.

93. Marson F. (1996) Acute fracture bone remodelling graft in the corticography knee 11: 12-14.

94. Wilke G, Gresham H, Steckler. (1997) Recent advances in the treatment of bone diseases with disease of a new electronic treatment. Topical external treatment. New Crew Surg 81A: 156-168.

95. McGinnem H, Sander-Brogan F. (1990) Compartment monitoring in tibial fractures. The pressure threshold for decompression. J Bone Joint Surg 78B: 99-101.

Chapter 22

COMPLICATIONS OF MICROSURGERY

Earl Owen

There should be few, if any, complications from any planned microsurgical technique, due to the trained microsurgeon's precise attitude to all the parameters that make up the refined knowledge, experience, skills and care involved in the meticulous art of microsurgery.

Microsurgery is defined as surgery performed under the magnified field of the operating microscope on living bodily tissues and tubal structures under 1 mm in outside diameter. It requires the surgeon to learn new hand steadying and finger "pen holding" positions, and skills to manipulate the specially designed microinstruments, microsutures and other equipment. Thus, it needs time for practice.[1]

Magnification for surgery began in the 1920s when two Swedish ear, nose and throat surgeons (Nylen and Holmgrem) looked through microscopes to operate on the ear ossicles. The French eye surgeon (Paufique) in Lyon used early Zeiss microscopes to perform the first corneal grafts after the second world war at the end of the 1940s. After that, some gynaecologists used Zeiss's OPMI 1 model microscopes to better view the cervix. It was not until the late

1950s when the American Julius Jacobsen began using Zeiss's first operating microscope (O.M.), that he and some research scientists devised a way of anastomosing blood vessels of 1 mm or less external diameter in experimental animals.[2]

After much training and skill acquisition, some brave research surgeons, from the field of transplantation immunology research, commenced kidney and liver transplants in rodents under low magnification glasses (Sun Lee, 1960). In 1963, neonatal surgery was extended initially by the author to tiny premature babies who had severe congenital defects using high magnification with one surgeon hand controlling the OPMI 1. This was a difficult surgery until the surgeon could be assisted by someone else able to observe the same magnified field and until both the surgeon and his assistant could use instruments designed specifically for the very small visual field. With design collaboration with Zeiss in Oberkochen and Keeler in London in 1964, the fully motorized OPMI 2 (Zeiss) for two surgeons, controlled by a foot pedal, and new microsurgical instrumentation (Keeler) allowed the author to perform three layer oesophageal reconstructions in premature infants with congenital oesophageal atresia.[3] Successful attempts to replant human amputated digits at the end of the 1960s and early 1970s followed (Tamai, Chang, Chen, Owen). The pioneer microsurgeons perfected the techniques to join minute arteries, veins, lymphatics, and all the body's ducts and tubes, helped by the advent of the Zeiss Double O.M., and foot controls, which allowed the microsurgeons to have an assistant view the same magnified fields.[4] The magnification, focusing and X/Y directing done without the surgeon taking his hands off his instruments, greatly speeded up their procedures.

BEFORE ATTEMPTING ANY CLINICAL MICROSURGERY

a) Get Proper Training

Before attempting any of the techniques to be described here in clinical cases, the surgeon should have had many months of experience with an O.M. One must know the microscope's anatomy and how to position it so one can sit comfortably but well supported at the lumbar spine, as these operations take considerable time and a well supported but relaxed position helps enormously. The optics are then adjusted to the surgeon's eyes for perfect stereoscopic vision. Much practice is needed to be able to use round bodied microinstruments with both hands in "penholder" finger grips (first described by Patkin) to accurately place 10/0 curved needles and then gently but firmly tie microknots. Such simple details as cutting threads particularly short will cut down scar formation.

b) Understand the Living Tissues

The secret to successful microsurgery is obvious when one sees living human tissue under intense magnification, as then one realizes that any tension on tissues stops or severely lowers that tissue's capillary circulation, which can only be seen under magnified vision. So you learn to see tissue with a new respect, conserve only viable tissue, and to tie knots gently. The least number of sutures, the less the eventual fibrous tissue of normal healing. The least tension in marrying up tissue edges, the more the capillary circulation in the area can work to promote normal healing. The gentler the surgeon, the less damage that surgeon does to the actual tissue he joins.

c) Learn the Secret to Avoid Complications

When tolerances are so minimal, such as when anastomosing a vein or artery with an internal bore of half a millimeter, one must end up with as widely open a bore as possible with as healthy a capillary circulation to its coapting edges as is technically possible. This will ensure easy initial healing, which avoids excess scar tissue formation, because, in no other form of surgery is it so important to state that SCAR TISSUE IS THE ENEMY! Therefore, the SECRET in avoiding complications is to AVOID MAKING SCAR TISSUE. Scarring in an anastomosis narrows the bore, or twists the edges, or slightly buckles the internal surfaces, allowing build up and blockage of tubal contents.

In training for microsurgery, the most effective way of getting this message across to trainees is to have them slit their experimental tubal anastomoses horizontally along the tube through the join, and examine that join FROM THE INSIDE (intimal surface an artery) to reveal the damage the surgeon himself has done to that tube.

d) Keep the Tissues Moist and Warm

Because micro-techniques require more time than normal general surgery, and one is looking at a small area, under intense and perhaps hot lighting, one may not realise how rapidly the tissues are drying out. A key to an infection-free surgery in long operations is to keep the tissues viable at maximal health, by keeping warm fluid occasionally sprayed in the area. The author has been frequently told that he appears to operate almost "under water", as he keeps the hydration and viability of the tissues in their normal wet environment.

Once armed with good training and months of practice on living tissue, preferably on rodents in a skills laboratory, one is ready to observe some microsurgical operations either directly or on videos or CDs. It is helpful to see these visual aids, as even the best films, done at close magnification by the experts, reveal some cellular damage that even the best microsurgeons do to living tissue.

THE ENEMIES THAT CAUSE COMPLICATIONS

It is the following basic wrongs that cause the complications of microsurgery.

a) Tissue Damaged Due to Drying

Tissue damaged due to drying out will not microheal correctly. Thus they will more readily become infected. Infection is more likely in a very long operation with the tissues exposed for long periods of drying out, or in the presence of spilled blood not washed out of the wound site during or at the end of the operation. Dryness is an enemy!

b) Tissues Opposed Under Tension

Tissues opposed under tension cannot have a good enough capillary blood supply to nourish their edges, due to the tension collapsing the small blood vessel and therefore will more readily result in the creation of excess scar tissues. All the scar tissues will contract in time, and this will narrow or close badly joined tubes. Tissue tension is an enemy!

c) Leaving Damaged Tissues in Wound

Tissues are actually quite delicate when seen at high magnification. So when doing a debridement of damaged tissue under magnification, one must clearly excise all the damaged tissue, leaving behind only viable and easy to heal edges. So debridement in microsurgery is very important. Leaving behind damaged tissue in wound is an enemy!

d) Causing Bleeding

Causing bleeding from very small blood vessels and capillaries is a real crime in microsurgery, as one can see any sized vessels starting to bleed under magnification, and can pick them up with a fine bipolar coagulator and stop the bleed. Bleeding from these small vessels can lead to small pools of blood gathering in the wound, which become a blood culture and allow infection to flourish. Even a small infection can wreck a fine microsurgical procedure. Bleeding is an enemy!

e) Introducing Infection

Sterilisation of the whole operative area and the parts to be joined using microsurgical techniques is very important. This means that one must remove all foreign bodies, dirt, blood, etc., flush out the whole area repeatedly, excise all the dead or about-to-be-dead material, prevent vessel bleeding, and put into the wound the very MINIMUM of surgical material such as sutures, silastic, metal, etc. That is because everything left in the site will act as a foreign body and develop fibrous tissue around it (the body always reacts that way), and these become an eventual scar, jeopardizing the result. All these are the hiding places for infection, and infection is the enemy!

THE MOST COMMON MICROSURGICAL OPERATIONS, COMPLICATIONS, AND THEIR PREVENTION

A) Digit and Limb Replantations and Partial Replantations

The complications are: bone failing to heal normally due to poor alignment; poor fixation with too large and clumsy metalwork; failure to get X-ray confirmation of fixation; infection; and vessel clotting. In joining bones, use the smallest possible but safe number of screws and adequate plates, and avoid using Kirschner wires through joints, particularly in hand and feet digits. Sterility is paramount! The use of thin, strong wires joining small long bones through fine bored holes is an excellent technique as compression can be applied which aids healing. The author always cut out some bone length, however small it may be, to allow all the other structures, arteries, veins, nerves, tendons, etc. to avoid tension in their own anastomoses. The author's record in removing bone in a severely crushed radius and ulnar forearm amputation injury involved removing what ended up as a total 8 cm of each major bone, to allow the removal of non-viable tissues and the then successful series of anastomoses of tension-free bones, vessels, tendons, nerves and skin. The other complications of hand surgery also apply in these replantation and transplantation cases.[5–8]

B) Anastomoses of Very Small Arteries

The common complications are: bleeding, clotting and narrowing. Always remember that arteries have a rapid laminar flow of contents, and the largest thrombocytes are mostly lateral, so the thrombocytes will accumulate at and distal to the flow if the anastomosis is in any way uneven. They will further build up as the eddy currents from irregular joins deposit more downstream "sticky" cells, thus eventually closing that vessel and ending what might have otherwise been a brilliant and complicated well planned reconstructive operation. So, the key is to do the vessel inflow anastomoses first and most meticulously. Do not tie any microsurgical knots tightly. Just gently oppose the vessel sides, as there will be tissue swelling occurring after the wound is closed up. Do not put in too many knots as that means too much suture material, and too much eventual scarring around them which could stenose the join. Do not take too long to do the anastomosis, as the small clamps on the artery, although they are supposed to have only a weakened spring mechanism, will inevitably damage the internal surface of the vessel being joined, the longer they are left on. Thus, slightly wider spacing of interrupted sutures tend to occur in anastomoses done by experienced microsurgeons, who then gently apply a little pressure on their join for a few minutes to stop any post-join bleeding.[9]

C) Anastomoses of Small Veins

The complications are: draining failure, bleeding, clotting and infection. These can be more difficult than joining arteries, as veins can be ragged edged, collapsed, and floppy. The key is to get one good stay suture in (which can be removed later). Then one can assess whether the vein has previously been twisted, when one starts again, and a new well placed first suture allows you to get in two good stay sutures. It may then be possible to use two or more short running sutures between the stays to rapidly join veins. Again, use gentle pressure when tying the knots. Do one more vein than you think is enough! The drainage of the site is crucial to a good result. Always flush out veins (and arteries of course) with a heparin solution before joining them.

D) Anastomosis of the Ureter

The complications are: tissue swelling, not enough drainage, leakage of stenosis, pain and infection. Treat this as an artery and be very meticulous and with the thinnest microsutures you can use, and use interrupted sutures. Remember that urine is not water; it can carry some sludge, and the pain from a block of debris in the ureter is very severe indeed, so be very careful NOT to NARROW these joins. If there is a gap in bringing the cut edges together, do not try joining the gap, as tension will jeopardise the join. In that case, do a bladder to ureter tubal reconstruction.[10]

E) Anastomoses of the VAS, and Epididymo-Vasostomies

The complications are: blockage, leakage, peristalsis loss, infection and pain. Vasectomy "reversal" is becoming more popular as divorce rate rises. After 5000 individual microreversal cases, the author has evolved a three-layer criss-cross technique that rarely closes down postoperatively. The internal bore of the average vas is only 2–3 human hairs in diameter and the "three" layers are actually mucosa, sub-mucosa, thick muscle and adventitia. The author freshens the ends generously, achieves a viable vas, and closes the inevitable gap between the ends (there was perhaps an enthusiastic vasectomist who took out a lot of vas length) by using 5/0 nylon to bring together the tissue above and below where the join is to be made until the two vas ends "kiss". These ends are then slightly separated with the use of a thin wedge of silastic coloured mm ruled background. This avoids any tension on the actual microanastomosis itself. With each end being considered as a clock face, the inside mucosal layer is joined with the finest interrupted sutures (10/0); the inner muscle layer with 9/0 or 8/0 interrupted; and a few 8/0 or 6/0 sutures used for the looser outer muscular and adventitial layer for extra strength, irrespective of the contrast in the width disparity between the two ends.[11]

Even if the long blocked (testicular) side of the vas and epididymis in a "vasectomy" reversal, which was really a tie off of the terminal epididymis, has become twice the lesser diameter of the distal (prostatic) vas end, the join ends up neat if tied gently, and the area is left tension-free and free of any bleeding points. In epididymovasostomy (E.V.) and congenital azospermia cases, a special technique of side-to-end join can be made to have some epididymal mucosa inside the vas bore to avoid leakage of a very difficult anastomosis.[12]

F) Anastomoses of the Fallopian Tube

Complications are: blockage, infection and adhesions. Compared with the vas, this tube is a low pressure conduit with fewer muscles. Whereas the vas inner layer, despite micro-psuedo-villi, is virtually smooth, this tube has two types of thickened mucosa, one glandular, and the other villous, and the wider ampullary section is by far the thinner muscled. All its tubular mucosa is more important than that of the vas, so it should have minimal or no sutures scarring. The technique to avoid failure here is to only place joining microsutures in the submucosal, muscle, and peritoneal layers in a preferred three-layer join. It is important to reunite the gap in the mesentery of the tube, and strengthen it, retaining the blood supply so there is no gap and no tension at all upon joining the tube itself. As smooth a peritoneal surface as is possible is reconstructed with buried fine sutures at the conclusion of the join on either side. All fine adhesions are removed (we use a fine cautery needle and fine serrated scissors). The previously packed away pelvic contents are washed with warm Hartmann's solution until the latter crystal clear (may need small bleeder attention) and replaced before closing the Pfannensteil incision, having ensured all the abdominal contents were restored to their anatomical positions.[13]

G) Anastomoses of Peripheral Nerves

The complications are: failure to work at all, neuromata formation, infection and pain. The most difficult anastomoses in mircrosurgery are those "tubes" containing very soft tissue, and living axonal material in axonal bundles (individual fascicles). These "tubes" are indeed soft and unwieldy. Severed fascicles need to be matched to their cut continuations, and some surgeons prefer to match groups of fascicles in bundles and join those larger collections together. The author prefers to do individual matched fascicle to fascicle anastomoses if possible.

In the author's experience, being meticulous about matching bundles, or (better) the individual fascicles, will prolong the operation, but improve the eventual result.

When a nerve is severed, axonal material initially oozes out (actually a protein nerve budding process attempting natural repair), and hundreds of coalescing buds form an observable lump wider than the thin layer of perineurium normally holding all these axons. When repairing cut nerves, the finest sutures (10/0, 11/0) are placed to attempt to hold only the perineurial layers, which demands that each soft little neuroma is carefully but swiftly cut off just before the suture is placed.

This technique is best performed with special sharp serrated scissors, and this is the key to a successful nerve reconstruction. Just placing larger sutures through the epineurium to join peripheral nerves is not microsurgery, and if done to pull nerve ends together to overcome a gap, is usually doomed to failure. Such a technique, however, is good only if in an emergency, there is no surgeon around skilled enough to do microsurgical primary repairs. Such a keeping together of the nerve ends allows a few weeks for healing of other severed structures, and then a secondary nerve repair may have a much better chance of a good result.

There must be minimal tension on nerve repairs, and the author insists upon individual fascicular anastomoses with preservation of the supporting nerve material which contains that nerve's blood supply. Usually, the layer deeper to the nerve is supplying its blood vessels.

With a minimally tense join using 10/0 sutures placed to do the least damage to the soft axonal layer, and only using three or four careful sutures per fascicle in a clean, well hydrated wound, one can expect a good result. The enemies here are tension, floppy soft tissue, and the state of the surrounding tissue damage, all of which can lead to fibrosis of the area due to avascularity or infection. The trap for the unwary here is to use too many sutures for fascicular nerve repair.

If there is going to be tension from too much nerve loss, then an immediate nerve graft must be considered, in accident cases as well as delayed repairs, provided one is skilled.

WARNING: Nerve repairs and nerve grafts are the most difficult forms of microsurgery and should preferably be performed only by skilled experienced microsurgeons. A delayed nerve repair by a top microsurgeon is preferable to an immediate repair by an unskilled enthusiast.[14]

Tension, unmatched fascicles, inadequate blood supply, stripping of the nerve back in a forlorn attempt to "gain length", swelling of the surrounding tissues and infection are all causes of eventual non-function of the join.

H) "Free Flaps"

Complications are: failure, swelling and infection. A free flap (FF) is made of some tissue (one or more of muscle, skin, bone, messentary, etc.) with its supplying blood vessels, and sometimes also with its nerve supply. All the complications previously mentioned for these individual structure's anastomoses apply, but with some additions.

The size, shape and bodily positioning of the FF must be well worked out prior to the operation. Obviously, the venous return from the flap does better if it is gravity-assisted and without any compression. Obviously, the larger the arterial supply (and consequently the greater need for sufficient venous return), the better chance the FF has of healing and functioning. These operations must be well planned by experienced microsurgeons. Sticking to safe and well tried, well described donor sites to a suitable FF end area allows for the best chance.

So, ideally, choose a large donor flap artery of sufficient length to join the FF to where it is needed, and at least one large but preferably more than one adequate vein to the dependent end of the FF. Do not attempt nerves in a FF unless a successful outcome is expected. There are the usual general complications possible at the donor area which may require split skin grafting or other plastic surgery procedures to overcome the tissue defect. Careful postoperative regimes are needed to keep the FF in the correct drainage position and avoid even light pressure or trauma. Bandages or dressings should be of overall gentle pressure but windows for observation should be allowed. Some surgeons forgo any covering of their FF in the first postoperative weeks. Developing haematoma beneath the FF, infection or other tissue damage, can cause swelling whereas slow arterial blockage can cause discolouration and coldness to the skin covering an FF. Essential to these graft's survival is the constant vigilance of the staff with adequate charting of measurable parameters, and swift attention to any sudden change of these signs by the microsurgical staff. By early warning, an FF that would be otherwise lost, can be reopened and saved.[15]

OTHER MICROSURGICAL OPERATIONS

Microsurgery is ideal for all forms of small animal surgical research utilising rats, guinea pigs, mice and rabbits sparingly. Only use animals in necessary research where there is no substitute for such experimentation in live bodies, and with all care and pain elimination. Such necessary work is far cheaper and faster than in traditional large animal research. In our laboratories, microsurgeons in training can perform a total limb transplantation in our rodent model in about two hours, or a rodent kidney transplant in about an hour, as there are only three anastomoses in the latter procedure. Appropriate protocols allow such rapid conclusion of new surgical research ideas in significant numbers to speed up introduction of innovations into human surgery.[16]

When the author began microsurgical procedures with excellent equipment, he realised that all surgical operations should be done with microsurgical principles in mind. The real pioneers in this field were planning free flaps (G. Ian Taylor),[17] infertility operations (Owen), neurosurgery (Yasargil, Millesi), and the extensive use of microsurgery for trauma reconstructions over 40 years ago. Microsurgery for small vessels and tubes and nerves is now well established and used in almost all specialties, and increasingly, in surgical research. Urologists can use microsurgery skills to conserve or graft nerves to preserve distal nerve function in total prostatectomies. Plastic and reconstructive and cancer surgeons use microsurgery in ever more complex reconstructive operations. The necessity to avoid complications by diligent adherence to the principles of microsurgery is becoming even more important as surgery enters an even smaller terrain of "miniature surgery". Microsurgery is only the beginning of the miniaturisation of surgery.[18]

REFERENCES

1. Owen E. (1976) The operating microscope isn't everything – A warning and a prediction. *J Bone Joint Surg [Br]* **58-B**(4): 397–398.

2. Jacobsen JH, Suarez EL. (1960) Microsurgery in anastomosis of small vessels. *Surg Forum* **11**: 243–245.

3. Owen ER, Slome P. (1966) Microsurgery. *Annuals of Royal College of Surgeons*, Physiology Report.

4. Owen ER. (1979) History of general microsurgery. In: Beale J (ed.) (Houghton Mifflin, San Francisco).

5. Komatsu S, Tamai S. (1968) Successful replantation of a completely cut-off thumb. *Plast Reconstr Surg* **42**: 374–377.

6. Owen E. (1975) Replantation of amputated extremities. *Langenbecks Arch Chir* **339**: 613–615 (German).

7. Lendvay PG, Owen ER. (1970) Microvascular repair of completely severed digit: Fate of digital vessels after six months. *Med J Aust* **2**(18): 818–820.

8. Dubernard JM, Owen ER, *et al.* (1999) Human hand allograft: Report on first six months. *Lancet* **353**: 1315–1320.

9. Overton J, Owen ER. (1970) The successful replacement of minute arteries. *Surg* **68**(4): 713–723.

10. Owen E. (1969) Microtechniques in organ transplantation. In: Wilkinson JL (ed.), *Recent Advances in Pediatric Surgery* (Churchill, London).

11. Owen ER. (1977) Microsurgical vasovasostomy: A reliable vasectomy reversal. *Aust N Z J Surg* **47**(3): 305–309.

12. Owen ER. (1992) La vaso-vasostomie microchirurgicale: une methode fiable de retablissement de la continuitě děfěrentielle. *Progres Urol* **2**: 477–483.

13. Owen ER, Pickett-Heaps AA. (1977) The microsurgical basis of fallopian tube reconstruction. *Aust N Z J Surg* **47**(3): 305–309.

14. Millesi H, *et al.* (1972) The interfascicular nerve grafting of the median and ulnar nerves. *J Bone Joint Surg* **54A**: 727–750.

15. Taylor GI, Ham FJ. (1976) The free vascularized nerve graft. A further experimental and clinical application of *Surg Plast Reconst.* **57**(4): 413–426.

16. Owen ER, Bryant K, Hopewood PR. (1983) Microsurgery: A new horizon in vetinary surgery. *Aust Vet J* **60**(4): 97–100.

17. Taylor GI, Miller GD, Ham FJ. (1975) The free vascularized bone graft: A clinical extension of microvascular techniques. *Plast Reconst Surg* **55**: 533–544.

18. Owen ER. (1982) W.I.S.D.O.M., a microsurgical philosophy. Editorial. *Int J Microsurg.*

Chapter 23

COMPLICATIONS OF PLASTIC AND RECONSTRUCTIVE SURGERY

Ivo Pitanguy, Henrique N. Radwanski
and Natale Ferreira Gontijo De Amorim

INTRODUCTION

In view of the range of tissue and anatomical regions that are encompassed by their work, from the manipulation of the integument, muscles and fascia, bone and cartilage to performing surgical procedures from the head down to the extremities, plastic surgeons can perhaps be seen as true general surgeons. Although their specialty is mostly restricted to the superficial layers of the body, in some cases the plastic surgeon is involved with other surgical areas that are not in their scope of work. However, with the increase in techniques and technology, different sub-specialties have developed within plastic surgery itself, and it is almost impossible for the plastic surgeon to claim familiarity with all aspects of the field of practice.

Complications in plastic surgery are rarely life-threatening. An expanding haematoma, an ischemic musculo-cutaneous flap or a localised infection are controllable with direct and immediate attention. In the vast number of cases, a complication will cause no more than an extended leave from work. Nevertheless, even a restricted skin necrosis may be a calamitous event when

739

it occurs following a face-lift. Unaesthetic scars, a desensitised flap or prolonged oedema may cause varying degrees of discomfort, although usually of a temporary nature.

This chapter will present and discuss the most frequent complications that may occur from an aesthetic or reconstructive procedure. It is not the intention of the authors to cover every single complication. When considered a consequence of complications, the unfavorable result in plastic surgery, secondary surgery, will also be addressed.

BASIC PRINCIPLES

As in all surgical specialties, complications in plastic surgery are avoided by adhering to three basic principles, careful preoperative diagnosis and planning, precise surgical technique, and diligent postoperative follow-up. When a complication is perceived, immediate attention and the necessary intervention will assure that the extent of the complication is limited.[1,2]

Surgery planning involves a discussion with the patient, so as to comprehend the complaint. At this stage, it is important to educate the patient and review all pertinent information together. Most complaints following plastic surgery for an aesthetic reason involve disappointment with the results. Popular magazines may induce unrealistic ideas regarding surgery, and these should be investigated to filter patients who do not clearly understand the end result of the operation. In all circumstances, a collaborative patient is always helpful when a complication occurs.

The limitations imposed by the anatomy and the surgeon's own aesthetic principles must be carefully discussed. An understanding of the person as a lucid body, one that is constantly interacting with his or her social and emotional environment, allows the surgeon to capture the true nature of these procedures. The location and extension of scars should be described and delineated, preferably with an ink pen. Preoperative photographs serve as a legal document as well as a means to demonstrate the results attained in the postoperative period.

Possible postoperative events (such as swelling, haematoma, delayed healing) should be anticipated, and the patient must be warned of possible prolonged non-surgical care. The risk of flap necrosis is substantially increased in smokers. Heavy smokers (over 10 cigarettes a day) must decrease the amount of CO_2 and nicotine intake, as these are well-known toxins.

In almost all cases, a plastic surgery procedure, either aesthetic or reconstructive, will be an elective operation, planned beforehand. Preoperative examinations are requested and checked. As a final precaution, it is imperative to acertain that the patient knows what to expect from the operation. A consent form is prepared for the specific procedure, where all relevant information and possible complications are described.

Good surgical technique includes limiting undermining, avoiding dessication by using moist towels over the dissected flaps, and precise haemostasis. As many procedures involve the advancement or rotation of flaps, the prevention of complications begins with a correct design of flap dimensions, with special attention to the pedicle. Excess tension on the flaps will cause some degree of vascular embarrassment, and this may be worsened if the patient has any previous disease which decreases perfusion. Sutures should be placed such that tension is removed from the most superficial layers. This assures good healing and prevents widening of the scars.

A keen observation is required to anticipate and institute early treatment of any complication. The signs and symptoms of an expanding haematoma (pain, acute swelling) may indicate a bleeding vessel, and emergency bedside drainage may be required. The surgeon should not hesitate to take the patient back to the surgical suite for a review of haemostasis. Insufficient perfusion of a flap should be verified early. If this is a microsurgical flap, a decision must be made as to whether a re-anastomosis will save the entire flap.

Necrosis is suspected when the capillary filling is slow or absent, and will be apparent in the first 12 hours postoperatively. As soon as tissue loss is evident, surgical debridement is instituted. This should be conservative to preserve viable tissues from the edges, thus allowing for secondary healing. It is remarkable how delicate tissues (such as in the facial regions) recover from localised necrosis, and what seems as large areas of tissue loss will eventually result in minimal scarring. Infection must be prevented by instituting appropriate antibiotic treatment and frequent changes of dressings.

SECONDARY AESTHETIC SURGERY

While addressing a secondary procedure in aesthetic surgery, three areas are considered particularly challenging. In the senior author's experience, facial surgery, rhinoplasty and body contouring have demanded the greatest creativity in approaching the unfavorable result. These are discussed in this chapter;

when pertinent, the most frequent causes of complications and how they can be avoided will be described.

The Face

Aesthetic surgery of the face demands the utmost from the plastic surgeon, from the technical and the creative aspect.[3–5] Initially, we will describe the more common complication of a rhytidectomy, and then describe the surgical techniques that are performed for facial rejuvenation.

The "round-lifting" technique has been adopted as the standard procedure when addressing the aging face. As in any technique, facial flaps are adequately undermined to loosen the skin for subsequent rotation, rather than simple traction. The pulling of flaps without precise criteria will result in anatomical dislocations, which causes surgical stigmas. The principle behind the round-lifting procedure is to place the flaps with no excessive tension, and in such a way as to maintain important anatomical parameters in position, thus avoiding the unaesthetic appearance of a rhytidoplasty.

The major complications from a face lift are an expanding haematoma, nerve injury and flap necrosis. Once diagnosed, it is imperative to control the complication, limiting the extension of tissue injury (Table 1).

Due to the relatively large area of undermining, blood collection under skin flaps is not uncommon. It has been noted that haematomas are more common in male patients. Haemostasis is carefully performed before the final

Table 1. Rate of Complications in Face-Lifting Procedures, in the Senior Author's Private Clinic

FACE LIFTING 1957 – 2003 7,868 cases	
COMPLICATIONS	**%**
Haematoma	3.0
Alopecia	0.4
Nerve lesion	0.1
Dehiscence	0.1

closure of the tissue. At this point, and for the next 24 h, the patient's blood pressure must be carefully monitored and controlled, avoiding peaks that may cause larger vessels to bleed. Pain and general discomfort are factors that may cause patient unrest and increased blood pressure, and are addressed with appropriate medication. Suction drains are usually placed and removed after 24–48 h.

Because it requires constant observation by medical and nursing staff a rhytidoplasty is not an outpatient procedure but requires inpatient stay of one or two days.

An expanding haematoma should be diagnosed as early as possible, to avoid vascular injury to the flaps. This event usually occurs in the first eight hours postoperatively. The senior author has described his approach, which is the removal of the blood clots at the bedside, and washing the area with cold saline. In his experience, this is an expedient manoeuvre that is usually sufficient to evacuate the haematoma. If bleeding persists, the patient should be taken to the surgical suite. Under sedation, the flap over the area should be elevated, blood clots removed and the blood vessel visualised and clamped (Fig. 1). A non-expanding haematoma (i.e. when no excessive tension exists on the flaps) is drained in the out-patient department, and might need several sessions of drainage over the first 10 days.[6]

Nerve injury in a face-lift is almost always temporary, as long as proper surgical planes are respected. It is quite common for the patient to complain of numbness over the dissected areas; normal skin sensation returns in one or two months. Motor nerve injury causes greater concern. The temporal (innervating the muscles of the forehead) and mandibular branches of the facial nerve (innervating the depressor anguli oris) are the two most frequently injured nerves. A triangular area at the temporal region has been termed "no-man's land" by the senior author. Here, the nerve becomes more superficial and is at greater risk, especially from the electrocautery and haemostasis should be done very carefully[7–9] (Fig. 2).

The lesion to the mandibular branch occurs secondary to trauma mainly from the cannula that is used to remove fatty tissue from the neck. This liposuction should be done gently, and limited to the area below the level of the mandible (Fig. 3).

Two direct causes of skin necrosis are dissection that is too superficial or excessive tension on the flaps. An untreated expanding haematoma will

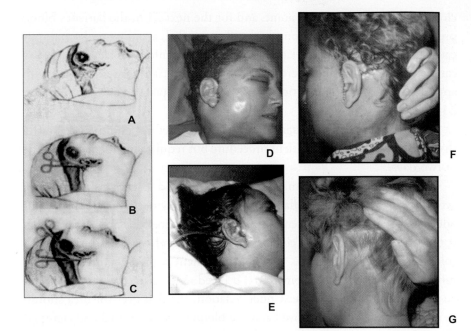

Fig. 1. [A–G] An expanding haematoma requires immediate attention. Bedside drainage may be performed to evacuate blood clots, thus avoiding vascular damage to the undermined flaps. This patient was submitted to drainage of an acute bilateral haematoma with removal of a few sutures at the bedside. No residual sequela is seen in the long-term postoperative period.

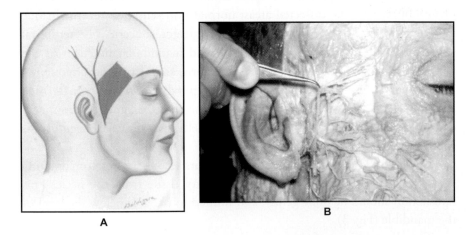

Fig. 2. [A, B] "No man's land" is an area where the frontal branch of the facial nerve is vulnerable to lesion. Haemostasis should be restricted in this area.

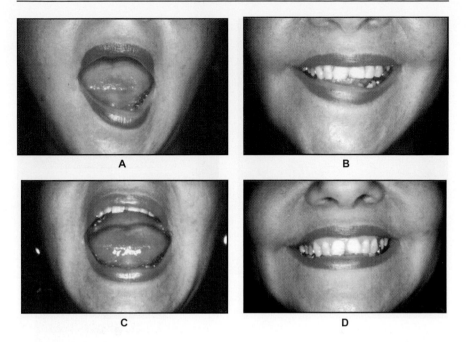

Fig. 3. [A–D] Paralysis of the mandibular branch of the facial nerve is noticeable during muscle dynamics. This is fortunately a rare occurrence, and usually subsides after a few weeks.

interrupt blood perfusion and lead to early tissue suffering. Indirect causes are insufficient blood circulation from pre-exisiting disease or more commonly, tobacco use. If poor perfusion is suspected, the surgeon should institute medication to increase blood flow. An established area of necrosis should be treated very conservatively, avoiding excessive debridement. Even a large area of necrosis will become a limited scar after the healing process is completed, usually after three to six months (Fig. 4).

Standard and secondary rhytidoplasty

Skin incisions for a facelift vary according to the extension of the procedure (i.e. an operation that involves undermining of the face alone or the neck region). The classic incision begins inside the temporal hairline, curves gently around the ear, follows in the retroauricular sulcus and finishes inside the cervical hairline. Incisions in the male patient may take advantage of the thick sideburn and be slightly inclined in the temporal region[10–15] (Fig. 5).

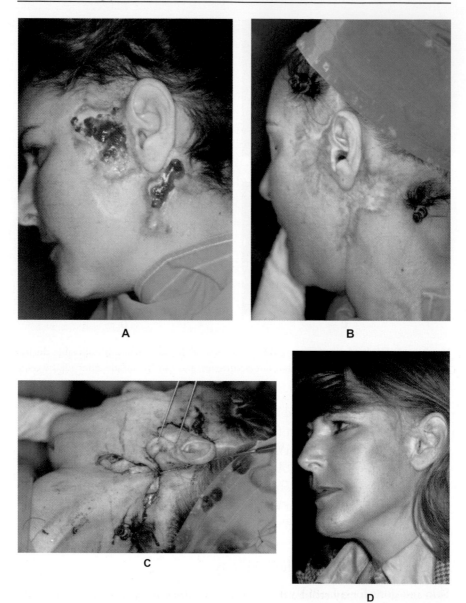

A

B

C

D

Fig. 4. [A–D] Necrosis of a skin flap following a face-lift, in a patient operated elsewhere. Treatment was conservative, with no debridement, and a secondary procedure was performed to resect remaining scars after healing was complete. The patient is seen one year following the last surgical procedure.

THE ROUND LIFTING

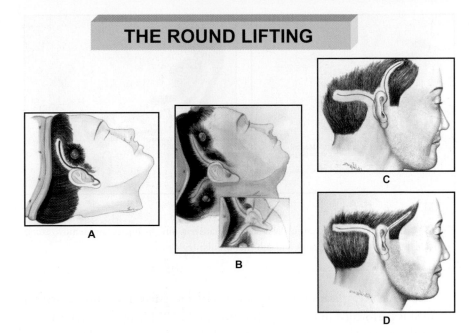

Fig. 5. [A–D] A face lift may demand one of several different incisions, which allows the surgeon a large margin for his creativity. Figure B shows the standard incision for a round-lifting rhytidectomy.

Skin dissection liberates the retaining ligaments (Fig. 6A). Excess fat is removed by liposuction, allowing for a more pleasant contour of the cervico-mandibular angle (Fig. 6B). Besides liberation retaining ligaments, excess fat is removed, allowing for a contour of the cervical-mandibular angle. Liposuction of the sub-mental region has brought a considerable improvement in the treatment of the heavy neck, with minimal incisions. (Before the advent of suction-assisted lipectomy, the heavy fatty neck[16] was usually corrected by an open approach, with wide undermining and the use of scissors for lipectomy. This may still be done when the surgeon encounters a very fatty neck.) Aspiration must be conservative to avoid excessive skeletonisation of the cervical-mandible angle. The treatment of medial platysmal bands is carried out under direct exposure when necessary. Approximation of diastasis is done with interrupted sutures, plicating down to the level of the hyoid bone.

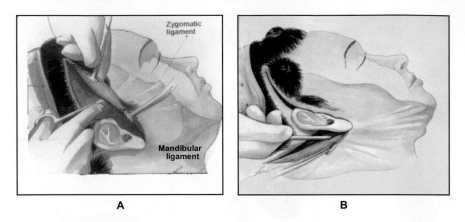

A   B

Fig. 6. [**A, B**] A small-bore cannula is used to liberate retaining ligaments and remove excess fat through liposuction of the neck and sub-mandibular regions.

Subsequently, plication of the superficial muscular aponeurotic system (SMAS) is performed in the same direction as the skin flaps, with repositioning of the malar fat pad. The durability of this manoeuvre is relative to the individual aging process. Tension on the musculo-aponeurotic system allows support of the subcutaneous layers, corrects the sagging cheek and reduces tension on the skin flap (Fig. 7).

Smas Plication and Malar Fat Pad Reposition

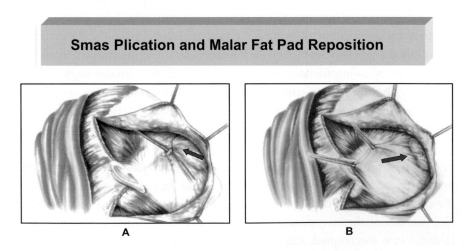

A   B

Fig. 7. [**A, B**] SMAS plication and malar fat pad repositioning.

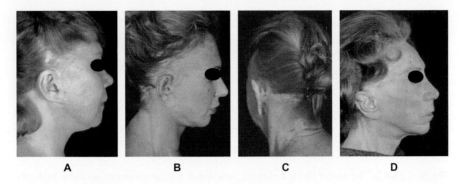

Fig. 8. [A–D] Stigmas of a rhytidectomy must always be avoided. Some of the most frequent examples are shown here: excessive elevation of the temporal hairline (i.e. sideburn), dislocation of the earlobe (known as the pixie-ear), a step-off of the cervical hairline and traction on the dissected flaps that are not correctly planned.

As previously mentioned, in the round-lifting technique, skin flaps are placed following a very precise vector of traction. Examples of flaps that have been pulled with no attention to the correct direction of traction, with consequent distortion of key anatomical landmarks, can be seen in Fig. 8.

The direction of traction of the facial or anterior flap is determined by a vector that connects the tragus to Darwin's tubercle of the ear, thus preserving the level of the sideburn. The cervical or posterior flap should also be pulled in an equally precise manner, in a superior and slightly anterior vector, preventing any visible interruption of the hairline. The S-shaped incision creates an advancement flap, that prevents a step-off in the cervical hairline, allowing the patient to wear her hair up without revealing the scar. Excessive tension that might cause widened and noticeable scars is avoided by this round-lifting technique (Fig. 9).

The effects of the round-lifting technique were studied by analysing the mechanical forces applied and the displacements produced. The method of finite elements was employed by a team of mechanical engineers; relevant equations were defined using a computer. Human skin was modeled as a pseudo-elastic, isotropic, non-compressible and homogeneous membrane, and a computational study of the fields of displacement and the tension to which the flaps are submitted during a rhytidoplasty demonstrated that the direction of traction creates areas of tension that can be either negative or positive.

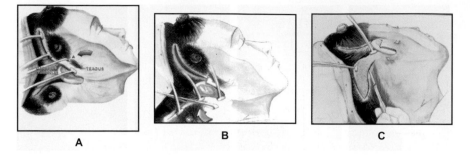

Fig. 9. [A–C] The round lifting technique establishes precise vectors of traction. In A, the facial flap is repositioned following a line that connects the tragus to Darwin's tubercle. In B, the vector of the cervical flap is slightly upwards, to avoid a step-off. In C, the italic-S advancement flap is shown.

These forces ultimately result in the correction of the signs of aging. In this study, the vectors described in the round-lifting technique addressed the main features that suffer distortion with aging while maintaining anatomical parameters. Although there were limitations due to the complexities of human skin (basic properties and individual variations) the study holds a close parallel to a real surgical procedure[17,18] (Fig. 10).

Secondary facial aesthetic surgery always presents with previous scars, and a decision should be made as to which are the most favorable incisions to correct specific areas. Variations of the incisions are chosen depending on the case,

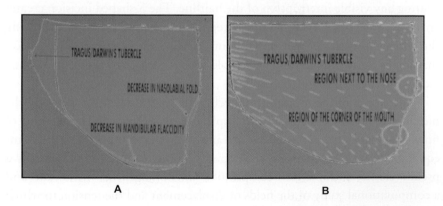

Fig. 10. [A, B] This computer model suggests that the most adequate direction of traction of the flaps is the one described by the round-lifting technique.

SECONDARY FACE-LIFTING

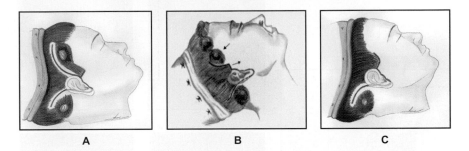

A   **B**   **C**

Fig. 11. [A–C] In secondary face-lifts, the surgeon should be versatile in alternative incisions.

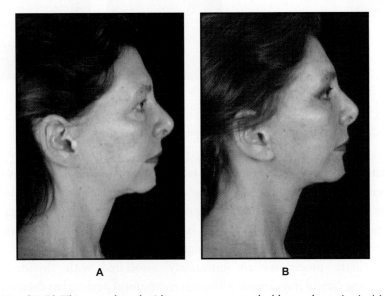

A   **B**

Fig. 12. [A, B] This secondary rhytidectomy was approached by an alternative incision, as demonstrated in Fig. 11B.

with the following goals in mind: treatment of loose skin and tissue flaccidity, resection of scars and maintenance of anatomical landmarks (Figs. 11 to 13).

In some cases, the surgeon will indicate correction of the signs of aging for the upper third of the face (i.e. the forehead). When the forehead is to be treated by the open approach using a coronal incision, it is fundamental

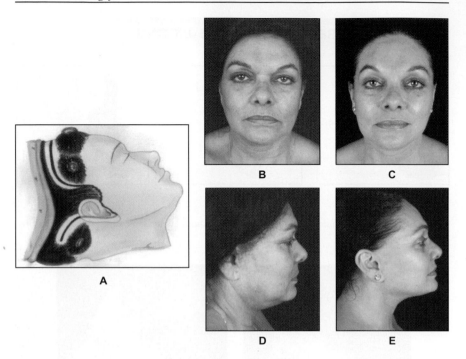

Fig. 13. [A–E] A combined pre-pilose facial incision with a coronal incision avoids a backwards displacement when performing a secondary rhytidectomy.

to first dissect, reposition and fix the facial and cervical flaps. This has been termed as the "block lifting technique", because the facial flaps are blocked before undermining and repositioning of the forehead (Fig. 14). An excessive elevation of the temporal and frontal hairline occurs when these parameters are not respected, resulting in visible signs of a rhytidectomy.[19–23]

Ancillary procedures are intimately associated with rhytidectomy, demanding careful indications. Although mechanical peeling has decreased in frequency, dermabrasion continues to be useful to treat marked facial creases in some patients. Currently, laser peeling can be associated with a facelift, as long as undermined areas are preserved. Chemical peeling is also a useful adjunct for correction of skin lines on the lips. However, this involves some social restrictions because of the prolonged erythema. Scarring of the perioral skin is a disagreeable complication from any of these procedures[24–29] (Fig. 15).

Blepharoplasty is usually indicated in primary facelifts. A common complication is lower eyelid ectropion, caused by excess removal of skin from the

FOREHEAD LIFTING

The "Blocking" Technique

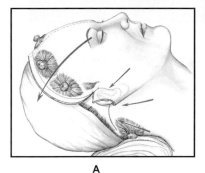

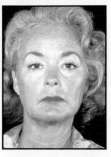

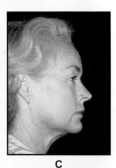

A

B

C

D

E

Fig. 14. [A–E] The blocking technique in a brow lift assures no anatomical alteration by initially positioning the dissected facial flaps before any traction is placed on the forehead.

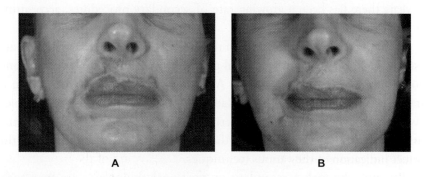

A

B

Fig. 15. [A, B] Any procedure that causes re-epithelialisation (either chemical, by abrasion or by laser) may cause secondary scarring. This patient presented with scars from a chemical peeling performed elsewhere one year previously. She was submitted to scar revision.

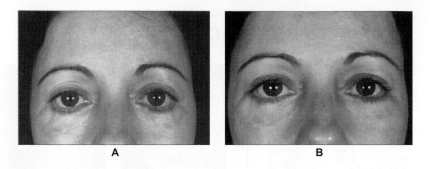

A   B

Fig. 16.   [A, B] Lower lid blepharoplasty may sometimes cause an ectropion, which must be correct by a canthoplasty.

lower lid. A transconjuntival approach for the treatment of lower eyelid fatty pouches together with a laser peel can avoid the frequent laxity of the lower eyelid due to the transcutaneous approach[30,31] (Fig. 16).

The Nose

The difficulties in performing rhinoplasty are of a surgical and artistic nature. With experience, each surgeon will learn the techniques that give the most satisfactory results in his hands. The aim is to produce predictable and constant results. It is the overall harmony of the face that should be ensured when planning for a rhinoplasty. In the senior author's experience, primary rhinoplasties still represent the great majority of patients. Nevertheless, over the last 10 years there has been a growing rate of secondary procedures, accounting for almost 30% of cases (Table 2).

The nose represents the center of the face, and is consequently of primary aesthetic importance. However, nasal physiology is equally fundamental, and should be corrected during surgery. An accurate diagnosis of its function is vital to an effective surgical plan. Radiological evaluation or more complex investigation may be required to determine functional alterations. Familiarity with the anatomy and function of the nose is a fundamental aspect in the correct indication of the various techniques.

Patients who seek a secondary or revisional rhinoplasty are frequently demanding and present a high degree of dissatisfaction. Many have already been submitted to multiple, successive procedures, which demands greater

Table 2. A Noticeable Increase in Secondary Rhinoplasty has been Observed Over the Last Two Decades

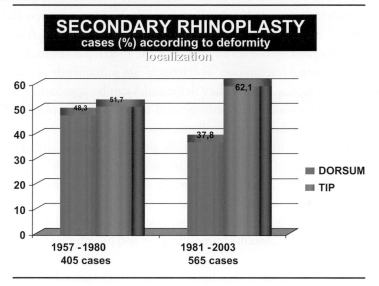

ability from the surgeon. The factors that should be carefully considered are time elapsed since the last procedure, alterations in anatomy, and the psychological disposition of the patient. Anxious patients can sometimes induce a less experienced surgeon to perform a secondary rhinoplasty for small alterations that would normally disappear with regression of residual swelling and natural accomodation of tissues. At least six months (ideally one year) following the last intervention should be allowed before the surgeon makes any decision to perform a revision rhinoplasty. An exception can be made for deformities due to inadequate osteotomies.

The management of postoperative nasal alterations is aided by classifying the observed deformity by regions. In our service, the following system of classification has been found to be useful: deformities due to inadequate or excessive resection of dorsum or nasal tip, incomplete or inappropriate fracture with step deformity or high placement of the osteotomy site, and stenosis of the internal nasal valve subsequent to inadvertently placed incisions affecting the flow of the nasal airways.

A revision of previous fractures is not always necessary, but is indicated when the patient presents a palpable step, a "green-stick" fracture, a severe deviation of the nasal skeleton or an "open roof" deformity. In rare cases, a secondary fracture may be performed in the early postoperative period (i.e. before completing six months). Its correction always requires a new fracture, which should be done lower than the existing line of fracture. A rounded osteotome, designed by the senior author, is the prefered instrument for this manoeuvre. External fractures or "in-fractures" are infrequently performed.

The great majority of secondary deformities can be approached through an intercartilaginous incision, routinely used in primary rhinoplasties. When performed correctly, this allows for all manoeuvres that may be necessary, such as resection of tissue, immobilisation of the nasal framework, and placement of grafts in any region of the nose. Other incisions may be used when they offer easier access to specific areas, or in the event of associated multiple incisions. In our view, open rhinoplasty is reserved for cases where precise preoperative diagnosis cannot be determined with simple inspection and palpation, or when the case demands absolute immobilisation and positioning of the skeletal framework (Fig. 17).

The internal nasal valves should be respected, with care taken to preserve the lining. The symmetry of the remaining alar cartilage should be maintained after resection of any excess. Maintaining the mucoperichondrial flap avoids later retraction and pinching of the nasal alae. When the patient presents with pinching of the nares on forceful inspiration, it reflects a lack of cartilaginous support, and the correction involves placing thin segments of cartilage to reconstruct the missing alar cartilage. Stenosis or constricting bands are corrected by z-plasties, mucosa grafting or other procedures that restore the diameter of the nasal valves.

The relationship between the dorsum and the tip is extremely important. A careful balance must be attained, and this often requires an addition rather than removal of tissues. Autologous cartilage is always used whenever grafting is necessary. Rejection, infection and excessive mobility are frequent complications of implants of any material besides autografts. The senior author prefers the use of cartilage from the concha harvested through a retroauricular access. The anterior and posterior perichondrium of the auricular cartilage are preserved, allowing for neochondrogenesis which avoids any aesthetic sequelae. Care should be taken to remove the cartilage in the form and size deemed adequate for the defect; subsequent shaping is performed with fine and delicate instruments.

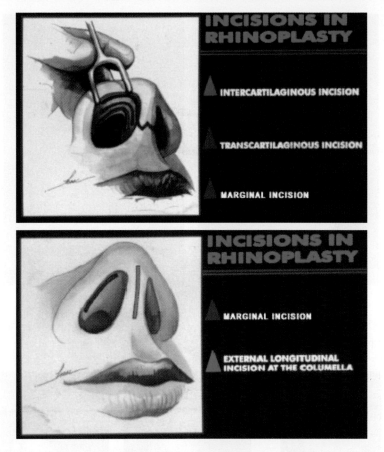

Fig. 17.   [A, B]   Different incisions may be indicated for primary as well as secondary rhinoplasty. It is always important to preserve the integrity of the internal nasal valves.

Tip surgery includes many different shapes of grafts. For small defects a triangular segment of cartilage may be adequate, while correction of the entire tip may require a "swallow wing" graft, a personal contribution described by senior author, providing a very pleasing finishing in overly resected noses (Figs. 18 and 19). Septal cartilage is more brittle and harder to mold correctly, and is obtained only with an associated septoplasty. Its use is reserved for reconstruction of a septal defect or as a support for the nasal tip. All grafts are fixed in place with sutures exiting through the skin; these are removed on the seventh postoperative day along with the protective cast. Defects situated between the tip and the columella may sometimes cause insufficient individuality of the

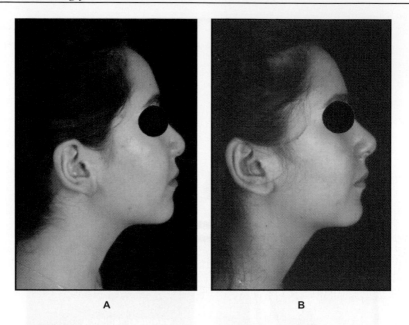

A   **B**

Fig. 18. [A, B] This secondary rhinoplasty was treated by placing cartilage grafts over the nasal tip, to increase the tip's projection.

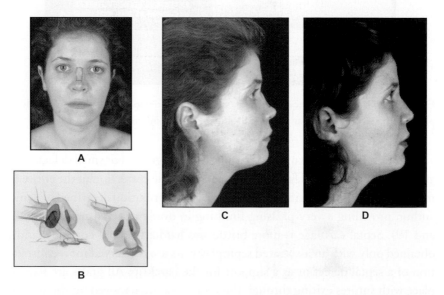

Fig. 19. [A–D] Excessive resection of the dorsum may result in a "saddle-nose" deformity, which will require grafting of autologous tissues. In this case, an appropriately shaped cartilage graft was obtained from the concha, and introduced through an intercartilaginous incision.

tip, despite an appropriate treatment of the dorsum and a pleasant aspect of the tip. These cases demand the placement of a graft to support and achieve a good projection of the tip and a greater definition of the columella. A small graft on the tip may be associated to increase tip distinctness. We routinely liberate the insertion of the depressor muscles with a curved, Fomon's scissors, thus giving greater individuality to the lower third of the nose (Fig. 20).

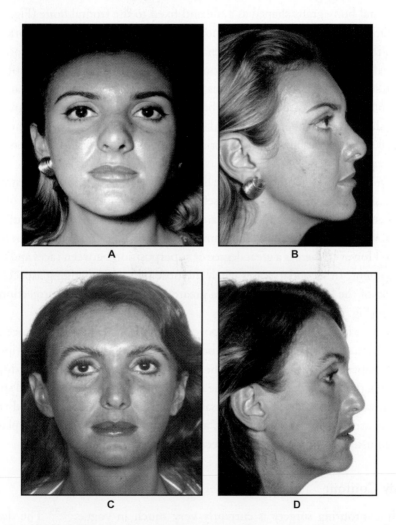

Fig. 20.   [A–D] Obtaining a pleasant balance between the tip and the dorsum was performed in this secondary rhinoplasty, by placement of cartilage grafts.

The resection of the dorsal hump is always done under direct vision, using a strong McIndoe scissors or a sharp osteotome. Alternatively, a rasp may be safer when the sugeon plans for a finer reduction of the dorsum. Opening of the nasal valves with resection of the excess upper lateral cartilages along its superior border is necessary whenever the profile remains irregular following treatment of the bony hump. Small defects of the dorsum are easily corrected by placing cartilage grafts shaped accordingly. Larger defects require the inclusion of a costal bony grafts shaped as a tile and fixed to the frontal bone (Fig. 21).

Despite adequate treatment of the osteocartilaginous nasal framework, the lower third of the bulbous nose often retains a residual "supra-tip" deformity marked by convexity of the tip region. This may be corrected by identifying and resecting the dermocartilaginous ligament, first described by the author in 1965. This structure, which has been identified in various ethnic groups, joins the dermis of the middle third of the nose to the junction of the two medial crura, extending anteroposteriorly to be incorporated in the membranous septum.[32,33]

During primary rhinoplasty, the ligament is routinely sectioned. A system of classification has proven to be useful in determining the thickness of the ligament. Strong Grade I ligaments, are usually present in negroid and bulbous noses, whereas thinner Grade III ligaments are more commonly found in finer noses. However, there is a great degree of superposition between races and type of ligament. In secondary cases when the nose presents a hanging aspect, the cutting of the ligament may confer a greater independence and projection of the tip (Fig. 22).

The external dressing is an important aspect of primary, and especially secondary, rhinoplasty and should be performed carefully. Several strips of sterile paper tapes are placed over the dorsum, starting from the root down. This will press the soft tissues over the nasal framework, preventing dead space and unwanted irregularity of the nasal profile. The tip is neatly covered with thinner strips of paper tape. Finally, a cast is cut from a thermolabile plastic and adjusted over the entire nose, decreasing postoperative oedema.

Body Contour

Body contouring surgery is currently very much in vogue.[34,35] The desire for an athletic body shape reflects today's competitive and fast-paced lifestyle. The rapidly burgeoning industry of health food and nutritional complements,

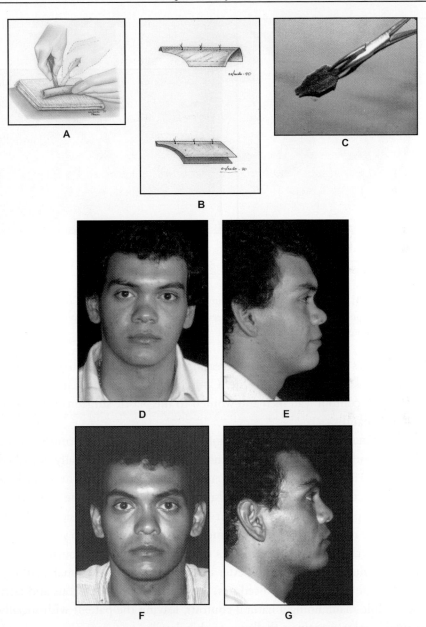

Fig. 21. [A–G] Greater increase in the dorsum may require a bony graft. A small section of a rib is prepared in the shape of a tile, with the necessary dimensions to project the dorsum. This young male patient was submitted to this procedure, secondary to a previous rhinoplasty performed elsewhere that resulted in a severe "saddle-nose" deformity.

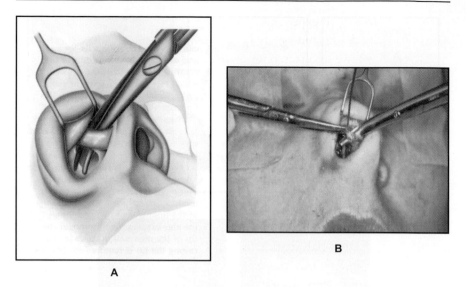

A   B

Fig. 22. [A, B] The dermocartilaginous ligament is situated over the nasal tip, and anchors the tip down; once it is liberated, the tip is seen to attain a slightly greater projection that is more harmonious to the tip-dorsum balance.

fitness centres and spas induce an increasingly large population to seek weight loss and a less sedentary way of life. Consequently, difficulties in defining a leaner body contour lead men and women to the plastic surgeon's office with greater demand.

Excisional techniques for correction of lipodystrophic deformities of the abdomen and trunk, and the upper and lower limbs, were initially described in the early 1960s and have evolved over the years. With the advent of suction-assisted lipectomy in the late 1970s, surgeons finally gained the capacity to "sculpt" the patient's body with greater finesse and minimal incisions, relegating the large removal of excess fat, by means of extensive scars, to very selected cases. Nevertheless, the basic precepts of excisional body contouring procedures continue to expand, with better understanding of functional anatomy. The ultimate goal of these procedures, to remove excess cutaneous and fatty tissue, while maintaining a natural contour, leaving the patient with socially acceptable scars, remains a challenge to this day.[36]

Body contouring surgery is a field where surgical creativity meets anatomical limitations, and where the highly motivated patient frequently encounters the surgeon's reluctance to perform surgery. Dissatisfaction may begin before surgery, as proper indication is perhaps the most important step to avoid an unhappy patient. The experienced surgeon should be able to perceive the patient's hidden desires and weigh the factors that may or may not be realistic.

The unfavorable results in body contouring surgery are always a source of frustration for the surgeon, yet revisions and touch-ups are fall-backs that are commonly performed with greater acceptance in this area of plastic surgery. True complications of any abdominal procedure may require the expertise of the reconstructive plastic surgeon (Fig. 23).

Indeed, body contouring presents the plastic surgeon with many conflicting issues. In today's aesthetically-aware society, patients are almost impelled to correct even the smallest deformity. Furthermore, the dichotomy between ideal form and opposing factors such as weight gain, skin flaccidity and the inevitable aging process become the source of personal frustration. On the other hand, increasing leisure time and sports activities result in the constant exposure of the body. Body contour deformities may involve aspects regarding the patient's psycho-social status and overall health, and the surgeon must always consider the possible benefits of a multidisciplinary team approach.

Although suction-assisted lipectomy has become a standard operation for the removal of localised excess fat, it should not be considered as a simple procedure. No more than 7% of the total body weight should be removed in one single session. When associated with other excisional surgery, areas that have been undermined must not be aspirated to avoid compromising the vascularity of the flap. This is particularly relevant when complementing an abdominoplasty with liposuction.

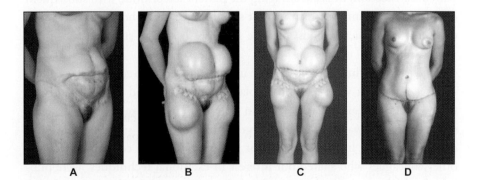

    A   B   C   D

Fig. 23. [A–D] In this case, following a gynecological procedure, the patient suffered loss of the superficial layer of the abdominal wall. Reconstruction may require the use of tissue expander for advancement of flaps. This was achieved and the flaps advanced successfully.

The grossly overweight patient, those with unrealistic expectations, or whose motivation is centered on the will of others should be discouraged from surgery. Although liposuction has greatly decreased the indications for dermolipectomies, skin cutaneous excess requires skin removal with the necessary implication of permanent scars, and this should be explained to the patient. Once the location and extension of final scars is described, it is helpful to draw these with a marker pen before surgery.

Our routine in preparing for surgery includes complete clinical and laboratory exams. When two or more simultaneous procedures are planned and a greater blood loss is expected autologous blood transfusion begins at least two weeks prior to surgery. A well-coordinated surgical team is essential to optimise the operative time. The anesthesiologists should be familiarised with the frequently long duration of the operation and the different stages of surgery, as some procedures require that the patient be placed in different positions.

Finally, it should be remembered that although these deformities may be treated by a single operation they sometimes demand more complex, combined procedures. Multiple or severe deformities, such as in patients who have undergone dramatic weight loss, will require a multistage plan. Body contouring in these cases should be considered a surgical program, consequently a second and even a third stage will be seen as part of the continuum. Above all, the full participation of the patient is to be stimulated. This is especially true in cases where more than one operation is indicated, the order of which is an important aspect to be decided. It is a good strategy to begin the surgical program by addressing those areas that present with the greater possibility of patient satisfaction, thus encouraging the patient to continue with subsequent operations. In summary, each patient should have his or her intimate desires evaluated and, wherever possible, the surgeon should be supportive of these motivations.

Excisional techniques that were in use over 40 years ago commonly resulted in large scars that widened and displaced with time, and whose final position was aesthetically unacceptable in many cases. For example, contouring of the abdomen was restricted to large deformities, with simple resection of excess tissues and limited concern for function. Personal contributions with other colleagues who shared our interest in excisional techniques, were published, which emphasised respect for the anatomy and the dynamics of areas presenting with contour deformities.[37–45]

These tenets, applied to trochanteric lipodystrophy and the "riding breeches" deformity, included limiting dissection to those tissues to be resected, curving incisions to camouflage scars better, and rotating the flaps rather than simply pulling on them. It was understood that direct traction leads to high tension, and when this is applied to the skin-dermis unit, will cause the well-known drawbacks of widened scars and distortion of sanatomy. In contrast, rotation implies a repositioning of the tissues. When this is done together with meticulous suturing in layers, which includes the superficial fascial system, tension is removed from the skin (Fig. 24).

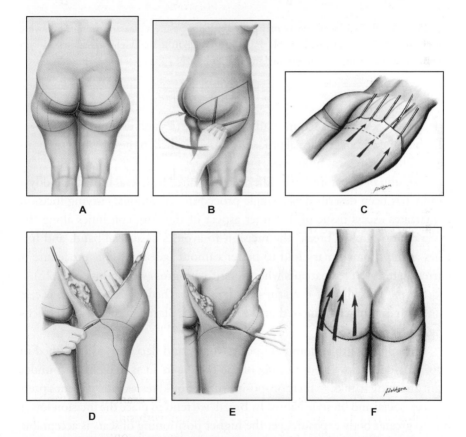

Fig. 24. [A–F] The "riding breeches" deformity is currently corrected by liposuction, sometimes in stages to allow for skin accommodation. The traditional, excisional approach, as described by the senior author, was based on a rotation, rather than pulling, of the dissected flaps, before resection of excess tissue.

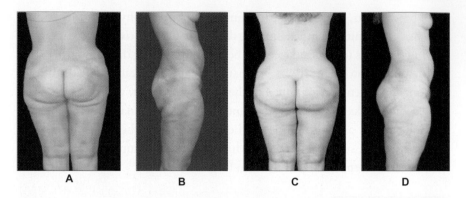

Fig. 25. [A–D] Excisional surgery may be indicated to assure a pleasant contour following liposuction. In this case, an unfavorable result of liposuction to the thighs was addressed with removal of excess tissue, as demonstrated in Figs. 24A–24F.

Some cases of liposuction result in irregularities and excess skin coverage. This may require an excisional procedure, as described in the era when suction-assisted lipectomy was unknown (Fig. 25).

Excision of upper limb flaccidity accompanied by lateral thoracic lipodystrophy has been described as a single procedure. A sinuous, curving incision demarcates excess tissue of the inner aspect of the arm, continues along the axilla taking care to "break" the incision to avoid a cicatricial band, and finishes at the submammary fold to better camouflage scars. This procedure is currently reserved for patients who present with gross weight loss (Fig. 26).

Simple flaccidity of the arm may be approached by resection of excess skin, with careful planning so that the final scar is placed in the bicipital sulcus (Fig. 27).

The approach to abdominal lipodystrophy and flaccidity, as described in 1967, includes a lower positioning of the final scars so as to be hidden under scanty bathing trunks.[38] Incision-positioning should respect the patient's preferences, social and lifestyle habits. In Brazil, we tend to place the incision lower due to greater body exposure, yet the higher positioning of scars is acceptable if this is planned with the participation of the patient.

The dissection of the abdominal wall is restricted to the central portion, leaving the flanks to be treated with liposuction. Plication of the rectus abdominis aponeurosis is done with inverted non-absorbable suture, without opening

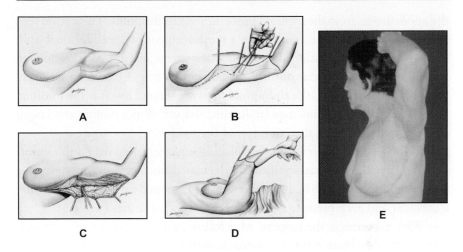

Fig. 26. [A–E] The thoraco-brachial dermolipectomy may still find an indication when treating excess tissue of the lateral chest and arm following massive weight loss.

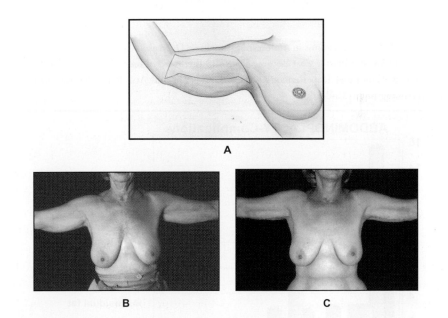

Fig. 27. [A–C] Simple laxity of the arm may require resection of excess tissue, as shown in the drawing.

the aponeurosis, from the xyphoid process down to the pubis. This causes tension towards the midline, resulting in a reinforcement of the abdominal wall. The umbilicus is repositioned through a transverse incision that, following tension on the flaps, is transformed into a smooth ring. Once they are ready for the final positioning, the abdominal flaps are rotated towards the midline, causing the lateral abdomen to be further shaped, thus avoiding the lateral dog-ears and decreasing the extension of the final scar.

It has been our observation that placing a plaster mold over a thick, soft dressing over the flap has significantly decreased our rate of serosanguinous collection. In the first 48 h, a small weight is positioned on this shield, so that a constant and even pressure is exerted over dissected tissues (Table 3).

With experience, the surgeon who follows these principles of excisional surgery should obtain a natural contour, with infrequent complications and acceptable final scars. A solid knowledge and respect for anatomy and a keen aesthetic sense cannot be overstressed. We have felt rewarded in these contributions by the high degree of patient satisfaction, and also by the results

Table 3.   Complications in Abdominoplasty have Decreased Considerably Since the Placement of a Plaster Cast Became Routine; the Steady Pressure Over the Undermined Abdominal Flap Remains for the First 48 h, and Avoids the Formation of Serosanguinous Collection

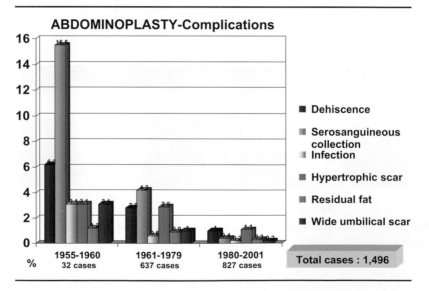

reported by colleagues who have comprehended these principles. Body contouring is often performed in association with other aesthetic procedures, and the preparation of an expert surgical team is essential.[46–48]

REFERENCES

1. Pitanguy I. (1996) Complications in aesthetic surgery: what experience has taught us over the years. *Lecture, 2nd International Symposium*, Eilat, Israel.
2. Pitanguy I. (1983) *Les Chemins de la Beauté. Un Maitre de la Chirurgie Plastique Témoigne* (J.C.Lattes, Paris).
3. Pitanguy I. (1979) The aging face. In: Carlsen L, Slatt B (eds.), *The Naked Face* (General Publishing, Ontario), p. 27.
4. Pitanguy I. (1991) Aging face surgery. In: Stucker FJ (ed.), *Plastic and Reconstructive Surgery of Head and Neck* (B.C. Decker, Philadelphia), p. 145.
5. Pitanguy I. (1993) Aging face surgery. *Symposium on Aesthetic Surgery of the Aging Face. A Major Course of the American Academy of Facial Plastic and Reconstructive Surgery*, March 3–7, Indianapolis, William H. Beeson (Course Director).
6. Pitanguy I, Ceravolo M. (1981) Hematoma postrhytidectomy: how we treat it. *Plast Reconstr Surg* 67: 526–528.
7. Pitanguy I, Ramos A. (1966) The frontal branch of the facial nerve: the importance of its variation in the face-lifting. *Plast Reconstr Surg* 38: 352–356.
8. Pitanguy I. (1980) Upper facial nerve anatomy and forehead lift. *Symposium on Problems and Complications in Aesthetic Plastic Surgery of the Face* (Monterrey, California), p. 45.
9. Pitanguy I, Ceravolo MP, Dègand M. (1980) Nerve injuries during rhytidectomy: considerations after 3203 cases. *Aesth Plast Surg* 4: 257–265.
10. Pitanguy I. (1967) La ritidoplastica: soluzione eclettica del problema. *Ediz Minerva Med* 22: 942–947.
11. Pitanguy I. (1984) The face. In: *Aesthetic Surgery of Head and Body* (Springer Verlag, Berlin), pp. 165–200.
12. Pitanguy I. (1987) Rhytidoplastik: perioperative richtlinien. *Laryngol Rhinol Otol* 66: 586–590.
13. Pitanguy I, Brentano JMS, Salgado F, Radwanski HN, Carpeggiani R. (1995) Incisions in primary and secondary rhytidoplasties. *Rev Bras Cir* 85: 165–176.
14. Pitanguy I, Radwanski HN, Amorim NFG. (1999) Treatment of the aging face using the "round-lifting" technique. *Aesth Surg J* 19: 3, 216–222.
15. Pitanguy I. (2000) Facial cosmetic surgery: a 30-year perspective. *Plast Reconstr Surg* 105: 1517–1526.

16. Pitanguy I, Salgado F, Radwanski HN. (1995) Submental liposuction as an ancillary procedure in face-lifting. *FACE* **4**(1): 1–13.

17. Pitanguy I, Pamplona DC, Giuntini ME, Salgado F, Radwanski HN. (1995) Computational simulation of rhytidectomy by the "round-lifting" technique. *Rev Bras Cir* **85**: 213–218.

18. Pitanguy I, Pamplona DC, Weber HI, Leta F, Salgado F, Radwanski HN. (1998) Numerical modeling of the aging face. *Plast Reconstr Surg* **102**: 200–204.

19. Pitanguy I. (1979) Frontalis-procerus-corrugator apponeurosis in the correction of frontal and glabellar wrinkles. *Ann Plast Surg* **2**: 422–427.

20. Pitanguy I. (1981) Indication for and treatment of frontal and glabellar wrinkles in an analysis of 3404 consecutive cases of rhitidectomy. *Plast Reconstr Surg* **67**: 157–166.

21. Pitanguy I. (1984) The forehead lift: problems and complications. Comments on chapter. In: Goldwyn RM (ed.), *The Unfavorable Result in Plastic Surgery*, 2nd edn. (Little, Brown and Co., Boston), Vol. 1, pp. 626–629.

22. Pitanguy I. (1984) Forehead lifting. In: *Aesthetic Surgery of Head and Body* (Springer Verlag, Berlin), pp. 202–214.

23. Pitanguy I, Radwanski HN. (1997) Rejuvenation of the brow. In: Matarasso SL, Matarasso A (eds.), *Dermatology Clinics* (W.B. Saunders, Philadelphia), Vol. 15, pp. 623–635.

24. Pitanguy I. (1978) Ancillary procedures in face-lifting. *Clin Plast Surg* **5**: 51–69.

25. Pitanguy I. (1968) Augmentation mentoplasty. *Plast Reconstr Surg* **42**: 460–464.

26. Pitanguy I. (1984) Chin problems. *Symposium on Problems and Complications in Aesthetic Plastic Surgery of the Face*, Toronto.

27. Pitanguy I, Muller P, Kauak L, Freitas L. (1988) Remodeling incisions of the earlobe. *Rev Bras Cir* **78**: 149–154.

28. Pitanguy I, Amorim NFG. (1997) Treatment of the nasolabial fold. *Rev Bras Cir* **87**: 231–242.

29. Pitanguy I, Soares G, Machado BH, de Amorim NF. (1999) CO_2 laser associated with the "round-lifting" approach. *J Cutan Laser Ther* **1**: 145–152.

30. Pitanguy I, Caldeira A, Alexandrino A. (1985) Blepharoplasty: personal experience with 4564 consecutive cases. *Ophthal Plast Reconstr Surg* **1**: 9–22.

31. Pitanguy I. (1988) Die operative behandlung des schweren unterlid-ektropiums mit einem transplantat aus haut und aperichondrium. *Klin Monatsbl Augenheilkd* **193**: 207–210.

32. Pitanguy I. (1965) Surgical importance of a dermocartilaginous ligament in bulbous noses. *Plast Reconstr Surg* **36**: 247–252.

33. Pitanguy I, Salgado F, Radwanski HN, Bushkin SC. (1995) The surgical importance of the dermocartilaginous ligament of the nose. *Plast Reconstr Surg* **95**: 790–794.

34. Pitanguy I. (1987) Body contour. *Am J Cosmet Surg* 4: 283–293.
35. Pitanguy I. (2000) Evaluation of body contouring surgery today: a 30-year perspective. *Plast Reconstr Surg* 105: 1499–1514.
36. Pitanguy I. (2001) Body contouring with excisions. In: Goldwyn RM, Cohen MN (eds.), *The Unfavorable Result in Plastic Surgery*, 3rd edn. (Lippincott Williams and Wilkins, Philadelphia), pp. 1158–1165.
37. Pitanguy I. (1964) Trochanteric lipodystrophy. *Plast Reconstr Surg* 34: 280–286.
38. Pitanguy I. (1967) Abdominal lipectomy: an approach to it through an analysis of 300 consecutive cases. *Plast Reconstr Surg* 40(4): 384–391.
39. Pitanguy I. (1972) Thigh lift and abdominal lipectomy. In: Goldwyn RM (ed.), *Unfavorable Results in Plastic Surgery* (Little Brown, Boston), p. 387.
40. Pitanguy I. (1973) Lipectomy, abdominoplasty and lipodistrophy of the inner side of the arm. In: Grabb W, Smith J (eds.), *Plastic Surgery: A Concise Guide to Clinical Practice*, 2nd edn. (Little Brown, Boston), pp. 1005–1013.
41. Pitanguy I. (1975) Abdominal lipectomy. *Clin Plast Surg* 2: 401–410.
42. Pitanguy I. (1975) Correction of lipodystrophy of the lateral thoracic aspect and inner side of the arm and elbow dermossenescence. *Clin Plast Surg* 2(3): 477–483.
43. Pitanguy I. (1977) Dermolipectomy of the abdominal wall, thighs, buttocks and upper extremity. In: Converse JM (ed.), *Reconstructive Plastic Surgery*, 2nd edn. (Saunders, Philadelphia), Vol. 7, pp. 3800–3823.
44. Pitanguy I. (1989) Thigh and buttock lift. In: Lewis JR (ed.), *The Art of Aesthetic Surgery* (Little Brown, Boston), Vol. 2, pp. 1060–1067.
45. Pitanguy I. (1995) Abdominoplasty: classification and surgical techniques. *Rev Bras Cir* 85: 23–44.
46. Pitanguy I, Cavalcanti MA. (1978) Methodology in combined aesthetic surgeries. *Aesth Plast Surg* 2: 331–340.
47. Pitanguy I. (1981) Combined aesthetic procedures. In: *Aesthetic Plastic Surgery of Head and Body* (Springer-Verlag, Berlin), pp. 353–359.
48. Pitanguy I, Ceravolo M. (1983) Our experience with combined procedures in aesthetic plastic surgery. *Plast Reconstr Surg* 71(1): 56–63.

Chapter 24

COMPLICATIONS OF MINIMALLY INVASIVE SURGERY

Rajesh Aggarwal, Shabnam Undre and Ara Darzi

INTRODUCTION

Minimal access surgical techniques are now considered to be the gold standard for biliary, anti-reflux and bariatric surgery.[1–3] This is mainly due to improved patient recovery with reduced pain, shorter hospital stay and a quicker return to normal daily activities.[4,5] This approach is also more cost effective to community healthcare once the initial investment in instruments and devices have been made.[6–8]

Following the first laparoscopic cholecystectomy, performed by Phillipe Mouret in 1987,[9] there were a large number of surgeons attempting this new technique. Indeed, many of the early operations were fuelled by strong public demand[10] and supported by commercial companies. However, it was not long before hospitals and surgical societies noted the increased rates of complications associated with these new techniques[11]; there were reports of bowel and aortic

Table 1.   Difficulties Associated with Laparoscopic Surgery

Long rigid surgical instruments amplify tremor
Reduced degrees of freedom
Fulcrum effect
Bimanual dexterity
2D to 3D visual ability — depth perception
Altered hand-eye-target axis

injury,[12,13] and even death in patients undergoing procedures which had been relatively risk free when performed in the traditional open manner.

The reason for the high rate of initial complications was the failure to recognise that the adoption of minimally invasive techniques for cholecystectomy required the surgeon to learn new skills (Table 1). Indeed, the skills acquired in open surgery have not led to an improved performance in the laparoscopic arena.[14] Hence all the surgeons were effectively novices in this field, regardless of their previous surgical experience. Furthermore, there was a learning curve associated with the acquisition of new skills, and many of the complications occurred due to a lack of initial training. Once a surgeon had passed beyond the learning curve, the complication rates were visibly reduced.[15]

This chapter aims to highlight the complications occurring from the introduction of minimal access surgery. It is divided into intraoperative complications, which may occur during any laparoscopic procedure, followed by a discussion of the physiological considerations with the patient, prior to obtaining consent for the operation. Specific complications related to biliary surgery are considered, along with the management strategies for bile duct injuries. This is followed by the reasons for conversion, culminating in a section on long-term complications of laparoscopic techniques.

INTRAOPERATIVE COMPLICATIONS

Due to the unconventional and unnatural surgical environment imposed by minimal access surgery, the majority of complications occur during the operative procedure. These are also the most serious, and can be divided into occurrence directly from the surgical procedure or from altered physiology due to an insufflated abdomen.

Complications of Access

The first major difference in performing a laparoscopic procedure, as opposed to open surgical techniques, is the need to enter the abdominal cavity through an incision no larger than 1–2 cm in length. This is achieved by incising through or around the umbilicus, and involves the use of either the Verres needle (Fig. 1) or Hasson port (Fig. 2) techniques.

The closed entry technique was developed by Janos Veress (1938) and involves a sharp needle entering into the peritoneal cavity. The surgeon makes an incision through the skin and subcutaneous fat, which is followed by grasping the anterior abdominal wall to lift it away from the underlying bowel. The device, which is no more than 2 mm in diameter and consists of a blunt hollow obturator inside a sharp needle, is then thrust through the remaining layers of

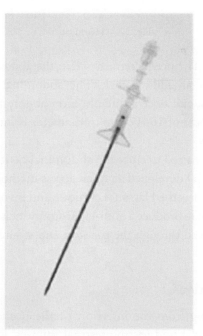

Fig. 1.   Veress needle.

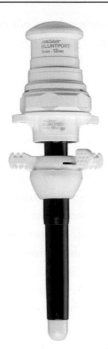

Fig. 2.   Hasson port.

the abdominal wall. The needle retracts when the abdominal cavity has been reached indicated by an audible click. The abdominal cavity is then insufflated with CO_2 gas, and once a suitable intra-abdominal pressure has been achieved, a sharp trocar of 10–12 mm in diameter is introduced blindly into the abdominal cavity.

To counteract the need to enter the abdominal cavity in a closed manner, Harrith Hasson (1971) developed an open access method of entry.[16] This has now been popularised as the Hasson technique and involves incising all layers of the abdominal wall to produce a mini-laparotomy incision. The blunt-ended port is then introduced through the incision and secured by two supporting sutures.

Vascular complications

Complications arising from the insertion of the primary port account for the majority of vascular and gastrointestinal injuries, leading to a mortality risk of 0.2%.[17] Vascular injuries are most catastrophic when they involve the great vessels that lie retroperitoneally, and require immediate conversion to laparotomy.[18] The estimated incidence of such major vascular injuries is 0.04–0.5%,[19] the wide variation possibly due to factors such as experience of the surgeon, difficulty of the cases and mode of access. The most common site of life-threatening injuries was the aorta (23%), followed by the vena cava (15%).[20]

In comparing the two methods of access, there are conflicting views on their safety. The closed technique is more popular,[21] although recent articles report that the Veress needle carries a higher risk of injury than the open technique.[22] A large Dutch review compared the incidence of major vascular injury in 489,335 patients operated upon using the closed technique, with that of 12,444 patients undergoing open laparoscopy.[23] The incidence of major vascular injury was 0.075% and 0% respectively.

A suggested alternative to the Veress needle is the use of optical access devices (Visiport, United States Surgical, Norwalk, CT, USA and Optiview, Ethicon Endosurgery, Cincinatti, OH, USA). These may provide a degree of safety by enabling the operator to insert a sharp but hollow trocar through the anterior abdominal wall with a laparoscope positioned within it. However, an FDA report of these two devices described 37 major vascular injuries and four resultant deaths.[24] Thus, the safety of these ports which are designed to protect vessels must be questioned.

Another important point is the time of diagnosis of a major vascular injury. Due to the retroperitoneal nature of the major vessels, it may not be until the end of the operation or even in the recovery room that the symptoms are manifested and the diagnosis made. Therefore, it is important to ensure that the laparoscope is introduced into the abdominal cavity in a vertical fashion to visualise any vascular or organ damage directly below the site of entry.

Vascular injury may also occur to the vessels of the abdominal wall, usually at the position of the accessory ports, and can lead to significant morbidity.[25] The injury may occur while inserting the accessory port, or at the end of the procedure when the incision is widened to remove tissue from the abdominal cavity. Such injuries may be a nuisance leading to leakage into the operative field or postoperative bruising. However, there is a possibility of continued haemorrhage once the port has been removed, which may require a return to the operating theatre. It is important to ensure visualisation of all incision sites while removing the ports at the end of the procedure. Persistent bleeding can be attended to by placing a heavy suture or balloon catheter to provide continued tamponade. The latter is introduced into the abdominal cavity through the bleeding trocar site wound, the balloon is inflated, and traction is placed on the catheter which is bolstered in place to keep it under tension. The balloon can be removed prior to patient discharge.

Gastrointestinal complications

Bowel injuries occur mostly during access, and seldom during dissection or adhesiolysis. The injury may occur with the open or closed techniques, and is more likely in a patient who has had previous abdominal surgery or peritonitis that has resulted in the fixation of the bowel to the undersurface of the anterior abdominal wall. The reported incidence of visceral injury is 0.083% with the closed technique and 0.048% with the open technique.[23] The bowel can be injured through penetration, and may be followed by insufflation if a Veress needle is used. An increased reading on the pressure gauge of the insufflating device is indicative of such an injury. However, the majority of bowel injuries remain undetected during the operation, presenting postoperatively as systemic upset, peritonitis, enterocutaneous fistulae or death.[26,27] Prevention begins by awareness of such injuries, trocar placement under direct vision, and additional care for patients with an increased likelihood of bowel adhesions.

Major Organ Damage

It is possible to damage any organ within the abdominal cavity, and this may occur during the insertion of ports or during the specified procedure. Bowel damage has been discussed, and the most common organs to be injured are liver, bladder and spleen.

Liver damage is generally regarded as a complication of laparoscopic cholecystectomy; it may also occur during laparoscopic fundoplication, right-sided nephrectomy or adrenalectomy. Such injuries tend to cause bleeding and can usually be managed through diathermy of the area, but may necessitate conversion. In a meta-analysis performed by Shea *et al.*, 112 of 1400 patients required conversion due to bleeding (8%).[28] Bleeding from the liver is more often a problem in patients suffering from liver cirrhosis, and reports are conflicting as to whether this is a contraindication to laparoscopic surgery.[29–31]

The general policy, in view of the advantages to the patient, is to have an expert surgeon who has a low threshold for conversion.

Bladder injury has a reported incidence of 0.5% in general surgical procedures, and 2% in gynaecology.[32] The introduction of laparoscopic hernia repair may also contribute to bladder injury with a recent review reporting eight cases from a total of 5203 repairs (0.2%).[33] Though rare, splenic injury may be a sequalae of either laparoscopic fundoplication,[34] or left sided adrenalectomy.[35]

Electrosurgical Injuries in Laparoscopy

The overall incidence of recognised electrosurgical injuries is between 1–2 patients per 1000 operations.[36] The majority of these injuries remain unrecognised at the time of operation, and involve an inadvertent perforation to the bowel. The main causes are inadvertent touching or grasping a tissue during current application, more so when the tip of the instrument is out of the laparoscopic field of view. Direct coupling between a portion of the intestine and a metal probe that is in contact with the active probe may also lead to injury. The injuries are more likely to occur when monopolar diathermy is used and bipolar diathermy should be recommended in anatomically crowded areas.

Nerve Damage During Laparoscopic Surgery

Intraoperative nerve injuries are generally noticed in the postoperative period. In the laparoscopic anti-reflux surgery, damage to the vagus nerve can present as severe intractable diarrhoea.[37] Similarly, laparoscopically assisted rectal resection is associated with a higher rate of pelvic nerve injury when compared to the open approach, leading to higher rates of male sexual dysfunction.[38]

A major morbidity from open inguinal hernia repair has been damage to the inguinal nerves and subsequent chronic groin pain. One study reported a 6% incidence of severe pain leading to restricted daily function following an open hernia repair.[39] Recent randomised controlled trials of laparoscopic versus open inguinal hernia repair have reported significantly lower rates of chronic inguinal pain,[40–42] and this may be further reduced in the laparoscopic group by using a large mesh without staple fixation.[43]

PHYSIOLOGICAL CONSIDERATIONS IN LAPAROSCOPIC SURGERY

During laparoscopic surgery, the intraabdominal pressure is maintained between 10–12 mm Hg, enabling the anterior abdominal wall to be lifted and visualisation of the necessary structures. In obese patients, it may be necessary to maintain a greater pressure to overcome the extra weight of the anterior abdominal wall. In physiological terms, the CO_2 pneumoperitoneum also places pressure on the abdominal organs and vessels leading to an increase in total peripheral resistance and subsequent central venous pressure. The Trendelenberg position adopted during surgery on the upper abdomen further exacerbates this situation be reducing venous return, cardiac output and blood pressure. These changes are insignificant in most individuals, but can lead to serious haemodynamic consequences in patients with underlying cardiac disease.

Patients with a compromised respiratory function are also vulnerable during laparoscopic surgery as the increased intraabdominal pressure can lead to respiratory embarrassment. Therefore, it may be necessary to reduce the intraabdominal pressure in these patients, to perhaps a value of 8–10 mm Hg. However, this can make the operation more difficult as the surgeon is performing under sub-optimal conditions, and has the propensity to lead to other procedure-specific complications.

A recent paper by Alijani *et al.* describes the technique of abdominal wall lift to counteract the unwanted respiratory and cardiac effects of positive pressure pneumoperitoneum.[44] This involves the creation of an intraabdominal workspace by elevating the anterior abdominal wall with an external mechanical lift device, and avoids the fall in cardiac output associated with standard insufflation techniques. However, the technique also makes it more difficult to perform the procedure, as evidenced by a greater number of errors when compared with the standard technique.

The anaesthetist and surgeon should also be aware of other complications related to the laparoscopic procedure such as gas embolism, pneumothorax and mediastinal emphysema, but further discussion is beyond the scope of this chapter.

BILIARY COMPLICATIONS

The spectrum of biliary complications varies from the common occurrence of perforation of the gallbladder and spilled gallstones to biliary leaks and the most serious of all, common bile duct injury.

Perforation of the gallbladder

The incidence is reported in the range of 10–40%, and occurs more frequently than during open cholecystectomy.[45] These rates are probably related to the experience level of the surgeon, and perhaps more importantly to the degree of inflammation.[46] The perforation of the gallbladder necessitates no more than a thorough washout at the end of the procedure, and the placement of the gallbladder in a bag prior to removal from the abdominal cavity. If the perforation is small, it may be possible to use a clip to seal it, preventing further leakage of bile.

The bile leak may be accompanied by a spillage of gallstones into the abdominal cavity. These should be removed intraoperatively and a thorough washout performed at the end of the procedure. However, any remaining stones are unlikely to cause major problems and it is not necessary to convert to an open procedure. A retrospective analysis of 10,174 laparoscopic cholecystectomies revealed that 581 cases (5.7%) were complicated by spilled gallstones, but only eight of these (1.4%) developed any serious postoperative complications.[47] The most frequently occurring complication is abscess formation, but small bowel obstruction, incarceration in a hernia sac, and trans-diaphragmatic migration have also been reported.[48] These diagnoses should be considered in any patient presenting with chronic abdominal sepsis following laparoscopic cholecystectomy, even if the original procedure was months or years ago. The treatment is based on clinical and radiological findings and may involve antibiotics, percutaneous drainage, or definitive surgical stone retrieval and abscess evacuation.

Biliary leak

A patient exhibiting a delayed recovery following laparoscopic cholecystectomy should undergo an ultrasound examination, which may confirm the presence

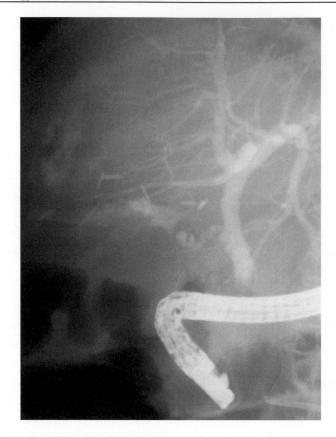

Fig. 3.   Endoscopic retrograde cholangiogram of an inadequately clipped cystic duct.

of a biloma, secondary to a biliary leak. The leak may originate from insufficient closure of the cystic duct stump (Fig. 3), or an aberrant accessory duct. The management of such a complication requires a multidisciplinary approach entailing an expert endoscopist, radiologist and surgeon to place a stent by ERCP, or a trans-abdominal drain. In severe cases leading to peritonitis, a laparotomy is the procedure of choice.

Bile duct injury

The majority of studies on open cholecystectomy reported bile duct injury rates of between 0.125% and 0.25%.[49,50] Bile duct injuries are serious complications, the incidence showing a marked rise to 2–4% after the introduction of laparoscopic cholecystectomy.[51–53] However, later series have shown this figure to return to 0.2–0.8%,[54–56] but it remains higher than in open surgery. The most recent review of 1522 cases revealed an incidence of 0.59%, while a questionnaire survey of 91,232 procedures in Brazilian centres reported a considerably lower incidence of 0.18%.[57] The higher rates in laparoscopic surgery have been attributed to the learning curve of inexperienced surgeons, inability to obtain good exposure of Calot's triangle and poor visualisation of the anatomy of the biliary tree when observed through a laparoscope. Learning curve studies have attempted to define a number of procedures beyond which bile duct injury is less common, but conflicting results have been reported.[26,58,59]

Injuries most commonly occur due to wrong identification of the common bile duct as the cystic duct and subsequent division (Fig. 4).[60,61] This may be due to an aberrant anatomical configuration, such as an unidentified cystic duct originating from the right hepatic duct leading to transaction of the hepatic duct. The more common situation of misidentification occurs when there is extensive inflammation within Calot's triangle. An intraoperative cholangiogram may enable clarification prior to the division of a structure, although one study of 46 bile duct injuries found that 11 of 16 cholangiograms were misinterpreted, and the injury type and severity was similar whether or not the cholangiogram had been performed.[62] Furthermore, a total of 80% of the injuries were noted postoperatively, with an average delay in diagnosis of ten days.

To be able to diagnose and manage a biliary injury, it is necessary to be aware of the strategies for classification. The Bismuth classification was developed prior to the advent of laparoscopic surgery and is still used.[63] More recently, the Strasberg,[64] McMahon,[65] Neuhaus[66] and Siewert[67] systems have been proposed. They vary in complexity and whether clinical and therapeutic aspects are incorporated, but essentially there is a gradation from accessory duct damage through to occlusion of the common bile duct.

It is generally accepted that the repair of a bile duct injury should be performed by an experienced biliary surgeon for the best results.[68] This implies that the patients operated upon by general surgeons should be transferred to a biliary centre for further management.[53] The procedure of choice for transection of the common bile duct is a biliary-enteric anastomosis such as a Roux-en-Y choledochojejunostomy, though a minor laceration may be sutured after insertion of a T-tube drain beside the anastomosis.

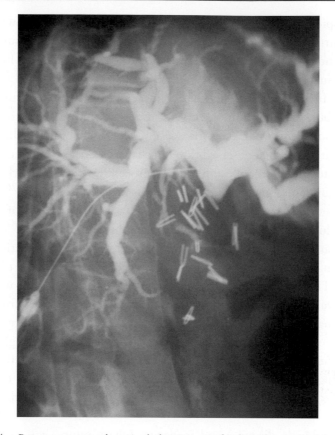

Fig. 4.   Percutaneous transhepatic cholangiogram of a clipped common bile duct.

If the complication is noted postoperatively, the initial procedure of choice is an endoscopic retrograde cholangiogram (ERC) to define the problem. If the injury is minor, such as an injury to an accessory duct, it is preferable to treat with placement of a biliary stent and repeat the ERC in six weeks time. Surgical intervention is warranted if the injury involves transection of a duct.

The incidence of a concomitant vascular injury in case of bile duct injury is very high, and may be due to aberrant anatomical configurations.[69] The management of the combined injury is unclear, ranging from intraoperative ligation to performing an angiogram prior to reconstruction.[70–72] Bile duct injury is a serious complication of laparoscopic cholecystectomy, and inadequate repair may lead to further complications such as secondary biliary cirrhosis, liver failure and death.[73]

Biliary stricture

A late complication of biliary surgery, biliary strictures may either be the result of reconstructive surgery or ischaemia caused by excessive use of electrocautery in the area of the common bile duct.[74] Its diagnosis is by cholangiography — MRI-based, endoscopic or percutaneous — and treatment is by balloon dilatation or biliary stenting.[75] Some authors suggest a surgical approach with a biliary-enteric anastomosis.[52]

CONVERSION TO AN OPEN PROCEDURE

The conversion to an open procedure is a standard risk of every laparoscopic operation, and must be communicated to every patient during the process of informed consent. Indeed, if the patient cannot tolerate an open procedure, they should not be offered a laparoscopic operation. Furthermore, the surgeon should possess the competency required to perform the procedure using an open approach.

The main reasons for conversion to an open procedure are bleeding from a major vessel, damage to a structure requiring repair of the laparotomy, or a procedure which is too difficult or dangerous to proceed with a laparoscopy. A further reason for conversion may be failure on the part of the patient to tolerate the laparoscopic procedure, in terms of low cardiorespiratory reserves.

LATE COMPLICATIONS OF LAPAROSCOPIC SURGERY

The immediate postoperative success of a laparoscopic surgery is by and large carried through to improved long-term outcomes for all patients. However, laparoscopic techniques have led to the development of new complications, which tend to present months or years after the initial surgery. The two most common, and most apparent, are related to the port-sites.

Port Site Herniae

Port site herniae develop when the fascia at either site is not closed adequately with sutures because of insufficient vision through the small incision and the risk of inadvertent injury to the tissues underlying the fascia. The reported incidence varies from 1–6%.[76] It is generally accepted that port-sites greater than 10 mm should undergo fascial closure, and this may lead to a reduction in the incidence of such herniae. Additionally, port site herniae may arise from postoperative wound infections or premature suture disruption. The sequalae of such hernia are as expected, comprising intestinal obstruction and incarceration. The management of this problem in the non-acute situation involves primary repair, with or without a prosthetic mesh.[77]

Port Site Metastases

Dobronte *et al.* were the first to describe this phenomenon, two weeks after a diagnostic laparoscopy for malignancy (Fig. 5).[78] Numerous cases have since been described for a variety of abdominal tumours[79]; a 1995 review reported a 4% incidence in patients with colorectal malignancies.[80] More recently, Ziprin *et al.* reviewed 27 studies, each with a minimum of 50 cases, and reported an overall incidence of only 0.71%.[81] This study has been corroborated by two others that reported incidence rates of 0.8%[82] and 0.6%.[83]

The aetiology is likely to be multi-factorial, including direct wound implantation, contamination of instruments, aerosolisation of tumour cells, surgical technique, excessive manipulation of tumour, and the effect of a

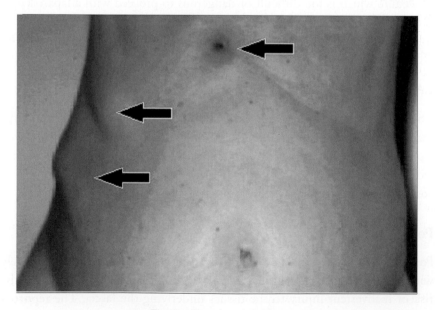

Fig. 5.   Port-site metastases.

hypoxic pneumoperitoneal environment.[79,81] Many techniques for prevention exist, but poor surgical technique with improper handling of the tumour is a frequent factor and one over which the surgeon has the most control. Furthermore, the surgeon must be trained and experienced in oncological laparoscopic surgical techniques.

Recurrence After Laparoscopic Hernia Repair

Inguinal hernia repair is a common operation, and currently both open and laparoscopic techniques are used. Patients treated with laparoscopic repair fare better in the early postoperative period,[40,42] however, the recurrence rates have been difficult to quantify due to the lack of long-term follow-up and small numbers of patients in each study. In a randomised trial (Liam *et al.*) of almost 1000 patients treated by laparoscopic or open inguinal hernia repair by recurrence rates at four years were found to be 4.9% and 10% respectively.[41] A more recent study of 1983 patients assigned to either laparoscopic or open repair reported recurrence rates of 10.1% versus 4.9% respectively at two year follow-up, concluding that the open technique is superior to laparoscopic hernia repair.[84] However, the rates of recurrence following repair of the recurrent herniae were similar (10% and 14.1% respectively).

The jury is still out regarding the place of laparoscopic inguinal hernia repair, and the National Institute for Clinical Excellence has advised surgeons in the UK to only perform the laparoscopic repair on bilateral and recurrent inguinal herniae.[85] Further studies are required prior to exclusive adoption of one or other technique.

CONCLUSION

Minimally invasive surgical techniques have rapidly gained acceptance and led to dramatic improvement in the morbidity and mortality of surgical procedures. However, the procedures have brought new complications, many of which are due to the surgeon's lack of knowledge and experience. While many of these complications are now rare, there is an exponential growth in the number and type of surgical procedures being performed laparoscopically. This is in tandem with new instruments and energy sources to aid the laparoscopic surgeon. Therefore it is more important than ever to ensure that the procedures are performed safely, with ongoing research to confirm superior patient outcomes when compared to traditional surgical methods.

References

1. Hinder RA, *et al.* (1994) Laparoscopic Nissen fundoplication is an effective treatment for gastroesophageal reflux disease. *Ann Surg* **220**: 472–481.
2. Lujan JA, *et al.* (2004) Laparoscopic versus open gastric bypass in the treatment of morbid obesity: a randomized prospective study. *Ann Surg* **239**: 433–437.
3. Vander Velpen GC, Shimi SM, Cuschieri A. (1993) Outcome after cholecystectomy for symptomatic gall stone disease and effect of surgical access: laparoscopic v open approach. *Gut* **34**: 1448–1451.
4. Soper NJ, Barteau JA, Clayman RV, *et al.* (1992) Comparison of early postoperative results for laparoscopic versus standard open cholecystectomy. *Surg Gynecol Obstet* **174**: 114–118.
5. Vitale GC, *et al.* (1991) Interruption of professional and home activity after laparoscopic cholecystectomy among French and American patients. *Am J Surg* **161**: 396–398.
6. Bosch F, Wehrman U, Saeger HD, Kirch W. (2002) Laparoscopic or open conventional cholecystectomy: clinical and economic considerations. *Eur J Surg* **168**: 270–277.
7. Delaney CP, Kiran RP, Senagore AJ, *et al.* (2003) Case-matched comparison of clinical and financial outcome after laparoscopic or open colorectal surgery. *Ann Surg* **238**: 67–72.
8. Sandbu R, Hallgren T. (2000) The economics of laparoscopic antireflux operations compared with open surgery. *Eur J Surg* **585**(Suppl): 37–39.
9. Mouret P. (1989) Presentation at Society of American Gastrointestinal Surgeons, Louisville, Kentucky.
10. The New Yorker. (2002) *Surgery Without Scars* (Conde Nast Publications, USA, 14-1-2002).
11. Southern Surgeons Club. (1991) A prospective analysis of 1518 laparoscopic cholecystectomies. *N Engl J Med* **324**: 1073–1078.
12. Brosens I, Gordon A, Campo R, Gordts S. (2003) Bowel injury in gynecologic laparoscopy. *J Am Assoc Gynecol Laparosc* **10**: 9–13.
13. Romain N, Michaud K, Brandt-Casadevall C, Mangin P. (2003) Fatal aortic injury during laparoscopy: report of two cases. *Am J Forensic Med Pathol* **24**: 80–82.
14. Figert PL, Park AE, Witzke DB, Schwartz RW. (2001) Transfer of training in acquiring laparoscopic skills. *J Am Coll Surg* **193**: 533–537.

15. Voitk AJ, Tsao SG, Ignatius S. (2001) The tail of the learning curve for laparoscopic cholecystectomy. *Am J Surg* **182**: 250–253.

16. Hasson HM. (1971) A modified instrument and method for laparoscopy. *Am J Obstet Gynecol* **110**: 886–887.

17. Nuzzo G, Giuliante F, Tebala GD, *et al.* (1997) Routine use of open technique in laparoscopic operations. *J Am Coll Surg* **184**: 58–62.

18. Nordestgaard AG, Bodily KC, Osborne RW, Jr, Buttorff JD. (1995) Major vascular injuries during laparoscopic procedures. *Am J Surg* **169**: 543–545.

19. Munro MG. (2002) Laparoscopic access: complications, technologies, and techniques. *Curr Opin Obstet Gynecol* **14**: 365–374.

20. Bhoyrul S, Vierra MA, Nezhat CR, *et al.* (2001) Trocar injuries in laparoscopic surgery. *J Am Coll Surg* **192**: 677–683.

21. Catarci M, Carlini M, Gentileschi P, Santoro E. (2001) Major and minor injuries during the creation of pneumoperitoneum. A multicenter study on 12,919 cases. *Surg Endosc* **15**: 566–569.

22. Mayol J, Garcia-Aguilar J, Ortiz-Oshiro E, *et al.* (1997) Risks of the minimal access approach for laparoscopic surgery: multivariate analysis of morbidity related to umbilical trocar insertion. *World J Surg* **21**: 529–533.

23. Bonjer HJ, *et al.* (1997) Open versus closed establishment of pneumoperitoneum in laparoscopic surgery. *Br J Surg* **84**: 599–602.

24. Sharp HT, *et al.* (2002) Complications associated with optical-access laparoscopic trocars. *Obstet Gynecol* **99**: 553–555.

25. Hurd WW, *et al.* (1993) Laparoscopic injury of abdominal wall blood vessels: a report of three cases. *Obstet Gynecol* **82**: 673–676.

26. Deziel DJ, *et al.* (1993) Complications of laparoscopic cholecystectomy: a national survey of 4,292 hospitals and an analysis of 77,604 cases. *Am J Surg* **165**: 9–14.

27. Wolfe BM, Gardiner BN, Leary BF, Frey CF. (1991) Endoscopic cholecystectomy. An analysis of complications. *Arch Surg* **126**: 1192–1196.

28. Shea JA, *et al.* (1996) Mortality and complications associated with laparoscopic cholecystectomy. A meta-analysis. *Ann Surg* **224**: 609–620.

29. Cuschieri A, *et al.* (1991) The European experience with laparoscopic cholecystectomy. *Am J Surg* **161**: 385–387.

30. Puggioni A, Wong LL. (2003) A meta analysis of laparoscopic cholecystectomy in patients with cirrhosis. *J Am Coll Surg* **197**: 921–926.

31. Yeh CN, Chen MF, Jan YY. (2002) Laparoscopic cholecystectomy in 226 cirrhotic patients. Experience of a single center in Taiwan. *Surg Endosc* **16**: 1583–1587.

32. Dalessandri KM, Bhoyrul S, Mulvihill SJ. (2001) Laparoscopic hernia repair and bladder injury. *JSLS* **5**: 175–177.

33. Tamme C, Scheidbach H, Hampe C, *et al.* (2003) Totally extraperitoneal endoscopic inguinal hernia repair (TEP). *Surg Endosc* 17: 190–195.
34. Granderath FA, Kamolz T, Schweiger UM, Pointner R. (2003) Failed antireflux surgery: quality of life and surgical outcome after laparoscopic refundoplication. *Int J Colorectal Dis* 18: 248–253.
35. Del Pizzo JJ, Shichman SJ, Sosa RE. (2002) Laparoscopic adrenalectomy: the New York-Presbyterian Hospital experience. *J Endourol* 16: 591–597.
36. Nduka CC, Super PA, Monson JR, Darzi AW. (1994) Cause and prevention of electrosurgical injuries in laparoscopy. *J Am Coll Surg* 179: 161–170.
37. Ukleja A, Woodward TA, Achem SR. (2002) Vagus nerve injury with severe diarrhea after laparoscopic antireflux surgery. *Dig Dis Sci* 47: 1590–1593.
38. Quah HM, Jayne DG, Eu KW, Seow-Choen F. (2002) Bladder and sexual dysfunction following laparoscopically assisted and conventional open mesorectal resection for cancer. *Br J Surg* 89: 1551–1556.
39. Callesen T, Bech K, Kehlet H. (1999) Prospective study of chronic pain after groin hernia repair. *Br J Surg* 86: 1528–1531.
40. Collaboration EH. (2000) Laparoscopic compared with open methods of groin hernia repair: systematic review of randomized controlled trials. *Br J Surg* 87: 860–867.
41. Liem MS, van Duyn EB, van der GY, van Vroonhoven TJ. (2003) Recurrences after conventional anterior and laparoscopic inguinal hernia repair: a randomized comparison. *Ann Surg* 237: 136–141.
42. Wellwood J, *et al.* (1998) Randomised controlled trial of laparoscopic versus open mesh repair for inguinal hernia: outcome and cost. *BMJ* 317: 103–110.
43. Macintyre IM. (1998) Does the mesh require fixation? *Semin Laparosc Surg* 5: 224–226.
44. Alijani A, Hanna GB, Cuschieri A. (2004) Abdominal wall lift versus positive-pressure capnoperitoneum for laparoscopic cholecystectomy: randomized controlled trial. *Ann Surg* 239: 388–394.
45. Sathesh-Kumar T, Saklani AP, Vinayagam R, Blackett RL. (2004) Spilled gall stones during laparoscopic cholecystectomy: a review of the literature. *Postgrad Med J* 80: 77–79.
46. Sarli L, Pietra N, Costi R, Grattarola M. (1999) Gallbladder perforation during laparoscopic cholecystectomy. *World J Surg* 23: 1186–1190.
47. Schafer M, *et al.* (1998) Spilled gallstones after laparoscopic cholecystectomy. A relevant problem? A retrospective analysis of 10,174 laparoscopic cholecystectomies. *Surg Endosc* 12: 305–309.
48. Shamiyeh A, Wayand W. (2004) Laparoscopic cholecystectomy: early and late complications and their treatment. *Langenbecks Arch Surg* 389: 164–171.

49. Andren-Sandberg A, Johansson S, Bengmark S. (1985) Accidental lesions of the common bile duct at cholecystectomy. II. Results of treatment. *Ann Surg* **201**: 452–455.

50. Roslyn JJ, *et al.* (1993) Open cholecystectomy. A contemporary analysis of 42,474 patients. *Ann Surg* **218**: 129–137.

51. Cameron JL, Gadacz TR. (1991) Laparoscopic cholecystectomy. *Ann Surg* **213**: 1–2.

52. Chapman WC, Halevy A, Blumgart LH, Benjamin IS. (1995) Post cholecystectomy bile duct strictures. Management and outcome in 130 patients. *Arch Surg* **130**: 597–602.

53. Way LW. (1992) Bile duct injury during laparoscopic cholecystectomy. *Ann Surg* **215**: 195.

54. Jatzko GR, Lisborg PH, Pertl AM, Stettner HM. (1995) Multivariate comparison of complications after laparoscopic cholecystectomy and open cholecystectomy. *Ann Surg* **221**: 381–386.

55. MacFadyen BV, Jr, Vecchio R, Ricardo AE, Mathis CR. (1998) Bile duct injury after laparoscopic cholecystectomy. The United States experience. *Surg Endosc* **12**: 315–321.

56. Rossi RL, Schirmer WJ, Braasch JW, *et al.* (1992) Laparoscopic bile duct injuries. Risk factors, recognition, and repair. *Arch Surg* **127**: 596–601.

57. Savassi-Rocha PR, *et al.* (2003) Iatrogenic bile duct injuries. *Surg Endosc* **17**: 1356–1361.

58. Moore MJ, Bennett CL. (1995) The learning curve for laparoscopic cholecystectomy. The Southern Surgeons Club. *Am J Surg* **170**: 55–59.

59. Scott TR, Zucker KA, Bailey RW. (1992) Laparoscopic cholecystectomy: a review of 12,397 patients. *Surg Laparosc Endosc* **2**: 191–198.

60. Branum G, *et al.* (1993) Management of major biliary complications after laparoscopic cholecystectomy. *Ann Surg* **217**: 532–540.

61. Davidoff AM, *et al.* (1992) Mechanisms of major biliary injury during laparoscopic cholecystectomy. *Ann Surg* **215**: 196–202.

62. Carroll BJ, Birth M, Phillips EH. (1998) Common bile duct injuries during laparoscopic cholecystectomy that result in litigation. *Surg Endosc* **12**: 310–313.

63. Bismuth H, Lazorthes F. (1981) *Les traumatismes operatoires de la voie biliare principale* (Masson, Paris).

64. Strasberg SM, Hertl M, Soper NJ. (1995) An analysis of the problem of biliary injury during laparoscopic cholecystectomy. *J Am Coll Surg* **180**: 101–125.

65. McMahon AJ, Fullarton G, Baxter JN, O'Dwyer PJ. (1995) Bile duct injury and bile leakage in laparoscopic cholecystectomy. *Br J Surg* **82**: 307–313.

66. Neuhaus P, *et al.* (2000) Classification and treatment of bile duct injuries after laparoscopic cholecystectomy. *Chirurg* **71**: 166–173.

67. Siewert JR, Ungeheuer A, Feussner H. (1994) Bile duct lesions in laparoscopic cholecystectomy. *Chirurg* **65**: 748–757.

68. Raute M, *et al.* (1993) Management of bile duct injuries and strictures following cholecystectomy. *World J Surg* **17**: 553–562.

69. Madding GF, Kennedy PA. (1972) Hepatic artery ligation. *Surg Clin North Am* **52**: 719–728.

70. Buell JF, *et al.* (2002) Devastating and fatal complications associated with combined vascular and bile duct injuries during cholecystectomy. *Arch Surg* **137**: 703–708.

71. Halasz NA. (1991) Cholecystectomy and hepatic artery injuries. *Arch Surg* **126**: 137–138.

72. Schmidt SC, Settmacher U, Langrehr JM, Neuhaus P. (2004) Management and outcome of patients with combined bile duct and hepatic arterial injuries after laparoscopic cholecystectomy. *Surgery* **135**: 613–618.

73. Sekido H, *et al.* (2004) Surgical strategy for the management of biliary injury in laparoscopic cholecystectomy. *Hepatogastroenterology* **51**: 357–361.

74. Hochstadetr H, *et al.* (2003) Functional liver damage during laparoscopic cholecystectomy as the sign of the late common bile duct stricture development. *Hepatogastroenterology* **50**: 676–679.

75. Costamagna G, Shah SK, Tringali A. (2003) Current management of postoperative complications and benign biliary strictures. *Gastrointest Endosc Clin N Am* **13**: 635–648, ix.

76. Di Lorenzo N, Coscarella G, Lirosi F, Gaspari A. (2002) Port-site closure: a new problem, an old device. *JSLS* **6**: 181–183.

77. Bowrey DJ, *et al.* (2001) Risk factors and the prevalence of trocar site herniation after laparoscopic fundoplication. *Surg Endosc* **15**: 663–666.

78. Dobronte Z, Wittmann T, Karacsony G. (1978) Rapid development of malignant metastases in the abdominal wall after laparoscopy. *Endoscopy* **10**: 127–130.

79. Curet MJ. (2004) Port site metastases. *Am J Surg* **187**: 705–712.

80. Wexner SD, Cohen SM. (1995) Port site metastases after laparoscopic colorectal surgery for cure of malignancy. *Br J Surg* **82**: 295–298.

81. Ziprin P, Ridgway PF, Peck DH, Darzi AW. (2002) The theories and realities of port-site metastases: a critical appraisal. *J Am Coll Surg* **195**: 395–408.

82. Hughes ES, McDermott FT, Polglase AL, Johnson WR. (1983) Tumor recurrence in the abdominal wall scar tissue after large-bowel cancer surgery. *Dis Colon Rectum* **26**: 571–572.

83. Reilly WT, *et al.* (1996) Wound recurrence following conventional treatment of colorectal cancer. A rare but perhaps underestimated problem. *Dis Colon Rectum* **39**: 200–207.

84. Neumayer L, *et al.* (2004) Open mesh versus laparoscopic mesh repair of inguinal hernia. *N Engl J Med* **350**: 1819–1827.

85. National Institute for Clinical Excellence. (2001) *Guidance on the Use of Laparoscopic Surgery for Inguinal Hernia* (NICE, London).

Chapter 25

COMPLICATIONS IN TRANSPLANTATION SURGERY

Konstantinos Vlachos, Thanos Athanassiou,
Nazar A. Mustafa, Vasillios E. Papalois
and Nadey S. Hakim

Organ transplantation is one of the major advances of the 20th century. The life saving replacement of the kidney, pancreas, liver, small bowel, heart and lung is the treatment of choice for end-stage organ failure. Continued progress in surgical techniques, organ procurement, preservation methods and immuno-suppression have contributed significantly to the progress of transplantation surgery, especially over the last two decades. However, post-transplant surgical complications are not rare and remain a challenge for the surgeon.

RENAL TRANSPLANTATION

Although the incidence of post-transplant surgical complications has fallen dramatically since the early days of renal transplantation, life and graft threat-ening situations still arise and early diagnosis with prompt treatment is crucial.

795

A remarkable number of innovative techniques have been used to salvage allografts, which would otherwise have been lost.

Vascular Complications

Vascular complications and their management are an important aspect of renal transplantation since their first description by Carrel who received the Nobel Prize in 1912 for his contribution to the field of transplantation surgery. The basic principle is to ensure adequate vascular supply for the kidney; therefore a lot of effort has been made to refine vascular surgical techniques and make them safe, and reliable.

Renal Artery Thrombosis

Renal artery thrombosis is an acute event that may occur intraoperatively or in the early postoperative period. It is the least common post-transplant vascular complication, with an incidence ranging from 0.9–3.5%.[1]

Arterial thrombosis may be extensive and involve the main renal artery or be limited to segmental arterial branches. Thrombosis of the main renal artery often results in allograft loss.

The possible causes of early arterial thrombosis include:

- Trauma to the donor artery during recovery or subsequent perfusion
- Poor surgical technique
- Torsion or kinking of the vessels
- Disparity in vessel size during anastomosis
- Dissection of a distal intimal flap
- Postoperative hypotension
- Hypercoagulable state
- Hyperacute or accelerated rejection
- Atherosclerosis of the donor or recipient vessels[2]

The clinical findings that suggest main renal arterial thrombosis are highly variable, from nearly asymptomatic to acute onset of allograft tenderness or gross haematuria. An acute change in urine output requires a radiographic assessment to exclude a graft-threatening vascular complication. The absence of arterial flow confirms the diagnosis of thrombosis. Duplex Doppler sonography, colour Doppler sonography, and renal scintigraphy can suggest the diagnosis but it should be confirmed by an angiography. The radiological findings vary, depending on the location and extent of the thrombus.

The allograft should always be explored, and successful thrombectomy with salvage has been reported on rare occasions. In segmental renal artery thrombosis, thrombolytic therapy with systemic heparin or streptokinase infusion may lead to recanalisation, but in most cases the allograft will be found infarcted and will require removal.

Transplant Renal Artery Stenosis

Renal artery stenosis (RAS) is the most common vascular complication in renal transplantation with incidence ranging between 1.6–12%.[3,4] However, its true prevalence remains unknown because reports vary depending upon the indications for renal angiography. When angiography was performed following a clinical suspicion the incidence was 1.5–5%.[5] In contrast, when postoperative angiography was performed on a routine basis, the incidence of radiographie stenosis was 25%. RAS can be detected post-transplant from a few months to years, but most cases are identified within 36 months following the transplantation.

Clinical findings that suggest RAS include poorly controlled hypertension, a decrease in the allograft function, and the appearance or change in the intensity of a bruit over the allograft. While these findings may be suggestive of the condition, they are of limited diagnostic value (positive predictive value of only 20% when clinical suspicion was investigated by renal angiography).[6]

The aetiology of RAS may include arterial damage during donor nephrectomy, faulty anastomotic suture technique, long vessels with angulation and stenosis after anastomosis, disparity in donor-recipient vessel size and the formation of atheromatous plaque in the recipient artery.[7] Stenosis at any location was encountered less frequently when an end-to-side (3.9%) rather than an end-to-end (9.7%) anastomosis was used.

Rejection has also been associated with stenosis, and histological changes associated with narrowing of wide renal arteries as well as complement and immunoglobulin deposits in the vessel wall of stenosed transplant renal arteries have been described.

Non-invasive screening methods for the diagnosis of transplant RAS (TRAS) include:

- Determination of peripheral plasma renin and the response to angiotensin-converting enzyme (ACE) inhibition
- Evaluation of the decline in glomerular filteration rate (GFR) by nuclear medicine scintigraphy after ACE inhibition
- Evaluation of the transplant renal artery with duplex colour sonography[6,8]
- Magnetic resonance angiography (MRA) is an accurate and non-invasive imaging modality that can clearly show the anatomy of the kidney blood supply with no risk of radiation or contrast allergies.
- CT scanning is used routinely in some centres to diagnose TRAS. It is reasonably accurate but the patient will be exposed to a relatively high radiation dose in addition to contrast complications.

The invasive screening methods to confirm TRAS include the use of intraarterial digital subtraction and conventional angiography. The criteria for performing an angiography should include hypertension that occurs suddenly or progressively, resistance to antihypertensive treatment, or hypertension co-existing with renal failure (rejection excluded). A decrease of >75% of the diameter of the artery and/or pressure gradient of >40 mmHg represents an angiographically significant RAS.[9]

The general principle is that when a lesion is angiographically demonstrable, it is functionally significant and should be treated. Percutaneous transluminal angioplasty (PTA) has been used since 1979,[7] and should be the initial step in the treatment of RAS; it carries an initial success rate of 50–80%. The procedure is usually carried out under mild sedation and rarely under general anaesthesia, using balloon catheters for dilatation. It can be easily repeated and results in minimal renal damage. The prevention of spasm and heparin therapy are essential to this treatment.

The possible complications of PTA are dissection, thrombosis, reversible renal failure, femoral artery pseudo-aneurysm and arterial perforation (7–28%).[10] Therefore, PTA should be carried out with the surgical staff on standby for immediate correction should any of these complications set in. The failure rates vary from 19–50%. Furthermore, graft loss as an immediate result of PTA may also occur, with an incidence of 0–20%.

The results of angioplasty depend on the condition of the distal vascular bed and the best results are achieved in patients with a post-stenotic dilation and the fewest arterial lesions. PTA with stent placement is a safe and effective treatment for TRAS associated with hypertension and renal dysfunction.

Surgical revascularisation should be considered for failed angioplasty or for lesions not amenable to angioplasty. The surgical techniques include:

- Resection of the stenotic segment with reanastomosis
- Transection of the transplant artery distal to the anastomosis and end-to-side reimplantation
- Bypass with autologous saphenous vein or Gore-Tex
- Open dilation
- Vein patch angioplasty

The immediate technical success rate of surgical correction is between 55–92%, with graft loss in up to 20% and a mortality rate of up to 5.5%.[11,12]

Other Renal Artery Complications

The use of extension grafts may be necessary to allow sufficient arterial length to permit a satisfactory anastomosis. They may also be obtained from another ABO-compatible adult donor, in which case the common and/or external iliac artery, and on occasion the carotid vessels, may be used. Pseudoaneurysm formation, stenosis, and occasionally, thrombosis of the extension graft may occur. The successful repair of a pseudoaneurysm of the extension graft has been reported. Infectious pseudoaneurysms can be associated with arterial rupture and usually require allograft nephrectomy, excision and ligation of the external iliac artery, and if necessary, an extra-anatomical bypass.[13]

Renal Vein Thrombosis

Renal vein thrombosis (RVT) is the only significant venous complication and usually occurs early in the postoperative period. Its incidence is reported to be 0.9–7.6%.[2] The major predisposing factors for RVT are:

- Poor surgical technique with stenosis of the venous anastomosis
- Kinking or angulation of the renal vein

- Postoperative hypovolemia and hypotension
- Hypercoagulable state
- Acute rejection
- Deep venous thrombosis

Renal vein compression by perinephric fluid collection.

RVT may present with clinical symptoms such as acute allograft swelling, pain, tenderness that gradually lead to oliguria and haematuria. The diagnosis is usually confirmed by ultrasound, DTPA renography and graft exploration. Venous Doppler examination of the renal vein has a high degree of accuracy in establishing the diagnosis.[8,14]

Re-exploration and thrombectomy is the immediate surgical approach when the diagnosis of RVT is suspected. The kidney can be salvaged only if re-exploration takes place very promptly. Late RVT (occurring over four weeks after transplantation) is usually a result of the propagation of deep iliac or femoral venous thrombosis into the renal vein.[15,16] Anticoagulation or use of intravenous streptokinase may be considered.[17]

The optimal treatment of RVT is prevention by precise surgical technique, ensuring adequate hydration and avoidance of postoperative complications, especially deep venous thrombosis and perinephric fluid collections.

Arteriovenous Fistulae

Although percutaneous allograft biopsy under ultrasound guidance is essential in the postoperative assessment of allograft dysfunction, it can be associated with potential complications such as arteriovenous fistula (AVF), arteriocalyceal fistula, iliac or mesenteric vascular lacerations, perirenal collections (haematoma), pseudoaneurysms, gross haematuria, and/or intra-abdominal organ injuries.

AVF is a well-recognised complication of biopsy in both the native kidney and renal allograft. It is a result of simultaneous injury to the walls of an adjacent artery and vein. The incidence of AVF is underestimated, because most small fistulas remain clinically silent, and is reported to be 1–10%.[18,19]

The risk factors are pre-existing hypertension and nephro-angiosclerosis. Other factors include accidental trauma, infection, local mycosis, rupture of an aneurysm, and technical problems during procurement. Angiography with selective embolisation is the treatment of choice in most cases. If this is not possible, it may be necessary to resect the fistula-bearing portion of the kidney.[20]

Urological Complications

The incidence of urological complications of renal transplantation ranges from 5–14%. Although rarely life threatening, they are associated with significant morbidity and possible long-term allograft dysfunction and loss.[21]

The last decade has witnessed a significant decrease in the incidence of urological complications, probably due to improved surgical techniques of ureteral implantation, better organ procurement techniques, careful preservation of the ureteric blood supply, and better diagnostic modalities.

The most common complications are ureteric obstruction and leakage. Others include vesicoureteric reflux, calculi, prostatic outflow obstruction, erectile dysfunction and complications related to post-transplant renal biopsies.

Obstruction

Urinary obstruction can occur at any stage, early or late after renal transplantation. The obstruction of the transplant kidney may be classified as being of either intrinsic or extrinsic origin. It may occur at the level of the ureterovesical junction, along the course of the transplant ureter or at the ureteropelvic junction. However, the most common site of ureteric obstruction is at the ureterovesical junction (63%), followed by the distal (13%), mid (13%), and proximal ureter (10%).[22]

Intrinsic ureteric obstruction is usually caused by ischaemia of the ureter leading to ureteric stricture.[23] This ischemia is usually the result of excessive dissection of the ureter itself or the renal hilum, which may compromise the ureteric blood supply, and usually occurs during organ retrieval or subsequent bench-work dissection.

Extrinsic ureteric obstruction may be caused by fluid collections, lymphoceles, haematomas or urinomas following urine leak; obstruction from tumour and peritransplant abscess is less common. Patients with a hypertrophic bladder wall, or with a high intravesical pressure, may develop obstruction of the ureter by the bladder itself.

The clinical presentation of obstruction include unexplained fall in urine output, graft dysfunction, urinary infection, and rarely, tenderness of the allograft. An ultrasound examination is essential to establish the diagnosis; the ultrasound findings associated with obstruction may include hydronephrosis and ureterectasis. Intravenous pyelography is contraindicated because of the deterioration in renal function associated with the obstructed allograft. A CT scan without contrast, although not showing the dynamic function of the kidney, may be helpful in visualising the collecting system and demonstrating the exact location of any fluid collections. Cystoscopy, retrograde ureterography and diuresis renogram also seem to be effective to provide the diagnosis. The F-15 renogram (administration of frusemide 15 min before the injection of isotopes) results in maximal urinary flow rates at the start of the renogram, decreasing the percentage of false positive results in dilated or poorly functioned systems. Percutaneous nephrostomy under ultrasound or CT guidance is another diagnostic modality. Following the placement of a percutaneous nephrostomy tube, further diagnostic studies as nephrostogram and pressure/flow may be undertaken to delineate the site, extent, and functional significance of the obstruction more precisely. Percutaneous nephrostomy may also allow decompression of the obstruction and stabilisation of renal function.[22,23]

Advances in minimally invasive endourological procedures can be applied to the transplant ureter. The intrinsic causes of obstruction, such as blood clots or oedema at the ureterovesical junction, may resolve spontaneously with either proximal diversion or stenting. However, other causes of intrinsic anatomic obstruction, such as ureteric stricture, may require more aggressive intervention. Ureteric obstruction due to a short-segment ureteric stricture may be amenable to balloon dilatation or endoureterotomy with long-term effectiveness reported to be 40–70%. The strictures at the ureteroneocystostomy appear to respond most favourably to endoluminal balloon dilatation. The length of the stricture, time following the transplant and, most importantly, the ureteric vascular supply appear to be the key factors determining the long-term effectiveness of endoscopic procedures.[24]

Stents are usually left in place for six weeks,[25] which is the interval required for complete ureteric muscular healing and return of peristalsis. Stenting is thought to provide scaffolding around which the ureter heals; on the other hand, all stents can cause irritation and inflammatory changes, which may impede healing or induce scar formation. Their routine prophylactic use during the transplant procedure has been controversial. The potential complications of internal stenting include infection, obstruction, encrustation, ureteral perforation, and stent migration.[26] Obstruction may still occur with a JJ stent in place, especially if it is a tight fit in the ureter and becomes kinked, blocking the internal lumen.

If endoscopic techniques are unsuccessful in treating obstruction, open surgical repair is indicated.[27] Any open repair should include inspection of the ureteroneocystostomy site for evidence of a haematoma or kinking of the intramural segment of ureter. If an ischemic distal ureter is found with adequate viable remaining length, a direct ureteric reimplantation may be possible. If the length is insufficient or the stricture is higher, an ipsilateral native ureterotransplant ureterostomy or native ureterotransplant pyelostomy and/or a Boari flap and psoas hitch may be the reconstructive method of choice either with an extraperitoneal or intraperitoneal approach. If there has been an infection in the vicinity of the ureter with fibrosis, the insertion of a ureteric catheter in the native ureter cystoscopically at the start of the procedure could be very helpful for the localisation of the native ureter. Pyeloureterostomy or ureteroureterostomy to the native ureter does not require native nephrectomy if the anastomosis of the transplant renal pelvis or ureter is performed end-to-side to the native ureter. If there is an insufficient, diseased, or an absent native ureter, a pyelovesicostomy and/or Boari flap may be necessary. Pyelovesicostomy and ureterocalicostomy have been described and vesicocalicostomy has been used when other reconstructive surgery had failed.[28]

Urine Leakage

Urine leak from the wound within the first few days of transplantation may arise from the calyceal system, renal pelvis, ureter, or bladder.[28] The reported incidence is 2–3%, and most cases of ureteric leakage (>75%) are associated with ureteric ischaemia. The incidence of urinary extravasation is not related to extremes of donor age, revascularisation, or preservation times, but seems to be more common in diabetics (6%).

The clinical signs and symptoms of urinary extravasation include graft tenderness or fullness, fever, and decreasing urine output.

Early leak of urine may indicate a blocked catheter; urinary obstruction due to catheter blockage will lead to stretching and opening up of suture line at the cystotomy wound or uretero-vesical anastomosis. In the early hours after renal transplantation, with early renal function, gentle washouts of the bladder should be attempted if the catheter is not draining adequately. If this fails the catheter should be changed and careful observations carried out to see if the drainage is restored, with cessation of urine leakage through the wound. Wound drainage fluid should be promptly analysed for urea and creatinine, and if these values are not comparable to the corresponding serum levels, a leak should be suspected.

Cystography should be performed next, with films obtained in anterior/posterior and oblique projections, both before and after bladder drainage.

An ultrasound may reveal hydronephrosis and/or a perinephric fluid. If a perinephric fluid collection is found, ultrasound-guided aspiration and biochemical analysis of the fluid may be helpful in the diagnosis of urinoma.

The management of small fistulae can vary from conservative treatment with placement of a simple uretheral catheter to adequate drainage with a percutaneous nephrostomy or internal stent, since most of them will heal spontaneously.[23] For larger leaks, percutaneous drainage may be initially attempted, but open operative repair and drainage are often required. The method of repair depends on the site of leak, the viability of the ureter, the usable ureteral length, and the bladder mobility. A necrotic distal ureter should be resected and a repeat ureteroneocystostomy attempted if an adequate length of ureter remains. If not, pyeloureterostomy or ureteroureterostomy to the native ureter should be performed.[29]

General Surgery Complications

Collections

Perinephric fluid collections of blood, lymph, serum or pus, of greater than 50–100 cc volume are detected in 20–50% of the renal transplant recipients on routine follow-up ultrasound examinations,[29] and seem responsible for a variety of complications such as the obstruction of the excretory tract, ipsilateral leg oedema and proteinuria.

Haematomas

Postoperative perirenal haematomas comprise 5–20% of all aspirated fluid collections. While small perirenal haematomas may be asymptomatic, larger haematomas can produce significant local wound and flank pain and cause ureteric obstruction. The ultrasound or CT findings of a large complex graft fluid collection support the diagnosis. Small haematomas can be treated conservatively while larger ones should be aspirated under ultrasound or CT guidance. Nevertheless, expanding haematomas may signal ongoing haemorrhage and require exploration for bleeding control.

Abscess

Recipients with fever, graft pain, tenderness and leukocytosis within the first few days to weeks after transplantation should be diagnosed as perirenal abscess. Most late peritransplant abscesses occur as a consequence of graft pyelonephritis. Ultrasound or CT-guided needle aspiration may confirm the diagnosis and permit percutaneous drainage. Although most of them are well localized and thick-walled, they may rupture into the peritoneal cavity and result in peritonitis. This serious complication carries significant morbidity and mortality. The surgical management of a peritransplant abscess includes drainage, antibiotics, and a judicious reduction in immunosuppression.

Lymphocele

The incidence of clinically significant lymphoceles is reported to be 0.6–18%.[30] Most lymphoceles present within the first 2–6 months following renal transplantation. Lymphocele formation is related to inadequate ligation of the lymphatics during iliac vessel dissection at the time of the transplant. They have also been associated with the use of anticoagulants, diuretics, and excessive steroid use. The diagnosis of a symptomatic lymphocele should be confirmed by ultrasonography and needle aspiration with chemical and bacteriological analysis. Percutaneous drainage resolves the problem most of the time; if not, open or laparoscopic drainage of the lymphocele in the peritoneal cavity is indicated.

Laparoscopic surgery has become widely accepted for the treatment of lymphoceles following kidney transplantation. The most common indications for open drainage are non-infectious wound complications and the high risk of vessel or ureter injury due to proximity to hilar structures.[31,32]

Miscellaneous

There are also a number of surgical complications related to the operation of renal transplantation and these include renal stones, gastrointestinal (GI) complications, hydrocele, spontaneous rupture of the kidney, femoral neuropathy and vesico-ureteric reflux.

Calculi

Renal transplant lithiasis is a relatively uncommon complication.[33,34] Calculi may have been present in the donor kidney or may develop after transplantation. Several predisposing conditions can lead to the formation of calculi, such as ureteric stricture, use of non-absorbable suture for the anastomosis, chronic infection, papillary necrosis, hypercalcemia due to hyperparathyroidism, hypophosphatemia, glucocorticoid administration, primary hyperoxaluria, and distal renal tubular acidosis. Stones can be diagnosed incidentally on routine post-transplant ultrasound, and usually require no treatment. However, intervention may be required when hydronephrosis or post-transplant infection occur, compromising the allograft function. The treatment options for transplant calculi include ureteric stents, endourologic techniques, and open surgery.[33] The position of the transplant kidney within the renal pelvis makes the treatment of renal calculi relatively simple by percutaneous nephrolithotomy or Extracorporeal Shockwave Lithotripsy (ESWL). However, ESWL is not the best option in poorly or non-functioning grafts because of impaired passage of fragments in such oliguric or anuric kidneys.

Gastrointestinal Complications

The recipients of renal grafts are at increased risk for GI complications, including erosive disease and GI bleeding. The selection of pharmacotherapy for GI conditions in patients with concomitant renal disease is complicated by three factors:

• Potential for a significant negative impact on renal function
• Requirement for dose alteration in renal insufficiency
• Potential for drug-drug interactions with concomitant medications

The clinical spectrum of GI complications range from non-specific signs of abdominal discomfort to life-threatening surgical emergencies.

With improved immunosuppressive regimes, especially those with low dose steroids, the incidence of GI complications such as duodenal ulcer with haemorrhage, and the complications of diverticular disease have decreased considerably. Furthermore, with improved medical regimes for upper GI disorders, operative intervention is now seldom required. Proton pump inhibitors appear to be the most suitable acid-suppressing therapy for patients with renal disease; recently developed drugs in this class (e.g., rabeprazole) may be the best choice for treatment of patients with both acid-related GI conditions and renal disease.

Hydrocele

A hydrocele on the side of the renal transplant is common if the cord has been ligated and divided. The prevention of this complication is by preservation of the cord, which also preserves fertility. The ureter must be placed posterior to the cord to avoid obstruction of the ureter. Hydrocoele infection secondary to a cutaneous b-haemolytic Group A Streptococcal infection has been also described in renal transplant recipients. Sepsis and renal failure are associated with this severe, life-threatening infection. Early diagnosis and treatment is crucial to optimise the outcome.[35]

Rupture

Spontaneous renal allograft rupture is an uncommon post-transplant complication secondary to RVT or acute vascular rejection. The condition usually presents within the first 10 days of operation as gross swelling at the site of transplantation and sometimes very severe haemorrhage. Immediate exploration is required; if the haemorrhage is not severe, it may be possible to salvage the kidney. The large fissures which are usually present on the surface of the kidney can be covered by synthetic haemostatic material such as Haemocel or Surgicel. Some of them can be primarily repaired but graft nephrectomy is frequently necessary after graft rupture.[36,37]

Femoral Neuropathy

Femoral neuropathy is probably due to the compression of the femoral nerve and its blood supply by a retractor at the time of operation. Although the femoral nerve is not exposed during a renal transplant operation, damage may result from cutting, stretching, compression, diathermy or devascularisation of the nerve.[38,39]

Vesicoureteric Reflux

Pre-existing vesicoureteric reflux as the cause of end-stage renal failure has a negative impact on the long-term survival of the transplanted kidney. Persistent infections with no other demonstratable pathology should be treated by surgery (reimplantation of the ureter or anastomosis to the native ureter).

PANCREAS TRANSPLANTATION

Pancreas transplantation is considered to be an effective therapeutic option for selected patients with Type I diabetes mellitus. The majority of cases are simultaneous kidney and pancreas transplants (SPK, 86%), followed by pancreas after kidney (PAK, 10%), and pancreas transplant alone (PTA, 4%). Current one and five year patient survival rates exceed 90% and 80%, respectively, without significant differences between the procedures. Pancreatic graft survival rates at one year are 84% for SKP, 73% for PAK, and 70% for PTA.[40]

The typical complications of major abdominal surgery can also occur after pancreas transplantation, such as:

- Prolonged ileus
- Bowel obstruction
- Cholecystitis
- Persistent gastroparesis
- Superficial and deep wound infection
- Fascial dehiscence

In addition, pancreatic grafts are also susceptible to a unique set of surgical complications mostly related to the exocrine secretions and the low microcirculatory blood flow of the gland. While the incidence of surgical complications has markedly decreased over the years, technical failures continue to be the leading cause of graft loss after pancreas transplant and result in major morbidity and mortality.[41]

Vascular Complications

Postoperative vascular complications following pancreas transplantation are the main concern of a transplant surgeon. The complexity of the vascular reconstruction of the graft and the low intra-parenchymal flow contribute to this serious problem. Furthermore, parenchymal pathology due to pancreatitis or rejection may increase the intrapancreatic vascular resistance to the point of causing secondary thrombosis of the main vessels.

Thrombosis, haemorrhage, mycotic pseudoaneurysm, AVF, and recipient lower extremity ischaemia following pancreas transplantation have all been described.

Thrombosis

Thrombosis is the most frequently observed surgical complication of pancreas transplantation. The rate of graft thrombosis is 6% in SPK, 7% in PAK, and 90% in PTA, nearly half of the non-immunological graft failures.[42] Usually, it is an early event that appears within the first two weeks after transplant in nearly 90% of the cases.[43]

Donor-related risk factors are age (above 45 years) and cause of death due to cerebrovascular events. The best bench reconstruction results are obtained by using donor iliac Y graft as opposed to an interposition graft between splenic and mesenteric artery. However, both these complicated reconstruction techniques are significant risk factors for arterial thrombosis. The presence of early graft pancreatitis is also a significant risk factor in solitary pancreas transplants.[43]

Low flow within the microvasculature of the pancreatic graft is partly responsible for thrombosis. The volume flow in the splenic artery of the pancreatic graft (when arterial reconstruction is done with the Y graft) is 10–15% of the volume flow in the splenic artery of the native pancreas of the recipient.[44] The low blood flow within the pancreatic graft can be decreased even further (leading to graft thrombosis) as a result of hypotension or inadequate anticoagulation.

The typical clinical presentation of pancreatic graft thrombosis in a patient with previously functioning graft is the sudden onset of hyperglycaemia. If the aetiology is portal vein thrombosis, haematuria is very common if the exocrine part of the pancreas is drained in the bladder and can be the only sign for grafts with poor endocrine function. If the pancreatic graft is bladder-drained, the disappearance or sudden decrease of urinary amylase may be diagnostic. Occasionally, the patient may complain of sudden onset of abdominal pain, especially after portal vein thrombosis that causes significant swelling of the thrombosed graft.

The presence of graft thrombosis can be easily confirmed by duplex ultrasonography while angiography may be occasionally used to establish the diagnosis.

Haemorrhage

Post-transplant bleeding can be treated conservatively with blood transfusion and correction of coagulopathy, but can lead to early relaparotomy. In a cohort of 142 pancreas transplant recipients, intra-abdominal bleeding resulted in 23 laparotomies (16%).[45] An important risk factor is the use of anticoagulation in pancreas transplant recipient at high risk for vascular thrombosis. Registry data suggest that massive bleeding has been responsible for graft loss in 0.2% of SPK, 0.3% of PAK, and 0% of PTA in the last five years.[40]

Mycotic pseudoaneurysm

Mycotic pseudoaneurysm is a rare but potentially fatal surgical complication and occurs as a consequence of intra-abdominal infection. It may present as generalised sepsis, unilateral iliac vein thrombosis, loss of distal pulses in the lower extremity, tenderness and pain, pulsatile mass, or massive intra-abdominal bleeding. This complication is so severe that graft pancreatectomy is almost always necessary.

Arteriovenous fistulas

AVF are usually localised at the site of the ligation of the mesenteric vessels but they can be a temporary consequence of a traumatic pancreatic graft biopsy. This complication can be successfully treated either conservatively with observation or with interventional radiological techniques, but may require surgical intervention.

Recipient distal ischaemia

Distal ischaemia of the recipient's limp has been described. The standard vascular surgical techniques can be successfully used for revascularisation and donor's iliac artery.[46]

Graft pancreatitis

Pancreatitis of the graft is a serious surgical complication that occurs in 2% of SPK, 3% of PTA and 2.5% of PAK and is responsible for graft loss usually when complicated by intra-abdominal infection (0.5%).[42] An increased serum amylase is common after pancreas transplantation and can be indicative of either asymptomatic or symptomatic pancreatitis with abdominal pain and distension.

This complication may be related to donor factors, such as haemodynamic instability and vasopressor administration, or to procurement and perfusion injury, as well as preservation and reperfusion injury. Graft pancreatitis can result in fistulae, fluid collections, pseudo-cysts or abscesses surrounding the pancreatic graft.

The diagnosis of graft pancreatitis is based on the presence of hyperamylasaemia in combination with radiological evidence by ultrasonography or CT scan of the pancreatic oedema and inflammation. Sometimes the diagnosis is made during explorative laparotomy based on findings of pancreatic oedema and saponification.

Patients with a diabetic neurogenic bladder can develop "reflux pancreatitis" from inadequate bladder emptying. The placement of Foley catheter and the use of octreotide can usually achieve the cure of this relatively common condition. However, on occasion, enteric conversion of the graft is needed for recurrent reflux pancreatitis.

Octreotide can also be effective as a prophylactic agent to decrease the incidence of technical complications by inhibiting the pancreatic graft exocrine secretion.[47]

Intra-abdominal Infections

The incidence of intra-abdominal infections following pancreas transplantation is about 10%.[48] Improved and standardised surgical technique, better bacterial and fungal prophylaxis, newer immunosuppressive protocols and mostly, more careful donor selection, have decreased these infections and reduced the rejection rate.

Pancreatitis caused by reperfusion injury, contamination and bacterial translocation from the donor duodenum, anastomotic leaks, and graft necrosis have all been associated with the development of infection. Furthermore, there is a significantly increased risk associated with older donor age, longer preservation time, older recipient age, enteric drainage versus bladder drainage, vascular graft thrombosis, and re-transplant versus primary transplant.[49] Intra-abdominal infections usually occur during the first 90 days following pancreas transplant with abdominal pain, distension, and obstruction.[49]

CT scan is the examination of choice, and CT-guided drainage of the fluid collection (for bacterial and fungal culture, evaluation of the creatinine and amylase levels) is a very valuable diagnostic and therapeutic tool. The perfusion of the graft should always be assessed by duplex ultrasonography.

Perioperative antimicrobial prophylaxis of the recipient must include fluconazole for fungal prophylaxis with the combination of imipenem or piperacillin with vancomycin. If the patient fails to respond to conservative management, surgical exploration should be carried out without hesitation. In most cases, multiple laparotomies may be necessary to control the infection. In over 50% of the cases graft pancreatectomy is indicated. Intra-abdominal infections leading to graft loss are considered as a relative contraindication to re-transplantation because of the high risk of recurrent infection.

Anastomotic Leak

Leaks of the duodenal anastomosis (bladder or enteric) following pancreas transplantation is a highly morbid complication. Anastomotic leaks are almost always complicated by intra-abdominal infection with the previously described serious implications. The incidence of duodenal leaks is about 10%.[50] The occurrence of early duodenal leaks is usually technical, whereas ischaemia, pancreatitis, rejection and cytomegalovirus (CMV) ulcers are responsible for late leaks.

For bladder-drained pancreases routine cystogram has a diagnostic sensitivity of 82% but abdominal CT scan with bladder contrast injection is the gold standard of the diagnosis with an accuracy of 96%. CT-guided drainage of the fluid collection is essential for the diagnosis and also an early attempt of conservative management. The presence of high amylase in the drained fluid or, elevated creatinine for bladder-drained graft, is suggestive of the diagnosis. Duodenal leaks can respond to conservative treatment with the insertion of a Foley catheter and drainage of any collections under ultrasound or CT guidance. For enterically-drained pancreases, surgical intervention and exploratory laparotomy with repair of the leak or the duodeno-enterostomy.

Complications Related to Bladder Drainage

The management of the exocrine pancreatic secretion after pancreas transplantation still remains controversial. Bladder drainage is a safe and well-established technique but can lead to urological or metabolic complications. The incidence of these complications can be up to 50%.[51] Minor urinary tract infections are quite common, and activated pancreatic enzymes[52] can lead to cystitis or urethritis.[53] In severe cases, patients may develop gross haematuria,[54] urethral stricture, or perforation of the bladder or duodenal segment. The continuous loss of fluids and bicarbonate leads to dehydration and metabolic acidosis. The tendency for volume depletion can cause or exacerbate pre-existing orthostatic hypotension. All recipients must increase fluid and salt intake and many require additional oral bicarbonate supplementation. Salt pills, flurocortisone, or acetazolamide are also prescribed and in some severe cases, patients require inpatient intravenous rehydration.

Minor leaks can be usually managed by Foley catheter drainage, but failure of conservative management mandates operative intervention consisting of either primary repair or enteric conversion.[55]

Because of the multiple complications of bladder drainage, the current surgical technique of pancreatic exocrine drainage, especially for SPK, consists in a side-to-side ileo-duodenostomy and several groups have documented the efficacy and safety of this approach.[56,57]

LIVER TRANSPLANTATION

Liver transplantation has become the treatment of choice for many patients with end-stage liver disease. The perioperative morbidity and mortality have decreased dramatically over the past two decades. Chronic liver failure secondary to cholestatic liver disease is the most frequent indication for liver transplant in adults while biliary atresia is the commonest cause in children.[58]

Despite these advances, there are several potentially lethal conditions that may complicate the immediate postoperative period. The failure of the graft to regain any useful metabolic activity is known as primary non-function, and almost uniformly requires retransplantation for any hope of survival. Lesser degrees of immediate dysfunction require experienced clinical judgment as to the probability of sustaining long-term patient survival.[59]

Vascular Complications

Vascular complications of liver transplantation, although not very common, are associated with a high level of morbidity, graft failure, and mortality. The most widely reported vascular complications related to the graft are those of the hepatic artery and its reconstruction, but complications of the portal vein, vena cava and others have also been described.

Hepatic artery complications

Thrombosis

Thrombosis of the hepatic artery occurs at a rate of 1.7–26%. It is also one of the most common causes of graft failure and mortality in the recipient, with a higher incidence in the paediatric group. Thrombosis of the hepatic artery showed an increase of around 5–6 fold when the donor hepatic artery was reconstructed using an interposition graft on the aorta above the celiac axis.

The common risk factors associated with hepatic artery thrombosis include small size of the artery (<3 mm), weight of the patient(less than 7 kg), and the use of an anastomotic site without a Branch patch or Carrel patch.[60] There has been no evidence of any association of donor arterial anomalies with hepatic artery thrombosis. Thrombosis may also be secondary to a low-flow state associated with intra-hepatic oedema usually seen with severe allograft rejection and the direct consequences of an immunological attack with associated vasculitis.[61]

The clinical presentation of hepatic artery thrombosis varies from an increase in serum transaminase levels, liver abscesses, biliary complications such as cholangitis, bile duct stenosis and necrosis, to liver dysfunction and finally failure. An impairment of the graft function was observed in patients with early hepatic artery thrombosis, whereas destruction of the biliary tract was more common in patients with late hepatic artery thrombosis.

The evidence of biliary tract complications should always raise the suspicion of hepatic artery thrombosis. The clinical presentation of biliary leak or obstructive biliary complications associated with intrahepatic strictures and biliary ectasia or bile leaks suggests ischaemia of the biliary tract. The impaired arterial inflow to liver graft preferentially affects the biliary tree because of its almost total reliance upon hepatic arterial blood supply.[62] A significant occurrence (47%) of hepatic artery thrombosis takes place within the first three days following orthotopic liver transplantation while 53% occurs 30 days or more post-transplant.[63]

The initial diagnosis of hepatic artery thrombosis is by Doppler ultrasonography of the graft vasculature combined with real time scanning (Duplex sonography), with a sensitivity of 92% for detection of hepatic artery thrombosis, immediately followed by angiographic evaluation.[64] Complications of hepatic artery thrombosis include haemorrhage associated with uncorrectable coagulopathy, acute hepatic encephalopathy and/or seizures, and the development of progressive multi-organ failure.

This condition requires rapid diagnosis and in most cases, urgent re-transplantation. Alternative therapy comprising recombinant plasminogen lysis with hepaticojejunostomy, liver abscess drainage and surgical thrombectomy has not been widely accepted, in part as a result of the high rate of subsequent biliary complications.[65]

Stenosis

Stenosis of the hepatic artery has been recognised as a complication of liver transplantation more recently. A high index of suspicion is necessary when patients present with unexplained abnormalities in liver function tests.[66]

The Doppler examination of the graft vasculature may demonstrate increased velocity in the region of the stenosis and flattened systolic peaks in the post-stenotic area, and should prompt an arteriogram.

The treatment of choice is PTA but when this fails the resection of the stenotic segment of the hepatic artery and re-anastomosis have reported good results.[67]

Portal vein complications

Thrombosis

Portal vein thrombosis is an uncommon cause for presinusoidal portal hypertension and reported in only 2–3% of recipients, although the true incidence is almost certainly higher because some patients may have an initially silent thrombosis.[61]

The risk factors include preoperative thrombosis of the hepatic portal vein, previous portacaval shunts, improperly flushed portal vein, size mismatch of the donor-recipient portal veins and anastomotic errors such as kinking, redundancy and "purse-stringing" narrowing of the portal vein. Portal vein thrombosis can be caused by one of three broad mechanisms: spontaneous thrombosis which develops in the absence of mechanical obstruction, usually in the presence of inherited or acquired hypercoagulable states, intrinsic mechanical obstruction because of vascular injury and scarring or invasion by an intrahepatic or adjacent tumour, extrinsic constriction by adjacent tumour, lymphadenopathy or inflammatory process. Usually, several combined factors result in portal vein thrombosis.

The consequences of portal vein thrombosis are mostly related to the extension of the clot within the vein. GI bleeding from the varices is the most frequent presentation.

Non-invasive imaging techniques are currently used for the screening of patients and the initial diagnosis of portal vein thrombosis. The invasive techniques are reserved for cases the non-invasive means are inconclusive, prior to percutaneous interventional treatment, or in the preoperative assessment of patients. The recanalisation of the portal vein with anticoagulation alone may not be consistent or appropriate in highly symptomatic patients. The catheterisation of the superior mesenteric artery (SMA) facilitates diagnosis as well as therapy by allowing the intra-arterial infusion of thrombolytic drugs in the same setting. Direct transhepatic portography allows precise determination of the degree of stenosis and extension within the portal vein, as well as pressure measurements.[68]

Thrombotic occlusions can be managed by mechanical thrombectomy or pharmacologic thrombolysis. The underlying occlusions because of organised or refractory thrombus, or fixed venous stenosis are best corrected by balloon angioplasty and stent placement. The advantages of mechanical thrombectomy include the potential to rapidly remove the thrombus without requiring pro-longed thrombolytic infusions, and reducing potential life-threatening com-plications of thrombolytic therapy. However, possible drawbacks include the risk of intimal or vascular trauma to the portal vein, which may promote recurrent thrombosis.[69,70]

The arterialisation of the portal vein, is being propagated as a technical possibility in liver transplant recipients with pre-existing portal vein throm-bosis, but cannot be recommended as a standard clinical procedure.

Hyperperfusion injury and arterial steal syndrome

Dysfunction of a small-for-size graft is an important clinical problem after living donor liver transplantation in adults. Portal hyperperfusion injury may be the cause, and the portal pressure should be measured when clinical suspi-cion arises. Splenic artery ligation is a technically simple procedure that can be applied for the prevention or treatment of such injury.[71]

Arterial steal syndromes (ASS) following orthotopic liver transplanta-tion (OLT) are characterised by arterial hypoperfusion of the graft caused by shifting of the blood flow into the splenic or gastroduodenal artery. It may present with elevated liver enzyme levels, impaired graft function, or cholesta-sis. Despite their potentially devastating consequences, such as ischaemic bil-iary tract destruction or graft failure, ASS has received little attention to date. Its incidence is similar to that of other vascular complications (5.9%). Untreated ASS may lead to serious complications in more than 30% of patients. The treatment consists of splenectomy, coil embolisation of the splenic or gastro-duodenal arteries, or reduction in splenic artery blood flow by administration of an artificial stenosis. Of the treatment options, banding the splenic artery is associated with the lowest complication rate. Banding also may be per-formed prophylactically in selected patients to prevent the development of this condition.[72]

Vena cava complications

Stenosis of the vena cava happens in less than 1% of liver transplants and may occur as a result of technically inadequate construction of either the infrahep-atic or suprahepatic vena caval anastomoses. The diagnosis is made by Duplex sonography and phlebography of the inferior vena cava. Its management consists of full anti-coagulation and long-term (3–6 months) administration of warfarin. Infrahepatic vena caval stenosis has also been successfully treated by transluminal balloon angioplasty.[73,74]

Hepatic vein complications

Patients who receive a liver transplant for Budd-Chiari syndrome are at risk of developing recurrent hepatic vein occlusion. The maintenance of long-term anticoagulation with warfarin has been recommended to avoid recurrence of the syndrome.[75,76]

Haemorrhage

Variceal haemorrhage

The intra-abdominal portosystemic collaterals present some of the most difficult technical challenges to the surgeon during liver transplantation. It was recently suggested that persistent portosystemic collateralisation remains even after successful grafting resulting in intra-abdominal or gastro-oesaphageal bleeding occasionally.[77,78]

Splenic artery aneurysms

The incidence of splenic artery aneurysm in patients with cirrhosis ranges from 7–17%. The rupture of the aneurysm is reported to result in significant morbidity and mortality. Definitive management can await liver transplant,[79,80] and it is recommended that all patients should undergo a four phase CT or MRA as part of the liver transplant evaluation and the identified splenic artery aneurysm should be embolised before or resected at transplantation.[81]

Mycotic pseudoaneurysm

Mycotic pseudoaneurysm is a rare but frequently devastating complication of liver transplantation.[82] Fewer than 50 cases have been reported in the literature and the overall incidence is between 0–5%.

Most authors advocate hepatic artery ligation, although some have reported encouraging results after resection and reconstruction.

Other complications

Intravascular cannulae

Venovenous bypass circuit entails the placement of cannulae into the lower vena cava via the saphenofemoral venous junction and into the portal vein for systemic and splanchnic decompression respectively during the anhepatic phase of the operation. Blood is returned to the systemic circulation via a cannula placed into the axillary vein. The complications related to these cannulation sites have been infrequent, limited primarily to haematomas, seromas, or localised abscesses.

Complex hepatic artery reconstruction

Complex hepatic artery reconstruction is technically challenging especially for split-liver and living related liver transplantation, but seems not to affect its long-term outcome.[83]

Biliary Complications

Biliary tract complications represent the main cause of morbidity following liver transplantation. Their incidence still remains stubbornly high at about 15% of the transplanted livers. Several factors have been implicated in their pathogenesis:

- Thrombosis of the blood vessels that supply the biliary epithelium is associated with necrosis of the associated bile ducts leading to strictures and leaks.
- Post-transplant bile composition is super-saturated with cholesterol. This may result in sludge and stone formation. Cyclosporin A may also inhibit bile salt production.
- The transplanted liver is a denervated organ, and it has been suggested that denervation of the biliary tract inhibits bile flow and perhaps alters bile composition.
- T tubes (used to protect duct-to-duct biliary anastomosis) as foreign bodies are prone to bacterial colonisation and forms a focus for the deposition of biliary sludge.

Diagnosis

The septic patient requires urgent investigation and prompt treatment because of the potentially lethal combination of infection and immunosuppression. The diagnosis consists of culturing of blood, urine, sputum, T tube bile and ascites fluid. Chest radiography and ultrasonography of the abdomen with percutaneous aspiration for microbiology are needed. Following ultrasonography or CT evaluation, a T tube cholangiogram is performed under antibiotic prophylaxis. For patients with a Roux-en-Y biliary anastomosis, a percutaneous transhepatic cholangiogram is necessary to visualise the biliary tree.

The most common biliary complications are:

Leakage

Bile leakage may occur from the biliary anastomosis or around the T tube at its insertion into the bile duct mostly due to faulty surgical technique. Usually this happens immediately after the operation or may be recognised during T tube cholangiography postoperatively. Such leaks can be managed with prolonged T tube drainage. However, most bile leaks may become apparent several days after the operation and present with biliary peritonitis or an infected collection. Although the area of the leak can be stented either endoscopically or percutaneously, surgical biliary reconstruction with excision of the stricture and re-anastomosis to a Roux loop of jejunum is the definitive treatment.

Bile leaks may also occur in the postoperative phase following liver biopsy, but this is almost invariably associated with prior obstruction and dilatation of the biliary tract. Ultrasonography before liver biopsy should guard against this complication.

Strictures

Transpapillary endoscopic and percutaneous transhepatic radiological interventions are both effective therapies for biliary complications associated with liver transplantation. They are complementary approaches that help avoid surgery for these complications.[84] Biliary reconstruction following living donor liver transplantation requires microsurgical techniques and can be performed as a direct end-to-end anastomosis. In most cases, endoscopic placement of an inside stent is useful for treating biliary stricture.[85,86]

Ischaemic-type biliary lesions are the most frequent cause of non-anastomotic biliary strictures in liver grafts, affecting about 2–19% of the patients after liver transplantation. They are characterised by bile duct destruction, subsequent stricture formation, and sequestration. The management is with repeated dilatations by endoscopic means,[87] failing which surgery is needed. Intrahepatic strictures are not usually amenable to surgical correction and re-transplantation may be the only long-term solution. For extrahepatic strictures surgical biliary reconstruction is possible and effective.

Lithiasis

Biliary stones may develop after liver transplantation and biliary-enteric anastomosis, in the absence of mechanical stricture, secondarily to bile stasis caused by functional disorder of the efferent jejunal loop. Hepatobiliary scintigraphy plays a central role in the diagnosis of such a disorder.[88]

Biliary casts usually develop in up to 18% of liver transplant recipients. Casts are associated with morbidity, graft failure, need for retransplantation and mortality. Proposed aetiological mechanisms include acute cellular rejection, ischaemia, infection and biliary obstruction but are more likely to develop in the setting of hepatic ischaemia and biliary strictures. Endoscopic and percutaneous cast extraction might achieve favourable results and should be attempted before surgical therapy.[89]

Cholestasis

Cholestasis due to the deposition of biliary sludge is the most common late postoperative biliary complication in liver transplant patients. The contributing factors include chronic rejection causing ischaemia of the biliary epithelium, prior presence of T tube and denervation of the biliary tract including the ampulla of Vater. The conservative treatment with ursodeoxycholic acid may solve the problem by increasing bile solubility. However, if the cholangiography demonstrates stenosis or dysfunction at the ampulla, endoscopic sphincterotomy is the intervention of choice.

Cholangitis

Concomitant inflammatory bowel disease had no detrimental influence on the outcome of liver transplantation in patients with primary sclerosing cholangitis. The course of inflammatory bowel disease is not altered after liver transplantation and immunosuppression including steroids does not prevent its exacerbations. Patients with primary sclerosing cholangitis and inflammatory bowel disease may have an increased risk of developing colorectal cancer after liver transplantation.[90]

The development of colorectal neoplasia is a serious threat to patients with inflammatory bowel disease and primary sclerosing cholangitis after liver transplantation. A long-term aggressive colonic surveillance and colectomy in selected high-risk patients with longstanding severe colitis is recommended.[91,92]

SMALL BOWEL TRANSPLANTATION

For over three decades, the small bowel was considered to be the forbidden organ in transplantation. Although it was one of the first to be grafted experimentally, it was the last to be transplanted successfully in humans. Only recently, with the introduction of effective immunosuppressive medications, can small bowel transplantation be considered a possible treatment for selected patients with intestinal failure.[93,94]

The technical aspects of procuring and transplanting the intestine were studied early in the century by Alexis Carrel and later refined by Lillehei and colleagues[95] at the University of Minnesota in 1955. Monchick and Russell[96] established a rat model for small bowel transplantation, which opened the door for investigators to explore the unidirectional immune phenomena as well as the physiologic function of the transplanted gut. Furthermore, the pioneering clinical work of the group at the University of Pittsburgh has allowed small bowel transplantation to become a clinical reality.[97]

The experience with small bowel transplantation under cyclosporine immunosuppression was encouraging, but ultimately proved to be unsatisfactory as graft loss to rejection continued to be inevitable. The success of human small bowel transplantation hinged on the advent of FK506 (tacrolimus), which has shown to be of great promise in liver and small bowel transplantation. The failure of early attempts in human small bowel transplantation made chronic total parenteral nutrition (TPN) the best option for treatment of intestinal failure[98]; however, long-term parenteral nutrition sometimes leads to severe liver impairment and it is under these conditions that small bowel transplantation has re-emerged as a potential treatment option for irreversible intestinal failure in selected patients.[99,100]

Approximately, 100 small bowel transplantations are performed per year worldwide, of which 38% are of the small bowel alone, 46% combined liver and small bowel transplantation, and 16% are a cluster.[101] Of the 800 patients transplanted so far, 50% show a survival rate up to 15 years post-transplant. Furthermore, over 80% of these patients are off parenteral nutrition, in good health and with good quality of life.[102,103]

Surgical Complications

Haemorrhage

When the indication for bowel transplantation is portal hypertension, in which previously attempted complex surgical procedures may have caused multiple adhesions, the risk of severe bleeding during the enterectomy is very high. Therefore it is essential to perform a preoperative embolisation to reduce the risk of bleeding.

In combined liver-intestine transplantations, poor postoperative hepatic function may cause also intraperitoneal haemorrhage. A second look laparotomy is mandatory in such cases.

Vascular complications

Arterial and venous thrombosis is uncommon, occurring in less than 4% of cases. Postoperative Doppler ultrasound can detect the vascular flow very easily. If thrombosis is detected by ultrasound, arteriography must be performed as an emergency. Urgent re-operation to ensure reperfusion could avoid graft loss.

Intestinal perforation

Intestinal or colonic perforation is not very common after small bowel transplantation. The clinical signs are not acute and the diagnosis is often difficult. Perforation can be the first symptom of rejection; intestinal perforation can also occur after small bowel biopsies.[104]

Sepsis

The prevention of graft rejection requires a high degree of immunosuppression, which contributes to frequent sepsis. Bacterial, fungal and viral infections have been reported to occur in small bowel transplants. Intravenous antibiotic prophylaxis and oral decontamination are used to prevent postoperative sepsis. Infectious diseases occur earlier in small intestine transplantation combined with colon transplantation, but their incidence is the same in isolated intestinal and combined intestinal-liver transplantation. Most episodes of bacterial infection may be related to bacterial translocation. Doppler ultrasound or CT scanning are helpful in detecting intra-abdominal sepsis which must be drained under their guidance or surgically if needed.

Enterocolitis

Ischaemia and bacterial proliferation can lead to enterocolitis or even more to necrotizing enterocolitis, with severe haemorrhage associated with peritoneal symptoms that may necessitate even the removal of the graft. The sudden onset of abdominal distension and pain, lack of bowel movement, and vomiting after closure of the diagnostic stoma months after transplantation can suggest the diagnosis of primary non-function of the graft due to enterocolitis. A plain abdominal X-ray can reveal pneumatosis intestinalis and angiography may exclude possible obstruction of large vessels. Upper GI endoscopy can show ulcerative enteritis usually with spontaneous perforations. Long cold ischaemia time and poor donor selection can cause this surgical complication.[105,106]

Stomal complications

The pathological examination of the mucosal biopsy specimen of the graft serves as the most important and fundamental method in current clinical diagnosis of rejection. It can reveal the characteristics of the rejection and its degree. The endoscopic surveillance gives a good view of the mucosa of the bowel graft and biopsy specimen can be taken precisely at the lesion sites. Therefore, stomas are very useful for performing biopsies. However, they can be complicated by local infection or by fluid loss that leads to local inflammation or electrolyte disorders. Stoma prolapse is not uncommon. When the clinical status of the patient is stabilised, the stoma should be closed.

HEART TRANSPLANTATION

Introduction

Heart transplantation has evolved from an experimental procedure to a widely accepted therapeutic option for the management of end-stage heart failure.[107] In the early 1960s, Lower and Shumway perfected the technique for orthotopic cardiac transplantation using cardiopulmonary bypass and demonstrated the long-term survival and function of the denervated heart. As a prelude to human cadaveric transplantation, Hardy performed a chimpanzee xenotransplant in 1964.[108] Although technically successful, the primate heart was too small to support the circulation. The first successful human heart transplant was performed on 3 December 1967, by Christian Barnard in South Africa.[109] The recipient survived for 18 days and eventually succumbed to pneumonia. Norman Shumway performed the first successful heart transplant in the US on 6 January 1968.[110]

In the 1970s the most significant clinical advances in heart transplantation were the development of the trans-venous right ventricular endomyocardial biopsy technique for monitoring allograft rejection (Caves) and the categorisation of a biopsy-grading system for quantifying rejection severity (Margaret Billingham).[111] It was not until cyclosporine was clinically introduced in the early 1980s that heart transplantation became common practice. Today, more than 250 centres worldwide perform heart transplants. During the last decade, immunosuppression has been further refined with the introduction of monoclonal antibody OKT-3, the use of steroid-free protocols, and the availability of tacrolimus.

Indications

Heart transplant candidates require an aggressive and thorough screening process. The indications for heart transplantation are end-stage heart failure (New York Heart Association Class III or IV symptoms and failure of maximal medical therapy) with a poor long-term prognosis.

The current indications for placing candidates on the waiting list are:

- Cardiogenic shock or low output state with reversible end-organ dysfunction requiring mechanical support
- Low output state or refractory heart failure requiring continuous inotropic support

- Advanced heart failure signs and symptoms (NYHA Class III or IV) with objective documentation
- Recurrent or rapidly progressive heart failure symptoms unresponsive to maximised vasodilators and a flexible diuretic program
- Severe hypertrophy or restrictive cardiomyopathy with NYHA Class IV heart failure or anginal symptoms

The contraindications to a heart transplant are the following:

- Active infection
- Recent malignancy
- Pulmonary hypertension with irreversibly high pulmonary vascular resistance (greater than 6 Wood units, or 3–4 Wood units during a vasodilator trial)
- Diabetes mellitus and evidence of significant retinopathy, neuropathy, or nephropathy
- Myocardial infiltrative or inflammatory disease
- Active peptic ulcer disease
- Any systemic illness that would limit life expectancy or compromise functional rehabilitation
- Significant severe pulmonary parenchymal disease
- Irreversible renal dysfunction
- Severe peripheral vascular or cerebrovascular disease
- Irreversible hepatic dysfunction or cirrhosis
- Documented medical non-compliance
- Active substance abuse (including tobacco)
- Untreated psychiatric illness

The indications for heart transplantation are similar in several respects for children and adults. A transplant is indicated for any child with end-stage heart disease whose condition is refractory to maximal medical therapy or other surgical intervention. Cardiomyopathy and complex congenital heart disease — with or without myocardial failure — are the two main diagnostic groups. There are no reliable predictors of poor survival for children with dilated cardiomyopathy or heart failure, and the decision to place them on the waiting list is a difficult one.[112,113] The most common clinical indication includes increasing heart failure despite maximal medical therapy. Some children are referred because of a congenital heart abnormality, before severe heart failure develops, when the natural history of the abnormality precludes long-term survival. Those with growth failure or cardiac cachexia should also be considered for a transplant. Importantly, children need a reliable caregiver to administer immunosuppression and other post-transplant care.

Retransplantation remains controversial as some recipients suffer progressive graft dysfunction. Despite maximal care after a heart transplant, chronic rejection and allograft coronary artery disease are the major factors affecting long-term survival. Retransplantation in this subgroup has a short-term survival similar to initial transplantation in critically ill patients. Limited donor organ availability and restrained financial resources complicate the issue of retransplantation.

Complications

Improvement in immunosuppression and post-transplant care have largely been responsible for the tremendous success, in both short- and long-term survival rates, of heart transplantation. One of the leading causes of death in the first year post-transplant is rejection.[114,115] Maintenance immunosuppression currently comprises cyclosporine, azathioprine, and prednisone; this triple-drug combination is designed to limit the toxicity of any one drug by allowing lower doses of several drugs. Most deaths in the first year are caused by acute rejection or infection. The development of these two problems is interrelated: insufficient immunosuppression may lead to acute rejection, whereas over-immunosuppression may result in opportunistic infections. Other complications include graft coronary artery disease, malignancy, and toxicity related to long-term drug therapy.

Rejection

Rejection has been classified as cell-mediated (most common) and antibody-mediated (also known as humoral or vascular). Chronic rejection has been renamed "allograft coronary artery disease", since it is actually a type of vasculopathy. The factors associated with an increased risk of rejection include human leukocyte (HLA) mismatches,[116] female gender and younger donor hearts,[117,118] non-O blood type,[119] panel reactive antibody screen greater than 10%,[120,121] positive donor-specific cross-match, OKT3 murine monoclonal antibody sensitisation, cytomegalovirus (CMV) infection,[122] and anti-HLA antibodies.[123] Large multi-centre trials have further identified female gender, HLA mismatches, and the use of female or younger donors as the highest risk factors for rejection.[124]

Infection

Immunosuppressed heart recipients are predisposed to life-threatening infections from a wide variety of common opportunistic organisms such as CMV and *Pneumocystis carinii*. Infection prophylaxis at our institution includes daily trimethoprim-sulfamethoxazole, acyclovir, and nystatin for three months post-transplant. Recipients require aggressive evaluation and a high index of suspicion for the development of infection as well as aggressive surveillance of potential infections.

Transplant Coronary Artery Disease

Transplant coronary artery disease (TCAD) was formerly referred to as chronic rejection, now recognised as a misnomer. Graft coronary artery disease may form quite rapidly post-transplant, or it may progress more slowly; the precise pathophysiology is unclear. It tends to affect the large epicardial coronary and smaller branch vessels in a diffuse fashion, rendering angioplasty or bypass surgery impossible. Graft atherosclerosis is the leading cause of death and complications after the first post-transplant year.[125] Since the transplanted heart is denervated, recipients do not develop angina and usually present with overt congestive heart failure or sudden death. Compared with non-transplant patients with coronary artery disease, transplant recipients display fewer proximal stenoses (76% vs. 100%) and more distal vessel occlusions (49% vs. 4%). The rapidity of disease progression is highlighted by the absence of collateral circulation in 92% of the transplant recipients.[126]

To monitor graft atherosclerosis, recipients undergo annual cardiac catheterisation. Developing strategies to prevent the graft coronary artery disease is one of the most important areas of research at many transplant centres. The treatment of angiographie TCAD using antiplatelet agents, aspirin, dicumarol, heparin, or fish oil has been ineffective.[127]

Coronary angioplasty, atherectomy, and bypass surgery have been performed in a limited number of cardiac transplant recipients. A multi-centre registry has retrospectively assessed the effects of coronary revascularisation on patient survival.[128] Coronary angioplasty has a high initial rate of success in treating discrete lesions (94%) but is associated with frequent procedural complications and a re-stenosis rate above 50%.

The only definitive therapy currently available for advanced multivessel TCAD is retransplantation. Elective retransplantation should be considered when the angiographic disease is severe or its rate of progression is life threatening or when extensive left ventricular dysfunction has developed. Unfortunately, survival following retransplantation is decidedly lower than initial transplantation. The registry data report an overall one year survival rate of only 55%.[129] Even selecting an ideal candidate yields a one year survival rate of 74%.[130] Accelerated TCAD is more likely to occur in retransplanted allografts.

Acute aortic dissection is a rare complication that occurs following orthotopic heart transplantation. Heart-transplant recipients with arterial hypertension and donor-related risk factors are prone to it and require careful follow-up.

Left atrial thrombosis in the absence of rheumatic heart disease and atrial fibrillation is a rare occurrence. Despite an uneventful postoperative course, sinus rhythm and normal contractility of the heart, large thrombi could be found several months following transplantation. Surgical thrombectomy could be performed under cardiopulmonary bypass.

Gastrointestinal Complications

GI complications are observed in 15–35% of transplant recipients, with mortality rates as high as 30%. Upper GI bleeding, usually due to peptic ulcer disease or haemorrhagic gastritis, accompanies the stress of cardiac surgery or high-dose corticosteroids frequently. Its incidence has decreased dramatically with the prophylactic use of H2-blockers.

Cholelithiasis is present in 30–40% of the transplant recipients and is twice as common as for age and gender-matched controls. Gallstones develop within two years in 2–17% of patients with normal pretransplant ultrasonography. The risk of morbidity and mortality from gallstone disease is high in cardiac transplant patients, particularly immediately after the procedure. Post transplant patients require annual ultrasound examinations to detect the onset of gallstone disease, and this risk is higher than in the general population. Furthermore, gallstones alone are an indication for cholecystectomy in the cardiac transplant patient. Although some advise a more aggressive management of asymptomatic patients, biliary colic or gallstone pancreatitis are not uncommon and many centres routinely recommend a laparoscopic cholecystectomy in clinically stable patients with gallstones.[131]

Pancreatitis ranges from 1.5–18% in heart transplant recipients. Cardiopulmonary bypass, vasopressor-mediated splanchnic vasoconstriction, and high-dose corticosteroids account for early postoperative pancreatitis. Nasogastric suction and TPN should be implemented and continued until symptoms and biochemical abnormalities resolve.[132]

Malignancy

The incidence of malignant tumours in transplant recipients ranges from 4–18% (average 6%), a 100-fold increase above the general population.[133] Heart transplant recipients are at particular risk for the development of cancers of the skin and lips, as well as lymphomas. Compared with kidney transplant recipients, cardiac transplant patients have a two-fold overall increase in neoplasia risk and a six-fold increase of visceral tumours. No relationship has been demonstrated between the type of maintenance immunosuppression and the risk of malignancy. The combination of immunosuppression and a history of prior smoking may account for the increased risk of developing lung cancer in heart transplant recipients.[134]

Results of Heart Transplantation

According to the International Society for Heart and Lung Transplantation Registry report, a total of 30,297 heart transplants in 257 transplant centres were done worldwide as of 15 February 1995.[135] The actuarial survival was 76% at one year, with about a 4% mortality rate per year thereafter over 12 years of follow-up. The survival has improved in the past 20 years; in the most recent era (1988 through 1994) the rates were 81% at one year and 73% at three years.

LUNG TRANSPLANTATION

Introduction

Over the last 15 years, lung transplantation has emerged as a successful therapeutic option for a number of patients with end-stage pulmonary parenchyma and vascular disease. The advances in recipient and donor selection, operative technique, and postoperative management have resulted in improved early survival. There are three surgical options, single lung (SLT), bilateral lung (BLT) and combined heart-lung (HLT) transplantation.

Experimental lung transplantation in animal models began in 1949 and subsequently when Henri Metras reported his initial experiences with left isolated lung transplantation in a canine model.[136] Following further laboratory investigations, Hardy performed the first human SLT in 1963 in a 58-year-old convict with squamous cell carcinoma of the left hilum and emphysema. The patient succumbed to renal failure and malnutrition 18 days after the procedure.[137]

By 1978, 31 transplants had been performed by more than 20 centres around the world. Only 20 patients survived more than a week, and 16 developed bronchial complications. While one patient lived for six months, more than half the deaths in those surviving 14 days were due to bronchial dehiscence.[138]

Following the advent of combined HLT in Stanford, USA, the Toronto Lung Transplant Group achieved the first long-term successes in unilateral pulmonary transplantation in 1983.[139] This was quickly followed by the proliferation of lung transplant programmes, such that by 1996 over 1,600 single lung implantations had been performed worldwide. Today, progress in surgical techniques and intensive care methods has reduced the mortality and morbidity of the procedure.

Indications

Currently, lung transplantation has a narrow and specific range of indications. Because pulmonary transplantation continues to develop, these indications may not be comprehensive, and may not apply in the future particularly with research into lung reduction surgery for emphysema and lobar transplantation. Generally, patients must have end-stage disease, refractory to conventional medical and surgical treatment. There are three possible lung transplant procedures to be considered for the potential recipient, the choice of which depends mainly upon the type of disease present.

Complications of Lung Transplantation

The complications of lung transplantation can be classified into three broad categories, surgical (of the operation itself), immunological, and complications due to the immunosuppressive agents used to prevent rejection, including infection, malignancy, and direct side effects of the medications.

Surgical Complications

Pulmonary artery obstruction

Pulmonary artery obstruction may occur as a result of anastomotic stenosis, kinking, or extrinsic compression. Persistent pulmonary hypertension and unexplained hypoxemia may be evident in these cases. Attention to anatomic factors, such as the length of the donor and recipient pulmonary artery and division of the pericardial attachments surrounding the donor pulmonary artery, as well as awareness of the potential for a flap wrapping the bronchial anastomosis to compress the adjacent anastomosis helps avoid these problems.

Left atrial anastomotic obstruction

Left atrial anastomotic obstruction can also occur due to faulty anastomotic technique or extrinsic compression by clot, pericardium or an omental flap. It results in more severe abnormalities than pulmonary artery obstruction, including marked pulmonary hypertension and ipsilateral pulmonary oedema. The diagnostic methods for these vascular anastomotic complications include routine intraoperative measurement of anastomotic gradients and TEE, which is particularly helpful in assessing the left atrial anastomosis. Postoperatively, the diagnostic measures include contrast angiography and ventilation/perfusion scanning. Reoperation and correction of the anastomosis is indicated if clinical compromise is apparent, which is particularly likely if there is significant left atrial anastomotic obstruction.

Haemorrhage

The underlying pulmonary disease of lung transplant recipients frequently leads to the formation of dense pleural adhesions and the hypertrophy of the bronchial circulation. These changes may promote haemorrhage following the removal of the recipient's native lung(s). Any degree of haemorrhage can be exacerbated by the anticoagulation necessary for cardiopulmonary bypass, which is required during some transplant operations. The incidence of major haemorrhage has been reduced by the use of aprotinin as a haemostatic and the use of a transverse incision rather than a median sternotomy in double lung transplant recipients, which allows better visualisation of the pleural surface and posterior mediastinum.[140]

Reimplantation response

The reimplantation response (morphologic, radiology, and functional changes that occur in a lung transplant in the early postoperative period) is the result of surgical trauma, ischaemia, denervation, lymphatic interruption, and other injurious processes (exclusive of rejection) that are unavoidable aspects of the transplant operation. The reimplantation response presents with the triad of worsened gas exchange, decreased lung compliance, and alveolar and interstitial infiltrates, typically most extensive in perihilar regions. The treatment is supportive, with mechanical ventilation, and diuretics and fluid-restriction as tolerated.

Pleural complications

Pleural space complications are not uncommon after lung transplantation, although they are usually of minor importance.

Pneumothorax

Pneumothorax may occur on either the side of a lung graft or on the side of a native lung. However, it is of greater concern when it arises from the lung graft because of the possibility of airway dehiscence communicating with the pleural space. More commonly, pneumothorax results from the rupture of a bulbous lesion in an emphysematous native lung after SLT. Conservative management with intercostal tube drainage is indicated.

Pleural effusions

Pleural effusions are common after lung transplantation, particularly when a large size disparity exists between the donor lungs and the thorax. Continued chest tube drainage following the primary procedure is not indicated as a preventive measure and may actually lead to secondary infection and empyema. Small-bore catheter drainage of persistent pleural effusions in lung transplant recipients is usually successful, but drainage is often prolonged and may require multiple catheter placements.[141]

Invasive measures, such as thoracentesis or tube drainage are indicated only for effusions complicated by a delayed pneumothorax, for enlarging effusions, or for large effusions that persist for more than four weeks postoperatively.

Empyema

Empyema is uncommon after lung transplantation. It is most frequently seen when a persistent pleural space due to a prolonged air leak, a chronic effusion, or an incompletely expanded lung is secondarily infected, usually with sputum flora. The management is initially conservative, with tube drainage and antibiotic therapy. In some cases, local drainage by rib resection or Eloesser flap will allow for adequate resolution. However, when the etiologic agent has a limited antimicrobial sensitivity (e.g., *B. cepacia* or *Aspercillus*) more aggressive measures such as transposition of muscle flaps or limited thoracoplasty to obliterate the space may be indicated.

Airway complications

Airway anastomotic complications are diagnosed by direct visualisation with flexible bronchoscopy.[142] Their presence also can be signalled by changes in follow-up spirometry indicative of unilateral mainstem bronchial obstruction.[143,144] Anastomotic narrowing due to granulation tissue can be treated with rigid bronchoscopy and surgical debrident, or with bronchoscopic N1):YAC laser ablation[145]; narrowing due to stricture formation can be managed with bronchoscopic dilatation or stem placement.[146]

Airway complications are significantly less common in the recent experience with lung transplantation. Bronchial ischaemia is the most common cause of postoperative airway complications. Airway ischaemia leads to mucosal ulceration, followed by progressive mural necrosis. Localised bronchomalacia is frequently present adjacent to this region, resulting in a spectrum of abnormalities ranging from anastomotic dehiscence to sub-mucosal fibrosis. Partial anastomotic dehiscence occurs followed by formation of granulation tissue and eventually some degree of anastomotic stenosis.

The overall incidence is 15–20%. Healing usually occurs without further treatment or secondary complication. In the remainder, the airway complication requires more specific management and may lead to secondary complications. Of these patients, 70% will require anastomotic dilatation or stent placement and 20% will develop a bronchopleural fistula that will require a tube and perhaps reoperation. Death due to sepsis or secondary infective complications occurs in 10% of the patients, who develop symptomatic airway complications.

In most cases, the treatment of airway complications is conservative. Significant granulations should be excised by rigid brochoscopy or laser excision, sometimes repeatedly, until healing is complete. The areas of granulation heal by fibrosis, which may cause anastomotic stenosis (more than 50%). These are amenable to dilatation by the rigid bronchoscope or by endobronchial balloon dilatation. Most of them will require the temporary placement of endobronchial stents for several months until sufficient remodeling of the fibrous tissue has occurred to create a stable anastomosis. Silastic self-retaining stents are used in most cases. Single lumen stents are used for most isolated lung transplant procedures, while the Y-type are useful for stenoses occurring after HLT or *en bloc* DLT.

Where free communication occurs between the anastomotic site and the pleural space or the mediastinum, reinflation of the lung by chest tube insertion and/or mediastinal drainage via a mediastinoscopy incision will usually result in healing. If there is complete dehiscence and massive airleak or mediastinal contamination, surgical revision is rarely possible because of the short length of donor bronchus. Urgent retransplantation has been successfully performed for these patients in some cases.

Cardiac and haemodynamic complications

Though relatively infrequent, both perioperative myocardial infarctions and cardiac arrests have occurred in lung transplant recipients.[147] More common cardiac and haemodynamic complications are atrial arrhythmias and episodes of systemic hypotension. Postoperative atrial arrhythmias, including atrial fibrillation and Flutter, are not unexpected given that atrial clamps are applied intraoperatively and that some handling of the heart is inevitable. Most convert spontaneously or with medical therapy, making the need for DC cardioversion infrequent.

Gastrointestinal complications

GI complications occurring early post-transplant include gastric ulcer perforation,[148] the development of a diaphragmatic hernia through the defect created to allow passage of the omental pedicle used to wrap the bronchial anastomosis, and the development of a prolonged paralytic ileus requiring nasogastric suction and parenteral nutritional support. A postoperative ileus developing in a transplant recipient may be potentiated by drug toxicities. GI complications occurring late may present atypically, resulting in delay in diagnosis and poorer outcomes.

A GI complication unique to patients with underlying cystic fibrosis (CF) is the development of a meconium ileus equivalent. In this syndrome, small bowel obstruction occurs, presenting with pain, distension, constipation, and bilious vomiting.[149]

Organ failure

This will present early during postoperative recovery, with poor gas exchange and delayed weaning from ventilation. The chest X-ray will show diffuse shadowing consistent with diffuse acute lung injury. Early organ failure may result from a long ischaemic time, poor organ preservation, or reperfusion injury. Supportive therapy is all that can be done pending an improvement in pulmonary function with the resolution of the X-ray appearances.

Infection

Bacterial pneumonia is common after lung transplantation as the lungs are continually exposed to the environment during the respiratory cycle. Sepsis can become overwhelming as a result of immunosuppression, and diagnosis and treatment with appropriate antibiotics must not be delayed. The bacteriological profile of recipients is observed preoperatively and donor lung lavage specimens are also investigated to provide early microbiological diagnoses and antibiotic sensitivities. All patients should receive prophylaxis against pneumocystis pneumonia with Co-Trimoxazole.

Oral fungal infection is prevented by the administration of Nystatin and Oraldene by mouth, but serious local or systemic infection with *Aspergillus* is of particular concern and may require treatment with toxic drugs such as Amphoteracin. Viral infections are also potentially life-threatening in the immuno-compromised patient. All patients receive prophylaxis against herpes virus infection with oral Acyclovir. CMV can be organ-transmitted and matching the recipient to donor for CMV status is certainly preferable. Prophylactic

CMV hyperimmune globulin may be given in cases of CMV mismatching, but severe disease, which usually develops in the fourth to eighth week postoperatively, may require intravenous Ganciclovir.

Rejection

The patients are maintained on Cyclosporine and Azathioprine regimes indefinitely, with Cyclosporine levels under constant review. Most patients experience one or two episodes of rejection. Significant rejection is characterised by pyrexia, worsening hypoxia and infiltrates on the chest X-ray. The diagnosis is often difficult as these symptoms and signs are also present in the adult respiratory distress syndrome and infection.

The lung graft must be continually monitored to detect sub-clinical rejection. Simple lung function tests are non-invasive and show a deterioration in both FEV1 and FVC in rejection. Transbronchial biopsy with a flexible bronchoscope used under radiological guidance is performed regularly to look for perivascular infiltrates of lymphocytes, which are diagnostic of rejection. Biopsies are performed at one week and one month post-transplant and at threemonthly intervals to one year. They are then taken at six-monthly intervals to the second year and yearly thereafter. Additional biopsies and lavage specimens may be obtained as clinically indicated to exclude infection or rejection. The biopsy of the heart is not required in combined heart-lung transplantation, as the rejection of the lung nearly always occurs first. Significant acute rejection must be treated with high dose pulsed intravenous Methylprednizolone for three days before repeat biopsy.

Obliterative bronchiolitis

The chronic rejection of the allograft is manifested as an organising obstruction of small airways with a surrounding lymphocyte infiltrate — obliterative bronchiolitis. About a third of long-term survivors develop this condition, which is characterised by a cough and progressive dyspnoea. It is unusual for obliterative bronchiolitis to present earlier than three months post-transplant, and patients undergo surveillance with lung function tests and transbronchial biopsy to detect it early. Obliterative bronchiolitis is more likely after repeated episodes of rejection, but bronchial ischaemia, viral infection and recurrent bacterial infection have all been implicated in the aetiology.[150] The treatment may take the form of augmented immunosuppression or total lymphoid irradiation, which is a more recent development. Retransplantation may be considered, but the results are not satisfactory.

Clinical results

Lung transplantation is an effective therapy in selected patients with end-stage pulmonary disease. A single, bilateral or combined heart-lung transplantation may be undertaken, depending on the clinical indication. The survival rates at one year were 66% following an SLT, 75% in BLT and 70% in HLT. At five years postoperatively, it was 50% following SLT, 60% each for BLT and HLT patients. Patients benefit considerably through improved quality of life and exercise tolerance.

POST-TRANSPLANT SURGICAL INFECTIONS

Solid organ transplantation has increased in frequency since the first human kidney was transplanted in 1954. The introduction of cyclosporine in 1980 remarkably improved the outcome of solid organ transplants, not only the graft function, but also prolonged patient survival.[151] Newer immunosuppressive agents like tacrolimus have even better results.

As immunosuppressive agents and graft survival have improved, infection and malignancy have become the main life-threatening complications following organ transplantation. As a result of the increased number of transplanted, and hence immunosuppressed people in the community, an increased incidence and spectrum of opportunistic infections is observed in this population.[152,153]

The diagnosis and treatment of infections in solid organ transplant patients is not an easy and straightforward process. The spectrum of pathogens causing infections and the symptoms are not the same as in non-transplant patients. The prevention, diagnosis and treatment of infection in this population requires a coordinated and integrated input from the transplant physicians, transplant surgeons, radiologists, pathologists and microbiologists.

Solid organ transplant patients tolerate infection badly and it is usually difficult to treat established infection. It is therefore vital to try to prevent them and to treat them promptly if they occur.

Surgeons have a great role in causing and preventing infection during transplant surgery. The adherence to strict asepsis during transplant surgery, competent surgical techniques and avoidance of haematomas and lymph collections reduces the chances of post-surgery infections.

The nursing of transplant patients plays a major role in prevention of infection. The nursing policies among hospitals vary from barrier nursing to ordinary wards, and consequently, the rate of post-transplant surgical infection also varies.

The general principles of prevention of surgical infections outlined early in this book, apply to transplantation surgery. However, extra effort should be made in the preoperative work up of the transplant patients to attain the best possible results.

Transplant candidates should be evaluated thoroughly prior to surgery and any identified infection should be treated; even asymptomatic infection can evolve into an overwhelming sepsis following transplantation. The sensitivity of the causative agents of infection to antimicrobial therapy should be documented for future use if needed. Patients with recurrent conditions like cholycystitis, diverticulitis or sinusitis should be treated surgically if necessary.

Patients predisposed to infections due to anatomical, metabolic or haematological problems should be identified and their need for prophylactic therapy assessed. Examples of such conditions are: Vesico-ureteric reflux, sinus obstruction, cardiac valvular abnormalities, intravascular clot, prosthetic biomaterials such as vascular grafts, artificial joints, dialysis access fistulae, or catheters.

Urinary catheters and intravenous lines should be avoided as much as possible before transplant and removed as early as possible after the transplant.

Different transplant centres follow varying protocols of antimicrobial prophylaxis prior to transplantation, depending on the type of transplant and the experience of each centre. Increasingly effective prophylactic and pre-emptive strategies are being developed to prevent the infectious consequences of immunosuppressive therapy. The cornerstone of this effort is the recognition that effective immunosuppressive strategies require an antimicrobial regime to make them safe and that such antimicrobial prophylaxis regime needs to be individualised to appropriately match the escalation and de-escalation of the immunosuppression.

Net State of Immunosuppression

The susceptibility of a transplant patient to infection is determined on one hand by his degree of immunosuppression and on the other, by exposure to pathogens either in the hospital or in the community. The degree of immuno-suppression or the **net state of immunosuppression** is the end result of a complex interaction of several factors.[154,155] It is the sum of any congenital, metabolic, operative, and transplant-related factors like

- Type, dose and duration of immunosuppressive agents
- Postoperative lymphocele, haematomas, devitalised tissues
- Cause of organ failure
- Comorbid conditions
- Infection with immuno-modulating viruses e.g., HIV
- Other causes of defective immune system

Timetable of Infection

Post-transplant infections tend to follow a regular predictable pattern within specific time frames.[151] The post-transplant period can be divided into three parts according to the susceptibly of the patient to different types of infectious agents.

The first six weeks post-transplant

The infections in this period are mainly due to surgery and hospitalisation or reactivation of infections already present in the recipient or transferred with the organ from the donor.

Transplantation surgery, like other types of surgery, can be followed by postoperative infective complication. Patients can develop urinary catheter related infection, pneumonia, surgical site infection, central venous line infection, ureteric stents related infections etc., and even nosocomial infections. Patients at a higher risk of nosocomial infection are those requiring prolonged ventilatory support, with diminished lung function, persistent ascites, stents of the urinary tract or biliary ducts and poorly revascularised graft tissue.[156,157]

Surgery and immunosuppression can reactivate infections already present in patients like sinusitis in CF patients who are receiving a lung transplant and urinary tract infection in patients with vesico-ureteric reflux who are receiving a kidney transplant. Infections can also be transferred from the donor and the classical example is hepatitis and CMV. These infections are avoidable by a good work up of both the transplant donor and recipient before surgery.

One to six months post-transplantation

During this period patients will be at high risk of opportunistic infections although some residual problems related to surgery can persist.

There is great variation in the incidence and type of opportunistic pathogens between different transplant centres and each centre has its own prophylaxis policy according to the prevalence of the pathogens in that specific centre.

Infections due to opportunistic pathogens include:

- *Pneumocystis jiroveci* (formerly *Pneumocystis carinii*) pneumonia
- Latent infections, such as protozoal diseases like toxoplasmosis, leishmaniasis and Chagas' disease[158]
- Geographic fungal infections, such as histoplasmosis, coccidioidomycosis, and rarely blastomycosis
- The viral pathogens, particularly the herpes group viruses but also CMV, hepatitis B and C
- Tuberculosis and increasingly non-tuberculous mycobacteria[159]

More than six months post-transplantation

Six months or more post-transplant, most patients recieve stable and relatively modest levels of immunosuppression. They are subject to community-acquired respiratory virus infection, particularly influenza and Pneumococcal pneumonia. Late infection can occasionally be related to the transplanted organ and there are some reports of infections originating from donated organs appearing months after the transplant.[160–162]

The patients with episodes of rejection who still need intensive immunosuppression will continue to be at high risk of opportunistic pathogens as in the first six months.

Evaluation of Transplant Patients with Suspected Surgical Infection

Transplantation surgery carries the same risk of surgical infection like other types of surgery, but the inflammatory response to infection is different due to immunosuppression. The suppression of the immune system leads to masking of clinical signs and symptoms of infection, which can progress silently to overwhelming sepsis. Furthermore, the transplantation surgery usually involves changes in the normal anatomy and hence changes the physical signs of infection. Because of this, and combined with the fact that transplant patients tolerate infection badly, surgeons should be very careful in assessing transplant patients with possible surgical infection.

Again, due to impaired immune response, routine laboratory investigations may be misleading and imaging and histological diagnosis must be considered. The threshold for advanced imaging like CT scanning and MRI should be low but this does not rule out preliminary X-rays and ultrasound scans. Cytology and histology obtained from the suspected site of infection is the only definitive answer to the question of diagnosis of infection.

Empirical antimicrobial therapy should be started as soon as infection is suspected and the choice of antibiotic should be considered carefully to cover the possible offended bacteria. Antibiotic therapy in transplant patients is a complicated issue as toxicity is common and interference and interaction with immunosuppressive agents is always a possibility.

Antibiotics can be used as the initial therapy but surgical intervention is frequently needed in surgical infections in transplant patients.

Some Examples of Lethal and Rare Post-Transplant Surgical Infections

Antifungal therapy is reasonably effective in treating invasive mycosis[162]; however in the transplant setting the usual dosages of Amphotericin B deoxycholate ranging between 1–1.5 mg/kg/day is frequently complicated by nephrotoxicity, precluding its continuation or necessitating a dosage reduction. In solid organ transplant recipients receiving Amphotericin B deoxycholate for aspergillosis, nephrotoxicity developed in 36% and dialysis was required in 18%.[163]

Although the role of surgery in treating invasive mycosis is not yet well defined,[164] surgery is used as an adjunct to antifungal therapy to prevent serious complications like massive haemoptysis in cases of angioinvasive fungi, e.g., aspergillosis and zygomycosis. It also helps in reducing the fungal burden facilitating medical treatment.[165] Early thoracic CT scans, along with aggressive medical and surgical approach to therapy, led to survival rates of 72% among neutropenic haematological patients with invasive aspergillosis.[166]

Surgery is considered a critical component of the management of another angioinvasive mycosis, zygomycosis. Lobectomy, brain abscess drainage and debridement are some times life saving procedures despite the high mortality.[167]

Combined surgical resection with antifungal therapy is the recommended therapeutic approach for phaeohyphomycosis. It is caused by dematiaceous or black pigmented fungi which are difficult to eradicate, even with prolonged antifungal therapy. Thus, for cutaneous and subcutaneous phaeohyphomycosis, complete, wide and deep margin resection should be performed.[168] Surgical resection, when feasible, is also recommended for central nervous system lesions due to phaeohyphomycosis.

Klein and his colleagues reviewed the management of hand and upper extremity infection in 911 cardiac transplant recipients at the Stanford University Medical Centre over a 30 years period. Thirteen heart transplant recipients were treated for infections of the hand and upper extremity on an inpatient basis, 10 (77%) required operative debridement, and three (23%) required more than one operative procedure. Furthermore, nine patients (69%) had bacterial infections, six (46%) had fungal infections [four of these (31%) had both bacterial and fungal infections], one (7.7%) had a mycobacterial infection, and one (7.7%) was not cultured. Hand and upper-extremity infections in transplant recipients frequently resulted in deep-space infections, tenosynovitis, and osteomyelitis. These are routinely managed by antibiotics, immobilisation, and limited incision and drainage. However, this study showed that in immunocompromised patients, these infections may be more aggressive, can be caused by more than one type of organisms and may require more emergent and active treatment.[169]

Another example of unusual pathogen presentation was published by El Khoury and his colleagues who described a case of post-menopausal tubo-ovarian abscess in a renal transplant recipient. It is an uncommon cause of infection in the female genital tract. The presentation included mild abdominal symptoms with rapid progression of peritonitis and surgical abscess that needed drainage.[170]

CONCLUSION

Transplantation surgery is a very challenging for both patients and surgeons. For the patients, transplantation is the start of a different life, free of the misery of a chronic disabling disease. This new life is not without problems and a high degree of compliance is needed to protect the patient and the graft. For the surgeons, transplantation is not only an operation that needs to be done skilfully, but the start of the life long care for their transplant patients. This often requires prompt diagnosis and intensive treatment of a variety of surgical and surgery related complications. It is a difficult task but the outstanding results of modern transplantation show that it is a task that is well worth the fight.

REFERENCES

1. Groggel GC. (1991) Acute thrombosis of the renal transplant artery: a case report and review of the literature. *Clin Nephrol* **36**(1): 42; Jordan ML, Cook GT, Cardella CJ. (1982) Ten years of experience with vascular complications in renal transplantation. *J Urol* **128**(4): 689–692.
2. Rijksen JF, *et al.* (1986) Vascular complications in 400 consecutive renal allotransplants. *J Cardiovasc Surg* **23**: 91.
3. Jordan ML, *et al.* (1996) Renal vascular hypertension in the transplant patient. In: *Renal Vascular Hypertension*. London: WB Saunders, pp. 267–285.
4. Huysmans FT, *et al.* (1987) Factors determining the prevalence of hypertension after renal transplantation. *Nephrol Dial Transplant* **2**: 34.
5. Erley M, Duda H, *et al.* (1992) Noninvasive procedures for diagnosis of renovascular hypertension in renal transplant recipients — A prospective analysis. *Transplantation* **54**(5): 863.
6. Sutherland RS, *et al.* (1993) Renal artery stenosis after renal transplantation: the impact of the hypogastric artery anastomosis. *J Urol* **149**: 980.
7. Dodd GD, *et al.* (1991) Imaging of vascular complications associated with renal transplants. *AJR* **157**: 449.

8. Lohr JW, *et al.* (1986) Percutaneous transluminal angioplasty in transplant renal artery stenosis: experience and review of the literature. *Am J Kidney Dis* **VII**(5): 363.

9. Benoit G, *et al.* (1987) Treatment of renal artery stenosis after renal transplantation. *Transplant Proc* **19**: 3600.

10. Shapira Z, *et al.* (1996) Revascularization for transplant renal artery stenosis. In: *Renal Vascular Disease* (WB Saunders, London), pp. 521–528.

11. Jordan ML, Cook GT, Cardella CJ. (1982) Ten years of experience with vascular complications in renal transplantation. *J Urology* **128**(4): 689–692.

12. Dophia NB, *et al.* (1991) Renal transplant arterial thrombosis: association with cyclosporine. *Am J Kidney Dis* **XVII**(5): 532.

13. Pluemecke C, *et al.* (1992) Renal transplant artery rupture secondary to Candida infection. *Nephron* **61**: 98.

14. Duckett T, *et al.* (1991) Noninvasive radiological diagnosis of renal vein thrombosis in renal transplantation. *J Urol* **146**: 403.

15. Merion RM, Calne RY. (1985) Allograft renal vein thrombosis. *Transplant Proc* **17**: 1746.

16. Delbeke D, Sacks GA, Sandier MP. (1989) Diagnosis of allograft renal vein thrombosis. *Clin Nucl Med* **14**: 415.

17. Chiu AS, Landsberg DN. (1991) Successful treatment of acute transplant renal vein thrombosis with selective streptokinase infusion. *Transplant Proc* **23**(4): 2297.

18. Brandenburg VM, Frank RD, Riehl J. (2002) Color-coded duplex sonography study of arteriovenous fistulae and pseudoaneurysms complicating percutaneous renal allograft biopsy. *Clin Nephrol* **58**(6): 398–404.

19. Merkus JWS, *et al.* (1993) High incidence of arteriovenous fistula after biopsy of kidney allograft. *Br J Surg* **80**: 310.

20. Schmid T, *et al.* (1989) Vascular lesions after percutaneous biopsies of renal allografts. *Transplant Int* **2**: 56–58.

21. Shoskes DA, *et al.* (1995) Urological complications in 1,000 consecutive renal transplant recipients. *J Urol* **153**(1): 18–21.

22. Jones JW, Hunter DR, Matas AJ. (1993) Successful percutaneous treatment of ureteral stenosis after renal transplantation. *Transplant Proc* **25**(I): 1038.

23. Dreikorn K. (1992) Problems of the distal ureter in renal transplantation. *Urol Int* **49**: 76.

24. Lang EK, Glorioso LW III. (1988) Antegrade transluminal dilatation of benign ureteral strictures: long term results. *AJR* **150**: 131.

25. Pozo Mengual B, *et al.* (2003) Ureteral stenosis after kidney transplantation: treatment with a self-expanding metal prosthesis. *Actas Urol Esp* **27**(3): 190–195.

26. Nicholson ML, *et al.* (1991) Urological complications of renal transplantation: the impact of Double J ureteric stents. *Ann R Coll Surg Engl* **73**: 316.

27. Motiwala HG, Shah SA, Patel SM. (1990) Ureteric substitution with Boari bladder flap. *Br J Urol* **66**: 369.

28. Cullman HJ, Prosinger M. (1990) Necrosis of the allograft ureter — Evaluation of different examination methods in early diagnosis. *Urol Int* **45**: 164.

29. Van Son JW, *et al.* (1986) Vesicocalicostomy as ultimate solution for recurrent urological complications after cadaveric renal transplantation in patient with poor bladder function. *J Urol* **136**: 889.

30. Malovrh M, *et al.* (1990) Frequency and clinical influence of lymphoceles after kidney transplantation. *Transplant Proc* **22**(4): 1423.

31. Fahlenkamp D, *et al.* (1993) Laparoscopic lymphocele drainage after renal transplantation. *J Urol* **150**: 316.

32. Fuller TF, *et al.* (2003) Management of lymphoceles after renal transplantation: laparoscopic versus open drainage. *J Urol* **169**(6): 2022–2025.

33. Caldwell TC, Burns JR. (1988) Current operative management of urinary calculi after renal transplantation. *J Urol* **140**: 1360.

34. Qazi YA, Ali Y, Venuto RC. (2003) Nephrolithiasis is an infrequent complication following renal transplantation and acquisition of a stone with the donor kidney is rare. *Ren Fail* **25**(2): 315–322.

35. Beiko DT, *et al.* (2003) Group A streptococcal hydrocele infection and sepsis in a renal transplant recipient. *Can J Urol* **10**(1): 1768–1769.

36. Finley DS, Roberts JP. (2003) Frequent salvage of ruptured renal allografts: a large single center experience. *Clin Transplant* **17**(2): 126–129.

37. Gill IS, *et al.* (1992) Clean intermittent catheterization and urinary diversion in the management of renal transplant recipients with lower urinary tract dysfunction. *J Urol* **148**: 1397.

38. Franz M, *et al.* (1992) Incidence of urinary tract infections and vesicorenal reflux: a comparison between conventional and anti-refluxive technique of ureter implantation. *Transplant Proc* **24**: 2773.

39. Penn I. (1994) The problem of cancer in organ transplant recipients: an overview. *Transplant Sci* **4**(l): 23–32.

40. Sutherland D, Gruessner A. International Pancreas Transplant Registry (IPTR): 2000 Midyear Update Report. University of Minnesota, Minneapolis, MN, USA.

41. Venstrom JM, *et al.* (2003) Survival after pancreas transplantation in patients with diabetes and preserved kidney function. *JAMA* **290**(21): 2817–2823.

42. Gruessner A, Sutherland DER. (1994) Pancreas transplants results in the United Network for Organ Sharing (UNOS) USA. Registry compared with non

USA-data in the International Registry. In Terasaki P, Cecka J, (eds.) *Clinical Transplants*. Los Angeles: UCLA Tissue Typing Laboratory, pp. 47–68.

43. Troppmann C, *et al.* (1996) Vascular graft thrombosis after pancreatic transplantation: univariate and multivariate operative and nonoperative risk factor analysis. *J Am Coll Surg* **182**(4): 285–316.

44. Papalois VE, Hakim NS, EL-Atrozy T, *et al.* (1998) Evaluation of the arterial flow of the pancreatic graft with Duplex-Doppler ultrasonography. *Transplant Proc* **30**(2): 255.

45. Troppman C, *et al.* (1998) Surgical complications requiring early relaparotomy after pancreas transplantation. *Ann Surg* **227**(2): 255–268.

46. Benedetti E, *et al.* (1997) Iliac reconstruction with arterial allograft during pancreas-kidney transplantation. *Clin Transplant* **1**: 459–462.

47. Benedetti E *et al.* (1998) A prospective randomized clinical trial of perioperative treatment with octreotide in pancreas transplantation. *Am J Surg* **175**(1): 14–17.

48. Benedetti E, *et al.* (1996) Intra-abdominal fungal infection after pancreatic transplantation: incidence, treatment and outcome. *J Am Coll Surg* **183**: 307–316.

49. Gruessner RWG, *et al.* (1997) The surgical risk of pancreas transplantation in the cyclosporine era: an overview. *J Am Coll Surg* **185**(2): 128–144.

50. Hakim N, Gruessner A, Papalois B. (1997) Duodenal complications in bladder-drained pancreas transplants. *Surgery* **121**(6): 618–624.

51. Hickey D, *et al.* (1997) Urological complications of pancreatic transplantation. *J Urol* **157**: 2042–2048.

52. Nghiem DD, Gonwa TA, Corry RJ. (1987) Metabolic effects of urinary diversion of exocrine secretions in pancreatic transplantation. *Transplantation* **43**: 70–75.

53. Tom WW, *et al.* (1987) Autodigestion of the glans penis and urethra by activated transplant pancreatic exocrine enzymes. *Surgery* **102**: 99–101.

54. Sollinger HW, *et al.* (1992) Indications for enteric conversion after pancreas transplantation with bladder drainage. *Surgery* **12**: 842–846.

55. Stephanian E, *et al.* (1992) Conversion of exocrinesecretions from bladder to enteric drainage in recipients of whole pancreatico-duodenal transplants. *Ann Surg* **216**: 663–672.

56. Van der Werf WJ, *et al.* (1998) Enteric conversion of bladder-drained pancreas allografts: experience in 95 patients. *Transplant Proc* **30**(2): 441–442.

57. West M, *et al.* (1998) Conversion from bladder to enteric drainage after pancreaticoduodenal transplantation. *Surgery* **124**(5): 883–893.

58. Kelly D, Sibal A. (2003) Current status of liver transplantation. *Indian J Pediatr* **70**(9): 731–736.

59. Marroquin CE, *et al.* (2003) Emergencies after liver transplantation. *Semin Gastrointest Dis* **14**(2): 101–110.

60. Imagawa DK, Busuttil RW. (1996) Technical problems: vascular. In: Busuttil RW, Klintmalm GB (eds), *Transplantation of the Liver*, 1st edn (WB Saunders Company, Philadelphia), pp. 626–632.

61. Samuel D, *et al.* (1989) Portal and arterial thrombosis in liver transplantation: a frequent event in severe rejection. *Transplant Proc* **21**: 2225–2227.

62. Northover JMA, Terblanche J. (1978) The importance of the blood supply to the bile duct in human liver transplantation. *Transplantation* **26**: 67.

63. Gunsar F, *et al.* (2003) Late hepatic artery thrombosis after orthotopic liver transplantation. *Liver Transpl* **9**(6): 605–611.

64. Flint EW, *et al.* (1988) Duplex sonography of hepatic artery thrombosis after liver transplantation. *AJR Am J Roentgenol* **151**: 481–483.

65. Stange BJ, *et al.* (2003) Hepatic artery thrombosis after adult liver transplantation. *Liver Transpl* **9**(6): 612–620.

66. Vivarelli M, *et al.* (2003) Repeated graft loss caused by recurrent hepatic artery thrombosis after liver transplantation. *Liver Transpl* **9**(6): 629–631.

67. Abad J, *et al.* (1989) Hepatic artery anastomotic stenosis after transplantation: treatment with percutaneous transluminal angioplasty. *Radiology* **171**: 661–662.

68. Helling TS. (1985) Thrombosis and recanalization of the portal vein in liver transplantation. *Transplantation* **40**: 446–448.

69. Uflacker R. (2003) Applications of percutaneous mechanical thrombectomy in transjugular intrahepatic portosystemic shunt and portal vein thrombosis. *Tech Vasc Intervent Radiol* **6**(1): 59–69.

70. Ott R, *et al.* (2003) Outcome of patients with pre-existing portal vein thrombosis undergoing arterialization of the portal vein during liver transplantation. *Transpl Int* **16**(1): 15–20.

71. Lo CM, Liu CL, Fan ST. (2003) Portal hyperperfusion injury as the cause of primary nonfunction in a small-for-size liver graft-successful treatment with splenic artery. *Liver Transpl* **9**(6): 626–628.

72. Nussler NC, *et al.* (2003) Diagnosis and treatment of arterial steal syndromes in liver transplant recipients. *Liver Transpl* **9**(6): 596–602.

73. Rose BS, *et al.* (1988) Transluminal balloon angioplasty of infrahepatic caval anastomotic stenosis following liver transplantation: case report. *Cardiovasc Intervent Radiat* **11**: 79–81.

74. Sullebarger, *et al.* (2003) Transjugular percutaneous inoue balloon mitral commissurotomy in a patient with inferior vena cava obstruction after liver transplantation. *Catheter Cardiovasc Intervent* **59**(2): 261–265.

75. Halff G, *et al.* (1990) Liver transplantation for the Budd-Chiari syndrome. *Ann Surg* **211**: 43–49.

76. Campbell DA, *et al.* (1988) Hepatic transplantation with perioperative and long term anticoagulation as treatment for Budd-Chiari syndrome. *Surg Gynecol Obstet* **166**: 511–518.

77. Navasa M, *et al.* (1993) Hemodynamic and humoral changes after liver transplantation in patients with cirrhosis. *Hepatology* **17**: 355–360.

78. Lata J, *et al.* (2003) Management of acute variceal bleeding. *Dig Dis* **21**(1): 6–15.

79. Nosaka T, *et al.* (2003) Varicose bleeding after liver transplantation in a patient with severe portosystemic shunts. *J Gastroenterol* **38**(7): 700–703.

80. Brems JJ, *et al.* (1988) Splenic artery aneurysm ruptures following orthotopic liver transplantation. *Transplantation* **45**: 1136–1137.

81. Ayalon A, *et al.* (1988) Splenic artery aneurysms in liver transplant patients. *Transplantation* **45**: 386–389.

82. Houssin D, *et al.* (1988) Mycotic aneurysm of the hepatic artery complicating human liver transplantation. *Transplantation* **46**: 469–472.

83. Soliman T, *et al.* (2003) The role of complex hepatic artery reconstruction in orthotopic liver transplantation. *Liver Transpl* **9**(9): 970–975.

84. Park JS, *et al.* (2003) Efficacy of endoscopic and percutaneous treatments for biliary complications after cadaveric and living donor liver transplantation. *Gastrointest Endosc* **57**(1): 78–85.

85. Hisatsune H, *et al.* (2003) Endoscopic management of biliary strictures after duct-to-duct biliary reconstruction in right-lobe living-donor liver transplantation. *Transplantation* **76**(5): 810–815.

86. Settmacher U, *et al.* (2003) Technique of bile duct reconstruction and management of biliary complications in right lobe living donor liver transplantation. *Clin Transplant* **17**(1): 37–42.

87. Abou-Rebyeh H, *et al.* (2003) Complete bile duct sequestration after liver transplantation, caused by ischemic-type biliary lesions. *Endoscopy* **35**(7): 616–620.

88. De Moor V, *et al.* (2003) Cholangitis caused by Roux-en-Y hepaticojejunostomy obstruction by a biliary stone after liver transplantation. *Transplantation* **75**(3): 416–418.

89. Shah JN, *et al.* (2003) Biliary casts after orthotopic liver transplantation: clinical factors, treatment, and biochemical analysis. *Am J Gastroenterol* **98**(8): 1861–1867.

90. Van de Vrie W, *et al.* (2003) Inflammatory bowel disease and liver transplantation for primary sclerosing cholangitis. *Eur J Gastroenterol Hepatol* **15**(6): 657–663.

91. Vera A, *et al.* (2003) Colorectal cancer in patients with inflammatory bowel disease after liver transplantation for primary sclerosing cholangitis. *Transplantation* **75**(12): 1983–1988.

92. Tachopoulou OA, *et al.* (2003) Hepatic abscess after liver transplantation: 1990–2000. *Transplantation* **75**(1): 79–83.

93. Shi LW, *et al.* (2003) Incisional hernia following orthotopic liver transplantation. *Transplant Proc* **35**(1): 425–426.

94. Heaton N, *et al.* (2003) Small-for-size liver syndrome after auxiliary and split liver transplantation: donor selection. *Transplantation* **9**(9): S26–S28.

95. Lillehei RC, *et al.* (1967) Transplantation of stomach, intestine, and pancreas: experimental and clinical observations. *Surgery* **62**: 721–741.

96. Monchik GJ, Russell PS. (1971) Transplantation of small bowel in the rat: technical and immunological considerations. *Surgery* **70**: 693–702.

97. Todo S, *et al.* (1995) Outcome analysis of 71 clinical intestinal transplantations. *Ann Surg* **222**: 270–282.

98. Veenendaal RA, *et al.* (2000). Clinical aspects of small-bowel transplantation. *Scand J Gastroenterol Suppl* **232**: 65–68.

99. Charbonnet P, *et al.* (1997) Small intestine transplantation. *Rev Med Suisse Romande* **117**(4): 337–341.

100. Abu-Elmagd K, Bond G. (2003) Gut failure and abdominal visceral transplantation. *Proc-Nutr-Soc* **62**(3): 727–737.

101. Muller AR, *et al.* (2003) Small bowel transplantation — current status and initial results. *Zentralbl Chir* **128**(10): 849–855.

102. Schroeder P, Goulet O, Lear PA. (1990) Small bowel transplantation: European experience. *Lancet* **336**: 110–111.

103. Tzakis A, Toclo S, Stand T. (1994) Intestinal transplantation. *Annit Rev Mcd* **45**: 79–91.

104. Jie Ding, *et al.* (2003) Postoperative endoscopic surveillance of human living-donor small bowel transplantations. *World J Gastroenterol* **9**(3): 595–598.

105. Mims TT, Fishbein TM, Feierman DE. (2004) Management of a small bowel transplant with complicated central venous access in a patient with asymptomatic superior and inferior vena cava obstruction. *Transplant Proc* **36**(2): 388–391.

106. Pascher A, *et al.* (2003) Late graft loss after intestinal transplantation in an adult patient as a result of necrotizing enterocolitis. *Am J Transplant* **3**(8): 1033–1035.

107. Rodeheffer R, McGregor C. (1992) The development of cardiac transplantation. *Mayo Clin Proc* **67**: 480–484.

108. Hardy J, *et al.* (1964) Heart transplantation in man: developmental studies and report of a case. *J Am Med Assoc* **118**: 1132–1137.

109. Barnard CN, *et al.* (1967) *S Afr Med J* **41**: 1271–1274.

110. Reitz BA. (1990) in Baumgartner WA *et al.* (eds), *Heart and Heart-Lung Transplantation* (Saunders, Philadelphia), pp. 1–14.

111. Caves P, *et al.* (1973) Percutaneous endomyocardial biopsy in human heart recipients. *Ann Thorac Surg* **16**: 325–329.
112. Lewis AB, *et al.* (1991) *Am J Cardiol* **68**: 365–369.
113. Addonizio LJ. (1992) *Prog Pediatr Cardiol* **1**: 72–80.
114. Kirklin JK, *et al.* (1988) *J Am Coll Cardiol* **11**: 917–924.
115. Hosenpud JD, *et al.* (1995) *J Heart Lung Transplant* **14**: 805–815.
116. Costanzo-Nordin MR. (1992) *J Heart Lung Transplant* **11**: S90–103.
117. Crandall BG, *et al.* (1988) *J Heart Lung Transplant* **7**: 419–423.
118. Renlund DG, *et al.* (1987) *Am J Med* **S3**: 391–398.
119. Lavée J, *et al.* (1991) *J Heart Lung Transplant* **10**: 921–930.
120. Kormos RL, *et al.* (1988) *Transplant Proc* **20**: 741–742.
121. Hammond EH, *et al.* (1990) *Transplantation* **50**: 776–782.
122. Normann SJ, *et al.* (1991) *J Heart Lung Transplant* **10**: 674–687.
123. Sociu-Foca N, *et al.* (1991) *Transplantation* **51**: 716–724.
124. Spiegelhalter DJ, Stovin PGI. (1983) *Statis Med* **2**: 33–40.
125. Hunt SA, *et al.* (2003) in Hurst, *et al.* (eds), *The Heart* (McGraw-Hill, New York).
126. Gao S, *et al.* (1988) Accelerated coronary vascular disease in the heart transplant patient: coronary angiographie findings. *J Am Coll Cardiol* **12**: 334–340.
127. Gao S-Z, Hunt S, Schroeder J. (1995) Accelerated graft coronary artery disease. In: Shumway SJ, Shumway NE (eds), *Thoracic Transplantation* (Blackwell Scientific, Cambridge, MA).
128. Halle A, *et al.* (1995) Coronary angioplasty, atherectomy, and bypass surgery in cardiac transplant recipients. *J Am Coll Cardiol* **26**: 120–128.
129. Hosenpud J, *et al.* (1998) The registry of the international society for heart and lung transplantation: fifteenth official report 1998. *J Heart Lung Transplant* **17**: 656–658.
130. Ensley R, *et al.* (1992) Predictors of survival after repeat heart transplantation. *J Heart Lung Transplant* **11**: S142–S158.
131. Richardson WS, *et al.* (2003) Gallstone disease in heart transplant recipients. *Ann Surg* **237**(2): 273–276.
132. Augustine S, *et al.* (1991) Gastrointestinal complications in heart and in heart-lung transplant patients. *J Heart Lung Transplant* **10**: 547–556.
133. Penn I. (1993) Incidence and treatment of neoplasia after transplantation. *Heart Lung Transplant* **12**: S328–S336.
134. Johnson WM, Baldrusson O, Gros TJ. (1998) Double jeopardy: lung cancer after cardiac transplantation. *Chest* **113**: 1720–1723.
135. Hosenpud JD, *et al.* (1995) *J Heart Lung Transplant* **14**: 805–815.
136. Métras D. Henri Métras. (1992) A pioneer in lung transplantation. *J Heart Lung Transplant* **11**(6): 1213–1215.

137. Hardy JD, *et al.* (1963) Lung homotransplantation in man: report of the initial case. *JAMA* **186**: 1065–1074.

138. Veith FJ. (1978) Lung transplantation. *Surg Clin North Am* **58**: 357–364.

139. Toronto Lung Transplant Group. (1986) Unilateral lung transplantation for pulmonary fibrosis. *N Engl J Med* **314**: 1140–1145.

140. De Hoyos A, Maurer JR. (1992) Complication following lung transplantation. *Sem Thorac Cardiovasc Surg* **4**: 132–146.

141. Marom EM, *et al.* (2003) Pleural effusions inlung transplantation. *Radiology* **228**(1): 241–245.

142. Shennib H, Massard G. (1994) Airway complications in lung transplantation. *Ann Thorac Surg* **57**: 506–511.

143. Anzeuto A, *et al.* (1994) Use of the flow-volume loop in the diagnosis of bronchial stenosis after single lung transplantation. *Chest* **105**: 934–936.

144. Neagos GR, *et al.* (1993) Diagnosis of unilateral mainstem bronchial obstruction following single-lung transplantation with routine spirometry. *Chest* **103**: 1255–1258.

145. Colt HG, *et al.* (1992) Endoscopic management of bronchial stenosis after double lung transplantation. *Chest* **102**: 10–16.

146. Dumon JE. (1990) A dedicated tracheobronchial stent. *Chest* **97**: 328–332.

147. Haydock DA, Trulock EP, Kaiser LR, *et al.* (1992) Lung transplantation: analysis of thirty-six consecutive procedures performed over a twelve-month period: Washington University Lung Transplant Group. *J Thorac Cardiovasc Surg* **103**: 329–340.

148. Hoekstra HJ, Hawkins K, de Boer WJ, *et al.* (2001) Gastrointestinal complications in lung transplant survivors that require surgical intervention. *Heart Lung* **88**(3): 433–438.

149. Littlewood JM. (1992) Gastrointestinal complications. *Br Med Bull* **48**: 847–859.

150. Novick RJ, Schafers HJ, Stitt L, *et al.* (1995) Recurrence of obliterative bronchiolitis and determinants of outcomes of 139 pulmonary retransplant recipients. *J Thorac Cardiovasc Surg* **110**: 1402–1414.

151. Fishman JA, Rubin RH. (1998) Infection in organ transplant recipients. *N Engl J Med* **338**: 1741.

152. Winston DJ, Emmanouilides C, Busuttil RW. (1995) Infection in liver transplant recipients. *Clin Infect Dis* **21**: 1077.

153. Rubin RH, Wolfson JS, Cosimi AB, Tolkoff-Rubin NE. (1981) Infection in the renal transplant recipient. *Am J Med* **70**: 405.

154. van den Berg AP, Klompmaker IJ, Haagsma EB, *et al.* (1996) Evidence for an increased rate of bacterial infections in liver transplant patients with cytomegalovirus infection. *Clin Transplant* **10**: 224.

155. Collins LA, Samore MH, Roberts MS, *et al.* (1994) Risk factors for invasive fungal infections complicating orthotopic liver transplantation. *J Infect Dis* **170**: 644.
156. Fishman JA. (2003) Vancomycin-resistant enterococcus in liver transplantation: what have we left behind? *Transplant Infect Dis* **5**: 109–111.
157. Hadley S, Karchmer AW. (1995) Fungal infections in solid organ transplant recipients. *Infect Dis Clin North Am* **9**: 1045.
158. Grossi P, Farina C, Riocchi R, Gasperina D. (2000) Prevalence and outcome of invasive fungal infections in 1,963 thoracic organ recipients. *Transplantation* **70**: 112.
159. Doucette K, Fishman JA. (2004) Non-tuberculous mycobacterial infection in hematopoietic stem cell and solid organ transplant recipients. *Clin Infect Dis* **38**: 1428.
160. Luppi M, Barozzi P, Schulz TF, *et al.* (2000) Bone marrow failure associated with human herpesvirus 8 infection after transplantation. *N Engl J Med* **343**: 1378.
161. Lake KD. (1995) Drug interactions in transplant patients. In: Emery RW, Miller LM (eds), *Handbook of Cardiac Transplantation* (Hanley and Belfus, Philadelphia), p. 173.
162. Linden PK. (2003) Amphotericin B lipid complex for the treatment of invasive fungal infections. *Expert Opin Pharmacother* **4**: 2099–2110.
163. Wingard JR, Kubilis P, Lee L, *et al.* (1999) Clinical significance of nephrotoxicity in patients treated with amphotericin B for suspected or proven aspergillosis. *Clin Infect Dis* **29**: 1402–1407.
164. Robinson LA, Reed EC, Galbraith TA, *et al.* (1995) Pulmonary resection for invasive Aspergillus infections in immunocompromised patients. *J Thorac Cardiovasc Surg* **109**: 1182–1197.
165. Singh N. (2000) Invasive mycoses in organ transplant recipients: controversies in prophylaxis and management. *J Antimicrob Chemother* **45**(6): 749–755.
166. Caillot D, Casasnovas O, Bernard A, *et al.* (1997) Improved management of invasive pulmonary aspergillosis in neutropenic patients using early thoracic computed tomographic scan and surgery. *J Clin Oncol* **15**: 139–147.
167. Singh N, Gayowski T, Singh J, Yu, VL (1995) Invasive gastrointestinal zygomycosis in a liver transplant recipient: case report and review of zygomycosis in solid-organ **transplant** recipients. *Clin Infect Dis* **20**: 617–620.
168. Clancy CJ, Singh, N. (1998) Dematiaceous fungi: chromoblastomycosis, mycetoma, subcutaneous and cutaneous phaeohyphomycosis, and non-invasive sinusitis. In: Yu VL, Merigan TC, Barriere SL (eds), *Antimicrobial Therapy and Vaccines* (Williams & Wilkins, Baltimore, MD), pp. 1095.

169. Klein Matthew B, Chang James. (2000) Management of hand and upper-extremity infections in heart transplant recipients. *Plast Reconstr Surg* **106**(3): 598–601.

170. El Khoury Joseph, Stikkelbroeck MML, Goodman Annekathryn, *et al.* (2001). Postmenopausal tubo-ovarian abscess due to pseudomonas aeruginosa in a renal transplant patient: a case report and review of the literature. *Transplantation* **72**(7): 1241–1244.

Chapter 26

COMPLICATIONS OF THE GASTROINTESTINAL ENDOSCOPIC PROCEDURES AND THEIR MANAGEMENT

David Westaby and Panagiotis Vlavianos

Considering the large number of endoscopic procedures performed and the importance given to the associated complications, it is surprising that there is a paucity of objective published data on this topic. Most of the reports on endoscopic complications are anecdotal and retrospective and often, what constitutes a complication is poorly defined. Furthermore, over the recent years the range of patients undergoing endoscopic procedures has changed, from screening procedures for perfectly healthy individuals to invasive procedures in patients with life threatening problems and a multitude of co-morbid conditions.

A complication has been variously defined as an incident occurring as a result of a procedure, which represents a deviation from the normal or ideal course, i.e., a negative outcome.

The complications associated with gastrointestinal (GI) endoscopic procedures can be divided into **general**, which can occur with any endoscopic procedure and **specific** for the type of the procedure.

While general complications include those associated with the risks of the sedation, analgesia and infection, specific complications include those associated with instrumentation.

Serious consideration should be given to proper evaluation of the indications and contraindications for any procedure, to prevent complications.

Finally, even after every possible precaution is taken, complications may arise in some patients and the endoscopist should have clear knowledge of their management.

In addition to the endoscopic sequelae conventionally described as complications, missed or inaccurate diagnosis should also be considered as a complication, but is not dealt with on this review.

GENERAL COMPLICATIONS

Complications Associated with Sedation and Analgesia, and Their Management

Background

Cardiopulmonary complications related to sedation and analgesia are the most common type of complication seen with diagnostic endoscopy and may account for over 50% of all reported complications in GI endoscopy (Tables 1 and 2).[1–4]

Table 1. Cardiopulmonary Complications of Upper GI Endoscopy

Frequency	0.005–0.5%
Mortality rate	0–0.05%

Rates differ depending on the population studied and length of follow up.[1–11]

Table 2.   Cardiopulmonary
Complications of Upper GI
Endoscopy

Cardiac Arrest
Respiratory Arrest
Transient Hypoxia
Aspiration Pneumonia
Pulmonary Embolism
Myocardial Infarction
CVA

As the number of elderly and high-risk patients subjected to endoscopic procedures increases, the number of cardiopulmonary complications rises in parallel. Sedation and analgesia may lead to respiratory depression, hypotension, cardiac or respiratory arrest and an inability to warn for excessive and dangerous instrumentation. The latter can lead to intense vagal stimulation or perforation. A judicious use of sedatives and analgesics is extremely important, especially in patients with chronic obstructive airways disease.

In one study, oxygen saturation was less than 80% in 7% of the pre-medicated patients undergoing gastroscopy.[5] Such desaturations may be lethal for patients with concomitant cardiovascular disease, although it is not clear how well desaturation correlates with myocardial ischaemia or the clinical outcome.

In a five-year prospective study from Norway,[6] with an overall complication and mortality rate of 0.14% and 0.04% respectively, non-fatal and fatal pulmonary complications occurred in 0.03% (2/7,314) of the patients undergoing a diagnostic upper GI endoscopy and in none of the 4,490 colonoscopy patients. Both fatalities occurred in patients with COPD. There were no cardiac complications documented in that series.

In a prospective British survey[7] of upper GI endoscopy in 36 hospitals involving 13,036 patients, the mortality rate for diagnostic endoscopy was 0.05% (1:2,000) and morbidity rate was 0.5% (1:200). At least five deaths resulted from cardiorespiratory complications during and after the diagnostic endoscopy. A further 36 instances of complication (11 pneumonia, six CVA, 19 MI) may have been related to the procedure, 67% of those occurring within seven days and the rest, within 30 days of the procedure. Only 11%

of the procedures were carried out without sedation, with or without a local anaesthetic. Furthermore, a clear link was established between the administration of local anaesthetic and the development of pneumonia after gastroscopy (10/11 patients with pneumonia, eight did not survive).

In a recent prospective German study[8] involving 110,469 OGD and 14,249 colonoscopies, the rate of cardiorespiratory complications were 0.005% and 0.01% respectively. The lower complication rate was attributed to only serious complications being recorded, improved monitoring and the participation of experienced gastroenterologists.

In another recent study[9] comprising 48% inpatients undergoing any type of endoscopic procedure, the extrapolated rate of occurrence of cardiovascular complications (defined as arrhythmia, chest pain or anginal equivalent, hypotension or myocardial infarction occurring within 24 h after endoscopy) was 308 (CI: 197–457) per 100,000 or one complication every 325 procedures, 2–70 times higher than previously reported. Independent risk factors were gender (male), modified Goldman score and the use of propofol. The Goldman score was developed and found to predict complications among patients undergoing surgery; it includes age, urgency of the procedure and evidence of cardiac arrhythmia, heart failure or hypoxia.

Management — recommendations

Cardiopulmonary complications occur relatively frequently during or after endoscopic procedures (Tables 1 and 2). Old age and co-existing heart or chest disease represent risk factors for these complications.

In patients with respiratory failure sedation is best to be avoided and endoscopy performed only if considered to have practical implications. Patients should be kept under close observation during and after an endoscopy.

The administration of benzodiazepines should be kept at a minimum and three minutes should elapse between doses. Benzodiazepines are eight times more potent when given with an opiod such as pethidine.[10] Therefore, it is important that the opioid is administered first followed by benzodiazepines at least one minute later so that their effect can be closely monitored. The endoscopist should be fully trained in basic and advanced life support and a resuscitation trolley should be immediately available. Benzodiazepine and opiod antagonists (Flumazenil 500 μg and Naloxone 400 μg) will counteract the action of the drugs given.

Routine oxygen supplementation may help counteract and pulse oximetry may detect the hypoxemia associated with sedation early; although most of the problems occur in high risk patients, some occur in low risk ones as well. The blood pressure should be routinely monitored in sedated patients.

Intravenous access with an indwelling plastic cannula should be established prior to the procedure and maintained until the patient has fully recovered. Local anaesthetic spayed into a vascular membrane is absorbed as quickly as if administered intravenously. Lignocaine is a respiratory depressant that can cause hypotension, bradycardia and cardiac arrest. These effects may be potentiated by benzodiazepines. Pharyngeal anaesthesia, combined with the presence of the endoscope is known to cause pulmonary aspiration.[11]

Risk of infection

Background

Infectious complications are extremely uncommon sequelae of GI endoscopic procedures. The most common type of infectious complications of endoscopy is thought to result from the endogenous microbial flora[12] gaining a portal entry, presumably because of mucosal trauma or instrumentation during the procedure. Patient to patient transmission, although understandably a cause of concern to the general public, is extremely rare.

(A) Risk of Endogenous Infections

Following diagnostic upper and lower GI endoscopy, the bacteremia rate is less than 4%. When observed, it is short lived (< 30 min), does not cause symptoms and the organisms most commonly recovered are from the oropharyngeal flora. Nevertheless, cases of endocarditis, meningococcemia, cerebral abcess, meningitis, retropharyngeal abcess, oesophageal abcess, perinephric abcess and empyema have been reported.

The risk can be higher following certain procedures. High-risk procedures include endoscopic sclerotherapy, endoscopic variceal ligation, oesophageal dilatation of benign and more commonly malignant strictures — especially when bougies rather than through the scope dilatation balloons are used — and percutaneous endoscopic gastrostomy (PEG) insertion. EUS is a relatively new procedure and infectious complications have been reported when performing FNA in a cystic lesion. ERCP-related infectious complications depend on the presence of an obstructed biliary system and pancreatic pseudocysts and will be discussed later in this review. Infectious complications are more common in cirrhotic or immunocompromised patients. Increased susceptibility to infection in cirrhosis has been attributed to impaired neutrophil chemotaxis, depressed levels of serum complement, B- and T- lymphocyte dysfunction, immunoglobulin defects and impaired reticuloendothelial system.

(B) Risk of Exogenous Infections

Patient to patient transmission of pathogens during endoscopy must be placed in the appropriate historical context to understand their relevance to infection control issues today.[13]

Hepatitis B: Prospective studies of patients who were exposed to an instrument contaminated with the hepatitis B virus (HBV) and seronegative patients, followed for up to one year after endoscopy, showed that despite inadequate disinfection, HBV transmission by endoscopy is extremely rare.

Hepatitis C: Although there have been a number of epidemiologic studies in which an association between endoscopy and the hepatitis C virus (HCV) seropositivity was found, there are difficulties in interpreting these studies. In fact, there are five published studies that demonstrate that the HCV is completely eliminated from contaminated endoscopes when accepted guidelines for cleaning and disinfection are followed.

HIV: There are no cases reported of endoscopic transmission of HIV.

Transmissible spongiform encephalopathies: To date no cases have been reported on the endoscopic tramsmission of CJD or other transmissible spongiform encephalopathies. **Variant Creutzfeldt-Jacob Disease** (vCJD) is a more recently recognised syndrome, believed to be caused by products containing the bovine spongiform encephalopathy (BSE) agent. No cases of endoscopic transmission have been reported.

Miscellaneous: Cases of salmonella transmission were last reported in 1987 but pseudomonas infection have been reported more recently and are associated with colonisation of water reservoir of the endoscopy equipment, and a failure to disinfect the elevator channel of the duodenoscope and dry the endoscope completely with 70% alcohol.

Recommendations

Protocols regarding endoscope disinfection should be adhered to very strictly. Local guidelines should be followed for the administration of antibiotic prophylaxis. In general, antibiotic prophylaxis is recommended when performing high-risk procedures in high-risk patients.

SPECIFIC COMPLICATIONS

Complications of Diagnostic Upper GI Endoscopy

Background

Major complication and death rates from diagnostic upper GI endoscopy are low, approximately 0.2–0.5% and 0.01–0.05% respectively, but can vary significantly depending on the patient population, the use of sedation and the endoscopic technique (Tables 3 and 4).[1–11]

Except for the complications associated with the use of sedation, a small risk of perforation and bleeding exists with diagnostic upper GI endoscopy. The perforation rate has been reported to be 0.03% following diagnostic upper GI endoscopy.[3] The predisposing factors to perforation include

Table 3.   Complications of Diagnostic   Upper   GI Endoscopy[1–11]

Morbidity:	0.13–0.5%
Mortality:	0.004–0.05%

Table 4.   Complications of Diagnostic Upper GI Endoscopy[1–11]

Cardiopulmonary
Perforation (0.03%)
Bleeding
Mallory-Weiss

the presence of anterior cervical osteophytes, Zenker's diverticulum, oeso-phageal strictures and malignancies. The mortality rate associated with oesophageal perforation is high, approximately 25%. The management of oesophageal perforation is discussed below.

Significant bleeding is a very rare complication of diagnostic upper GI endoscopy and usually occurs following a biopsy. The risk of haemorrhage may be increased (0.8%) in patients with previous gastric surgery.[14] Of the 15 patients identified in this study, two required a laparotomy, six were trans-fused and the rest necessitated only observation. It is more likely when throm-bocytopenia and/or coagulopathy is present but appears to be safe when platelets are above 20,000.

Mallory-Weiss tears occur in < 0.1% of diagnostic endoscopies and are usually not associated with significant bleeding.

Complications of Therapeutic Upper GI Endoscopy

Background

A 2004 report of the National Confidence Enquiry into Patient Outcome and Death[15] (NCEPOD) investigated the deaths occurring after a ther-apeutic endoscopy in hospitals in England, Wales and Northern Ireland. There were 3,669 deaths among 128,563 therapeutic procedures performed in 263 hospitals (overall mortality 3%). The overall therapeutic upper GI endoscopy mortality rate was 5% (PEG tube related mortality not included).

Complications of upper gastrointestinal dilatation

The most commonly observed complications of stricture dilatation are perfo-ration, pain, haemorrhage and bacteraemia/sepsis.[4,15] The risk of perforation varies from as low as 0.4% for a benign oesophageal stricture to as high as 10% when dilating a malignant one. The risk of bleeding has been shown to be 0–0.7%.[6,7,15] As discussed earlier, oesophageal dilatation is a high risk pro-cedure for bacteraemia and prophylactic antibiotics should be administered to moderate/high risk patients.

Benign oesophageal strictures: Although older studies[3] report a very low risk from dilatation of a benign stricture of approximately 0.4%, in a recent British survey,[7] perforation following dilatation of 554 benign strictures occurred in six patients (1.1%), half of whom did not survive.

The recently published NCEPOD survey showed a perforation rate of 2% following the dilatation of a benign stricture and 4.3% following dilatation (and stent insertion in 20% of the cases) of a malignant stricture in 2,945 patients who were audited prospectively. Two day mortality was 0.7%.

Achalasia dilatation: Achalasia dilatation carries a cumulative perforation risk of 2% but risk as high as 7% has been reported.[4] Risk may be minimised by using a graded dilatation technique, starting with a 30 mm balloon. Non-responders should then undergo dilatation to 35 mm and very rarely to 40 mm. Avoiding inflation pressure greater than 11 psi may be associated with fewer complications. Prolonged post-dilatation chest pain occurs in up to 15% of the patients. Gastro-oesophageal reflux, a relatively common problem after oesophageal myotomy, is a problem in only 5% of the patients.[16,17]

Malignant oesophageal strictures: The risk of perforation for dilating malignant oesophageal strictures is much higher than for benign strictures, approximately 10%.[4] Dilatation of a radiation stricture carries a risk of 2–6.5% and is not higher than the risk of dilating malignant strictures that did not receive radiation.[18,19]

Gastric outlet obstruction: The reported perforation rate is relatively low, from 0–6.7%. It appears as though perforations occur with attempts to dilate the gastric outlet to greater than 15 mm.[20]

Complications of gastric polypectomy

There is a relatively high risk of bleeding, up to 7.2% following this procedure[21] but in the majority of the cases the haemorrhage can be dealt with endoscopically and major complications occur only in 1.4% of the patients.

Complications in the treatment of upper GI malignancies

With the recent progress in the treatment of upper GI malignancies with chemo- and/or radiotherapy, endoscopic methods are currently used either as an emergency procedure or as palliation following treatment failure.

Thermal methods to apply heat energy directly to the tumour (argon plasma coagulation, laser, bipolar cautery) carry a major complication risk, approximately 10% including bleeding, perforation and fistula formation.[4]

Photodynamic therapy (PDT) is a relative recent treatment method, most commonly used in the treatment of early oesophageal neoplasia/high grade dysplasia. Complications include bleeding, perforation, fistulae, strictures, atrial fibrillation and sun photosensitivity.[22,23]

The insertion of **endoprostheses** in the form of self expandable metal stents are increasingly used in the management of malignant GI diseases, usually following treatment failure, to re-establish luminal patency. Post-stent deployment, and major complications (haemorrhage, perforation, aspiration) are relatively rare (3.3–7.5%).[4,24,25] Non-life threatening complications are common (20–40%) and include stent migration, blockage from food bolus or tumour in/over growth and these can usually be dealt with endoscopically. Pain is much less of a problem than it used to be with the previously used plastic stents and is present in 15% of the cases.

Oesophageal stents carry a higher risk of complication and lesser chance of acceptable palliation than gastroduodenal stents.[25]

Diagnosis and management of complications associated with upper GI endoscopy

Oesophageal perforation

Oesophageal perforation is the most feared complication of upper GI endoscopy, common between various — mainly therapeutic — endoscopic procedures in the upper gastrointestinal tract.

Accurate diagnosis and effective treatment of oesophageal perforation depends on early recognition of clinical features and clinical interpretation of diagnostic imaging. The most important factor determining the outcome is timing of diagnosis; if diagnosis is delayed more than 24 h, the mortality rate rises steeply from 10–25% to 40–60%.[26,27] This is because of the anatomical configuration and location of the oesophagus, which provides easy access to the mediastinum for bacteria and the digestive enzymes.

Despite advances in surgery, anaesthesia, postoperative care, hyperalimentation and the introduction of powerful antibiotics during the last two decades, leading to a substantial improvement in the outcome of oesophageal perforation, there is controversy regarding the best initial treatment of instrumental perforations. Most patients undergo emergency primary repair but favourable results have also been achieved with conservative management.[27]

In general there are three main signs and symptoms of oesophageal perforation[28]: pain, fever and emphysema (subcutaneous or mediastinal) but these can vary considerably resulting in delayed diagnosis. Crepitance, leucocytosis and pleural effusion may be present.

Ideally, most upper GI therapeutic procedures are performed under X-ray screening and the injection of contrast at the end of the procedure may demonstrate small leaks. The index of suspicion should be high following therapeutic procedures and a gastrografin swallow should be performed for persistent pain even in the absence of surgical emphysema. This may not reveal the leak either and clinical signs should alert the physician to ensure that the patient is not fed orally and begin broad spectrum antibiotics.

Non-operative management of oesophageal perforations should be considered if the perforation is circumscribed and drains well into the oesophagus, signs and symptoms of septicaemia are absent, the perforation is not in the abdominal cavity, not accompanied by obstructive oesophageal disease and not in the neoplastic tissue. If the conservative approach is chosen, even a slight deterioration in the patient's general condition should prompt a repeat of the gastrografin swallow and an immediate switch to surgical management.[29]

Since mortality increases steeply if the diagnosis of oesophageal perforation is made after 24 h, attempts have been made to improve the outcome of conservative management. In small non-controlled trials, the insertion of a covered (metal and more recently plastic) oesophageal stent in association with adequate drainage of the thoracic cavity showed promising results.[30] The insertion of a metal covered stent should also be considered in frail patients with malignant oesophageal disease.

Complications of endoscopic haemostasis

Background

Endoscopic haemostasis of non-variceal bleeding has been shown to significantly reduce rebleeding, the need for surgical intervention and ultimately mortality. A recently published meta-analysis[31] of 16 studies including 1,673 patients showed that although adrenaline injection alone is beneficial, the addition of a second therapeutic procedure further reduced rebleeding, emergency surgery and survival. This was regardless of the type of the second endoscopic procedure and although the benefit was more evident in patients with actively bleeding ulcers (Forrest Ia or Ib), the odds of rebleeding was 0.62 (95% CI: 0.31–1.22) in patients with non-bleeding visible vessel (Forrest IIa). A larger sample size is required to demonstrate a statistically significant effect. Complications included induction of massive bleeding requiring surgery (three patients), gastric wall necrosis (three patients) and perforation (four patients). These complications appeared with further injection and thermal methods and the two latter ones were more frequent in the combined (6/558) and not the adrenaline treatment group (1/560). The induction of bleeding occurred exclusively in the adrenaline-only group (5/560).

The treatment of **variceal bleeding** has undergone extensive investigation over the years and endoscopic variceal banding[34] has been established as the long-term treatment of choice. However, pharmacological treatment in the setting of acute bleeding or for long-term prophylaxis is also shown to be effective.

Management

Patients with severe/recurrent gastrointestinal haemorrhage are best managed by a multidisciplinary team of surgeons, gastroenterologists and radiologists, ideally in a high dependency area. The value of basic fluid resuscitation, to maintain normal haemodynamic parameters and adequate urinary output, should not be underestimated. If the initial endoscopic treatment fails to stop the haemorrhage surgical exploration or in high-risk patients, radiological embolisation should be carried out. If only temporary haemostasis is achieved and bleeding recurs, the therapeutic options include repeated endoscopic therapy, embolisation or surgery. The choice of treatment may be difficult and should depend on the available expertise, the condition of the patient and the haemodynamic and endoscopic findings. Furthermore, ulcers larger than 2 cm in diameter associated with hypotension when bleeding recurs, may be less likely to respond to repeat endoscopic therapy.[32] Treatment with high dose omeprazole has been shown to further reduce the incidence of rebleeding following dual endoscopic therapy.[33]

Variceal banding is associated with a 25% risk of rebleeding and can cause mucosal ulceration, oesophageal strictures, bacterial peritonitis and pulmonary infections. However, the extent of incidence is lower than with endoscopic sclerotherapy. The adherence to proper technique and banding protocol, including airways protection if necessary, and allowing at least a week between banding sessions for treatment-induced ulcers to heal, the use of sucralfate and protein pump inhibitors and prophylactic use of antibiotics reduce the likelihood of complications. If bleeding persists, a TIPS or surgery should be considered.

Complications of Percutaneous Endoscopic Gastrostomy (PEG) Tube Insertion

Background

A 1% incidence of immediate PEG-related mortality has been reported, but 30-day mortality is higher, at approximately 7%,[35,36] (Tables 5 and 6) indicating that the patient condition is often poor.

The aforementioned NCEPOD report[15] comprising 16,648 patients who had undergone a PEG procedure showed a 30-day mortality rate of 6%; of these

Table 5. Complications of Percutaneous Endoscopic Gastrostomy (PEG)[4,15,35,36]

Procedure Related Mortality	1%
30-Day Mortality	7%
Major Complications	0.4–8.4%

Table 6. Complications of Percutaneous Endoscopic Gastrostomy (PEG)[4,15,35,36]

Infection
Bleeding
Ileus
Internal Organ Injury
Tumour Seeding
Early PEG Tube Dislodgement
Late PEG Tube Dislodgement

43% died within one week. In 19% of the patients, the NCEPOD advisors considered the procedure futile. These data are in agreement with previous reports and stress the importance of an in-depth assessment for the indication of a PEG feeding tube as well as the need to adhere to strict procedural protocols.

The major complications associated with a PEG tube insertion occur in 0.4–8.4%[4,15,35,36] of the patients and include infection, bleeding, ileus, injury of internal organs and tumour seeding. Infectious complications include wound infections, abcess, necrotising fasciitis and aspiration pneumonia. Pneumoperitoneum has been reported in up to 38% of the patients following PEG tube insertion and is totally benign.

Management — recommendations

The prophylactic use of antibiotics has been shown to reduce the peristomal wound infections significantly and should be used routinely. Specific mention should be made of necrotising fasciitis which albeit rare is fatal in 30–70% of the cases. A high index of suspicion is required for the diagnosis and its treatment includes surgical debridement and antibiotics.

Bleeding can result from injury to gastric or abdominal wall vessels. The risk of bleeding is much higher if portal hypertension is present and collateral circulation has developed. Insertion of the PEG tube under or following ultrasound guidance is recommended.

Injury to internal organs such as the liver or colon can occur. Numerous reports of colo-gastro-cutaneous fistulae exist in the literature. These can remain silent until the original tube is replaced. Prompt removal of the tube is recommended as the fistula should heal within hours.

Feeding tubes can migrate and become impacted in the abdominal wall, the buried bumper syndrome. It is believed to be the result of excessive traction on the internal PEG bolster and results in resistance to flow through the tube and immobility of the tube. The treatment involves replacement of the tube with a new one. This can be very difficult sometimes, especially if the bumper is not visible endoscopically. If possible, a guide wire should be passed through the tube, the tract dilated and the tube subsequently pulled through endoscopically or pushed percutaneously. Alternatively, radial incisions can be made using an endoscopic knife to facilitate visualisation and grasping of the tube. Finally, on rare occasions a mini laparotomy may be required. If in doubt, an endoscopic ultrasound may provide information regarding the exact position of the bumper and facilitate removal.

Several reports have raised concerns of potential tumour seeding at the PEG site in patients with head and neck cancer. Fluoroscopic percutaneous feeding tube insertion may be preferable in these patients.

Early (within 10–15 days) tube dislodgement, before the formation of a mature fistulous tract, can result in peritonitis and may need a laparotomy. Late tube dislodgement is a relatively common occurrence in non-cooperative patients; a Foley catheter should be immediately inserted if possible to maintain tract patency. Care should be taken to avoid duodenal obstruction from distant Foley migration. Contrast injection and fluoroscopic checking can be used if there are doubts on the correct placement of the tube.

PEJ tube insertion is increasingly used, especially in the intensive care setting, to minimise the risk of aspiration. This involves a smaller diameter extension tube inserted through a standard PEG and positioned endoscopically at the distal duodenum/proximal jejunum. An estimated 91% reduction in the risk of aspiration against the propensity to block or migrate back in the stomach justifies the use of this tube in selected patients.

Complications of Colonoscopy

Background

Major complication and death rates from diagnostic and therapeutic colonoscopy have been reported in the region of 0.2–0.02% and 2–0.05% respectively[15,37] (Tables 7 and 8). These consist of bleeding, perforation, myocardial infarction and cerebrovascular accidents.

In considering the complications associated with colonoscopy, one should differentiate between **diagnostic vs therapeutic** colonoscopy, **younger vs older**

Table 7. Complications of Diagnostic and Therapeutic Colonoscopy[37–47]

	Diagnostic	Therapeutic
Morbidity	0.2%	2%
Mortality	0.02%	0.05%

Table 8.   Complications of Diagnostic
and Therapeutic Colonoscopy[37–47]

Cardiorespiratory	0.3%
Abdominal Pain	0.9%
Bleeding	0.2–2.3%
Perforation	0–0.3%
Post-polypectomy Syndrome	0.5–1.2%
Spleenic Rupture	
Intra-abdominal	
Haemorrhage	

patients, with or without **co-morbid diseases** and **asymptomatic vs symptomatic** individuals (i.e., screening colonoscopy or investigation of symptoms or findings from other tests like FOBT, flexible sigmoidoscopy, Ba enema or virtual colonoscopy). Finally although we may have accurate data for **immediate** post-procedural complications, **late complications** may still be underestimated because of under reporting. Furthermore, the definition of complications may vary among centres.

In a prospective study[38] of screening colonoscopy in 3,196 asymptomatic subjects (96.8% men, mean age 63 years, no active cardiac or pulmonary disease but 20% IHD, 8% previous CVA/TIA, 20% DM and 8.5% COPD), with polypectomy of at least one polyp performed in 53.8% of the group, there were no perforations and bleeding occurred in 0.22%, always associated with a polypectomy. The interval between the polypectomy and the onset of clinically apparent haemorrhage ranged from 1–16 days post-procedure. In all, there were **0.56% major complications** using strict criteria including 0.12% of the patients suffering an MI/CVA within nine days of the procedure. There was one death from a witnessed cardiac arrest two days after the colonoscopy. The colonoscopy itself was carried out without problems. Abdominal pain lasting > 2 hrs occurred in 0.8% of the patients and pain resulting in termination of the procedure in 0.9%. When only the complications of a diagnostic procedure were considered, the overall complication rate was 0.1%.

In another recent large scale survey from Germany[8] where only serious complications were considered (defined as needing intervention), there were 0.02% complications among 82,416 colonoscopies, 0.005% requiring surgery after a perforation had occurred, 0.001% bleeding episodes at biopsy sites, 0.01% cardiopulmonary complications and one death (mortality 0.001%) after surgery for a perforation. In the same study there were 0.36% complications out of 14,249 polypectomies, 0.26% bleeding, 0.06% perforation and 0.007% mortality (one patient died post-surgery from persistent bleeding).

Minor colonoscopic complications include vasovagal events and transient oxygen desaturation during the procedure, abdominal pain during or after the procedure and post-colonoscopy minor GI bleeding.

Rare complications include splenic rupture,[39] tearing of mesenteric vessels with intra-abdominal haemorrhage, acute appendicitis,[40] snare entrapment and ensnarement of adjacent normal bowel.[41]

In a British study comparing colonoscopic success, the diagnostic yield and complications in patients over and less than 80 years old[42] it was shown that the caecal intubation and complication rates were similar between the two groups and the main difference was a much higher detection rate of colorectal cancer in the older group (20% vs 7.4%).

Diagnosis and management of colonoscopic complications

The recognition of **factors associated with an increased risk of complications** may be used to decrease unfavourable outcomes. Pre-procedure history and physical examination may show an increased risk of cardiovascular, bleeding or other complications.

Benefit risk ratio should be considered in patients with co-morbidity and extra care taken with respect to bowel preparation and sedation. Severe electrolyte disturbances can occur in elderly patients or in those with renal or congestive heart failure. Minimal sedation should be used during the procedure. In the aforementioned British study,[42] significantly lower quantities of midazolam and meperidine were used in the older group. Adherence to proper technique during the procedure and injection of saline or epinephrine to raise the polyp before a polypectomy is performed, particularly for large, right-sided sessile polyps, may reduce the risk of bleeding and decrease the depth of thermal injury.[43] Mini snare resection of very small polyps without electrocautery, instead of hot-biopsy may decrease the risk of bleeding and perforation. Polyp size has been shown to be related to the risk of post-polypectomy bleeding (7% and 16% risk of bleeding when removing polyps greater than 10 mm and 20 mm respectively).[44] Although there are no prospective studies due to small numbers, it is believed that certain diagnoses including acute pseudo-obstruction, ischaemic colitis, severe inflammatory bowel disease, malignancy, steroid use and radiation colitis increase the risks of colonoscopy.

Colonoscopic perforation: The perforation rate during diagnostic or therapeutic colonoscopy vary between 0–0.3%.[38,45–47] The perforation could be due to mechanical trauma, barotrauma or as a result of a therapeutic procedure. Early symptoms are persistent abdominal pain and distention, and signs of peritonitis develop later. Plain abdominal X-ray in an upright position may demonstrate free air under the diaphragms but, if in doubt, abdominal CT scanning is recommended.[48]

Surgical consultation should be obtained if a free perforation is suspected. While surgical repair is often required, non-surgical management may be appropriate in some individuals; patients with silent perforation or signs of localised peritonitis without sign of sepsis who continue to improve with conservative management may avoid surgery. This includes bowel rest, intravenous fluids and antibiotics, and serial clinical examinations to detect early clinical deterioration.

There is a significant increase in morbidity and mortality with delayed diagnosis and treatment; the morbidity and mortality of the operative treatment of patients with colonic perforation has been found to correlate with the time to repair and surgical technique. Primary closure or resection and anastomosis are associated with lower morbidity and mortality than a diverting colostomy.[49,50] The post-polypectomy coagulation syndrome occurring due to a transmural burn in 0.51–1.2% should be considered in patients presenting with signs of localised peritonitis 1–5 days post-polypectomy, especially for sessile right sided polyps.[45,46] Free peritoneal air is absent and management is conservative.

Post-polypectomy haemorrhage: Acute post-polypectomy haemorrhage is often immediately apparent and amenable to endoscopic therapy. If a residual polyp stalk is present, this can be snared and the bleeding vessel coagulated. If this is not possible or no stalk is present, initial injection with adrenaline solution (1:10,000) will usually stop the bleeding, the area will be visualised better and thermocoagulation or hemoclips can be applied. If the bleeding persists, angiographic embolisation should be considered and surgery is the final option.[51,52]

Complications of Flexible Sigmoidoscopy

The perforation rate following a sigmoidoscopy is very low, between 0.01–0.004%.[53,54] Bleeding occurs very rarely unless a polypectomy was performed, in 0.006% of the patients. Besides discomfort, the most common complication of flexible sigmoidoscopy is vasovagal reaction, occurring in about 1% of patients.[53]

Complications of ERCP

As with other endoscopic procedures, the reported rates of complications of ERCP vary depending on study design, case mix, definition of complications and length of follow up. The average complication rate varies from 5–16% and mortality from 0.1–1.0% (Tables 9 and 10).[55–59] Recent studies have graded complications according to their severity as advocated by Cotton *et al.*[60] thereby facilitating comparison between different centres. The NCEPOD report in 2004[15] showed an ERCP-associated mortality of 2% but importantly it was thought that in 68% of the patients the procedure was futile due to the presence of liver metastasis and lack of biliary obstruction.

Table 9. Complications of ERCP[55–59]

Morbidity	5–16%
Mortality	0.1–1%

Table 10. Complications of ERCP[55–62]

Type	Frequency
Pancreatitis	5% (2–9%)
Haemorrhage	0.76–3.2%
Perforation	0.3–3.8%
Cholangitis	1–5%
Cholecystitis	0.5%
Cardiopulmonary	1–2.4%

The most common complication following an ERCP was sepsis (including post-ERCP pancreatitis related) followed by respiratory problems. A relatively high perforation rate in 2% of the cases was directly attributable to ERCP and haemorrhage in 4%.

Post-ERCP pancreatitis

Post-ERCP pancreatitis is one of the commonest ERCP related complications occurring in about 5% of the patients but with a wide variation in the reported series. It has recently become increasingly clear that there are patient and procedure related factors for post-ERCP pancreatitis. Multivariate analyses have shown that young age, female gender, suspected sphincter of Oddi dysfunction (SOD), prior post-ERCP pancreatitis, absence of chronic pancreatitis, pancreatic duct injection, pancreatic sphincterotomy, balloon dilatation of the sphincter, difficult or failed cannulation and pre-cut sphincterotomy for access in the bile duct are definitely related to increased risk of pancreatitis. The absence of CBD stones, normal serum bilirubin, pancreatic acinarization, pancreatic duct brush cytology, pain during ERCP and low endoscopy volume may be related, while non-dilated CBD, pancreas divisum, periampullary diverticulum, allergy to contrast media, prior failed ERCP, intramural contrast injection, biliary sphinctetomy, SOD manometry and therapeutic versus diagnostic ERCP do not seem to be associated with an increased risk. Standard endoscopic sphincterotomy does not increase the risk of pancreatitis.[55–63]

If one takes a critical look on the above, a profile of the high-risk patient for post-ERCP pancreatitis emerges: younger age, female gender, recurrent abdominal pain with no biliary obstruction present (suspected stones or SOD) and a history of recurrent or post-ERCP pancreatitis. More importantly, severe pancreatitis occurs almost exclusively in such patients.[57,63] Therefore, it is important that the risk factors are assessed prior to an ERCP and alternate procedures considered (MRCP, EUS, intraoperative cholangiogram) for high risk patients.

Strategies for avoiding post-ERCP pancreatitis

The best strategy to avoid post-ERCP pancreatitis is careful patient selection. Diagnostic ERCP should be avoided and alternative imaging investigations

(USS, MRCP, EUS) should be used to diagnose the pancreatico-biliary pathology.

Once an ERCP is performed, the insertion of a pancreatic stent is indicated in high-risk patients. This is shown to significantly decrease the risk of pancreatitis by approximately a factor of three, and virtually eliminate the risk of severe or necrotising pancreatitis with an odds ratio of 11.5 times lower.[64] Pancreatic stent insertion should be performed by an operator familiar with the technique, since in most studies the failure rate for pancreatic stent insertion ranges from 5–10% and it is conceivable that this confers a risk for pancreatitis.[65] The same study showed that insertion of a pancreatic stent was always successful, even in patients with small, tortuous ducts, when small caliber guide wires (0.018 inch) and short (2–3 cm), small diameter (3–4 Fr) stents were used. Following stent insertion pancreatic ductal and parenchymal changes have been observed in one to two thirds of the patients. Although most of these changes resolve spontaneously, the long-term outcome has not been thoroughly investigated. However, these changes were shown when 5–7 Fr stents were inserted, often for a relatively long time. Unflanged, longer, 3 Fr stents with a single duodenal pigtail have been shown to be associated with lower frequency of ductal changes.[63] These, if still present on an abdominal radiograph, should be removed endoscopically in two weeks.

Pharmacologic prevention of post-ERCP pancreatitis has been investigated in many studies,[63] but the results have been rather disappointing. Nitroglycerine either sublingually or transdermally, diclofenac as a rectal suppository post-ERCP, gabexate, a protease inhibitor, administered as a 6–12 h continuous infusion and somatostatin (but not octreotide) in a 12 h infusion may be effective. Their use has not been generally adopted because of several problems with the published trials. Inclusion of low risk patients, unclear definition of pancreatitis, high rate of pancreatitis in the control groups, large number of patients needed to treat to prevent an episode of pancreatitis and high expense are some of the problems encountered.

Haemorrhage

Haemorrhage is primarily a complication related to endoscopic sphincterotomy. Post-endoscopic sphincterotomy bleeding has been reported in 0.76–3.2%[54–57] of the patients. Moderate haemorrhage (up to four units of blood transfused) occurs in 0.9% and severe haemorrhage (necessitating the transfusion of five or more units of blood, angiography or surgery) occurs in 0.5% of the patients.[61] In approximately half the cases, clinical recognition of haemorrhage is delayed for 1–10 days after the endoscopic sphincterotomy.[59,61] The presence of coagulopathy, active cholangitis before the procedure, anticoagulant therapy within three days of the procedure, the endoscopist's case volume, precut sphincterotomy and observed bleeding during the procedure were shown to be independently associated with haemorrhage on a multivariate analysis.[58,59,61] The fact that post-endoscopic sphincterotomy risk of bleeding is related to the operator's experience and bleeding during the ERCP should reflect less precise control of the incision, or less effective endoscopic control of bleeding during the procedure. The relatively high percentage of delayed haemorrhage probably indicates inadequate coagulation rather than transection of an aberrant arterial branch. Should haemorrhage be noticed during or following an endoscopic sphincterotomy, it can often be stopped by injection of 1:10,000 adrenaline solution and or electrocautery. If bleeding does not stop or recurs, angiographic embolisation or surgery may be necessary.

Perforation

The incidence of perforation for ERCP has been reported between 0.3–3.8%.[56,59,61] Three types of perforation have been described: guide-wire induced perforation, periampullary perforation during sphincterotomy and perforation at a site remote from the papilla. Stent-related perforations have also been reported.[66] The risk factors for perforation are pre-cut sphincterotomy, intramural injection of contrast and Bilroth II gastrectomy. The perforation site is usually retroperitoneal. Prompt recognition and treatment with biliary and duodenal drainage, ensuring that the patient does not eat or drink anything, and administering broad spectrum antibiotics, results in clinical resolution without the need for surgical intervention in the majority (up to 86%) of the cases.[60,61,67,68]

Cholangitis and other infectious complications

This complication has generally been reported below 1% and it usually follows failed drainage in an obstructed system. In a prospective Danish study with a

30-day follow up, cholangitis was found in 5% of the patients post-ERCP.[56] Multivariate analysis showed that stent insertion was the single important risk factor for this complication. Combined percutaneous-endoscopic procedures have also been shown to predispose to cholangitis on a univariate analysis.[61]

Newly diagnosed cholecystitis occurs in 0.5–0.7% usually following endoscopic sphincterotomy.[56,61] In a European prospective trial of endoscopic balloon dilatation versus endoscopic sphincterotomy for the removal of bile duct stones, acute cholecystitis occurred in 7/71 (10%) patients in the sphincterotomy group who were followed up for six months.[69]

Cholangitis following ERCP for malignant hilar strictures (Klatskin tumours) deserves special mention. A randomised prospective trial comparing unilateral versus bilateral teflon stents, reported similar relief of jaundice but a lower rate of cholangitis in the unilateral stent group.[70] MRCP can be used in this setting to direct to the ductal system most suitable for drainage.[71] It is recommended that filling of all the intrahepatic segments should be avoided and attempts be made to drain all the filled segments.[72,73] More recently, self expandable metal stents have been used for malignant hilar strictures.[74,75] These appear to improve biliary drainage and decrease the risk of cholangitis and the need for biliary re-intervention but a randomised controlled trial is required to confirm it.

One has also to bear in mind when dealing with this type of tumour that surgical option should always be considered before an endoscopic intervention is attempted, even on a jaundiced patient, since currently surgeons are more successful in aggressively treating even the relatively advanced disease.[76]

Cardiorespiratory and thromboembolic complications

Significant cardiopulmonary complications have been reported in 1–2.4% of the patients[55,56,58,59,61] within 30 days of the procedure. These include atrial fibrillation, tachycardia with and without hypotension, chest pain, myocardial infarction, pneumonia and respiratory insufficiency.

Thromboembolic complications occur in up to 0.7% of the patients, including cerebrovascular events, TIA and thrombosis in upper and lower extremities. If the overall condition of the patients undergoing an ERCP is taken into account, these complications may not be as common as expected.

Complications of Endoscopic Ultrasound

In the recent years, endoscopic ultrasound (EUS) has seen a big expansion of its use and applications in diagnosing and staging GI and non-GI malignancies, aspirating fluid from cystic collections and obtaining samples for cytology of solid lesions in close proximity to the GI lumen.

Most studies that assess the complications related to this procedure are retrospective but there are a few prospective ones. The overall reported morbidity and mortality range from 0–5% and 0–1% respectively, most complications occurring following fine needle aspiration (FNA) (Tables 11 and 12).

In a recently published large prospective study from Denmark[77] of 3,324 patients, of whom 670 (20.2%) underwent an FNA for histological assessment, complications during or immediately after the procedure occurred in 10 (0.3%). Fifty percent of the complications (five patients) were oesophageal perforations in patients with oesophageal cancer and in two, following dilatation. The remaining complications included one mild pancreatitis, two patients with hemiparesis occurring during the procedure and one case each of post-procedural bleeding and myocardial infarction. The last two patients had undergone an FNA and did not survive (mortality 0.06%).

Table 11.   Complications of EUS[72–80]

Morbidity	0–5%
Mortality	0–1%

Table 12.   Complications of EUS[72–80]

Perforation	0–03%
Infection	0–1%
Pancreatitis	0–2%
Bleeding	0–1.3%
Cancer Seeding	
Bile	
Peritonitis	

Perforation

A survey of 86 physicians on cervical oesophageal perforation during EUS reported 16 perforations among 43,852 (0.03%) with one death (0.002% mortality).[78] The majority (94%) of the perforations occurred in patients over 65 years, and in those with a radial-scanning echoendoscope (15 of 16 patients). Furthermore, 44% of the patients had a history of difficult intubation during a prior endoscopic procedure, and 12 (75%) cases were because of physician inexperience (less than one year's experience in upper EUS or trainees). Two of the surviving 15 patients required surgical intervention.

Both oesophageal cancer and strictures have been independently linked to an increased incidence of oesophageal perforation[79] and recommendations vary from no touch to stepwise dilatation or use of mini probes.

Duodenal perforations have been reported during EUS examinations, but their overall incidence has not been studied.

Infectious complications

The frequency of bacteremia as a complication of EUS and EUS-FNA has been prospectively studied in three separate trials, none of which included rectal EUS.[80–82] These studies collectively included over 250 patients and no statistically significant difference was found in the frequency of bacteremia when compared with that seen at upper GI endoscopy. A single case of streptococcal sepsis has been reported among 327 lesions undergoing EUS-FNA in a patient with a pancreatic serous cystadenoma, despite prophylactic antibiotics.[83] The patient recovered with further antibiotic therapy.

Mediastinal cysts appear to be at risk of infection during EUS-FNA, either from bacterial or fungal organisms and can lead to mdiastinitis.[84] There have been isolated reports of retroperitoneal abcesses after EUS-guided celiac plexus block.[85] There have been no reports of perirectal abcesses following transrectal FNA. From the existing evidence it can be concluded that prophylactic antibiotics are not recommended for FNA of solid masses and lymphnodes. EUS-FNA of cystic lesions, especially mediastinal, appears to carry an increased risk of infection (< 1%) and therefore prophylactic antibiotics should be given prior to the procedure, and for a short duration.

Pancreatitis

The reported rate of pancreatitis following FNA of pancreatic lesions range from 0–2%.[83,86]

Haemorrhage

The reported incidence of bleeding following FNA varies between 0–1.3%. Occasional deaths from bleeding have been reported. Over a 13-month period, one study specifically evaluated extra luminal haemorrhage occurring among 227 patients undergoing EUS-FNA.[87] The overall rate was 1.3%.

Other rare complications reported following EUS-FNA include cancer seeding of the fine needle track following FNA of a malignant lesion[88] and bile peritonitis.[89] EUS-guided celiac plexus blockade or neurolysis carries a small risk of major complications comparable to the one associated with percutaneous blockade or neurolysis.

REFERENCES

1. Freeman ML. (1994) Sedation and monitoring for gastrointestinal endoscopy. *Gastrointest Endosc Clin N Am* **4**: 475–499.
2. Benzamin SB. (1996) Complications of conscious sedation. *Gastrointest Endosc Clin N Am* **6**: 277.
3. Silvis SE, Nebel O, Rogers G, Mandelstam P. (1976) Results of the 1974 American society for gastrointestinal endoscopy survey. *JAMA* **235**: 928.
4. (2002) Complication of upper GI endoscopy. Standards of practice committee of the American society for gastrointestinal endoscopy. *Gastrointest Endosc* **55**: 784–793.
5. Hart R, Classen M. (1990) Complications of diagnostic gastrointestinal endoscopy. *Endoscopy* **22**: 22–23.
6. Reiertsen 0, Skjoto J, Jacobsen CD, Rosseland AR. (1987) Complications of fiberoptic gastrointestinal endoscopy five years' experience in a central hospital. *Endoscopy* **19**: 1–6.
7. Quine MA, Bell GD, McCloy RF, *et al.* (1995) Prospective audit of upper gastrointestinal endoscopy in two regions of England: safety, staffing and sedation methods. *Gut* **36**: 462–467.
8. Sieg A, Hachmoeller-Eisenbach U, Eisenbach T. (2001) Prospective evaluation of complications in outpatient GI endoscopy: a survey among German Gastroenterologists. *Gastrointest Endosc* **53**: 620–627.

9. Gangi S, Saidi F, Patel K, *et al.* (2004) Cardiovascular complications after GI endoscopy: occurrence and risks in a large hospital system. *Gastrointest Endosc* **60**: 679–685.

10. Ben-Shlomo I, Abd-El-Khan H, Ezry J, *et al.* (1990) Midazolam acts synergistically with fentanyl for induction of anaesthesia. *Br J Anaesth* **64**: 45–57.

11. (1991) Pulmonary aspiration during emergency endoscopy in patients with upper gastrointestinal haemorrhage. *Crit Care Med* **19**: 330–333.

12. Nelson DB. (2003) Infectious disease complications of GI endoscopy: Part I, endogenous infections. *Gastrointest Endosc* **57**: 546–556.

13. Nelson DB. (2003) Infectious disease complications of GI endoscopy: Part II, exogenous infections. *Gastrointest Endosc* **57**: 695–711.

14. Domellof L, Enander L-K, Nilsson F. (1983) Bleeding as a complication to endoscopic biopsies from the gastric remnant after ulcer surgry. *Scand J Gastroenterol* **18**: 951–954

15. Scoping our practice. The 2004 report of the National Confidential Enquiry into Patient Outcome and Death.

16. Wehrmann T, Jacobi V, Jung M, *et al.* (1995) Pneumatic dilatation in achalasia with a low-compliance balloon: results of a 5-year prospective evaluation. *Gastrointest Endosc* **42**: 31–36.

17. Eckardt VF, Kanzler G, Westermeier T. (1997) Complications and their impact after pneumatic dilatation for achalasia: prospective long-term follow-up study. *Gastrointest Endosc* **45**: 349–353.

18. Swaroop VS, Desai DC, Mohandas KM, *et al.* (1994) Dilation of esophageal strictures induced by radiation therapy for cancer of the oesophagus. *Gastrointest Endosc* **40**: 311–315.

19. Ng TM, Spencer GM, Sargeant IR, *et al.* (1996) Management of strictures after radiotherapy for oesophageal cancer. *Gastrointes Endosc* **43**: 584–590.

20. Kuwada SK, Alexander GL. (1995) Long term outcome of endoscopic dilation of non-malignant pyloric stenosis. *Gastrointest Endosc* **41**: 15–17.

21. Muehldorfer SM, Stolte M, Martus P, *et al.* (2002) Diagnostic accuracy of forceps biopsy versus polypectomy for gastric polyps: a prospective multicentre study. For the Multicenter Study Group "Gastric Polyps". *Gut* **50**(4): 465–470.

22. Overholt BF, Panjehpour M, Haydek JM. (1999) Photodynamic therapy in Barrett's oesophagus: follow-up in 100 patients. *Gastrointest Endosc* **49**: 1–7.

23. Maier A, Tomaselli F, Gebhard F, *et al.* (2000) Palliation of advanced esophageal carcinoma by photodynamic therapy and irradiation. *Ann Thorac Surg* **69**: 1006–1009.

24. Dumonceau J-M, Deviere J. (1999) Self expandable metal stents: oesophageal stents. *Baillere's Clin Gastroenterol* 13: 109–119.

25. Lindsay JO, Andreyev HJN, Vlavianos P, Westaby D. (2004) Self-expanding metal stents for the palliation of malignant gastroduodenal obstruction in patients unsuitable for surgical bypass. *Aliment Pharmacol Ther* 19: 901–905.

26. Brinster CJ, Singhal S, Lee L, *et al.* (2004) Evolving options in the management of esophageal perforation. *Ann Thorac Surg* 77(4): 1475–1483.

27. Gupta NM, Kaman L. (2004) Personal management of 57 consecutive patients with esophageal perforation. *Am J Surg* 187: 58–63.

28. Nair LA, Reynolds JC, Parkman HP, *et al.* (1993) Complications during pneumatic dilatation for achalasia or diffuse oesophageal spasm. Analysis of risk factors, early clinical characteristics, and outcome. *Dig Dis Sci* 38: 1893–1904.

29. Altorjay A, Kiss J, Voros A, Bohak A. (1997) Non-operative management of esophageal perforations: Is it justified? *Ann Surg* 225(4): 415–421.

30. Siersema PD, Homs MYV, Haringsma J, *et al.* (2003) Use of large diameter metallic stents to seal traumatic non-malignant perforations of the oesophagus. *Gastrointest Endosc* 58(3): 356–361.

31. Calvet X, Vergara M, Brullet E, *et al.* (2004) Addition of a second endoscopic treatment following epinephrine injection improves outcome in high-risk bleeding ulcers. *Gastroenterology* 126: 441–450.

32. Lau JYW, Sung JJY, Lam Y-H, *et al.* (1999) Endoscopic retreatment compared with surgery in patients with recurrent bleeding after initial endoscopic control of bleeding ulcers. *N Engl J Med* 340: 751–756.

33. Lau JYW, Sung JJY, Lam Y-H, *et al.* (2000). Effect of intravenous Omeprazole on recurrent bleeding after endoscopic treatment of bleeding peptic ulcers. *N Engl J Med* 343: 310–316.

34. Laine L, Cook D. (1995) Endoscopic ligation compared with sclerotherapy for treatment of esophageal variceal bleeding. A meta-analysis. *Ann Intern Med* 123: 280–287.

35. Larson DE, Burton DD, Schroeder KW, DiMango EP. (1987) Percutaneous endoscopic gastrostomy. Indications, success, complications and mortality in 314 consecutive patients. *Gastroenterology* 93: 48–52.

36. Mathus-Vliegen LM, Koning H. (1999) Percutaneous endoscopic gastrostomy and gastrojejunostomy: a critical reappraisal of patient selection, tube function and the feasibility of nutritional support during extended follow-up. *Gastrointest Endosc* 50: 746–754.

37. Complications of colonoscopy. (2003) Statement of the standards of practice committee of the American society for gastrointestinal endoscopy. *Gastrointest Endosc* 57: 441–445.

38. Nelson DB, Mc Quaid KR, Bond JH, *et al.* (2002) Procedural success and complications of large scale screening colonoscopy. *Gastrointest Endosc* **55**: 307–314.

39. Janes SEJ, Cowan IA, Dijkstra B. (2005) A life threatening complication after colonoscopy. *BMJ* **330**: 889–890.

40. Hirata K, Noguchi J, Yoshikawa I, *et al.* (1996) Acute appendicitis immediately after colonoscopy. *Am J Gastroenterol* **91**: 2239–2240.

41. Nivatvongs S (1986). Complications in colonoscopic polypectomy: an experience with 1555 polypectomies. *Dis Colon Rectum* **28**: 825–830.

42. Arora A, Singh P. (2004) Colonoscopy in patients 80 years of age and older is safe, with high success rate and diagnostic yield. *Gastrointest Endosc* **60**: 408–413.

43. Norton ID, Wang L, Susan AL, *et al.* (2002) Efficacy of colonic submucosal saline solution injection for the reduction of iatrogenic thermal injury. *Gastrointest Endosc* **56**: 95–99.

44. Zubarik R, Mastropietro C, Lopez J, *et al.* (1999) Prospective analysis of complications 30 days after outpatient colonoscopy. *Gastrointest Endosc* **50**: 322–328.

45. Nivatvongs S. (1986) Complications in colonoscopic polypectomy: an experience with 1555 polypectomies. *Dis Colon Rectum* **28**: 825–830.

46. Macrae F, Tan K, Williams C (1983) Towards safer colonoscopy: a report on the complications of 5000 diagnostic or therapeutic colonoscopies. *Gut* **24**: 376–383.

47. Waye J, Lewis B, Yessayan S. (1992) Colonoscopy: a prospective report of complications. *J Clin Gastroenterol* **15**: 347–351.

48. Stapokis J, Thickman D. (1992) Diagnosis of pneumoperitoneum: abdominal CT vs. upright chest film. *Comput Assist Tomogr* **16**: 713–716.

49. Gedebou TM, Wong RA, Rappaport WD, *et al.* (1996) Clinical presentation and management of iatrogenic colonic perforations. *Am J Surg* **172**: 454–458.

50. Vincent M, Smith LE. (1983) Management of perforations due to colonoscopy. *Dis Colon Rectum* **6**: 61–63.

51. Sorbi D, Norton I, Conio M, *et al.* (2000) Post-polypectomy lower GI bleeding: descriptive analysis. *Gastrointest Endosc* **51**: 690–696.

52. Parra-Blanco A, Kaminaga N, Kojima T, *et al.* (2000) Hemoclipping for post-polypectomy and post-biopsy colonic bleeding. *Gastrointest Endosc* **51**: 37–41.

53. Ashley, *et al.* (2001) Achieving quality in flexible sigmoidoscopy. *Am J Med* **111**: 649.

54. Anderson ML, Pasha TM, Leighton JA. (2000) Endoscopic perforation of the colon: lessons from a 10-year study. *Am J Gastroenterol* **95**: 3418–3422.

55. (2003) Complications of ERCP. The standards of practice committee of the American society for gastrointestinal endoscopy. *Gastrointest Endosc* **57**: 633–638.

56. Christensen M, Matzen P, Schulze S, Rosenberg J. (2004) Complications of ERCP: a prospective study. *Gastrointest Endosc* **60**: 721–731.

57. Vandervoot J, Soetikno RM, Tham TCK, *et al.* (2002) Risk factors for complications after performance of ERCP. *Gastrointest Endosc* **56**: 652–656.

58. Masci E, Toti G, Mariani A, *et al.* (2001) Complications of diagnostic and therapeutic ERCP: a prospective multicenter study. *Am J Gastroenterol* **96**(2): 417–423.

59. Loperfido S, Angelini G, Benedetti G, *et al.* (1998) Major early complications from diagnostic and therapeutic ERCP: a prospective multicenter study. *Gastrointest Endosc* **48**: 1–10.

60. Cotton PB, Lehman G, Vennes J, *et al.* (1991) Endoscopic sphincterotomy complications and their management: an attempt at consensus. *Gastrointest Endosc* **37**: 383–393.

61. Freeman ML, Nelson DB, Sherman S, *et al.* (1996) Complications of endoscopic biliary sphincterotomy. *N Engl J Med* **335**(13): 909–918.

62. Freeman ML, DiSario JA, Nelson DB, *et al.* (2001) Risk factors for post-ERCP pancreatitis: a prospective, multicenter study. *Gastrointest Endosc* **54**: 425–434.

63. Freeman ML, Guda MD. (2004) Prevention of post-ERCP pancreatitis: a comprehensive review. *Gastrointest Endosc* **59**: 845–864.

64. Singh P, Sivak MV, Agarwal D, *et al.* (2003) Prophylactic pancreatic stenting for prevention of post-ERCP acute pancreatitis: a meta-analysis of controlled trials (abstract). *Gastrointest Endosc* **57**: AB89.

65. Freeman ML, Overby C, Qi D. (2004) Pancreatic stent insertion: consequences of failure and results of a modified technique to maximize success. *Gastrointest Endosc* **5**: 8–14.

66. Rashdan A, Fogel E, McHenry L, *et al.* (2003) Pancreatic ductal changes following small diameter long length unflanged pancreatic stent placement (abstract). *Gastrointest Endosc* **57**: AB213.

67. Howard TJ, Tan T, Lehman GA, *et al.* (1999) Classification and management of perforations complicating endoscopic sphincterotomy. *Surgery* **126**: 658–665.

68. Enns R, Eloubeidi MA, Mergener K, *et al.* (2002) ERCP-related perforations: risk factors and management.*Endoscopy* **34**: 293–298.

69. Bergman JJGHM, Rauws AAJ, Folckens P, *et al.* (1997) Randomised trial of endoscopic balloon dilation versus endoscopic sphincterotomy for removal of bileduct stones. *Lancet* **349**: 1124–1129.

70. De Palma GD, Galloro G, Siciliano S, *et al.* (2001) Unilateral versus bilateral endoscopic hepatic duct drainage in patients with malignant hilar biliary obstruction: results of a prospective, randomized and controlled study. *Gastrointest Endosc* **53**: 547–553.

71. Hintze RE, Abou-Rebyeh H, Adler A, *et al.* (2001) Magnetic resonance cholangiopancreatography-guided unilateral endoscopic stent placement for Klatskin tumours. *Gastrointest Endosc* **53**: 40–46.

72. Sherman S. (2001) Endoscopic drainage of malignant hilar obstruction: is one biliary stent enough or should we work to place two? *Gastrointest Endosc* **53**: 681–684.
73. Chang WH, Kortan P, Haber GB. (1998) Outcome in patients with bifurcation tumours who undergo unilateral versus bilateral hepatic duct drainage. *Gastrointest Endosc* **47**: 354–362.
74. Peters RA, Williams SG, Lombard M, *et al.* (1996) The management of high-grade hilar strictures by endoscopic insertion of self-expanding metal endoprostheses. *Endoscopy* **28**: 10–16.
75. Cheng JLS, Bruno MJ, Bergman JJ, *et al.* (2002) Endoscopic palliation of patients with biliary obstruction caused by non-resectable hilar cholangiocarcinoma:efficacy of self-expandable metallic Wallstents. *Gastrointest Endosc* **56**: 33–39.
76. De Groen PC, Gores GJ, LaRusso NF, *et al.* (1999) Biliary tract cancers. *N Engl J Med* **341**: 1368–1378.
77. Mortensen MB, Fristrup C, Holm FS, *et al.* (2005) Prospective evaluation of patient tolerability, satisfaction with patient information and complications in endoscopic ultrasonography. *Endoscopy* **37**: 146–153.
78. Das A, Sivac MV Jr., Chak A. (2001) Cervical esophageal perforation during EUS:a national survey. *Gastrointest Endosc* **53**: 599–602.
79. Adler DG, Jacobson BC, Davila RE, *et al.* (2005) ASGE guideline: complications of EUS. *Gastrointest Endosc* **61**(1): 8–12.
80. Barawi M, Gottlieb K, Cunha B, *et al.* (2001) A prospective evaluation of the incidence of bacteremia associated with EUS-guided fine-needle aspiration. *Gastrointest Endosc* **53**: 189–192.
81. Levy MJ, Norton ID, Wiersema MJ, *et al.* (2003) Prospective risk assessment of bacteremia and other infectious complications in patients undergoing EUS-guided FNA. *Gastrointest Endosc* **57**: 672–678.
82. Janssen J, Konig K, Knop-Hammad V, *et al.* (2004) Frequency of bacteremia after linear EUS of the upper GI tract with and without FNA. *Gastrointest Endosc* **59**: 339–344.
83. Williams DB, Sahai AV, Aabakken L, *et al.* (1999) Endoscopic ultrasound guided fine needle aspiration biopsy: a large single center experience. *Gut* **44**: 720–726.
84. Wildi SM, Hoda RS, Fickling W, *et al.* (2003) Diagnosis of benign cysts of the mediastinum: the role and risks of EUS and FNA. *Gastrointest Endosc* **58**: 362–368.
85. Hoffman BJ. (2002) EUS-guided celiac plexus block/neurolysis. *Gastrointest Endosc* **56**(Suppl): S26–S28.

86. Gress F, Michael H, Gelrud D, *et al.* (2002) EUS-guided fine needle aspiration of the pancreas: evaluation of pancreatitis as a complication. *Gastrointest Endosc* **56**: 864–867.
87. Affi A, Vasquez-Sequeiros E, Norton ID, *et al.* (2001) Acute extraluminal haemorrhage associated with EUS-guided fine needle aspiration: frequency and clinical significance. *Gastrointest Endosc* **53**: 221–225.
88. Shah JN, Fraker D. (2004) Melanoma seeding of an EUS-guided fine needle track. *Gastrointest Endosc* **59**: 923–924.
89. Chen HY, Lee CH, Hsieh CH. (2002) Bile peritonitis after EUS-guided fine-needle aspiration. *Gastrointest Endosc* **56**: 594–596.

Chapter 27

COMPLICATIONS OF INTERVENTIONAL RADIOLOGICAL PROCEDURES

Gabriel Conder and Wady Gedroyc

INTRODUCTION

Over the last 40 years many clinical problems requiring surgical intervention have been responding to minimally invasive procedures under imaging guidance (Table 1).

Significant advantages in terms of patient morbidity or mortality can be gained using radiological intervention rather than conventional surgical methods, which in turn leads to financial savings for healthcare services. For example, the classical treatment for renal artery stenosis was surgical reconstruction; however, percutaneous transluminal angioplasty[2] can be done as a day case or an overnight stay with similar results and has become the treatment of choice.

The expansion in the variety of different interventional radiological procedures has lead to an increase in the percentage of examinations, from 1% in 1989 to 5% in 1997, leading to an increase in the workload of these departments.[3]

Table 1. Clinical Problem, Surgical Treatments and Interventional Radiology Alternatives[1]

Clinical Problem	Surgical Solution	Interventional Radiology Solution
Acute abdomen	Laparotomy	Image guided drainages
Hydro- and pyonephrosis	Surgical nephrostomy	Percutaneous nephrostomy
Nephrolithiasis	Surgical nephrolithotomy	Percutaneous nephrolithotomy
Malignant biliary obstruction	Surgical choledochoenterostomy	Percutaneous biliary drainage and stent placement
Undiagnosed mass lesions	Open biopsy	Image guided biopsy
Peripheral vascular disease	Endarterectomy, bypass	PTA, stent placement
Upper gastrointestinal bleeding due to varices	Surgical portocaval shunt creation	Transjugular intrahepatic portosystemic shunt creation
Renal artery stenosis	Endarterectomy, bypass	PTA, stent placement
Feeding difficulties	Surgical gastrostomy	Percutaneous gastrostomy
Peripheral or pulmonary arteriovenous malformations	Surgical resection	Embolisation, ablation
Uterine leiomyoma	Hysterectomy, myomectomy	Embolisation, ablation
Sub-arachnoid haemorrhage due to aneurysm	Craniotomy and aneurysm clipping	Coil embolisation
Hepatic tumours	Hepatic resection	Ablation

With the increasing utilisation of interventional radiology services by surgical and other clinical teams it is important for the referring clinicians to understand the potential complications, to aid the choice of treatment and allow for early detection and treatment of complications.

While all interventional radiological procedures carry the risk of specific complications there are general considerations applicable to most of these procedures. Often, the failure of the clinicians to consider these factors while organising a procedure results in delay or cancellation of the intervention. Some of these factors, such as the pregnancy status of a woman about to undergo an X-ray procedure, are already familiar to clinicians. In addition, they should be familiar with the risk of complications in using iodinated

X-ray contrast in patients with iodine allergy, atopic asthma or on metformin for diabetes before requesting IVU or contrast enhanced CT.

The factors specifically related to interventional radiological procedures include risk of bleeding that is associated in varying degrees with any interventional procedure. A patient's full blood count and clotting should be checked prior to an anticipated intervention, ideally early enough to allow for the correction of clotting or platelet abnormalities. That the patients may be taking anti-coagulants is also a possibility that must not be ruled out.

Complications, delay and cancellation of the intervention due to these general factors can generally be avoided with timely recording of history, examination and laboratory investigation, and proper liaison with the interventional radiologists. They would far rather be involved in the planning of a procedure than to have a poorly prepared or inappropriate patient arrive in the interventional room.

GASTROINTESTINAL INTERVENTIONAL RADIOLOGY

Gastrointestinal Stenting

Colorectal stenting

Patients with colonic obstruction secondary to malignant disease can be treated radiologically with a self-expanding metal stent relieving the obstruction for elective single-stage surgery with a primary end-to-end anastomosis or as a primary palliative procedure.

The technique involves having the sedated patient in the left lateral position and a stiff guide wire passed through the stricture. A self-expanding stent is then placed with the stricture at its midpoint. The technical success rate is between 90–100%[4–7] with shorter stays and fewer complications compared with surgically treated patients.[5]

Significant complications occur in less than 10% of the patients, and include bowel perforation, stent migration and sepsis.[4,7–10,11] Uncovered stents have a lower risk of migration[9] and the risk of perforation can be reduced by the use of self-expanding rather than balloon dilated stents. In palliative stenting re-obstruction with tumour is a delayed complication[9,10] although repeat stenting is feasible.

Minor self-limiting complications are seen and include minor rectal bleeding and self-limiting abdominal discomfort.[4,6–8]

Oesophageal stenting

In patients with dysphagia due to oesophageal stenosis (usually secondary to inoperable malignancy but occasionally due to benign causes such as caustic ingestion) endoluminal stenting has become the treatment of choice. It has been shown to be more effective than radiotherapy, chemotherapy or endoscopic laser ablation in malignant dysphagia.[12,13] Covered stents can be used to treat fistulas between the oesophagus and the respiratory tree.[14]

Radiological insertion is similar in technique to that of colonic stents. Under sedation and pharyngeal anaesthesia, a catheter is passed orally. The stenosis can be delineated by injecting water soluble contrast and a guide wire passed through. The stent can then deployed, usually self-expanding, although a balloon may be necessary. The results are good with rapid improvement in dysphagia scores.[12,14–16]

A significant complication of the procedure is stent migration, particularly if the stent is placed across the gastro-oesophageal junction. The problem of migration is more marked in plastic covered stents.[12,17,18] The use of uncovered metal stents of the second generation covered stents that have flared proximal portions, such as the Flamingo Wallstent and Ultraflex, reduce the incidence of migration.[12,17,18] In contrast, uncovered stents have a higher incidence of blockage due to tumour growth,[12,17] which can be treated by re-stenting or endoscopic laser therapy.

Further significant post-procedure complications include perforation, oesophago-respiratory fistula formation, haemorrhage, food impaction, benign strictures secondary to the mechanical effects of the stent, pain and fractures of stent wires.[15,16,18–20]

A complication that can cause the patient significant distress following stenting is severe gastro-oesophageal reflux which can be refractory to treatment with proton pump inhibitors and sleeping in the head-up position.[16,18]

Percutaneous Feeding Tube Placement

Percutaneous gastrostromies and gastrojejunostomies are indicated in the management of patients unable to gain adequate nutrition orally. The common indications are proximal occlusion such as in head and neck cancers as well as oesophageal tumours. In these cases feeding tube placement can be elective in anticipation of occlusion. Dysphagia due to causes not directly related to occlusion, such as mucositis following radiotherapy or neural compromise, can also be treated this way. The additional calorific uptake in these patients can lead to increased quality of life.[21] Another indication for these procedures is palliation of the vomiting that can occur in gastric outlet or a more distal obstruction. A dual lumen gastrojejunostomy can aid some patients with feeding through the distal jejunal port and aspiration of secretions through the proximal gastric port. A radiological placement is associated with fewer major complications than endoscopic or surgical placement.[22]

The procedure is usually carried out under local anaesthetic. The colon can be identified by contrast taken orally or by an NG or NJ tube the preceding day. The liver should be delineated by ultrasound to confirm that it does not lie between the puncture site and stomach. The stomach is then distended with gas and punctured under fluoroscopic or CT guidance. Generally the stomach is anchored with ties to the anterior abdominal wall, gastroplexy, which reduces the risk of leakage of gastric contents into the peritoneum. A guide wire is then inserted into the stomach, and the jejunum if required, and the feeding tube passed over it and secured.

Mortality is low (< 1%) and one study of 400 feeding tube placements reported only one procedure-related death.[23] Serious complications include haemorrhage, peritonitis due to leakage of gastric content, and colonic injury, which is a cause of peritonitis.

Haemorrhage is rare[23] but is more likely in those with uncorrected clotting disorders or portal hypertension. Spillage of gastric content and subsequent peritonitis may be reduced by gastroplexy. Ascites increases the risk of peritonitis and elective paracentesis may reduce that risk.[23] Other infective complications that have been reported include local cellulitis, requiring adequate hygiene and antibiotics, and hepatic abscess following an inadvertent puncture.[23]

A common complication is the accidental dislodgement of the tube. If the tube has been *in situ* for more than two weeks it may be possible to recannulate the track under fluoroscopic guidance. As with primary feeding tube placement, a confirmation of an endoluminal placement with water-soluble contrast is vital to avoid the severe peritonitis associated with accidental intraperitoneal feeding. Often the tube can be partially withdrawn and the port holes can lie in the percutaneous tract resulting in apparent leakage; it can usually be repositioned easily. Patient and staff education plays a key role in preventing inadvertent dislodgement of feeding tubes.

HEPATOBILIARY INTERVENTIONAL RADIOLOGY

Transjugular Intrahepatic Portosystemic Shunt

Since the first clinical use of a transjuguar intrahepatic portosystemic shunt (TIPS) in 1982[24] the procedure has been used increasingly for the management of portal hypertension and its complications (Table 2). It involves the percutaneous manufacture of an artificial shunt between the right or left portal veins and one of the hepatic veins through the liver parenchyma. The

Table 2.   Indications for TIPS[25]

Accepted

Acute variceal bleeding refractory to medical and endoscopic treatments or not amenable to endoscopic therapy

Recurrent variceal bleeding in Child's class C patients who are resistant or intolerant of conventional medical or endoscopic therapy

Promising

Refractory ascites or hepatic hydrothorax

Hepatorenal syndrome

Budd-Chiari Syndrome and veno-occlusive disease

Not Indicated

Initial therapy of acute variceal bleed

Initial therapy to prevent recurrent haemorrhage after first variceal bleed

Prevention of recurrent variceal bleeding refractory to conventional treatment in Child's class A and B patients

Prevention of first variceal bleed

Prior to live transplantation of reduce operative morbidity

Hepatopulmonary syndrome

procedure can be performed without general anaesthesia although it may be required for airway protection in some patients.

The preparation for a TIPS procedure consists of a Doppler ultrasound scan to confirm the patency of the portal and hepatic venous systems. Tense ascites, if any, should be drained electively. The nature of the patient group indicates that coagulopathy is very common and platelets of < 60000 and an INR of >1.8 should be considered for correction; intravenous antibiotics are generally used.

The procedure involves gaining central venous access, via the right internal jugular vein preferably, and catheterisation of a hepatic vein. A wedged hepatic venogram to localise the portal venous system is performed and a puncture needle advanced. A guide wire is advanced into the mesenteric or splenic veins. The tract is dilated with an angioplasty balloon and an expandable stent deployed to a diameter of approximately 10 mm. An embolisation of varices can be done via the TIPS.

While the procedure-related mortality is approximately 1–2%,[25,26] the one year mortality is high, between 24–54% [26] as is the complication rate. The most common significant complications are shunt dysfunction and hepatic encephalopathy.

Shunt dysfunction is defined as occlusion or stenosis (>50% narrowing) with an associated portosystemic gradient of greater than 12 mmHg. It is often asymptomatic and associated with clinical consequences in only a quarter of cases,[25] usually variceal rebleeding or recurrent ascites. Dysfunction secondary to thrombosis is generally an acute post-procedure event, occurring in 10–15% of the cases.[27,28] Technical errors in stent placement, such as stent retraction or the use of a very short endoprostheses, can be factor in thrombosis. Other aetiological factors include bile duct injury,[29,30] but in most cases no causes are found. In acute thrombosis patency can be re-established radiologically, although there is risk of the clot being dislodged with a resultant pulmonary embolus.[26]

Stent occlusion is a more delayed complication occurring over 30 days following the procedure[26,29] and is usually due to pseudointimal hyperplasia at the hepatic venous end of the shunt or the intraparenchymal portion of the tract.[31] The reported incidence is up to 78%.[26]

Active surveillance is important owing to the fact that stent dysfunction is often asymptomatic. An ultrasound scan to detect thrombosis should be performed within 24 h of the procedure.[25,26] This will also pick up other early complications such as haemoperitoneum, hepatic haematoma and hepatic infarction. The suggested ongoing surveillance program is a repeat scan at six weeks, three months, six months and one year. Any clinical evidence of stent dysfunction should lead to an urgent ultrasound. However, ultrasound may be a good positive predictor of dysfunction but is a poor negative predictor and TIPS venography remains the gold standard, to be performed in any case of clinical evidence or dysfunction even in the case of a normal ultrasound. If a stenosis is found the stent can be decompressed at this time.[25,26] Owing to ultrasound being a poor screening tool coupled with the catastrophic consequences or a variceal re-bleed, some authorities recommend six monthly venograms for the first three years.[32]

In the event of dysfunction a percutaneous a recannulation can be attempted in the case of TIPS stenosis. If this fails a new TIPS may be inserted and failing that, a surgical shunt can be considered.

There is ongoing research in the prevention of stent dysfunction including use of covered stents, anti-platelet derived growth factor and brachytherapy.[25]

The other major complication of TIPS is hepatic encephalopathy which has a multifactorial aetiology, predominately related to bypassing the liver by portal blood flow through the TIPS and the increased bioavailablity of gut-related toxins that the liver would normally filter out from the systemic circulation. The incidence of new or worsening encephalopathy following TIPS has been reported as 20–31%.[26,33] The pre-procedure risk factors for post-TIPS encephalopathy include pre-TIPS encephalopathy, increased age, low albumin, low post-TIPS portosystemic gradient, severe underlying liver disease and non-alcoholic cirrhosis.[25]

The treatment of post-TIPS hepatic encephalopathy includes the treatment of any co-existent medical pathology, such as infection, a low protein diet, lactose and the use of antibiotics such as metronidazole and vancomycin. In a minority of patients (<10%) the encephalopathy is resistant to medical treatment and TIPS reduction, modification or occlusion may be necessary. Liver transplantation may be an option.

A less common complication of TIPS procedures is stent infection. Early infection can result from seeding at the time of insertion[34] or from technical complications at the time, such as a bile leak.[34–36] Late infection, months to years after the primary placement is often related to revision or stenosis treatment of the TIPS. The pathogens reported include *S. Aureus,* Gram-negative enteric organisms as well as organisms of relatively low pathological potential.[34] Fungal pathogens are also reported in the literature.[37,38]

As TIPS-related infection is often due to pathogens of low virulence, medical therapy can be successful in treatment. Unlike some endoprostheses, a TIPS stents cannot be removed without resorting to liver transplant.

Armstrong and Macleod suggested a definition for TIPS infection[34] — sustained bacteraemia in a patient with a TIPS, with or without ultrasound evidence of TIPS thrombus, with no other source of infection identified after thorough investigation. A "sustained bacteraemia" is defined as two or more blood cultures positive for the same organisms, the cultures separated by seven or more days.

Although a fever should always raise suspicion of infection, low grade fever has been reported[26] within 48 h following a TIPS insertion which usually resolves spontaneously. There is often a transient post-insertion rise in transaminases, again the levels rapidly return to baseline. Another usually transient finding following TIPS is a haemolytic anaemia that is seen 10–15% of the patients and generally resolves within a month. As this haemolysis can cause jaundice, it can raise concerns that the patient's liver disease is decompensating. The diagnosis of post-TIPS haemolysis is based a drop in haemoglobin and haptoglobin levels with a raised reticulocyte count and no accompanying autoimmune markers of haemolysis.[26]

Another more serious cause of post-TIPS jaundice is the creation of a biliary-shunt fistula.[26,35,36] Such a fistula can result in sepsis, especially with Gram-negative organisms, cholangitis, shunt thrombosis and haemobilia. The successful closure of biliary-shunt fistulae has been reported following the insertion of temporary biliary stent placement, sphincterotomy and a course of broad spectrum antibiotics[36]; however it may be necessary to occlude the TIPS shunt and place a new one.

There are a number of vascular complications associated with TIPS. Haemorrhage will always be a concern in patients with chronic liver disease and portal hypertension. Perforation of the portal vein with an associated intraperitoneal bleed is one of the more frequent vascular complications.[39–41] Such perforations have been treated with compression with an angioplasty balloon,[40] insertion of a covered stent,[39,41] or the insertion of a parallel TIPS shunt.[41] Acute intrahepatic haematoma is another haemorrhagic complication.[42] Fistulae have been reported between the portal vein and intrahepatic arteries, manifest on ultrasound by pulsitile TIPS blood flow. It can be treated by arterial embolisation.[43] The inherent sudden haemodynamic changes that occur with the placement of a TIPS shunt can lead to cardiopulmonary failure.[25]

Poor placement or migration of TIPS stents can lead to vascular complications. These include cardiac perforation,[44,45] formation of an aortoatrial fistula leading to right heart failure,[46] tricuspid valve regurgitation[47] and inferior vena cava stenosis.[48]

Misplacement of TIPS shunts so that they lie in the extrahepatic portal venous system can lead to increased technical complexity in a subsequent liver transplant, sometimes requiring venous reconstruction with an associated increased in transfusion requirements.[49,50] The incidence is higher when the radiologist is less experienced in the procedure[50] and careful radiological examination with CT and possibly venography is recommended prior to liver transplantation.

Percutaneous Transhepatic Cholangiography and Biliary Drainage

Percutaneous transhepatic cholangiography (PTC) is a diagnostic procedure that delineates biliary anatomy and pathology by the percutaneous puncture of a biliary radicle and subsequent instillation of iodinated contrast. Improvements in other diagnostic procedures such as ERCP, ultrasound and magnetic resonance pancreatography mean that this investigation is less common than previously.

Percutaneous transhepatic biliary drainage (PTBD) is a therapeutic procedure for patients with biliary obstruction, usually malignant in nature. A similar puncture is performed as in PTC and a guide wire passed into the biliary tree to allow insertion of a stent that allows biliary drainage either externally or internally, past any obstruction, into the duodenum.

The complication rates for PTC with a fine (21G) needle are low with a major complication rate of less than 2%.[51] These include haemorrhage, cholangitis, bile leakage, sepsis, renal injury and pneumothorax. Haemorrhage is the most serious complication in both PTC and PTBD.[52] Coagulopathy is a relative contraindication, and if efforts at correcting it fail, the procedure can proceed if it is judged that inaction would carry more risk than a haemorrhage.

PTBD carries all the same complications of PTC but the tract through the liver parenchyma is of greater diameter. This factor combined with *in situ* retention of a stent or drain means that some of these risks are greater in CTBD (PTBD?) and there are complications seen in PTBD that are not seen in PTC.

There is a small, but significant mortality rate of 1.6–2.6% associated with PTBD.[51–53] These procedure-related deaths are most commonly related to haemorrhage or sepsis.[52,53] The risk of haemorrhage is related to the number of independent, percutaneous passes attempted to canulate the biliary tree. Hamlin *et al.* recommended a single puncture with a thin, sheathed needle. If this was initially unsuccessful the needle was withdrawn to a sub-capsular position before being advanced again, minimising the number of liver capsule punctures necessary.[52] Embolising the liver parenchymal tract, with autologous clot, coils or Gelfoam was also recommended.[52] Serious haemorrhage, which occurs in 1.5–4.5% of cases,[51–53] can be treated by tamponading the hepatic tract with a large bore biliary catheter or hepatic artery catherisation and embolisation.[54]

Haemobilia is the most common haemorrhagic complication, occurring in 10–16% of the cases.[52,53] It often resolves spontaneously but can cause obstruction. The treatment involves hourly irrigation with 10 ml normal saline for 12–24 h (in heavy haemobilia) after which clots should lyse spontaneously.[53]

One of the frequent indications for PTBD is the drainage of an obstructed, infected biliary system and it is not surprising that infection and sepsis are well documented complications of the procedure. Any percutaneous biliary intervention should be covered with appropriate antibiotics. A transient fever and leukocytosis are relatively common, 10–16%,[52,53] and usually resolve with medical therapy. Systemic sepsis was found to be a less common, at 2.5–3.5% but a more serious complication. These infective complications are usually associated with infected bile[53] and samples should be obtained for microbiological analysis, at the time of the procedure. Some centres[53] found that a two-stage internal drainage resulted in reduced incidence of severe sepsis as well as increased chances of completing internal drainages in technically difficult patients. The two-stage internal drainage involves initial decompression of the obstructed biliary system with drainage followed by conversion to internal drainage into the duodenum 3–5 days later.

Delayed cholangitis is a frequent infective complication of PTBD, particularly when clamping an external drainage catheter as part of the change over from external to internal drainage. In one study[53] this was found to occur in 63% changeovers. The treatment is by unclamping the external drainage catheter and once the patient condition has stabilised, the external catheter is exchanged for a wider bore and re-clamped with a lower incidence of recurrent cholangitis (11%).

Other infective complications include hepatic abcesses, extra-hepatic abcesses as well as peritonitis.

In malignant biliary obstruction PTBD is often a palliative intervention and patients may be discharged into the community with the drainage *in situ* and there is high incidence of complications with Mueller's group[53] reporting 62 complications in 40 patients. Cholangitis, tube dislodgement and catheter occlusion by tumour, debris or bile encrustation were the main reported community complications. The group found that the incidence of complications in these patients appeared to correlate with the degree of family or nursing care received by the patients. Another group[52] had found that long-term external drainage catheters occluded in virtually all patients, needing exchange every 2–3 months on an average. The symptoms of an occluded drainage catheter include increasing alkaline phosphatase, worsening jaundice and bile drainage around the catheter to the skin.

Imaging Guided Liver Biopsy

Percutaneous liver biopsy is a vital tool in the diagnosis of both diffuse hepatic disease, such as suspected cirrhosis, and focal liver abnormalities such as neoplasia. Many centres perform liver biopsies for diffuse hepatic disease "blind", without imaging guidance however there is growing utilisation of imaging to guide sampling especially in technically difficult patients, such as the obese. Focal lesion sampling is routinely carried out under guidance. Most liver biopsies are carried under ultrasound guidance, avoiding the need for exposure of patient and radiologist to ionising radiation. However CT can be used for focal lesions that are not visible on ultrasound and the multi-planar imaging capability of the MRI means that lesions that are difficult to access by ultrasound or CT, for example sub-diaphragmatic lesions, can be sampled using MRI guidance.[55]

The procedure has a low complication rate at >2%.[54,56,57] Sixty percent of the complications present within two hours of the biopsy and 96% within the first day.[58,59] The main, serious complication being intraperitoneal haemorrhage usually presenting as pain, and sometimes with the clinical evidence of shock. Haemorrhage may be the result of laceration secondary to respiration during the biopsy or to penetration of the hepatic artery or portal vein branches.[57] While haemorrhage is usually self limiting, hepatic artery angiography and embolisation may sometimes be necessary. There is an increased risk of bleeding in the elderly, and in patients with more than three biopsy passes, cirrhosis or liver cancer.[59,60] Small hepatic haematomas are common, even in patients without symptoms, larger ones often presenting with pain, tachycardia and hypotension.[61,62] Generally haematomas can be managed conservatively. A delayed haemorrhagic complication is haemobilia (Fig. 1) that usually presents about a week following the procedure with gastrointestinal bleeding, pain and jaundice.[59,63] The procedure mortality is low at 0.1–0.01%.[57,64]

As is the case with all hepato-biliary interventions, a relatively high proportion of patients will have coagulopathies and there are two possible approaches to liver biopsy. Transjugular liver biopsy avoids puncturing the liver capsule and under fluoroscopic guidance, is via the right internal jugular vein and the hepatic veins. The liver parenchyma is then sampled through the hepatic vein walls. Thus the biopsy tract in the liver leads back to the vascular system, rather than into the abdominal cavity. This method can only be used to diagnose diffuse liver disease and not to sample focal hepatic lesions. It also carries the risks of central venous access such as pneumothorax, venous laceration, cardiac arrhythmias, intrahepatic fistula formation (Fig. 2), transient Horner's syndrome and liver capsule perforation.[57] The reported mortality rate for transjugular liver biopsy is 0.1–0.5%.[57] The transjugular approach can also be used in patients with massive ascites, morbid obesity are a part of a TIPS procedure.[57]

The second method is the plugged liver biopsy. It involves passing the biopsy needle through a plastic sheath with a haemostatic valve. Following the biopsy, the needle is removed leaving the sheath in place. The sheath is slowly withdrawn and the transhepatic tract embolised with coils.[65] As this is a guided technique, usually using ultrasound, it allows the sampling of focal

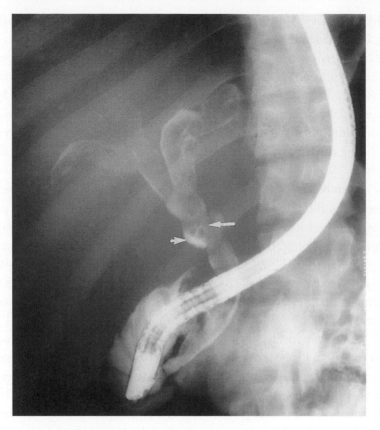

Fig. 1.   An ERCP following a liver biopsy demonstrating haemobilia. Contrast (short arrow) is seen to outline clot (long arrow) within the biliary tree.

lesions and is quicker than the transjugular approach. The complication rates between the two methods are similar.[66]

Although transient bacteraemia is reported in up to 13.5% of percutaneous liver biopsies[67] there are no clinical consequences. However, clinical sepsis can occur rarely in those with biliary obstruction and cholangitis.

Twenty-five percent of the patients have right upper quadrant or right shoulder pain following liver biopsy. This mild and brief — severe, ongoing pain raised concerns for more serious complications.[57]

Other rare complications include pneumothorax, pneumoperitoneum, pneumoscrotum, haemothorax, subcutaneous emphysema, biliary ascites,

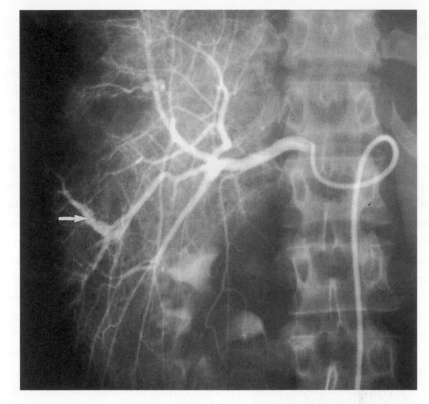

Fig. 2. A selective hepatic angiogram demonstrating arteriovenous fistula (arrowed) following a liver biopsy.

biliary peritonitis, carcinoid crisis, subphrenic abscess, pancreatitis due to haemobilia and needle breakage.[59,62,68]

URINARY TRACT INTERVENTIONAL RADIOLOGY

Percutaneous Nephrostomy

Since the first percutaneous nephrostomy was reported in 1955[69] the technique has become one of the mainstays in the management of supravesicular urinary tract obstruction. It can be used as a temporary measure, to relieve the obstruction caused by ureteric calculi prior to a definitive intervention. It can be a long-term therapy, often palliative, if caused by malignancy or other poorly responsive cases such as radiotherapy. Infection or suspected infection in an obstructed kidney is an indication for an emergency nephrostomy, even more so if there is coexisting uraemia.[70] Another less common indication for nephrostomy is the treatment of urinary fistula.[70,71] Although the results for this indication have been variable the technique has been successful, especially where the fistula has been complicated by a degree of urinary tract obstruction.[70]

The procedure in generally carried out under local anaesthetic and sedation. The pelvicalyceal system is punctured either under direct ultrasound guidance or fluoroscopically if it is opacified with an intravenous injection of iodinated contrast. Once a puncture is performed a guide wire is passed into the ureter, if possible, and a tract dilated. An 8–12 Fr catheter can then passed over the wire and secured. After the initial percutaneous drainage a ureteric endoprostheses can be inserted via the nephrostomy tract. This involves passing a guide wire past any ureteric obstruction, the balloon dilatation of the obstruction and the placing of an endostent. Ureteric endostent placement can be carried out as a one part procedure, at the time of initial nephrostomy, or as a two part intervention some days later.[72]

Overall the complication and mortality rates of percutaneous nephrostomy are low[70–72] and considerably lower than that of surgical nephrostomy.[73] As with much of interventional radiology, one of the main concerns in the percutaneous insertion of a nephrostomy is the risk of haemorrhagic complications. Significant haemorrhage (requiring transfusion, endovascular intervention or surgical intervention) is rare, 0.01–0.7%,[70,72,74,75] usually due to pseudo-aneurysms, arteriovenous fistulae or arteriolar damage. Severe haemorrhagic complications include retroperitoneal haemorrhage[72] and massive haemorrhage via drainage tubes due to direct renal artery branch injury. These can usually be treated by angiographic embolisation although nephrectomy or partial nephrectomy may be necessary as a last resort. In one case direct injury of a major renal artery was treated by embolisation of the vessel via the misplaced percutaneous nephrostomy tube.[76] In this case the nephrostomy tube was known to have transfixed the renal pelvis but was only as it was being withdrawn, with loss of the tamponading effect of the catheter, that severe haemorrhage became apparent. This report recommended that in cases of known renal pelvis transfixation the catheter should be withdrawn with a guide wire *in situ* so that in case of a haemorrhage a large bore catheter can be reinserted as tamponade.

Mild, self-limiting, haematuria is very common immediately following a percutaneous nephrostomy that many do not regard it as a complication.[70] However significant haematuria can result in clot retention leading to nephrostomy obstruction and subsequent catheter exchange.

Peri-nephric haematomas are fairly frequent[70] but rarely require anything further than conservative management.[77]

It is imperative to pay attention to any coagulopathy to reduce the incidence of haemorrhagic complications. In one study of 303 patients it was found that a platelet count of $<100,000/mm^3$ was associated with a significant ($P < 0.01$) increase in the need for blood transfusion.[71] Patient attention to temporary apnoea and avoidance of punctures are also suggested as a means of lowering the risk of haemorrhage.[70] The presence or absence of hydronephrosis, trocar size and needle size were not found to correlate to the incidence of haemorrhage.[71]

Many nephrostomy procedures are carried out for infected, obstructed upper renal tracts and it is no surprise that sepsis is a well recognised complication.[70–72,78,79] Bacteriuria is an inevitable consequence of a longstanding placement of a percutaneous nephrostomy but is usually asymptomatic.[80] Asymptomatic bacteraemia has been reported during nephrostomy tube manipulation and changeovers.[81] Interestingly, in this study no difference was found in the incidence of bacteraemia between the group given prophylactic antibiotics and the control group. Other studies using antibiotic coated nephrostomy catheters found no advantage in terms of infection.[82] Despite this finding many groups recommend appropriate antibiotic prophylaxis at the time of the procedure.[71,72] Although an emergency percutaneous nephrostomy can lead to a rapid clinical improvement in patients with an infected, obstructed system,[83] exacerbation of sepsis by nephrostomy can occur.[70] Some groups recommend minimalising intervention, such as anterograde nephrostogram or ureteric stent placement, while dealing with infected systems.[70,72] Therefore, the ureteric stent, if required in a case of pyonephrosis, should be done as a two part procedure.

Other infective complications include cellulitis at the drainage site, perinephric abscesses and splenic abscesses.[71,78,84]

Catheter complications included accidental extraction of the catheter, catheter kinking or blockage and urinary by-pass of the catheter. These can be treated with re-insertion or change of catheters.[71] The use of locking pigtail catheters leads to a reduction in the accidental displacement of drainage catheters.[71]

Other reported complications include placement of drainage tubes through the bowel, pneumothorax, pneumonia, pleural effusion, transient urinary peritonitis, biliary peritonitis, tumour seeding along the nephrostomy tract, air embolism and arteriovenous malformation formation.[70,71,79,85–90]

Renal calculi can be treated with a combined radiological/urological procedure, percutaneous nephrolithotomy. This procedure requires a general anaesthetic and the role of the radiologist is to perform a guided calyceal puncture, often aided by the retrograde instillation of contrast into the pelvicalyceal system. A nephrostomy tract is then dilated, usually to a much wider bore than is used for therapeutic nephrostomies (28 Fr vs. 10 Fr), and the urologist can use this tract to remove the calculi endoscopically.

The complication profile of this procedure is similar to that of a standard nephrostomy. The wider tract contributes to a higher incidence of significant haemorrhage related to percutaneous nephrolithotomy (PCNL) when compared with simple nephrostomy. The reported rates of haemorrhage requiring blood transfusion following PCNL range from 1–23%.[91–97] This compares with a reported rate of 0.4% in a series of 516 nephrostomies.[70] The reported rate of haemorrhage in PCNL requiring radiological endovascular intervention or surgical intervention ranges from 0.3–2.3%. An increased incidence of significant haemorrhage in PCNL was reported in cases with multiple punctures and renal pelvis perforation.[91] One study reported a significant ($P < 0.05$) drop in the incidence of haemorrhage requiring transfusion in patients whose nephrostomy tracts were dilated with a balloon rather than sequential dilators.[98] A recent development that may also lessen haemorrhagic complication has been the introduction of the mini-PCNL[99] in which smaller (e.g., 13 Fr) tracts are dilated, although the stone load and size may lead to conversion to a standard PCNL.

A rare delayed complication in PCNL cases is the development of calyceal infundibular stenosis[100,101] which can be treated with endoscopic dilatation but can progress to infundibular obliteration. Stone granulomata, where fragments of calculi migrate into the renal tract walls to cause an inflammatory reaction, have been reported in urinary tract and pelviureteric junction stenosis.[99]

Ultrasound Guided Renal Biopsy

Histological analysis of renal tissue is vital in planning the treatment of dysfunction in both native and transplanted kidneys. Ultrasound guided renal biopsy allows samples to be taken with a high rate of histological success with low complication rates.[102–105] A literature review[106] of 19,459 percutaneous renal biopsies (1951 to 1990) showed a complication rate of less than 11%, despite the fact that many were not ultrasound guided. Ninety per cent of these complications were self limiting and the mortality (0.08%) and nephrectomy (0.06%) rates were low. Recent studies have confirmed low rates of serious, mainly haemorrhagic, complications. The rates of complications requiring intervention in these studies range between 0.4–2.7%.[102–105] The complication rates have been reported to be significantly higher ($P < 0.001$) in native kidney biopsies, compared to grafts. The likely reason is the increased technical difficulty in native biopsies owing to the increased depth of the organ and greater organ movement with breathing compared to a renal graft. However in the study that reported this finding, the increase in complication rates was confined to minor complications such as self limiting macrohaematuria and small perinephric haematomas.[103]

Some studies have suggested that increased rates of haemorrhagic complications may be associated with the use of larger 14G needles rather than 18G[103] while another found that elevated creatinine levels ($>300 \, \mu mol/l$) lead to a significant increase in the incidence of haemorrhagic complications. Tang *et al.* recommended the use of desmopressin pre- and post-biopsy to help reduce the incidence of bleeding on these patients with renal function impairment. In the case of renal transplant biopsy, a study of 1,129 graft biopsies found that three resulted in transplant nephrectomies for haemorrhage. All three were found to be in the throes of acute rejection on histological examination.[107] Another study has reported that nephrectomies in native kidneys due to post-biopsy were invariably associated with severe parenchymal disease.[104] These findings that "inflamed" kidneys are at higher risk of haemorrhage than "normal" uninflamed ones. Other serious complications include peritonitis due to bowel perforation but are rare.[104]

The most common clinical complication following biopsy is mild haemorrhage, either a self limiting haematuria or small perinephric haematomas with a reported incidence of 4.5%.[102] Post-biopsy arterio-venous fistulae are common on Doppler studies (5%) and angiography (15–19%) (Fig. 3) but rarely cause clinical complications.[102,104]

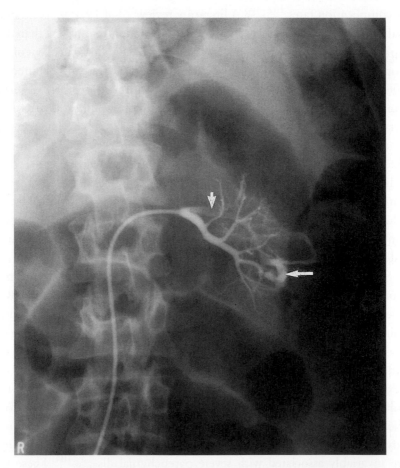

Fig. 3. A selective renal angiogram, following a renal biopsy, demonstrating an arteriovenous fistula (long arrow). Note the early venous filling (short arrow).

ARTERIAL ENDOVASCULAR INTERVENTIONAL RADIOLOGY

Puncture Site Complications

Any endovascular intervention requires a vascular puncture and all have similar potential complications at the puncture site. The most common site for arterial access is the common femoral artery and the incidence of serious complications here is low (0.5%), compared with other punctures; for example, the axillary artery shows a higher rate at 1.7%.[108]

The most common complication at the puncture site is haemorrhage with a reported incidence of up to 20%. If defined as an area of induration greater than 5 cm in diameter, the incidence falls to >2%; local haematoma requiring transfusion or surgical intervention is very rare.[108] The reported risk factors include bleeding diathesis, hypertension, the use of transluminal angioplasty balloons, inadequate puncture site compression following the procedure and patient weight.[109,110] Endovascular procedures such as stent insertion may utilise heparin to reduce the risk of thrombosis and over heparisation should be considered in incidences of post-procedure haemorrhage. In these cases, the correction of the coagulopathy with protamine sulphate can be carried out. In femoral artery puncture, a haemorrhagic complication that should be considered in post-angiogram patients with severe thigh and pelvic pain, even without clinical evidence, is a retroperitoneal haemorrhage, which is especially a risk in a high puncture above the inguinal ligament. In any patient with these symptoms, especially with an associated drop in haemoglobin, the diagnosis should be suspected and an urgent CT scan considered. Another local vascular complication is the formation of a pseudoaneurysm at the puncture site. The reported incidence of this complication has grown,[108,111] partly due to more accurate non-interventional diagnosis and partly due to more complex interventions involving larger punctures and catheters.[109,111,112] The incidence is reported as approximately 1–2% although most heal spontaneously.[108,112] The risk factors for the formation of a pseudoaneurysm include a very brief manual compression of the puncture site, aberrant punctures that make compression more difficult, obesity, larger catheters and heparinisation.[108,109,111,112] Clinically, they can present as a pulsitile mass, but the absence of pulsitility does not exclude the diagnosis. Local pain is a common complaint and referred pain and neurological deficit from nerve compression is a recognised complication.[113] The Doppler ultrasound is very accurate in diagnosing this complication at puncture sites and an ultrasound guided graded compression of the neck of the pseudoaneurysm sac or guided injection of thrombin are effective methods of therapeutic thrombosis within the sac. These minimally invasive methods have largely replaced by more invasive methods of treatment, such as angiographic coiling or surgery.[111,114] Further reported vascular complications of the puncture site include arterio-venous fistula formation, stenosis formation and local thrombosis with the associated risk of embolisation.[109,115] The punctured vessel can be damaged when contrast or a guide wire is forced through a misplaced puncture needle causing a local dissection.

Non-vascular puncture site complications involve damage to local structures such as nerves[109,113] and local sepsis[109] which is rare but can be serious.[116,117]

General and Catheter Related Complications of Endovascular Intervention[109]

Arterial endovascular interventional radiology[109] involves the needle puncture of the arterial system, typically via the common femoral artery, followed by a guide wire and a combination of dilators, catheters and interventional devices (e.g., angioplasty balloons and stents) passed into the arterial system. The passage of these devices into the arterial tree inevitably leads to the potential for complications. Technical complication and equipment failures include lost or fractured guide wires, catheters knotted during manipulation, angioplasty balloons rupturing, misplaced stent deployment and the tangling of guide wires and catheters with internal structures such as cardiac valves. These complications have become less frequent with improved quality of interventional equipment and radiologist experience. Most of these complications are recognised rapidly during the procedure and often corrected with further intervention, such as snaring lost guide wires or their fragments. On occasion, it may be necessary for open surgical treatment of these complications.

Vascular injuries remote from the initial puncture site can occur secondary to catheter or guide wire manipulation as well as by the intramural injection of contrast or saline. The most frequent injury of this type is the dissection of the tunica intima from the tunica media. The tunica intima can then form a flap which leads to the occlusion of the vessel. Such dissections can be treated radiologically with angioplasty used to appose the intima to its normal position.[118] The vessels can be perforated by catheter or guide wire manipulation and forced injection into a small calibre vessel in which the catheter is wedged.

One of the potentially disastrous complications of arterial endovascular intervention is compromise of the blood supply of various end organs. This may be caused by arterial dissection, spasm, thrombosis, rupture as well as by embolic events. The effect of interruption of blood supply can be variable ranging from no clinical effect and transient symptoms through to permanent disability and death. The natural history of these events depends on the vascular territory involved. The cerebral, renal and coronary territories are particularly vulnerable with potentially disastrous consequences of vascular compromise. Other territories, such as the hepatic, are more robust. Vasodilators and heparin can be administered to avoid spasm and thrombosis during intervention.

There are a number of causes of embolism occurring during an angiography. A thrombus can form at the puncture site or the catheter tip and embolise. Foreign material such as air, ruptured angioplasty balloons or threads of gauze can also be a cause of embolic complications. Scrupulous technique including regular catheter flushing to prevent thrombus formation and check for air in injection systems helps minimise the risk.

Endovascular intervention in atheromatous arteries runs the risk of distal cholesterol emboli.[119] Catheter and guide wire manipulation within such diseased vessels can release cholesterol from atheromatous plaques. These can range in size from those large enough to occlude vessels outright to microemboli of 150—200 μm. Showers of these microemboli can lead to the rare multiple cholesterol emboli syndrome if they reach a certain threshold. Pathologically, this is characterised by a progressive, ascending thrombosis.[119] This usually presents within minutes of the procedure usually with lower limb pain and often initially preserved pulses. A frequent finding is livedo reticularis, a blue mottled rash of the lower trunk and limbs (Fig. 4). The progressive thrombosis of arterioles can lead to ischaemia of the bowel, muscles, kidneys and pancreas giving rise to complications including pancreatitis, renal failure, rhabdomyolysis and ischaemic bowel. There is no specific therapy and the mortality is greater than 90%.[119]

A rare iatrogenic complication in any endovascular procedure is the injection in error. This complication can be due to the injection of incorrect doses

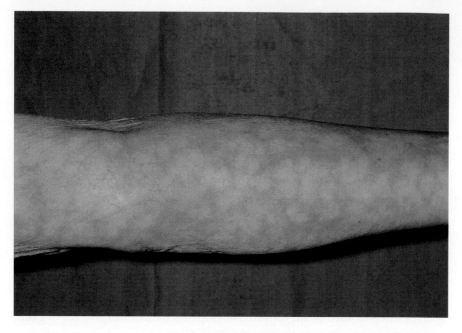

Fig. 4.   Livedo reticularis.

of correct medication, such as heparin or injection of the wrong drug. Catastrophic consequences have resulted from the mistaken injection of cleaning fluid. These complications can be prevented by meticulous checking prior to injection and prompt removal of the cleaning fluid from the procedure trolley once the puncture site has been sterilised.

Complications of Angioplasty and Stent Placement

Since the first report of percutaneous angioplasty in 1964,[120] angioplasty and endovascular stent placement have become first line treatments for stenotic vascular lesions,[2] while endoluminal stents are increasingly used in abdominal aortic aneurysms, particularly in patients who are poor surgical risks.[121]

Angioplasty involves routing a guide wire through the stenosis and a balloon catheter passed over it to traverse the narrowing and inflated with contrast to open up the obstruction. Vascular stents consist of cylindrical metal meshwork that can be placed across a stenosed segment in a similar fashion to angioplasty balloon. Some self expand while other deploy an angioplasty balloon. Within weeks there is a growth of endothelial cells over the stent incorporating it into the vascular wall. Stents for large vessels, such as for aortic aneurysms, often require a surgical arteriotomy, under a general anaesthetic. Angioplasty and stenting can be used in non-arterial endovascular situations such as venous stenosis or stenosis in dialysis arterio-venous fistulae.

All the complications of diagnostic angiography apply to these truly interventional techniques. Owing to the larger catheters used, puncture site complications such as haematoma of false aneurysm formation can be more prevalent without good post-procedure care of the site.

The patients undergoing angioplasty are often elderly with multiple co-morbidities and often develop medical complications, especially if they are undergoing emergency angioplasties for critical ischaemia. A study of 1,377 peripheral angioplasties found a 30 day mortality rate of 1.3%, rising to 4.9% in those with critical ischaemia.[122] The majority of the deaths in these patients were caused by bronchopneumonia with myocardial infarction as the next most frequent cause of death. The reported rate of complications following angioplasty ranges from 4–18%[122] but the rates of serious angioplasty complications requiring surgical intervention, such as emergency bypass, embolectomy, amputation or nephrectomy is lower, in the range of 2–4%.[122,123] The most common (2% of the cases) but serious complication is the occlusion of the treated vessel due to thrombosis, dissection due to the guidewire and the angioplasty balloon inflation. These complications may be treated with thrombolytics, endovascular treatment or surgical bypass. The risk of these iatrogenic acute ischaemic events is higher in the renal arteries and distal to the popliteal artery[122,123] as well as in patient undergoing angioplasty for critical ischaemia rather elective angioplasty for claudication.[122] Subintimal angioplasty is a process where an obstructed length of artery is bypassed by the deliberate subintimal dissection of the vessel followed by angioplasty of the dissection tract to create a new lumen. This process is not associated with increased frequency of complications.[122] The amputation rate following peripheral angioplasty is low (0.6%) but in 1,377 procedures this complication was not seen in angioplasty cases for claudication or graft complications, but was a feature in 2.2% of angioplasties for critical limb ischaemia.

A rare, potentially fatal, complication of angioplasty is arterial rupture, which has been reported in 0.4% of renal artery stenosis dilatation.[123] Local pseudoaneurysm formation is another reported complication. Both these complications can be amenable to endovascular treatment.

Embolic events are a potential complication with a reported incidence of 3–5%.[109] However, clinically significant embolic events are less common but can be serious leading to critical lower limb ischaemia, renal impairment or failure[124] and ischaemic bowel.

Angioplasty balloon rupture is a complication that is decreasing in frequency with improvement in its design over the years. The risks of a rupture include embolisation of the fragments, damage to vessel walls from rough edges of the fragmented balloon, and that to extract the irregular balloon an arteriotomy may be necessary.

Angioplasty is increasingly being supplemented by endovascular stent placement in which a metal meshwork stent is placed across a stenosis, as in renal artery stenosis,[2] or across an aneurysm or pseudoaneurysm, as is increasingly seen in the treatment of abdominal aortic aneurysms.[121] Stent placement has all the potential complications of angiography and angioplasty, but there are specific considerations with stent placements. These include mismatching of vessel and stent size increasing the risk of stent migration of embolisation, misplacement of the stent and thrombosis. The placement of a prosthetic device within the body always runs the risk of infection being implanted, either at the time of the procedure, primary infection, or at a later time secondary to bacteraemia. Such infective complications are rare, but have been reported. It may become necessary for the surgical removal of the stent to resolve the sepsis.[125,126]

One complication unique to the use of endovascular stents in the treatment of aneurysms is the formation of endoleaks. An endoleak refers to the persistent bleeding outside the graft but within the aneurysm sac or adjacent vessels in which the graft is deployed.[121,126] Endoleaks are classified by the origin of the persistent blood flow (Table 3), and can be diagnosed with the use of contrast enhanced spiral CT or formal angiography. Early endoleaks (onset of less than 30 days) can be initially treated by a period of observation and if they persist, treatment, usually endovascular, is considered. Late endoleaks, or those that occur after 30 days should be treated without the period of observation.[121] Endoleaks of types I to IV have been associated with vascular rupture, other causes of arterial rupture include separation of the graft modules and failure of the graft wall.[127]

In the endovascular treatment of aneurysms, covered stents are deployed and these can obstruct the side branches leading to risk of ischaemic damage.

Table 3.   Types of Endoleak[121]

Type of Endoleak	Description	Probable Cause	Relationship to Device	Treatment Alternatives
Type I	Distal or proximal attachment endoleak	Improper graft sizing or vessel measurement	Device related	Cuff placement
				Embolisation
		Vessel wall irregularities		Secondary endograft
				Open repair
Type II	Branch flow endoleks	Reperfusion via adjacent vessels, e.g. lumbar arteries	Not related to device	Conserviative
				Embolisation
				Laparoscopic ligation
		Inadequate identification of feeder vessels or graft placement		
		Anticoagulants		
Type III	Mid-graft or modular endolecks	Improper docking of graft sections	Device related	Secondary endograft
		Graft tear or perforation		
Type IV	Blushing through graft fabric	Excessive porosity of graft cover or prolonged anticoagulation	Device related	Conservative

For instance, in the treatment of abdominal aortic aneurysms the inferior mesenteric artery is often occluded by the stent deployment. In such circumstances it must be established first that the coeliac axis and superior mesenteric arteries are not severely diseased as ischaemic injury to the bowel may result from inferior mesenteric artery occlusion.

Therapeutic Endovascular Embolisation

The deliberate therapeutic occlusion of blood vessels by selective catheter injection of foreign material is the mainstay of many endovascular treatments. Common indications include acute haemorrhage, benign tumours such as uterine fibroids, malignant tumours as a preoperative or palliative measure, vascular malformations, pseudoaneurysms and priapisms. The technique involves an initial high quality diagnostic angiogram to precisely locate the vessel to be embolised. The offending vessel is then selectively catheterised and embolic material injected. A multitude of agents have been used as embolic material including metal coils, detachable balloons, gel foams including PVA particles, absolute ethanol and super glue.

As can be anticipated in this type of therapy, one of the potentially serious complications is the inadvertent misplacement of embolic material in the incorrect vessels leading to ischaemia and infarction. Normal vessels may also be compromised despite the correct placement of embolic material if there is propagation of thrombus beyond the target. Operator experience and impeccable technique are the best defence against such complications.

Although in some cases, such as tumours, the technique is designed to utilise tissue infarction, there are times when unintended or excessive tissue necrosis can occur even with the correct placement of embolic material.[128,129] In acute bowel haemorrhage embolisation can be an effective treatment but ischaemic injury can result in bowel infarction or stricture formation.[130] As with all interventional procedures there is a risk of local or systemic infection but is a further cause for concern because foreign material that can act as a focus of infection is instilled combined with the presence of infarcted and necrotic tissue.[130] This is further complicated by post-embolization syndrome,[131] a triad of pain, pyrexia and leucocystosis, which is seen in approximately 40% of the procedures. The syndrome may be related to tissue necrosis and can lead to concern regarding infection owing to the pyrexia and raised white cell count.

A recognised complication of embolisation procedures is renal failure due to massive tissue necrosis and dehydration[109] as well as any direct compromise of the renal vasculature associated with the intervention.

Specific complications may be associated with the embolisation of specific organs or lesions. Pulmonary embolisation may inadvertently occur during treatment of arterio-venous shunts as the embolic material can travel from the arterial system into the systemic venous system and on into the pulmonary arterial tree. Embolic infarction of endocrine tumours can lead the release of active hormones leading to complications secondary to a sudden increase in the blood levels of these hormones. A minimally invasive treatment of uterine fibroids, the embolisation of the uterine artery, can result in the sloughing off of sub-endometrial fibroids into the uterine cavity. This can be a delayed complication and may require surgical treatment.[132] Care must be taken in the embolisation of bronchial arteries for haemoptysis as the artery of Adamkiewitz, which supplies much of the thoracic spinal cord, has a variable origin near that of the bronchial arteries; it goes without saying that the accidental embolisation of this artery is a catastrophe.

VENOUS INTERVENTIONAL RADIOLOGY

Venous Filter Placement

Although the first line treatment of venous thrombosis remains anti-coagulation, initially with heparin or a low molecular weight derivative and then warfarin, there are occasions when the placement of a venous filter is indicated. One indication would be recurrent thrombosis or embolism despite adequate anti-coagulation or thrombo-embolic disease in patients who cannot be anti-coagulated, such as those with active gastrointestinal haemorrhage.

The filter is a meshwork of wires that expand from the vascular catheter once deployed. Following this, struts impact onto the vein walls and endothelialisation occurs to permanently fix the filter in place. Thus any emboli get caught in the mesh and cannot progress into the pulmonary vasculature. Typically the filter is placed in the inferior vena cava via a femoral vein puncture for the treatment of distal deep venous thrombosis. Caval filter use in other veins, such as the superior vena cava, has also been reported.[133]

Insertion of caval filters is associated with a low rate of serious complications, with a retrospective study of 1,765 of filter placements showing a serious, procedure related, complication rate of 0.3%.[134] These complications include deployment of filters in inappropriate places, stent migration and haemorrhagic complications from both venous and arterial injuries.

There are more delayed complications related to caval filter use. Although the filter is meant to prevent pulmonary embolic disease, the above study reported an incidence of post-filter pulmonary embolism of 2.7%. Indeed the filter itself has been reported as a focus of thrombus formation leading to caval obstruction.[134,135] Such a complication should be suspected in patients with filters *in situ* who develop bilateral leg swelling. Other complications include filter migration in both cranial and caudal directions, with a reported incidence of 6% and fracture of filter struts (usually asymptomatic).[135] To function properly it is necessary for the struts of the filter to abut the vein walls to allow the filter to anchor. However, these struts may erode and damage local structures, including erosion through the caval wall, and once this occurs the filter components can damage other structures. Such damage has been reported to the aorta, iliac arteries, lumbar arteries and gastro-intestinal structures.[135–137]

The placement of a meshwork of wires in the venous system can be an efficient way to trap emboli but unfortunately that is not all that can become entrapped within. A major iatrogenic complication following filter placement is that subsequent endoluminal venous intervention can result in the tangling of guide wires and catheters in the filter. Classically this is seen in the clinical placement of central venous lines with the "J" tip of the guide wire becoming enmeshed in the filter.[138] This can result in the migration of the filter, particularly within two weeks of placement before the filter is incorporated into the caval wall. Caval wall damage and fracture of the strut are also reported. Usually the situation can be rectified using an endoluminal snare but may require surgical intervention; needless to say prevention is a far better option. Common sense measures such as making sure all involved in the patient care are aware that the filter is *in situ* is at the forefront of this prevention. Generally the right internal jugular or subclavian vein punctures place the guide wire closer to the filter and the incidence of entrapment is higher in a right sided rather than a left sided approach.[138] An *in vitro* study[139] showed that the use of a straight rather than J-wire prevented entanglement and can be utilised clinically. Finally the fluoroscopic placement of the caval filters can be considered to prevent the complication.

MISCELLANEOUS INTERVENTIONAL RADIOLOGICAL PROCEDURES

Vertebroplasty

Vertebroplasty,[140,141] first described in 1987, is a radiological technique for the treatment of intractable back pain due to vertebral fractures. The aetiology of the fractures can be malignancy, osteoporosis and benign tumours such as aggressive haemangiomas. Using CT or biplane fluoroscopy guidance a bone biopsy needle is passed into the affected vertebral body via a vertebral pedicle. Continued imaging guidance is used to inject a polymethylmethacrylate (PMM) surgical cement into the vertebral body, thereby reinforcing it. Significant pain relief is seen in 70–90% of the patients, with an improvement usually seen within 24 h.

The most common serious complication associated with the procedure is leakage of cement from the vertebral body. The implications of such leaks depend on which route of leakage occurs. Serious complications can occur with leakage into the epidural space, leading to spinal cord compression which is a neurosurgical emergency. The leakage of cement into the exit foramina of the spine can lead to nerve root compression, which can be treated by intercostals steroid injections but may require surgery. Despite these potential complications serious neurological compromise is rare. In a study of 868 procedures[141] there were 15 cases of epidural leakage but only three cases of neuralgia were reported and none of spinal compression. Cement pulmonary embolism following leaks into paravertebral veins and can be fatal,[142] again a rare complication; in the series of 868 cases two incidences, both asymptomatic, were documented. Leaks into the adjacent inter-vertebral disks usually have no clinical implications but there is evidence that it may increase the risk of collapse of adjacent vertebral bodies. To minimise the risk of cement leak many recommend interosseous venography once the vertebral body has been punctured to demonstrate the position of the needle tip and delineate the site of the draining veins. In addition, the cement should be opacified with barium or metal powders and the cement injection closely monitored for evidence of leakage.

Another rare complication is infection and a strict aseptic technique is required to combat it. In addition, some use prophylactic intravenous antibiotics, while others use antibiotics mixed with the cement. Occasionally a pyrexia and temporary increase in pain sets in following the procedure due to the polymerisation process of the PMM cement.

Although the use of PMM cement has resulted in allergic reactions and hypotension in its use in orthopaedic surgery but this problem is rarely seen in vertebroplasty as the cement volumes used are much lower.

Radiological Ablations

A number of radiological techniques have been developed for the percutaneous ablation of abnormal solid tissue including hepatic and renal tumours, uterine fibroids as well as haemangiomas.[143,144] The tumours ablated can be malignant, such as hepatocellular and renal cell carcinoma or benign, such as hepatic adenomas. The ablation methods include percutaneous instillation of chemicals, including ethanol or acetic acid and thermal techniques. These targeted thermal injuries can be induced using focused high energy ultrasound beams, radiofrequency ablation, cryoablation, the percutaneous placement of laser fibres within lesions and the placement of electrodes for microwave ablation. Ultrasound, CT or MRI can be used to guide placement of fibres or catheters into lesions, however MRI has the advantage that thermal changes, representative of tissue destruction, can be detected due to changes in the tissues T1 weighting.[145] This allows real time thermal mapping of the ablated tissue and termination of the procedure once the target has been sufficiently ablated or if adjacent structures appear to be at risk. Other imaging techniques lack this advantage as well as the multi-planar imaging capabilities of MRI. High-energy ultrasound ablations differ from the other types of radiological ablation in that there is no need for a percutaneous puncture, and therefore complications associated with punctures are avoided.

Generally the types of complications that can occur are similar between the different forms of ablation procedure performed. These include abcesses forming in the necrotic post-ablation tissue, infarction of normal tissue, haemorrhage and damage to adjacent structures and organs. This last complication can result in biliary strictures and fistulae as well as gall bladder and bowel injuries. In the liver, thrombosis of the portal vein has been seen following hepatic ablations. A further delayed but serious complication that has been reported is seeding of a malignant tumour along the tracts of percutaneous punctures and many centres instil absolute alcohol into these tracts at the end of the procedure to lessen this risk.[145]

Less serious reported complications include skin burns, tenderness, post-procedure pyrexia, pleural effusions, pneumothorax, small haematomas and in the case of liver ablations derangement of liver function tests.

As might be expected, increasing lesion size is associated with increasing incidence of complications, especially if attempted as a single procedure rather than a staggered series of procedures. Although broadly the different methods have similar types of complication some do have different incidences of these complications. One review of liver ablation[144] found that methods such as percutaneous chemical ablations or cyroablation carried a higher incidence of complications when compared with interstitial laser photocoagulation.

REFERENCES

1. Becker GJ. (2001) 2000 RSNA Annual Oration in Diagnostic Radiology. *Radiology* **220**: 281–292.
2. Weibull H, Bergqvist D, Bergentz SE, *et al.* (1993) Percutaneous transluminal renal angioplasty versus surgical reconstruction of atherosclerotic renal artery stenosis: a prospective randomised study. *J Vasc Surg* **18**: 841–850.
3. Conoley PM. (2000) Productivity of radiologists in 1997: estimates based on analysis based on resource-based relative value units. *Am J Roentgenol* **175**: 591–595.
4. Mainar A, Tejero E, Maynar M, *et al.* (1996) Colorectal obstruction: treatment with metallic stents. *Radiology* **198**: 761–764.
5. Binkert C, Ledermann H, Jost R, *et al.* Acute colonic obstruction: clinical aspects and cost-effectiveness of preoperative and palliative treatment with self-expanding metallic stents — a preliminary report. *Radiology* **206**: 199–204.
6. de Gregorio M, Mainar A, Tejero E, *et al.* (1998) Acute colorectal obstruction: stent placement for palliative treatment — results of a multicenter study. *Radiology* **209**: 117–120.
7. Mainar A, de Gregorio M, Tejoro E, *et al.* (1999) Acute colorectal obstruction: treatment with self-expandable metallic stents before scheduled surgery — results of a multicentre study. *Radiology* **210**: 65–69.
8. Saida Y, Sumiyama Y, Nagao J, Takese M. (1996) Stent endoprostheses for obstructing cancers. *Dis Colon Rectum* **39**: 552–555.
9. Young WC, Soo SD, Ho WS, Sung KC, *et al.* (1998) Malignant colorectal obstruction: treatment with a flexible covered stent. *Radiology* **206**: 415–421.
10. Dauphine C, Tan P, Beart R, *et al.* (2002) Placement of self-expanding metal stents for acute malignant large-bowel obstruction: a collective review. *Ann Surg Oncol* **9**: 574–579.
11. Camunez F, Echenaguisa A, Simo G, *et al.* (2000) Malignant colorectal obstruction treated by means of self-expanding metallic stents: effectiveness before surgery and in palliation. *Radiology* **216**: 492–497.

12. Adam A, Ellul J, Watkinson A, *et al.* (1997) Palliation of inoperable esophageal carcinoma: a prospective randomised trial of laser therapy and stent placement. *Radiology* **202**: 344–348.

13. Cwikiel M, Cwikiel W, Albertsson M. (1993) Palliation of dysphagia in patients with malignant esophageal strictures. Comparisons of results of radiotherapy, chemotherapy and stent placement. *Acta Oncol* **38**: 75–79.

14. McGrath J, Browne M, Riordan C, *et al.* (2001) Expandable metal stents in the palliation of malignant dysphagia and oesophageal-respiratory fistulae. *Irish Med J* **94**: 270–272.

15. Cwikiel W, Tranberg K, Cwikiel M, Lillo-Gil R. (1998) Malignant dysphagia: palliation with esophageal stents — long-term results in 100 patients. *Radiology* **207**: 513–518.

16. Song HY, Do YS, Han YM, *et al.* (1994) Covered, expanded esophageal metallic stent tubes: experiences in 119 patients. *Radiology* **193**: 689–695.

17. Knyrim K, Wagner H-J, Bethge N, *et al.* (1993) A controlled trial of an expansile metal stent for palliation of esophageal obstruction due to inoperable cancer. *New Engl J Med* **329**: 1302–1307.

18. Sabharwal T, Hamady M, Chui S, *et al.* (2003) A randomised prospective study of the Flamingo Wallstent and Ultraflex stent for palliation of dysphagia associated with lower third oesophageal carcinoma. *Gut* **52**: 922–926.

19. Watkinson A, Ellul J, Entwisle K, *et al.* (1995) Esophageal carcinoma: initial results of palliative treatment with covered self expanding endoprostheses. *Radiology* **195**: 821–827.

20. Farrugia M, Morgan R, Latham J, *et al.* (1997) Perforation of the esophagus secondary to insertion of covered Wallstent endoprostheses. *Cardiovasc Intervent Radiol* **20**: 470–472.

21. Lopez M, Robinson P, Madden T, Highbarger T. (1994) Nutritional support and prognosis in patients with head and neck cancer. *J Surg Oncol* **55**: 33–36.

22. Wollman B, D'Agostino H, Walus-Wigle J, *et al.* (1995) Radiologic, endoscopic and surgical gastrostomy: an institutional evaluation and meta-analysis of the literature. *Radiology* **197**: 699–704.

23. Ho S, Marchinkow L, Legiehn G, *et al.* (2001) Radiological percutaneous gastrostomy. *Clin Radiol* **56**(11): 902–910.

24. Colapinto R, Stronell R, Birch S. (1982) Creation of a portosystemic shunt with a Gruntzig balloon catheter. *CMAJ* **126**: 267–268.

25. Ong J, Sands M, Younossi Z. (2000) Transjugular intrahepatic portosystemic shunts (TIPS): a decade later. *J Clin Gastroenterol* **30**: 14–28.

26. Boyer TD. (2003) Transjugular intrahepatic portosystemic shunt: current status. *Gastroenterology* **124**: 1700–1710.

27. LaBerge J, Somberg K, Lake J, *et al.* (1995) Two-year outcome following transjugular intrahepatic portosystemic shunt for variceal bleeding: results in 90 patients. *Gastroenterology* **108**: 1143–1151.

28. Jalan R, Forrest E, Stanley A, *et al.* (1997) A randomized trial comparing transjugular intrahepatic portosystemic stent-shunt with variceal band ligation in the prevention of rebleeding from esophageal varices. *Hepatology* **26**: 1115–1122.

29. Saxon R, Barton R, Keller F, Rosch J. (1995) Prevention, detection and treatment of TIPS stenosis and occlusion. *Sem Intervent Radiol* **12**: 375–383.

30. Saxon R, Mendel-Hartvig J, Corless C, *et al.* (1996) Bile duct injury as a major cause of stenosis and occlusion in transjugular intrahepatic portosystemic shunts: comparative histopathologic analysis in humans and swine. *J Vasc Intervent Radiol* **7**: 487–497.

31. Jalan R, Stanley A, Redhead D, Hayes P. (1997) Shunt insufficiency after transjugular intrahepatic portosystemic stent-shunt: the whens, whys, hows and what should we do about it? (editorial) *Clin Radiol* **52**: 329–331.

32. Sanyal A, Freedman A, Luketic V, *et al.* (1997) The natural history of portal hypertension after transjugular intrahepatic portosystemic shunts (comment) *Gastroenterology* **112**: 889–898.

33. Zuckerman D, Darcy M, Bocchini T, Hildebolt C. (1997) Encephalopathy after transjugular intrahepatic portosystemic shunting: analysis of incidence and potential risk factors. *Am J Roentgenol* **169**: 1727–1731.

34. Armstrong P, Macleod C. (2002) Infection of transjugular intrahepatic portosystemic shunt devices; three cases and a review of the literature. *Clin Infect Dis* **36**: 407–412.

35. Willner I, El-Sakr R, Werkman R, *et al.* (1998) A fistula from the portal vein to the bile duct: an unusual complication of transjugular intrahepatic portosystemic shunt. *Am J Gastroenterol* **93**: 1952–1955.

36. Mallery S, Freeman M, Peine C, *et al.* (1996) Biliary-shunt fistula following transjugular intrahepatic portosystemic shunt placement. *Gastroenterology* **111**: 1353–1357.

37. Darwin P, Mergner W, Thuluvath P. (1998) Torulopsis Glabrata fungemia as a complication of a clotted transjugular intrahepatic portosystemic shunt. *Liver Transpl Surg* **4**: 89–90.

38. Schiano T, Atillasoy E, Fiel M, *et al.* (1997) Fatal fungemia resulting from an infected transjugular intrahepatic portosystemic shunt stent. *Am J Gastroenterol* **94**: 709–710.

39. Owen R, Rose J. (2000) Endovascular treatment of a portal vein tear during TIPS. *Cardiovasc Intervent Radiol* **23**: 230–232.

40. Kim J-K, Yun W, Kim J-W, *et al.* (2001) Extrahepatic portal vein tear with intraperitoneal haemorrhage during TIPS. *Cardiovasc Intervent Radiol* **24**: 436–437.

41. Petit P, Lazar I, Chagnaud C, *et al.* (2000) Iatrogenic dissection of the portal vein during TIPS procedure. *Eur Radiol* **10**: 930–934.

42. Fickert P, Trauner M, Hausegger K, *et al.* (2000) Intra-hepatic haematoma complicating transjugular intra-hepatic portosystemic shunt for Budd-Chiari syndrome associated with anti-phospholipid antibodies, aplastic anaemia and chronic hepatitis C. *Eur J Gastroenterol Hepatol* **12**: 813–816.

43. Pattynama P, van Hoek B, Kool L. (1995) Inadvertent arteriovenous stenting during transjugular intrahepatic portosystemic shunt procedure and the importance of hepatic artery perfusion. *Cardiovasc Intervent Radiol* **18**: 192–195.

44. Prahlow J, O'Bryant T, Barnard J. (1998) Cardiac perforation due to Wallstent embolization; a fatal complication of the transjugular intrahepatic portosystemic shunt procedure (comment). *Radiology* **207**: 551.

45. McCowan T, Hummel M, Schmucker T, *et al.* (2000) Cardiac perforation and tamponade during transjugular intrahepatic portosystemic shunt placement. *Cardiovasc Intervent Radiol* **23**: 298–300.

46. Sehgal M, Brown D, Picus D. (2002) Aortoatrial complicating transjugular intrahepatic portosystemic shunt by protrusion of a stent into the right atrium: radiologic/pathologic correlation. *J Vasc Intervent Radiol* **13**: 409–412.

47. Linka A, Jenni R. (2001) Migration of intrahepatic portosystemic shunt into right ventricle: an unusual cause of tricuspid regurgitation. *Circulation* **103**: 161–162.

48. Turnes J, Garcia-Pagan J, Ginzalez-Abraldes J, *et al.* (2001) Stenosis of suprahepatic inferior vena cava as a complication of transjugular intrahepatic portosystemic shunt in Budd-Chiari patients. *Liver Transpl* **7**: 649–651.

49. Mazziotti A, Morelli M, Grazi G, *et al.* (1996) Beware of TIPS in liver transplant candidates. Transjugular intrahepatic portosystemic shunt. *Hepato-Gastroenterology* **42**: 1606–1610.

50. Clavien P, Selzner M, Tuttle-Newhall J, *et al.* (1998) Liver transplantation complicated by misplaced TIPS in the portal vein. *Ann Surg* **227**: 440–445.

51. Burke DR. (1997) Percutaneous transhepatic cholangiography: major complications. *J Vasc Intervent Radiol* **8**: 677–681.

52. Hamlin J, Friedman M, Stein M, Bray J. (1986) Percutaneous biliary drainage: complications of 118 consecutive catheterizations. *Radiology* **158**: 199–202.

53. Mueller P, van Sonnenburg E, Ferruci J. (1982) Percutaneous biliary drainage: technical and catheter related problem in 200 procedures. *Am J Roentgenol* **138**: 17–23.

54. Morgan R, Jackson J, Adam A. (2001) Interventional techniques in the hepato-biliary system. In: Grainger R, Allison D, Adam A, Dixon A (eds.), *Diagnostic Radiology: A Textbook of Medical Imaging* (Harcourt Publishers Ltd., London), pp. 1307–1332.

55. Bremer C. (2003) Interventional magnetic imaging. In: Reimer P, Parizel P, Stichnoth FA. (eds.), *Clinical MR Imaging. A Practical Approach*, 2nd edn. (Springer, Berlin), pp. 575–576.

56. Nazarian L, Feld R, Herrine S, *et al.* (2000) Safety and efficacy of sonographi-cally guided random core biopsy for diffuse liver disease. *J Ultrasound Med* **19**: 537–541.

57. Bravo A, Sheth S, Chopra S. (2001) Current concepts: liver biopsy. *N Engl J Med* **344**: 495–500.

58. van Leeuwen D, Wilson L, Crowe D. (1995) Liver biopsy in the mid-1990s: questions and answers. *Sem Liver Dis* **15**: 340–359.

59. Piccinio F, Sagnelli E, Pasquale G, Giusti G. (1986) Complications following percutaneous liver biopsy: a multicentre retrospective study on 68,276 biopsies. *J Hepatol* **2**: 165–173.

60. Janes C, Lindor K. (1993) Outcome of patients hospitalized for complications after outpatient liver biopsy. *Ann Intern Med* **118**: 96–98.

61. Raines D, Van Heertum R, Johnson L. (1974) Intrahepatic haematoma: a com-plication of percutaneous liver biopsy. *Gastroenterology* **67**: 284–289.

62. Van Thiel D, Gaveler J, Wright H, Tzakis A. (1993) Liver biopsy: its safety and complications as seen at a liver transplant centre. *Transplantation* **55**: 1087–1090.

63. Lichtenstein D, Kim D, Chopra S. (1992) Delayed massive haemobilia following percutaneous liver biopsy: treatment by embolotherapy. *Am J Gastroenterol* **87**: 1833–1838.

64. Bellavia R, Haaga J, Herbener T. (1998) Liver biopsy. In: Gazelle S, Saini S, Mueller P (eds.), *Hepatobiliary and Pancreatic Radiology: Imaging and Intervention* (Thieme, Stuttgart).

65. Allison D, Adam A. (1988) Percutaneous liver biopsy and track embolisation with steel coils. *Radiology* **169**: 261–263.

66. Dick R, McCormick P, Sawyer A. (1989) Comparison of plugged percutaneous versus transjugular liver biopsy in 55 patients with compromised clotting. British Society for Gastroenterology (London), meeting April 1989.

67. Reddy K, Schiff E. (1997) Complications of liver biopsy. In: Taylor MB (ed.), *Gastrointestinal Emergencies*, 2nd edn. (Williams & Wilkins, Baltimore), pp. 959–968.

68. Ruben R, Chopra S. (1987) Bile peritonitis after liver biopsy: non-surgical management of a patient with an acute abdomen: a case of report with a review of the literature. *Am J Gastroenterol* **82**: 265–268.

69. Goodwin W, Casey W, Woolf W. (1955) Percutaneous trocar (needle) nephrostomy in hydronephrosis. *J Am Med Assoc* **157**: 891–894.

70. Stables D, Ginsberg N, Johnson M. (1978) Percutaneous nephrostomy: a series and review of the literature. *Am J Roentgenol* **130**: 75–82.

71. Farrell T, Hicks M, Marshall E. (1997) A review of radiologically guided percutaneous nephrostomies in 303 patients. *J Vasc Intervent Radiol* **8**: 769–774.

72. Kaskarelis I, Papadaki M, Malliaraki N, *et al* (2001) Complications of percutaneous nephrostomy, percutaneous insertion of ureteral endoprosthesis, and replacement procedures. *Cardiovasc Intervent Radiol* **24**: 224–228.

73. Gonzalez-Serva L, Weinerth J, Glenn J. (1977) Minimal mortality of renal surgery. *Urology* **9**: 253–255.

74. von der Recke P, Nielsen M, Pedersen J. (1994) Complications of ultrasound guided nephrostomy. A 5 year experience. *Acta Radiol* **35**: 452–454.

75. Peene P, Wilms G, Baert A. (1990) Embolization of iatrogenic renal haemorrhage following percutaneous nephrostomy. *Urol Radiol* **12**: 84–87.

76. Cowen N, Traill Z, Phillips A, Gleeson F. (1998) Direct percutaneous transrenal embolization for renal artery injury following percutaneous nephrostomy. *Br J Radiol* **71**: 1199–1201.

77. Merine D, Fishman E. (1989) Perirenal haematoma following catheter removal. An unusual complication percutaneous nephrostomy. *Clin Imaging* **13**: 74–76.

78. Soper J, Blaszczyk T, Oke E, *et al.* (1988) Percutaneous nephrostomy in gynaecologic oncology patients. *Am J Obstet Gynecol* **158**: 1126–1131.

79. Lee W, Patel U, Patel S, Pillari G. (1994) Emergency percutaneous nephrostomy: results and complications. *J Vasc Intervent Radiol* **5**: 135–139.

80. Cronan J, Marcello A, Horn D *et al.* (1989) Antibiotics and nephrostomy tube care: preliminary observations. Part I. Bacteriuria. *Radiology* **172**: 1041–1042.

81. Cronan J, Marcello A, Horn D, *et al.* (1989) Antibiotics and nephrostomy tube care: preliminary observations. Part II. Bacteremia. *Radiology* **172**: 1043–1045.

82. Barbaric Z, Davis R, Frank I, *et al.* (1976) Percutaneous nephrostomy in the management of acute pyohydronephrosis. *Radiology* **118**: 567–573.

83. Reinberg Y, Moore L, Lange P. (1989) Splenic abscess as a complication of percutaneous nephrostomy. *Urology* **34**: 274–276.

84. Nosher J, Ericksen A, Trooskin S, *et al.* (1990) Antibiotic bonded nephrostomy catheters for percutaneous nephrostomies. *Cardiovasc Intervent Radiol* **13**: 102–106.

85. Lopes NA, Tobias-Machado M, Juliano R, *et al.* (2000) Duodenal damage complication percutaneous access to the kidney. *Sao Paulo Med J* **118**: 116–117.

86. Morris D, Siegelbaum M, Pollack H, *et al.* (1991) Renoduodenal fistula in a patient with chronic nephrostomy drainage: a case report. *J Urol* **146**: 835–837.

87. Kontothanassis D, Bissas A. (1997) Biliary peritonitis complicating percutaneous nephrostomy. *Int Urol Nephrol* **29**: 529–531.

88. Oefelein M, MacLennan G. (2003) Transitional cell carcinoma recurrence in the nephrostomy tract after percutaneous resection. *J Urol* **170**: 521.

89. Kellett M. (2001) Interventional uroradiology. In: Grainger R, Allison D, Adam A, Dixon A (eds.), *Diagnostic Radiology: A Textbook of Medical Imaging* (Harcourt Publishers Ltd. London), pp. 1693–1716.

90. Cadeddu J, Arrindell D, Moore R. (1997) Near fatal air embolism during percutaneous nephrostomy placement. *J Urol* **158**: 1519.

91. Stoller M, Wolf J, St Lezin M. (1994) Estimated blood loss and transfusion rates associated with percutaneous nephrolithotomy (comment). *J Urol* **152**: 1977–1981.

92. Lee W, Smith A, Cubelli V, *et al.* (1987) Complications of nephrolithotomy. *Am J Roentgenol* **148**: 177–180.

93. Roth R, Beckmann C. (1988) Complications of extracorporeal shock wave therapy lithotripsy and percutaneous nephrolithotomy. *Urol Clin North Am* **15**: 155–166.

94. Patterson D, Segura J, Leroy A, Benson R, May G. (1985) The etiology and treatment of delayed bleeding following percutaneous lithotripsy. *J Urol* **133**: 447–451.

95. Kessaris D, Bellman G, Padalidis N, Smith A. (1995) Management of haemorrhage after percutaneous renal surgery. *J Urol* **153**: 604–608.

96. Sacha K, Szewczyk W, Bar K. (1996) Massive haemorrhage presenting as a complication after percutaneous nephrolithotomy (PCNL). *Int Urol Nephrol* **28**: 315–318.

97. Gremmo E, Ballanger P, Dore B, Aubert J. (1999) Haemorrhagic complications during percutaneous nephrolithotomy. Retrospective studies in 772 cases. *Progres Urol* **9**: 460–463 (in French).

98. Davidoff R, Bellman G. (1997) Influence of technique of percutaneous tract creation on incidence of renal haemorrhage. *J Urol* **157**: 1229–1231.

99. Wong M. (2001) An update on percutaneous nephrolithotomy in the management of urinary calculi. *Curr Opin Urol* **11**: 367–372.

100. Weir M, D'A Honey R. (1999) Complete infundibular obliteration following percutaneous nephrolithotomy. *J Urol* **161**: 1274–1275.

101. Parsons J, Jarrett T, Lancini V, Kavoussi L. (2002) Infundibular stenosis after percutaneous nephrolithotomy. *J Urol* **167**: 35–38.
102. Tang S, Li J, Lui S, *et al.* (2002) Free-hand, ultrasound-guided percutaneous renal biopsy: experience from a single operator. *Eur J Radiol* **41**: 65–69.
103. Preda A, Van Dijk L, Van Oostaijen J, Pattynama P. (2003) Complication rate and diagnostic yield of 515 consecutive ultrasound-guided biopsies of renal allografts and native and native kidneys using a 14-gauge biopty gun. *Eur Radiol* **13**: 527–530.
104. Furness P, Philpott C, Chorbadjian M, *et al.* (2003) Protocol biopsy of the stable renal transplant: a multicentre study of methods and complication rates. *Transplantation* **76**: 969–973.
105. Hergesell O, Felten H, Andrassy K, *et al.* (1998) Safety of ultrasound-guided percutaneous renal biopsy — retrospective analysis of 1090 consecutive cases. *Nephrol Dial Transpl* **13**: 975–977.
106. Schow D, Vinson R, Morrisseau P. (1992) Percutaneous renal biopsy of the solitary kidney: a contraindication? *J Urol* **147**: 1235–1237.
107. Wilczek H. (1990) Percutaneous needle biopsy of the renal allograft. A clinical safety evaluation of 1129 biopsies. *Transplantation* **50**: 790–797.
108. Spies J, Berlin L. (1998) Complications of femoral artery puncture. *Am J Roentgenol* **170**: 9–11.
109. Jackson J, Allison D, Hemingway A. (2001) Principles, techniques and complications of angiography. In: Grainger R, Allison D, Adam A, Dixon A (eds.), *Diagnostic Radiology: A Textbook of Medical Imaging* (Harcourt Publishers Ltd., London), pp. 149–184.
110. Cragg A, Nakagawa N, Smith T, Berbaum K. (1991) Hematoma formation after diagnostic angiography: effect of catheter size. *J Vasc Intervent Radiol* **2**: 231–233.
111. Fellmeth B, Roberts A, Bookstein J, *et al.* (1991) Postangiographic femoral artery injuries: nonsurgical repair with US guided compression. *Radiology* **178**: 671–675.
112. Katzenschlager R, Ugurluoglu A, Ahmedi A, *et al.* (1995) Incidence of pseudoaneurysm after diagnostic and therapeutic angiography. *Radiology* **195**: 463–466.
113. Colville R, Colin J. (1998) Median nerve palsy after high brachial angiography. *J R Soc Med* **91**: 387.
114. Etemand-Rezei R, Peck D. (2003) Ultrasound guided thrombin injection of femoral pseudoaneurysms. *Can Assoc Radiol J* **54**: 118–120.
115. McIvor J, Rhymer J. (1993) 245 transaxillary arteriograms in artiopathic patients: success rate and complications. *Clin Radiol* **45**: 390–394.

116. Resnik C, Sawyer R, Tisnado J. (1987) Septic arthritis of the hip: a rare complication of angiography. *Can Assoc Radiol J* **38**: 299–301.

117. Young N, Chi KK, Ajaka J, *et al.* (2002) Complications with outpatient angiography and interventional procedures. *Cardiovasc Intervent Radiol* **25**: 123–126.

118. Murphy T, Dorfman G, Segall M, Carney W. (1991) Iatrogenic arterial dissection: treatment by percutaneous transluminal angioplasty. *Cardiovasc Intervent Radiol* **14**: 302–306.

119. Palmer F, Warren B. (1988) Multiple cholesterol emboli syndrome complicating angiographic techniques. *Clin Radiol* **39**: 519–522.

120. Dotter C, Judkins M. (1964) Transluminal treatment of arteriosclerotic obstruction: description of a new technique and a preliminary report of its application. *Circulation* **30**: 654–670.

121. Uflacker R, Robinson J. (2001) Endovascular treatment of aortic aneurysms: a review. *Eur Radiol* **11**: 739–753.

122. Axisa B, Fishwick G, Bolia A, *et al.* (2002) Complications following peripheral angioplasty. *Ann R Coll Surg Engl* **84**: 39–42.

123. Gardiner G, Meyerovitz M, Stokes K, *et al.* (1986) Complications of transluminal angioplasty. *Radiology* **159**: 201–208.

124. Hoffman O, Carreres T, Sapoval M, *et al.* (1998) Ostial renal artery stenosis angioplasty: immediate and mid-term angiographic and clinical results. *J Vasc Intervent Radiol* **9**: 65–73.

125. DeMaioribus C, Anderson C, Popham S, *et al.* (1998) Mycotic renal artery degeneration and systemic sepsis caused by infected renal artery stent. *J Vasc Surg* **28**: 547–550.

126. Woodburn K, May J, White G. (1998) Endoluminal abdominal aortic aneurysm surgery. *Br J Surg* **85**: 435–443.

127. Bernhard V, Mitchell R, Matsumara J, *et al.* (2002) Ruptured abdominal aortic aneurysm after endovascular repair. *J Vasc Surg* **35**: 1155–1162.

128. Rosenkrantz H, Bookstein J, Rosen R, *et al.* (1982) Postembolic colonic infarction. *Radiology* **142**: 47–51.

129. Huang L, Cheng Y, Huang C, *et al.* (2003) Incomplete vaginal expulsion of pyoadenomata and focal bladder necrosis after uterine artery embolization for adenomyosis: a case report. *Human Reprod* **18**: 167–171.

130. Klatte E, Becker G, Holden R, Yune H. (1987) Embolisation procedures. In: Ansell G, Wilkins RA (eds.), *Complications in Diagnostic Imaging* (Blackwell Scientific Publications, London), pp. 148–158.

131. Hemingway A, Allison D. (1988) Complications of embolization: analysis of 410 procedures. *Radiology* **166**: 669–672.

132. Braude P, Reidy J, Nott V, *et al.* (2000) Embolization of uterine leiomyomata: current concepts in management. *Human Reprod Update* **6**: 603–608.

133. Spence L, Gironta M, Malde H, *et al.* (1999) Acute upper extremity deep venous thrombosis: safety and effectiveness of superior vena caval filters. *Radiology* **210**: 53–58.

134. Athanasoulis C, Kaufman J, Halpern E, *et al.* (2000) Inferior vena caval filters: review of a 26 single-centre clinical experience. *Radiology* **216**: 54–66.

135. Ferris E, McCowan T, Carver D, Mcfarland D. (1993) Percutaneous inferior vena caval filters: follow up of seven designs in 320 patients. *Radiology* **188**: 851–856.

136. Feezor R, Huber T, Welborn M, Schell S. (2002) Duodenal perforation with an inferior vena caval filter: an unusual cause of abdominal pain. *J Vasc Surg* **35**: 1010–1012.

137. Woodward E, Farber A, Wagner W, *et al.* (2002) Delayed retroperitoneal arterial hemorrhage after inferior vena cava (IVC) filter insertion: case report and literature review of caval perforations by IVC filters. *Ann Vasc Surg* **16**: 193–196.

138. Strieb E, Wagner J. (2000) Complications of vascular access procedures in patients with vena caval filters. *J Trauma Injury Infect Crit Care* **49**: 553–558.

139. Kaufman J, Thomas J. (1996) Guide-wire entrapment by inferior vena cava filters: in vitro evaluation. *Radiology* **198**: 71–76.

140. Peh W, Gilula L. (2003) Percutaneous vertebroplasty: indications, contraindications, and technique. *Br J Radiol* **76**: 69–75.

141. Gangi A, Guth S, Imbert J, *et al.* (2002) Percutaneous vertebroplasty: indications, techniques and results. *Radiographics* **23**: e10.

142. Chen H, Wong C, Ho S, *et al.* (2002) A lethal pulmonary embolism during percutaneous vertebroplasty. *Anesth Anal* **94**: 1060–1062.

143. Goldberg SN, Ahmed M. (2002) Minimally invasive image guided therapies for hepatocellular carcinoma. *J Clin Gastroenterol* **35**(Suppl 2): S115–S129.

144. Garcea G, Lloyd T, Aylott C, *et al.* (2003) The emergent role of focal liver ablation techniques in the treatment of primary and secondary liver tumours. *Eur J Cancer* **39**: 2150–2164.

145. Dick E, Joarder R, De Jode M, *et al.* (2003) MR-guided laser thermal ablation of primary and secondary liver tumours. *Clin Radiol* **58**: 112–120.

Chapter 28

PSYCHIATRIC COMPLICATIONS RELATED TO SURGICAL PROCEDURES

Justin L. Dwyer and Steven Reid

The importance of psychological factors in the management of surgical patients has been highlighted in a report by a joint working party of the Royal College of Surgeons of England and the Royal College of Psychiatrists.[1] Surgery is a traumatic event and these factors have considerable potential in affecting its outcome. Preoperative psychological morbidity, as well as making the assessment of presenting symptoms and surgical risks more difficult, increases the risk of postoperative complications such as delirium, cognitive impairment and functional disability. The changes in surgical practice, with increasing use of day surgery and the reduced length of hospital admissions, have further highlighted the need to consider these issues. This chapter aims to outline the important aspects of the preoperative assessment related to psychiatric illness, present an overview of the psychiatric complications that may occur following surgery, and describe their management.

Box 1   General Points on the Assessment of Patients Presenting with Emotional Distress and Psychiatric Illness

- Evaluation of current mental state and coping style.
- Previous history of psychiatric illness — often a useful guide to the current diagnosis, and may indicate the most appropriate treatment.
- Collateral history from those who know the patient well — particularly important where the patient is unable to give a history.
- Details of personal circumstances and social support.
- Past history of risk behaviour — including deliberate self-harm and suicide attempts, as well as threats or aggression toward others.

Common Psychiatric Terminology

- **Adjustment disorder** — a maladaptive reaction or difficulty in coping following an identifiable stressor such as surgery. This may occur in the short or long-term e.g., social withdrawal following stoma surgery.
- **Anxiety** — an unpleasant emotional state with the expectation of something untoward happening. It is usually associated with autonomic arousal leading to symptoms such as sweating, palpitations and tremor.
- **Depression** — abnormally low mood that is experienced by the patient as pervasive, persistent and painful. It is associated with negative and pessimistic thinking.
- **Somatization** — a process in which emotional distress is experienced and communicated in physical terms.
- **Psychosis** — refers to more severe forms of mental illness in which there is a fundamental impairment of reality-testing i.e., an inability to distinguish between subjective experience and reality. Psychotic symptoms often have a bizarre quality and include delusions and hallucinations.
- **Delusions** — abnormal beliefs that are fixed, false, not amenable to reason and that are out of keeping with the patient's social and cultural background.
- **Hallucinations** — perceptions experienced in the absence of an external stimulus, such as "voices". They are also experienced as originating in the outside world, and can occur in any sensory modality. Visual hallucinations should raise the possibility of organic illness such as delirium and alcohol withdrawal.

PREOPERATIVE ASSESSMENT

Psychiatric illness may lead to miscommunication, inaccurate diagnosis and potentially inappropriate surgery, and poor postoperative adjustment. Therefore, the evaluation of the current mental state in patients being considered for surgery is essential. The ability to comply with postoperative management, especially important in transplantation surgery where immuno-suppressants are required, may affect the decision to proceed with the surgery, and should be included in the preoperative assessment. The assessment should also take account of the personal circumstances of the patient, their illness and the surgical procedure itself, as these factors will affect their response. Surgery affecting body parts with significant emotional and symbolic meaning (e.g., head and neck, breast, testes) raise specific concerns and anxiety about potential disfigurement.

The preoperative assessment should include the documentation of psychotropic medication and the risk of interaction with the anaesthetic and postoperative drugs (Table 1). Most drugs can be continued safely until the time of surgery and resumed postoperatively once oral tolerance is established; in some cases discontinuation of psychotropic medication may be appropriate. Due to their propensity for interactions with other drugs it is recommended that a specific class of antidepressants, monoamine oxidase inhibitors, are withdrawn two weeks before general anaesthesia. This should be done in consultation with the psychiatrist, taking into account the risk of a deteriorating mental state.

Anxiety Disorders

Preoperative anxiety occurs frequently, and while education and reassurance are usually sufficient, some patients may require specific treatment if the symptoms are disabling or interfere with the management. Anxiety symptoms can be psychological, physical, or a mixture of both. Somatic complaints associated with anxiety, such as palpitations, chest pain, tachypnoea and gastrointestinal disturbance may be difficult to distinguish from organic illness; severe anxiety may lead to refusal of treatment. There is some evidence that preoperative anxiety is associated with a poor outcome and increased risk of complications following surgery.[2] Blood and needle phobias are common but are readily managed with psychological treatment, such as graded exposure.[3] Where the symptoms are

Table 1.   Potential Anaesthetic Interactions with Psychotropic Drugs*

Drug	Anaesthetic Interactions	Notes
Antidepressants		
Selective serotonin reuptake inhibitors (SSRI)	Prolongs action of ropivacaine	Check bleeding time as spontaneous bleeding has been reported
Tricyclics	Cause hypertension when used with adrenaline Arrhythmias	Patients on tricyclics may not require anticholinergics during anaesthesia Tricyclics reduce the seizure threshold
MAOI	Hypertensive crises with pethidine and indirectly-acting sympathomimetics (e.g. curare)	Requires strict postoperative adherence to restricted diet
Mood stabilisers		
Lithium	Toxic levels reached with dehydrated patients, on diuretics or those in heart failure	Requires careful monitoring of pre- and postoperative serum levels
Carbemazapine	Accelerates recovery from non-depolarising muscle relaxants	
Antipsychotics	May enhance hypotensive effects	Discuss with psychiatrist if cessation considered
Anxiolytics		
Benzodiazepines	Enhanced sedative effect	Be aware of potential for withdrawal syndrome if usual dose stopped
Buspirone	Does not potentiate sedative or muscle relaxant effect of anaesthesia	

*For further details refer to the manufacturer's information.

severe, specialist psychological treatment may be indicated; in the short term management with benzodiazepines usually provides rapid symptomatic relief. Diazepam (5–10 mg per day, orally) and lorazepam (1–2 mg per day, orally) are commonly used. Due to their potential to cause physical dependence and withdrawal symptoms, these drugs should be used at the lowest effective dose for the shortest period of time (a maximum of four weeks).

Drug and Alcohol Misuse

Up to 20% of male inpatients have alcohol-related problems, and alcohol misuse contributes to 20–25% of all general hospital admissions[4] with young male patients being the group at highest risk.[5] The detection of substance misuse is often difficult due to concealment but drug withdrawal, particularly delirium tremens, is not uncommon in patients admitted for elective surgery. A physical examination may reveal evidence of the stigmata of chronic alcohol and other drug misuse. Laboratory investigations, including the mean red cell volume (MCV), gamma-glutamyl transpeptidase (γ-GT) and aspartate transamainase (AST) are also useful in the identification of alcohol misuse.

Mood Disorders

The assessment of mood disorders in a medical setting can be difficult as patients commonly present with unexplained physical complaints rather than reported low mood. However, it is important to recognise mood disorders because depression is associated with increased postoperative morbidity and mortality, as well as difficulty in adhering to the treatment. The detection and management of depression is discussed in detail later.

Psychotic Disorders

Individuals with psychotic disorders are at particular risk of relapse following a stressful event such as surgery, and a careful assessment and monitoring of the mental state preferably involving a mental health specialist, is important. Patients currently experiencing psychotic symptoms may be unable to consent to treatment (*vide infra*). Special nursing arrangements such as close observation and a single room may be help reduce agitation and minimise risk.

Somatoform Disorders

Somatoform disorders (also called functional or hysterical disorders) are syndromes characterised by a preoccupation with physical symptoms, which occur either in the absence of, or disproportionate to the underlying organic disease. They are chronic disorders and should be distinguished from the ubiquitous, and more acute, process of somatization where psychological factors present as physical symptoms. The differential diagnosis may be problematic with such patients, since the surgical diagnosis is dependent upon the history and physical symptoms and a failure to recognise somatoform disorders may lead to unnecessary or inappropriate surgery. Factitious disorders present a further challenge involving patients who present with physical symptoms and signs that have been simulated or fabricated with no apparent motivation other than to adopt the sick role. The most frequently reported scenario is Munchausen's syndrome where the patient, usually male, makes multiple, often dramatic presentations to different hospitals using different names. However, the majority of the cases of factitious disorder (over 90%) involve young, female patients often working in medical settings.[6] Given the deception involved and the difficulty in engaging patients with factitious disorder, it is a challenge to establish its prevalence; however, it is almost certainly underdiagnosed. The diagnosis is particularly difficult during the initial assessment, although suspicion may be aroused by inconsistencies in the history, and discrepancy between symptoms and signs. Key to its identification is an awareness of the common features and an appropriate index of suspicion.

Personality Disorders

In the surgical ward, patients with personality disorders may present with challenging and unreasonably demanding behaviour. Sudden and dramatic mood changes, deliberate self-harm, and acts regarded as manipulative can lead to alienation of the patient from the clinicians as well as divisions amongs the clinical team itself. Its management requires a consistent and co-ordinated approach with clearly set boundaries, and the involvement of a mental health specialist, if possible.

POSTOPERATIVE COMPLICATIONS

Delirium

Delirium is an acute, reversible syndrome characterised by fluctuating cognitive impairment. It is a common cause of disturbed behaviour postoperatively, and often passes undetected and therefore poorly managed. Most studies on the prevalence of delirium have been carried out in medically unwell inpatients with estimates of 20–30%.[7–10] Follow up studies on hospitalised patients suggest that less than half of the patients with delirium have fully recovered from it by the time of discharge. A number of risk factors have been identified (Box 2).

The core feature of delirium is a global impairment of cognitive functioning particularly affecting orientation and memory. Attention may be impaired on a continuum from clouding of consciousness to coma. The symptoms typically fluctuate over time and worsen at night. Impaired attention, and disturbed thought processes may reflect in incoherent speech. Other symptoms include disturbed behaviour, social withdrawal, fluctuating mood and perceptual abnormalities.[11] Illusions and hallucinations are common, and visual hallucinations are particularly suggestive of delirium. The patient may also experience fleeting persecutory delusions, typically believing that the staff and other patients are conspiring against them. Delirium can present at any time during admission, but appears more commonly in the first week, often on the third day, postoperatively.[12]

Box 2   Risk Factors for Delirium[8,10]

- Age > 70 years old
- Alcohol misuse
- Pre-existing cognitive impairment
- Cardiac and hip fracture surgery
- Abnormal serum potassium, sodium or glucose
- High Blood Urea Nitrogen–Creatinine (BUN/Cr) ratio
- Visual impairment
- Malnutrition

Although frequently undetected, the diagnosis of delirium is important because of its associated morbidity and mortality. The diagnosis is made on the basis of the clinical features mentioned above, and should be suspected in any patient who presents acutely with disturbed behaviour or a sudden change in mood or personality. Its detection is aided by routine cognitive assessment on admission, using brief scales such as the Mini-Mental State Examination[13] to identify deteriorating cognitive function and provide a baseline measurement (Box 3).

Box 3   The Mini-Mental State Examination[13]

Scoring instructions: Add points for each correct response. A score below 28 indicates abnormal cognitive function.

ORIENTATION

1. What is the   Year?
                         Season?
                         Date?
                         Month?

2. Where are we?   Country?
                         County?
                         Town?
                         Hospital?
                         Floor?   (Score 0–10)

REGISTRATION

3. Name three objects, taking one second to say each.
    Then ask the subject to repeat all three after you
    have said them. Repeat the answers until patient
    learns all three (up to six trials).   (Score 0–3)

ATTENTION AND CALCULATION

4. Serial sevens (beginning with 100 count
    backwards by 7–93, 86, 79, 72, 65). Alternatively,
    spell WORLD backwards.   (Score 0–5)

(Continued)

(*Continued*)

RECALL

5.   Ask for names of three objects learned in Q.3.   (Score 0–3)

LANGUAGE

6.   Point to a pencil and a watch. Have the patient
     name them as you point.   (Score 0–2)

7.   Have the patient repeat "No ifs, ands or buts."   (Score 0–1)

8.   Have the patient follow a three-stage command:
     "Take this paper in your right hand, fold it in half,
     and put it on your knee".   (Score 0–3)

9.   Have the patient read and obey the following:
     "CLOSE YOUR EYES".   (Score 0–1)

10. Have the patient write a sentence of his or her
     choice. (The sentence should contain a subject
     and an object, and should make sense.)   (Score 0–1)

11. Have the patient copy a design of intersecting
     pentagons. (The sides and angles should be
     preserved, with a central diamond.)   (Score 0–2)

                                                        Total /30

The two notable differential diagnoses for delirium are a psychotic illness such as schizophrenia, and dementia. Schizophrenia is not associated with obvious cognitive impairment and visual hallucinations are less common. Dementia has a gradual onset and lacks the markedly fluctuating course of delirium. However, delirium often presents in pre-existing dementia. There are numerous causes, the most common being prescribed medication and acute infection. However, it is important to be aware that alcohol withdrawal which occurs due to hospital admission may also lead to delirium (Box 4).

An attempt should be made to prevent the development of delirium, and if possible, patients should be screened on admission, for risk factors such as substance misuse or cognitive impairment. The early identification of problems such as dehydration, malnutrition, polypharmacy and drug dependence is crucial. A recent intervention study that actively managed cognitive

Box 4   Some Causes of Delirium

- Intoxication with drugs — e.g., alcohol, illicit drugs, sedative hypnotics, opiates, steroids, cimetidine, anticonvulsants, anticholinergic agents
- Withdrawal syndromes — alcohol, sedative hypnotics, barbiturates
- Metabolic causes — hypoxia, hypoglycaemia, hepatic, renal or pulmonary insufficiency, disorders of fluid and electrolyte balance, endocrine disorders
- Infections
- Head trauma
- Epilepsy — ictal, interictal, postictal
- Vascular disorders — cerebrovascular, cardiovascular
- Vitamin deficiency — thiamine, nicotinic acid, B12

impairment, sleep deprivation, immobility, visual and hearing impairment and dehydration significantly reduced the incidence of delirium in elderly inpatients.[14] Once delirium has developed, the mainstay of management is the investigation and treatment of the underlying cause. This may be difficult in some cases, particularly where insight is impaired and behaviour is disturbed. Managing the environment is essential for reducing the risk of harm to the patient and others. Such interventions will also reduce demands on the patient's impaired cognition. Environmental measures include placing the patient in a side room off the open ward, away from the exit and in clear view of the nursing station. Orienting cues such as clocks and calendars, photos of family, and signs indicating the name of the ward, and members of staff are helpful. Where practical, ensure that the same member of staff nurses the patient. This will be of value in orienting the patient and monitoring the changes in their mental state. Drug treatment may be necessary for managing symptoms of delirium but it should be done carefully because antipsychotics and benzodiazepines can worsen the condition. They should be prescribed using a fixed dosing regimen rather than an "as required" basis. Antipsychotics are commonly used and are effective with a rapid onset of action. Haloperidol (1–10 mg/d) is effective, has few anticholinergic adverse effects, minimal cardiovascular side effects and is available in oral and intramuscular formulations. New antipsychotics, such as olanzapine and risperidone are being used with increasing frequency in clinical settings as they have an improved toxicity profile.[15] Benzodiazepines are used when antipsychotics are ineffective or cause unacceptable adverse effects. They are the treatment of choice when delirium is associated with withdrawal from alcohol or sedatives. In delirium tremens, associated with alcohol withdrawal, chlordiazepoxide (or diazepam) should be prescribed in a reducing regimen. In other situations, oral, intramuscular, or intravenous lorazepam may be given up to once every four hours. The general measures such as supplemental oxygen[16,17] may also be effective. A regular review of the management of delirium and the underlying causes should continue for the duration of the admission; the patient's legal status should be reviewed if detention or treatment without consent is necessary.

Depression

The diagnosis of depression in surgical patients presents a challenge. Postoperatively, depressive symptoms occur frequently and it is not always clear when they merit clinical attention. Furthermore, depression often presents with somatic complaints such as fatigue, poor sleep, and reduced appetite, but these symptoms are almost universal following surgery. There is also a common and misleading perception that depression is an understandable psychological reaction to surgery. Although diagnosis may be difficult, its recognition and appropriate treatment is important, as postoperative depression is associated with impaired recovery, prolonged hospital admission, and increased mortality.

Depression has been identified in 10–15% of medical and surgical inpatients; it may also occur as a psychological reaction to the surgical procedures themselves. Surgery is a stressful life event and is often associated with feelings of loss of control and fear of the future. A prior history of depression certainly makes the patient more vulnerable. The factors related to surgery that may increase the risk of depression include an unsuccessful outcome, chronic pain, wound infection, and malignancy. Depression may also occur as a specific consequence of physical illness or its treatment. It may be the sole presenting symptom of an underlying disease (e.g., carcinoma of the pancreas) and this should be considered especially in patients presenting with depression for the first time in later life. The role of prescription medicines in causing depression is frequently highlighted and merits consideration in assessment, although a direct cause-effect relationship has been definitively established for only a few drugs (Box 5).

Box 5   **Physical Illnesses and Drugs Commonly Associated with Depression**

Physical illnesses associated with depression
Intracranial

- Tumours
- Parkinson's disease
- Huntington's disease
- Cerebrovascular disease
- Encephalopathies
- Head injury
- Multiple sclerosis

Extracranial

- Malignancy
- Endocrine disorders
- Infections (e.g., hepatitis B, infectious mononucleosis)

Drugs associated with depression

- Antihypertensives — reserpine, clonidine, propanolol, nifedipine
- Antiarrhythmics — digoxin, procainamide
- Anti-parkinsonian — L-dopa, amantadine
- Cytotoxic agents — interferons, vincristine
- H2-blockers — cimetidine
- Hormonal agents — corticosteroids, anabolic steroids, oral contraceptives
- Anticonvulsants — barbiturates, carbamazepine, vigabatrin
- Antiretroviral agents — nevirapine, efavirenz

In distinguishing depressive disorders from adjustment reactions postoperatively, the severity and duration of symptoms are important. Feelings of despondency or anger are short-lived and transient in adjustment reactions. Although somatic symptoms such as weight or appetite change, insomnia, and fatigue or energy loss may be poor indicators of depression in the physically ill, taking account of all depressive symptoms whether or not they may be attributed to an underlying physical problem is beneficial and does not

Box 6   Signs of Depression in the Postoperative Patient

- Fearful or depressed appearance
- Social withdrawal or decreased talkativeness
- Psychomotor retardation or agitation
- Depressed mood
- Non-reactive affect
- Diurnal variation of mood
- Loss of enjoyment or interest in life
- Brooding, self-pity or pessimism
- Feelings of worthlessness or excessive or inappropriate guilt
- Feelings of helplessness
- Feeling a burden
- Recurrent thoughts of death or suicide
- Thoughts that the illness is a punishment
- Frequent crying

The presence of three or more of these symptoms for at least two weeks is indicative of a depressive illness.

lead to overdiagnosis. It is important to ask about thoughts of self-harm in the assessment of depression in the physically ill. Chronic physical illness — in particular, cancer, HIV and AIDS, renal disease, and chronic pain — is associated with an increased risk of suicide, especially in the elderly (Box 6).

Patients presenting with depressive symptoms may benefit from both support and clear information about their physical state, leading to reduced fear and uncertainty. Once the diagnosis has been established, the management should include prompt treatment with antidepressants. There is often a reluctance to use antidepressants in patients with physical illness to avoid complications in the treatment and subsequent adverse effects or drug interactions. However, a systematic review of 18 studies concluded that treatment with antidepressants (including tricyclic antidepressants and selective serotonin reuptake inhibitors) in depression associated with a range of physical illnesses was well-tolerated and led to significant improvements, when compared with either placebo or no treatment[18] There are a number of basic principles to consider while prescribing an antidepressant:

- Discuss likely outcomes with the patient, e.g., gradual relief from depressive symptoms over several weeks.
- Antidepressants do not cause physical dependence.
- Prescribe a dose of antidepressant (after titration, if necessary) that is recognised as effective.
- The antidepressant will need to be taken for at least 4–6 months to prevent any relapse of depression.
- Antidepressants must be taken regularly as prescribed and not just when the patient is feeling low.

The prescription of a particular antidepressant should be considered in the context of an assessment of the individual patient. There has been a shift in prescribing patterns with increased use of SSRI and newer antidepressants instead of tricyclics because of improved tolerability. Some examples of frequently used antidepressants are provided in Table 2.

In some cases, the severity of the depression may warrant a referral to a psychiatrist. This is indicated by a lack of response to antidepressant treatment, the presence of suicidal thoughts or acts of deliberate self-harm, the presence of psychotic symptoms, and a refusal to eat or drink. In situations where a patient's life is endangered by profound weight loss or severe dehydration, and a rapid therapeutic response is required, electroconvulsive therapy (ECT) may be beneficial. The use of ECT may have declined in recent years but it remains an effective treatment for severe depression.

SURGICAL SPECIALTIES

Transplantation Surgery

The advances in medicine and surgery have dramatically improved the life expectancy and quality of life of transplant recipients. Despite these changes, transplantation surgery remains a major life event, and patients face a number of stressors, both medical and psychological, that may have a profound impact on their postoperative outlook. Furthermore, as procedures have become more

Table 2. Selected Antidepressants

Antidepressant	Licensed Doses	Adverse Effects	Notes
Amitriptyline	30–200 mg/d optimum range for depression is 150–200 mg; amitriptyline has analgesic properties at lower doses	Sedation; postural hypotension; dry mouth, constipation, urinary retention, blurred vision; sexual dysfunction; arrhythmias	Cardiotoxic in overdose; may interact with SSRIs, alcohol, and antimuscarinics
Fluoxetine	20 mg/d	Nausea, dyspepsia, diarrhoea, insomnia, agitation, sexual dysfunction	Inhibitor of cytochrome enzymes; long half life 14 days
Citalopram	20–60 mg/d	As for fluoxetine but agitation and insomnia less common	Few interactions; liquid formulation available
Sertraline	50–200 mg/d	As for fluoxetine but agitation and insomnia less common	Inhibitor of cytochrome enzymes
Paroxetine	20–50 mg/d	As for fluoxetine but sedation more common; extrapyramidal symptoms may occur although rare	Inhibitor of cytochrome enzymes; liquid formulation available
Venlafaxine	75–375 mg/d	Nausea, insomnia, dry mouth, sweating, headache, sexual dysfunction	Few interactions; slow release preparation available
Mirtazapine	15–45 mg/d	Increased appetite, weight gain, drowsiness	Few interactions; nausea and sexual dysfunction are relatively uncommon

routine, patients who would have been excluded from transplantation because of psychiatric illness are now often considered to be suitable for treatment.

Psychiatric illness, particularly depression and anxiety, is common in patients awaiting transplantation surgery. A preoperative mental state examination allows for the identification of previously unrecognised disorders as well as recognising the patients at risk of non-compliance following surgery.[19] Delirium is the most common post-transplant psychiatric complication.[20–23] Along with the risk factors mentioned earlier, corticosteroids and immunosuppressants are well known precipitants of delirium. Depression is also common with the incidence as high as 60% during the first year post-transplant.[24] In particular, patients who are poorly compliant with treatment should always be assessed for depression. Mood disorders that develop secondary to infections, metabolic disturbances and adverse drug effects e.g., ciclosporine, corticosteroids should also be considered.[25] As with depression, anxiety disorders occur frequently and may interfere with the ability to understand treatment recommendations and, consequently compliance.[24] Agitation, fear, and insomnia are the usual presenting features. However, it should be noted that heart transplant patients do not experience the cardiac symptoms of anxiety, tachycardia and palpitations because the heart is denervated. Fear of graft rejection may lead to anxious ruminations, and patients may go to disproportionate lengths to protect the graft, engaging in highly restrictive lifestyles, and frequently presenting with somatic complaints attributed to rejection. Transplant support groups may be assist patients by making them feel less isolated and identifying alternative ways of coping. Specialist psychological treatment is a treatment option when support alone does not work.

Cardiac Surgery

There is a well-recognised association between coronary heart disease and psychological morbidity, particularly depressive illness. The prevalence of major depression in patients with coronary heart disease is 17–22%,[26] and for many of these patients, depression develops into a chronic illness. In a 12-month follow-up study, over 50% of the patients identified as depressed following coronary catheterisation and angiography but were left untreated remained depressed.[27] Anxiety symptoms are often encountered in coronary heart disease, and cardiac surgery in particular is a recognised precipitant of anxiety disorders. Patients may become preoccupied with concerns about the amount and type of stress they will be able to manage, especially with regard to sexual activity. Sexual dysfunction is a frequent postoperative complaint.

The use of pacemakers and implantable defibrillators is also a risk factor for psychological problems. Polypharmacy is also common because the patients are typically elderly, with multiple medical problems.[28] Although the quality of life may be improved, anxiety is experienced immediately after implantation. This is often associated with fear of accidental discharge and frequent shocks, panic attacks and imagined "phantom" shocks.[29]

Cardiac rehabilitation, a mainstay of treatment following cardiac surgery, usually includes an element of psychological support and offers a valuable opportunity for the identification of emergent psychiatric illness. The treatment of anxiety disorders will include anxiolytic medication, cognitive and behavioural therapies, and support groups.

ENT Surgery

The psychological effects of head and neck surgery are dependent upon a number of factors. The patient may be confronted with a life-threatening illness, difficulties with speech, vision or hearing postoperatively, and the surgery itself is potentially disfiguring. Facial disfigurement may lead to patients complaining of an inability to recognise themselves or extreme social withdrawal.[30] Although the majority of patients adapt successfully, they typically experience a longer and more complicated postoperative course. Defects in speech, swallowing, and hearing may cause significant distress, but also make the assessment of mental state more difficult. This inability to communicate may result in frustration and anger, with consequent "acting out", physical aggression and striking out at staff.[31] In tracheotomy patients who present with features of anxiety or panic, hypoxia secondary to intermittent airway obstruction is an important differential diagnosis.[32]

Plastic and Reconstructive Surgery

A psychosocial evaluation is an essential component of the preoperative assessment in patients seeking plastic surgery. Unrealistic expectations must be identified as along with the risk factors for a poor outcome and dissatisfaction.

Patients going through major life crises, and in particular relationship diffi-culties, merit further exploration about their motivation and expectations of surgery. Psychiatric disorders, if suspected, may require specialist referral and treatment before surgery is considered.

The preoperative diagnosis is of particular importance because body dys-morphic disorder (or dysmorphophobia) is the most common psychiatric disorder associated with requests for plastic surgery. The defining feature of the body dysmorphic disorder is a preoccupation with an imagined or slight defect in appearance that the patient regards as markedly abnormal, and which leads to clinically significant distress or impairment in functioning. The preoccupa-tion is usually an overvalued idea in some patients it may be delusional. Body dysmorphic disorder often occurs in association with depression or substance misuse. Patients frequently have a history of obsessive-compulsive disorder and may present with repetitive checking, grooming, and picking behaviour.[33] The treatment is difficult, in part because patients usually lack insight into the ill-ness. There is some evidence of the benefit of cognitive behavioural therapy and SSRI, and antipsychotic medication may be effective in patients with delusional beliefs.

Amputations

The loss of a limb is both cosmetically and functionally disabling. When it occurs in the context of a longstanding illness such as complicated diabetes or those with vascular disease, an amputation may provide welcome relief from chronic pain and infection. However, dealing with the grief and loss for the amputated limb, and adjusting to a significant alteration in body image may lead to denial and depression. The incidence of major depression is reported to be 34–50% in patients following amputation, with no significant difference in the prevalence between surgical or traumatic amputees.[34,35] The precipitating circumstances should be considered however, as related traumatic experiences such as episodes of violence, death of kin, or an accident may be of greater significance than the amputation itself.[36]

Phantom limb phenomena, the persistence of pain or sensations as if the limb were still present, has been reported in as many as 38% of patients post-amputation.[36–38] There are several theories of the pathophysiology of phantom limb pain, but these are not widely agreed upon. The cause is likely to be multifactorial, which would explain the wide variability in the effects of treatment. Pre-amputation pain is a notable risk factor for the development of phantom limb pain. Its symptoms range from localised pain including stabbing, shooting, cramping, or burning sensations to more complex experiences of aberrant proprioception. Phantom limb pain is often missed if not specifically queried and may lead to patients becoming agitated and confused. There has been little systematic study of the relationship between phantom pain and psychiatric disorder but, unsurprisingly, denial and depression are considered to be related to a poor outcome.[36] However, in one small study, no relation was found between the experience of phantom pain and emotional distress.[38] The broad range of drug treatments used for phantom pain may be indicative of their equivocal effect. Anticonvulsants such as carbamazepine and gabapentin, and tricyclic antidepressants have reportedly been of benefit. In cases where a stump neuroma is suspected, surgical intervention may be effective.

Stoma Surgery

Stoma surgery, the temporary or permanent surgical opening of the intestine, colon or ureter to the abdominal wall, is performed to manage a range of diseases including congenital malformation, inflammatory bowel disease, cancer, and trauma. The association with a reduction or loss of bowel control makes the stoma a frequent source of embarrassment or shame, and consequent psychological distress. Approximately 25% of stoma patients experience clinically significant postoperative psychological symptoms.[39] Anxiety states are common, and often associated with a fear of unpleasant odours or leakage and soiling. Patients may become socially withdrawn, avoiding public places, and deleterious effects on marital and sexual relationships are frequently reported. A past history of depression or anxiety, the presence of misinformed or unusual beliefs about stomas, and postoperative physical complications are all associated with the development of psychological morbidity, and these factors should be explored before and after surgery. Specialist stoma nurses have an invaluable role in the identification and management of such problems, and if necessary referral for psychiatric assessment is recommended.

Breast Cancer Surgery

The high prevalence of psychological morbidity following surgery for breast cancer has been repeatedly demonstrated, with prevalence rates of 30–40% for depression and anxiety in the year following mastectomy.[40] A range of treatments are now available, including radical or modified radical mastectomy, lumpectomy; in addition, chemotherapy or bone marrow transplantation may be suggested. The radical nature of some surgical procedures is generally considered as a significant factor in the psychological effects of treatment because of their threat to a woman's sense of self-esteem and femininity. However, studies have found little difference in the incidence of depression or anxiety following treatment between women who undergo breast conservation surgery and those who undergo mastectomy.[41] Due consideration should also be given to the role of adjuvant treatments, such as corticosteroids and chemotherapy in precipitating changes in the mental state.

Urological Surgery

The primary psychological issues specific to urological surgery are those relating to anxiety about the loss of attractiveness and libido, impotence, and anorgasmia. Erectile dysfunction is a common complication of urological surgery, and is a significant contributor to anxiety, depression and other psychiatric disorders, but may also be secondary to these. Although the emotional state is important in impotent men, vascular, neurological, and endocrine causes, either alone or in combination, need to be considered. Erectile dysfunction is also an adverse effect of many drugs including alcohol. Previously, the mainstays of management comprised mechanical devices, intracavernous injections and psychological treatment, but in the last five years these have all been superseded by the use of the phosphodiesterase inhibitor, sildenafil. Studies have demonstrated the efficacy of this drug, which enhances penile smooth muscle relaxation, in 70% of men with erectile dysfunction from organic, psychogenic, and mixed causes.[42] However, psychological factors must be considered as they often affect the outcome of treatment even when a predominant physical cause has been demonstrated.

INFORMED CONSENT AND COMPULSORY TREATMENT

In most situations where psychiatric complications present following surgery patients are able to provide an informed consent for the treatment or clearly possess the capacity to refuse it. In some instances, particularly where the patient presents a risk of harm to himself or others, there may be uncertainty about the responsibility and ability of the hospital staff to provide treatment. A typical example would be a patient presenting with postoperative delirium, requiring ongoing treatment but who is hostile, abusive, and refuses to co-operate. Unlike most aspects of medicine, medico-legal issues do not cross national boundaries and the following relates to the law in England and Wales. In other jurisdictions guidance should be sought from the hospital legal department.

In the UK, the Mental Health Act (1983) provides for the legal detention and treatment of persons with mental illness. This applies to situations where admission is considered necessary in the interest of their health or safety, or for the protection of others, but they are unable or unwilling to consent to such an admission. The Act does not allow for the detention and treatment of patients in the case of physical illness, although it may be used where physical illness contributes to mental disorder e.g., the use of thyroxine in mental disorder caused by hypothyroidism.

Where the Mental Health Act does not apply, either because there is no mental disorder present or in emergency situations where there is insufficient time to implement it, treatment without consent may only be given under common law. This is dependent on the assumption that the patient lacks the capacity to decide whether or not to accept medical treatment. That is, the patient is unable to comprehend and retain the necessary information pertaining to their treatment, and weigh the information in the balance, balancing the risks and benefits, so as to make a choice. All registered medical practitioners are considered qualified to make an assessment of capacity.[43] However, if there is concern about the presence of mental disorder, a psychiatric assessment will be necessary. Postoperatively, treatment in the absence of consent is most commonly required in an acute emergency, e.g. delirium, and may involve restraint or sedation treatment. Under common law, treatment should always be the minimum necessary, and the need for such treatment should be reviewed regularly. The reasons for using common law and an appraisal of the patient's capacity must be clearly documented. If the situation is likely to persist in the long term or more serious treatment is required, the hospital's legal department should be consulted.

REFERENCES

1. Royal College of Surgeons of England & Royal College of Psychiatrists. (1997) Report of the Working Party on the Psychological Care of Surgical Patients. Council Report CR55. London: Royal College of Surgeons of England/Royal College of Psychiatrists.
2. Perski A, Feleke E, Anderson G *et al.* (1998) Emotional distress before coronary bypass grafting limits the benefits of surgery. *Am Heart J* **136**: 510–517.
3. Hellstrom K, Fellenius J, Ost LG. (1996) One versus five sessions of applied tension in the treatment of blood phobia. *Behav Res Ther* **34**: 101–112.
4. Lloyd GG, Chick J, Crombie E. (1982) Screening for problem drinkers among medical inpatients. *Drug Alcohol Depend* **10**: 355–359.
5. Barrison IG, Viola L, Mumford J *et al.* (1982) Detecting excessive drinking among admissions to a general hospital. *Health Trends* **14**: 80–83.
6. Turner J, Reid S. (2002) Munchausen's syndrome. *The Lancet* **359**: 346–349.
7. Rogers MP, Liang MH, Daltroy LH *et al.* (1989) Delirium after elective orthopaedic surgery: risk factors and natural history. *Int J Psychiatry Med* **19**: 109–121.
8. Inouye SK, Charpentier PA. (1996) Precipitating factors for delirium in hospitalized elderly persons. Predictive model and interrelationship with baseline vulnerability. *JAMA* **275**: 852–857.
9. Levkoff S, Cleary P, Liptzin B, Evans DA. (1991) Epidemiology of delirium: an overview of research issues and findings. *Int Psychogeriatr* **3**: 149–167.
10. Marcantonio ER, Goldman L, Orav EJ *et al.* (1998) The association of intraoperative factors with the development of postoperative delirium. *Am J Med* **105**: 380–384.
11. Liptzin B, Levkoff SE. (1991) An empirical study of delirium subtypes. *Br J Psychiatry* **161**: 843–845.
12. Inouye SK, Viscoli CM, Horwitz RI *et al.* (1993) A predictive model for delirium in hospitalized elderly medical patients based on admission characteristics. *Ann Intern Med* **119**: 474–481.
13. Folstein MF, Folstein SE, McHugh PR. (1975) "Mini-mental state". A practical method for grading the cognitive state of patients for the clinician. *J Psychiatr Res* **12**: 189–198.
14. Inouye SK, Bogardus ST Jr., Charpentier PA *et al.* (1999) A multicomponent intervention to prevent delirium in hospitalized older patients. *N Engl J Med* **340**: 669–676.
15. Sipahimalani A, Masand PS. (1997) Use of risperidone in delirium: case reports. *Ann Clin Psychiatry* **9**: 105–107.

16. Gustafson Y, Brannstrom B, Berggren D *et al.* (1991) A geriatric-anesthesiologic program to reduce acute confusional states in elderly patients treated for femoral neck fractures. *J Am Geriatr Soc* **39**: 655–662.

17. Aakerlkund LP, Rosenburg J. (1994) Postoperative delirium: treatment with supplementary oxygen. *Br J Anaesth* **72**: 286–290.

18. Gill D, Hatcher S. (1999) A systematic review of the treatment of depression with antidepressant drugs in patients who also have a physical illness. *J Psychosom Res* **47**: 131–143.

19. Rocca P, Cocuzza E, Rasetti R, Rocca G, Zanalda E, Bogetto F. (2003). Predictors of psychiatric disorders in liver transplantation candidates: logistic regression models. *Liver Transpl* **9**: 721–726.

20. DiMartini A, Fitzgerald MG, Magill J *et al.* (1996) Psychiatric evaluations of small intestine transplantation patients. *Gen Hosp Psychiatry* **18**: 25S–29S.

21. Craven J. (1990) Psychiatric aspects of lung transplant. *Can J Psychiatry* **35**: 759–764.

22. Trzepacz PT, Brenner R, Van Thiel DH. (1989) A psychiatric study of 247 liver transplantation candidates. *Psychosomatics* **30**: 147–153.

23. Phipps L. (1991) Psychiatric aspects of heart transplantation. *Can J Psychiatry* **36**: 563–568.

24. Dew MA, Roth LH, Schulberg HC *et al.* (1996) Prevalence and predictors of depression and anxiety-related disorders during the year after heart transplantation. *Gen Hosp Psychiatry* **18**: 48S–61S.

25. Shapiro PA, Fornfeld DS. (1989) Psychiatric outcome of heart transplantation. *Gen Hosp Psychiatry* **11**: 352–357.

26. Carney RM, Rich MW, Tevelde A *et al.* (1987) Major depressive disorder in coronary artery disease. *Am J Cardiol* **60**: 1273–1275.

27. Hance M, Carney RM, Freedland KE, Skala J. (1996) Depression in patients with coronary heart disease. A 12-month follow-up. *Gen Hosp Psychiatry* **18**: 61–65.

28. Pinski SL, Trohman RG. (1995) Implantable cardioverter-defibrillators: implications for the nonelectrophysiologist. *Ann Intern Med* **122**: 770–777.

29. Fricchione GL, Olson LC, Vlay SC. (1989) Psychiatric syndromes in patients with the automatic internal cardioverter defibrillator: anxiety, psychological dependence, abuse, and withdrawal. *Am Heart J* **117**: 1411–1414.

30. Dropkin MJ, Malgady RG, Scott DW *et al.* (1983) Scaling of disfigurement and dysfunction in post operative head and neck patients. *Head Neck Surg* **16**: 559–570.

31. Bronheim H, Strain JJ, Biller HF. (1991) Psychiatric aspects of head and neck surgery. Part II: Body image and psychiatric intervention. *Gen Hosp Psychiatry* **13**: 225–232.

32. Basawaraj K, RifkinR, Seshagiris D, *et al.* (1990) The prevalence of anxiety disorders in patients with chronic obstructive pulmonary disease. *Am J Psychiatry* **147**: 200–201.
33. Phillips KA. (1996) Body dysmorphic disorder: diagnosis and treatment of imagined ugliness. *J Clin Psychiatry* **8**: 61–65.
34. Kashani JH, Frank RG, Kashani SR, *et al.* (1983) Depression among amputees. *J Clin Psychiatry* **44**: 256–258.
35. Cansever A, Uzun O, Yildiz C, *et al.* (2003) Depression in men with traumatic lower part amputation: a comparison to men with surgical lower part amputation. *Mil Med* **168**: 106–109.
36. Lundberg SG, Guggenheim FG. (1986) Sequelae of limb amputation. *Adv Psychosom Med* **15**: 199–210.
37. Shukla GD, Sahu SC, Tripathi RP, Gupta DK. (1982) Phantom limb: a phenomenological study. *Br J Psychiatry* **141**: 54–58.
38. Fisher K, Hanspap RS. (1998) Phantom pain, anxiety, depression, and their relation in consecutive patients with amputated limbs: case reports. *Br Med J* **316**: 903–904.
39. White CA, Hunt JC. (1997) Psychological factors in post-operative adjustment of stoma surgery. *Ann R Coll Surg* **79**: 3–7.
40. Maguire GP, Lee EG, Bevington DJ *et al.* (1978) Psychiatric problems in the first year after mastectomy. *Br Med J* i: 963–965.
41. Fallowfield LJ, Baum M, Maguire GP. (1986) Effects of breast conservation on psychological morbidity associated with diagnosis and treatment of early breast cancer. *Br Med J* **293**: 1331–1334.
42. Goldstein I, Lue TF, Padma-Nathan H *et al.* (1998) Oral sildenafil in the treatment of erectile dysfunction. *N Engl J Med* **14**: 1397–1404.
43. British Medical Association & Law Society. (1995) Assessment of Mental Capacity: Guidance for Doctors and Lawyers. London: British Medical Association.

Chapter 29

MEDICO-LEGAL ISSUES

Victoria J. Mansell and Martin A. Mansell

INTRODUCTION

The interaction between the doctor and a patient is one of the most direct of all human relationships and this is most true of the patient with their surgeon. No other field of medical activity has such a direct link between cause and effect, with an equal potential for immense benefit or fatal catastrophe. Through the ages, all civilisations have honoured the "successful" doctor, with the downside that incompetent or dangerous practitioners are liable to face the wrath of an aggrieved patient and society. The rising tide of medical litigation in the US and the UK is simply the modern expression of the age-old desire to punish a bad practitioner, although it is now fuelled by the availability of sometimes-questionable data on surgical outcomes and, what the doctor usually perceives to be, rapacious lawyers. However, our litigation-prone attitude in the West is no more than a reflection of the immense clinical responsibility that doctors have always carried which, in due course, will find worldwide expression, adapted to the relevant ethical, cultural and legal systems. Practitioners outside Europe should not delude themselves that the current epidemic of medical

negligence litigation is a matter for the English-speaking countries, alone —
it will soon be coming to a court near you!

This chapter briefly reviews the principles of medical ethics that have led
to the legal systems which are in place today, summarises modern approaches
to information gathering and risk management and describes the practical
issues for the surgeon when litigation occurs.

MEDICAL ETHICS: A SUMMARY

Codes of ethical behaviour have existed since the earliest times and are usually
based on a combination of values derived from religion and society. There
has always been intense interest in the behaviour of doctors because of the
privileged role they hold in society. Involvement in matters of life and death
are everyday events for the doctor and it is no surprise that issues of probity,
financial behaviour and personal conduct should be considered fair game for
those who consider themselves best placed to comment on and regulate the
doctors' behaviour. This is, of course, quite separate from the rigorous scrutiny
of clinical judgement, which is a continuing part of good medical practice.
The codes of medical ethics can be briefly summarised as:

a. Virtue-based Ethics

   This idea was first developed by Aristotle in 4 BC and suggests that an action
   is right only if it is what a "virtuous agent" would do in the circumstances.
   Virtue, by this definition, allows humans to "flourish" emphasising, for
   example, that if an act is generous then it is likely to be good, and therefore
   to be encouraged. Although it is a useful way to bring together a number of
   aspects of human behaviour that are generally thought to be desirable, one
   major disadvantage is that it is ultimately based on an individual persons
   interpretation of what they consider as beneficial for them. Many regard
   this as vague and difficult to analyse and therefore of limited relevance to
   the behaviour of modern societies.

b. Duty-based Ethics

   By this definition, for an action to be correct it must be in accord with a
   moral principle determined either by God or reason. Certain acts such as
   lying, cruelty, violence, robbery etc. are forbidden under all circumstances
   and this approach usually involves a list of prohibitions, rather like the Ten

Commandments. Although it is helpful in deciding what you should not do, it gives little guidance when there are a number of possible alternative courses of action, which is usually the case in difficult clinical situations. In those societies whose legal principles rest heavily on religious law there is likely to be increasing conflict between traditionalists and those who would seek to translate the religious writings of the past to be relevant to the needs of a complex and rapidly-changing modern society.

c. Utilitarianism

By this approach an action is right if it leads to the best consequences, which are those where happiness is greatest. It is the consequences of the action that matter, thereby bringing an important modification of the simpler religious type of prohibition in which some acts are always forbidden, no matter what benefits they may produce. It is a simple concept that is helpful in providing quick answers to a wide range of common clinical dilemmas; simply do that which will maximise happiness/benefit to most people. However, it does not take us much further with the conflict between the wishes of the individual and the society in which they live, nor does it help define what really is the "best" outcome; the doctor can only rely on his perception of what is likely to the best outcome.

Current Ethical Principles

The above ethical systems have been crystallised in the last 20 years into four major ethical principles that can guide our thinking:

1. Respect for patient autonomy

It is the responsibility of the doctor and other healthcare professionals to give the patient all the necessary information to allow them to make the best decision given their personal, religious and cultural circumstances. The old fashioned paternalistic approach ("as your doctor I know best and this is what you should do") is now both outmoded and unacceptable.

2. Beneficence

This refers to the moral importance of doing good to others, especially patients. There will usually be no conflict between this principle and respect for a patient's autonomy, but problems are inevitable if a patient wishes to follow a particular path that is clearly not in their own best interest.

3. Non-maleficence

All doctors will try to avoid causing harm to their patients but there is no form of intervention, medical or surgical that does not carry the potential for predictable or unpredictable complications. Doctors who have faced the wrath of an aggrieved patient or their lawyer may well be reluctant to offer meaningful advice to future patients taking the view "Here are the facts — you decide". Although this reaction is understandable, it leaves the patient open to guidance from various uninformed sources and reduces the likelihood of them reaching the right decision. There is a fine line between respect for a patient's autonomy and allowing them to draw from the doctor's clinical experience.

4. Justice

There will always be a large gap between the potential benefits of medical developments and the resources required to make them real. The doctor's responsibility is towards multiple patients under his care. There are always uncertainties in any risk/benefit analysis and the easy way out is to treat the patient to the maximum, whatever the uncertainty, until the money runs out. However, it is wrong for doctors to negate this aspect of their responsibilities and it provides a powerful argument to support the need for doctors to be heavily involved in health-system management; if the doctors do not accept this responsibility it is likely to be assumed by non-clinical managers whose decisions will be less acceptable.

THE PROFESSION OF MEDICINE

The medical profession calls for a long and arduous training, typically involving considerable personal sacrifice, to make an important contribution to the general well being and quality of life of one's fellow men and women. The profession retains a monopoly on its services based on a rigorous series of qualifications, apprenticeships and postgraduate training. In the opinion of the authors, the profession is monitored and regulated by its senior and more experienced members, rather than lay or state appointees who lack both personal and specialist knowledge of what is involved.

At the moment, professional regulation in the UK is the responsibility of the General Medical Council, which has summarised the duties and responsibilities of the doctor in a number of guidelines. Good medical practice means that the well-being of the patient is the doctor's primary concern and this involves respect for patient autonomy, maintaining a high clinical standard of practice and avoiding the inevitable conflicts of interest which present themselves. Confidentiality, allowing the patient to make informed decisions on their care, and acting in their best interests when this is not possible, are important hallmarks of a responsible practitioner. Beyond the individual patient there are wider obligations to society, encompassing diverse subjects such as communicable disease, genetic testing, medical research and reproductive medicine.

The relationship between doctor and patient is central to good medical practice and has wide variations in different societies depending on their religious, moral, financial and political circumstances.

The traditional, paternalistic approach has a priestly background, which assumes that the greater knowledge and experience of the doctor places him or her in the ideal position to decide what is in the best interests of the patient. The patient's own views and values are of little importance, and any considerations of patient autonomy are ignored; it often results in advice or command based on a combination of factual evidence and value judgements that are of the doctor's rather than the patient. This seems reasonable in cases where patients do have considerable faith in their doctor's advice and are happy to accept it. On the flip side, it places a heavy burden on the doctor. Furthermore, the differences in clinical practice worldwide are the surest possible indication that hard facts on the "best treatment" are often not available. In these circumstances the doctor must be prepared to take a pragmatic approach and it is a matter of individual judgement on how much information should be communicated to the patient.

The informative model is at the opposite end of the spectrum and assumes that the patient has the intelligence and interest to receive complicated information about their possible treatment, to enable complete autonomy in their decision. The disadvantage is that the role of the doctor is reduced to a mere technician and there may be little or no detailed discussion with the patient.

The deliberative or interpretive model casts the doctor in the role of teacher or counsellor who has the time and expertise to present detailed, necessary information to the patient and allow them to reach their own conclusion, following an in-depth discussion of all the issues that are involved. Although this may appear as the ideal compromise, it requires an intelligent and articulate patient who is able to "speak the same language as their doctor". Given the rather unique position of the doctor in society this scenario seems rather unusual, to us.

Each practitioner will develop his own individual approach to these issues and the only thing that can be stated with certainty is that no single approach can be deemed best for every category of patient. Effective clinical management requires the doctor to be flexible in his attitudes and behaviour, while maintaining the bedrock values of professional practice that have been described above. Of course, the conflict between the legitimate needs of the state and society with the best interests of the patient cannot be ignored but "...in a changing world the ultimate realities remain".

CONFIDENTIALITY

The doctor must maintain the confidential nature of his relationship with the patient and this applies to intimate personal details volunteered by the patient, information revealed by the physical examination and the results of all investigations that are performed. Confidentiality is a cardinal principle in almost all moral codes of medical ethics, which has its roots in respect for patient autonomy; the only person to decide what information may or may not be released is the patient himself. Although the consequentialist approach would suggest that disclosure of information can be justified if it will have significant benefits for the common good, in practice it is only permissible in well defined circumstances, although these certainly range over the entire spectrum of clinical practice. Inappropriate disclosure of personal or medical details can have devastating consequences for the patient and the clinician should have a detailed understanding of what can be disclosed and the appropriate circumstances for such a disclosure. Attempting to reach ad hoc decisions about these complex legal and ethical issues without considerable forethought is a clear recipe for disaster.

The patient must also understand that modern surgical treatment is almost never the result of their surgeon working in isolation. A multi-disciplinary team is involved which includes other doctors, nurses, technicians, social workers etc., all of whom owe the same duty of confidentiality to the patient as does the lead surgeon. It is usually impossible to try and limit the access of other team members to "need to know" information; the provision of inadequate information is one of the surest ways to make a potential medical mistake actually come to pass. In practice, most patients do not have a problem in talking frankly to the surgeon's associates provided time is taken adequately to explain their important role.

Although maintenance of strict patient confidentiality is usually seen as being in the public interest there are many circumstances in which disclosure of potentially sensitive information is required by the law. Examples include notification of certain communicable and venereal diseases, termination of pregnancy, registration of births and deaths, reproductive medicine, living-related organ transplantation and fitness to drive. The disclosure of information when a crime has been committed is often a particularly difficult area; if a serious criminal offence, involving serious injury or death, has been committed, disclosing information that would help identify the culprit, to the police is imperative and the doctor has little to fear from the Court. On the other hand, the identification of a patient involved in a minor, civil offence may well be hard to justify, unless there is a real concern that a more serious offence is likely to follow. Discussing such a case with a senior colleague is good practice and it may be wise to involve the legal advisors to the hospital and/or the defence organisation. The disclosure of positive HIV status to a partner presents particular problems; a discussion with the patient often leads to an agreement to disclose, but this is not always the case and the doctor may need to act in the best interests of the patient's partner in these cases.

In many countries patients have a right to see their medical records and this will usually include case notes, medical reports, correspondence with other doctors, data stored on the computer and the personal file held by Social Services. The written medical notes are the single most important document recording an inpatient or outpatient course of treatment, and their significance cannot be over emphasised when it comes to dealing with litigation. In general terms, diagnostic and follow-on notes must be written legibly, concisely, dated and signed without the use of confusing abbreviations. Humour and unnecessary personal comment are best avoided and they appear in bad taste if ever examined in open court. Many hospitals now send a copy of the outpatient letter to the patient as well and a delicate balance needs to be maintained by the doctor writing it. Sufficient detail must be included to explain the range of possible and probable diagnoses but inclusion of sensitive or speculative information may well cause unnecessary anxiety to the patient. With this country's current emphasis on preservation of patient rights and the threat of legal action, we advocate a rather bland and generalised letter containing minimal information and, unfortunately minimal useful advice for the doctor who receives the letter.

The Data Protection Act requires that information in medical records be accurate, relevant, maintained only for approved purposes, for the minimum necessary time and not disclosed to any unauthorised persons. Patients (or more accurately "data subjects") are entitled to receive a description of the information, along with the origin of that information and to demand correction of any inaccuracies. The police cannot demand to see a patient's medical records although a senior judge or coroner can do so. The disclosure of information to the patient's employer will always require specific and detailed consent.

RESEARCH

Continuing progress in medical care is achievable only through research and this theme must run through the clinical practice of all healthcare professionals. To recognise the importance of "evidence based medicine" has become a cornerstone of modern medical practice which has been led by the work of the Cochrane Collaboration in a large and increasing number of countries throughout the world. In this context "research" means an ongoing evaluation of treatments, both old and new, and it is a sobering fact that much of what we regard as "conventional therapies" have never had their effectiveness examined and confirmed according to objective scientific principles. Of course, many surgical interventions that we regard as standard practice have their basis in centuries of clinical experience and a logic that is self evident, even to the most jaded medical statistician. However, times change and a continuing evaluation of traditional treatment is as important as that required for a radical and innovative surgical procedure.

As discussed below, even the most repetitive and routine operations require their effectiveness to be repeatedly verified against new therapies which become available and it has been suggested that every patient should be regarded as a potential subject in a clinical study. Although this represents an ideal situation, it does indicate how the doctor must continuously re-examine all areas of his clinical practice to confirm its effectiveness as objectively as possible. The randomised clinical trial provides the gold standard for such evaluation and is usually based on a comparison of "best treatment" with "new treatment". The use of a placebo group, which represents "no treatment", is often both impractical and unethical but has a limited place in situations where no effective therapy is considered available for a particular illness. There is a clear conflict between the doctor's perception of the best treatment for a particular patient and their random allocation in a controlled trial, which seems unlikely to ever be completely resolved. Randomised clinical trials are immensely difficult to plan and complete because of the problems in obtaining proper randomisation of subjects. It is common for the results of such studies to be partially or completely invalidated because of significant differences between the patient groups.

Because of these considerations, major clinical trials can only be initiated and completed by large pharmaceutical companies or governments. Adequate patient recruitment usually requires the trial to be conducted in multiple centres, which introduces uncertainties because of fundamental differences in routine clinical practice, both regionally and nationally. There is also an important global angle to the problem; most of the diseases requiring investigation in the Western world, such as atheroma and cancer, involve an ageing population, while those in the developing world are related to public heath issues such as infection and nutrition. A recently publicised example is the development of complex anti-HIV therapy, which will be applicable only to countries with sophisticated healthcare systems. It is easier to carry out such studies in developing countries, where the burden of HIV is very great, although the therapeutic advances that are achieved are unlikely to be applied to that particular patient population. Once the study has been completed, important ethical questions such as, are the study subjects to be cast aside to the minimal or non-existent care which is usually the norm in the poorer countries, arise.

Even in countries with adequate resources, medical research leads to difficult ethical questions. Large sums of money are involved in new drug development and the widespread adoption of a new therapy usually brings considerable financial rewards. The doctor involved must preserve his financial integrity and maintain reasonable professional fees for patient recruitment and completion of the study. Most importantly, ownership of the data and publication rights should rest with the lead doctors rather than the drug company; even negative or adverse results need to be published so that other investigators can benefit from it and literature bias can be minimised.

Surgical research often depends on the application of new technology and this usually requires rigorous preliminary evaluation in the experimental animal, however unpalatable this may be to some. The patient who is being offered an innovative operation must have a very clear understanding of the potential risks and uncertainties, and comprehensive information should be obtained before consent. Adequate insurance must be in place if a new product is involved, to deal with unforeseeable side effects. All planned research must be scrutinised by a properly constituted and competent Research Ethics Committee. There is a long list of research scandals, the effects of which have done immense harm to the achievements of medical science and these can only be prevented by adherence to the irritatingly complex and bureaucratic principles outlined above.

CONSENT

Even to touch a person, by law, constitutes battery, indicating the importance of the rigorous procedures involved in obtaining informed consent for a surgical operation. In simple terms, consent is only valid if it is informed, provided by a mentally competent person and is voluntary.

Information

Most cases that lead to surgical litigation do so because the patient has an unreasonable expectation of the benefits claimed for the operation. This is usually accompanied by a poor perception of the risks involved. All operations have their own well-documented complications and side effects and it would seem sensible that these are listed on the consent form, with a note being made to indicate that they have been specifically mentioned. For example, consent for a percutaneous needle biopsy of the kidney may include the risks of pain, haemorrhage, blood transfusion, arterial embolisation or even nephrectomy, with a simple note to record that these possibilities have, at least, been discussed. Recognised complications of transurethral resection of the prostate include urinary incontinence and retrograde ejaculation and it takes no more than a moment for these to be recorded either in the notes or on the consent form. Obtaining informed consent is an important matter which cannot be delegated to the most junior member of the surgical team; clearly, the person advising the patient must either be performing the operation themselves or possess sufficient experience to offer a true description of what may go wrong. By adopting this simple procedure, a significant number of otherwise vexatious legal claims, which are based on the patient's statement "I wasn't told about the risk of this problem when I signed the form," can be avoided.

There is some uncertainty about the details of the complication that need to be discussed. For a simple hernia repair, few would list problems such as pain at the operation site, a sore throat from the endotracheal tube or the need for postoperative chest physiotherapy if the patient is a smoker, because these are common to most similar operations. However, the uncertainty arises in the context of rare complications such as wound infection and dehiscence, intestinal damage from a misplaced suture, synergistic gangrene or even death from a DVT and pulmonary embolism. In English law, Sidaway (1994) offers some guidance; this case involved a patient undergoing neck surgery who was not specifically warned about the chance of spinal cord damage, which had a minuscule risk in the literature and, indeed, had never happened in the extensive clinical experience of the senior neurosurgeon who was operating. By the prevailing standard of Bolam (1957) the fact that a "responsible body" of neurosurgical opinion would not have warned their patients about this very rare complication should have provided an adequate defence. Indeed, this principle was broadly supported when the case was appealed, although there was some support for the "prudent patient test" which applies in the USA; according to this standard the doctor can be considered negligent if he withholds any information which the prudent patient would wish to know. In these litigious days it is better to give the patient too much rather than too little information, although no doctor likes to scare their patient by the perceived risks of a procedure so much that they deny themselves its immense benefits.

Competence

The capacity for a patient to arrive at a competent decision regarding their treatment depends on three main qualities:

- Good understanding and communication must be present so that they can comprehend the information given and express their decisions about the treatment clearly.
- They must have adequate mental capacity and short-term memory to retain this information along with sufficient reasoning ability.
- Finally, they must have a personal set of values to provide a framework in which their reasoning and conclusions can be formulated. This does not entail a conventional set of religious or societal beliefs and the patient's autonomy has to be respected at all times.

If a patient is judged incompetent because of a mental disorder or inability to communicate, the decision will often be based on the course of action that is thought to serve the best interests of the patient. In Scottish law, there is provision for a proxy to make decisions on behalf of an incompetent person but this is not yet a universal feature of legal systems in the UK or elsewhere. There is increasing interest in advance directives ("living wills") if the patient is aware that they are suffering from a relentlessly progressive disease such as cancer or dementia which will cause an inevitable failure of reasoning or capacity with time. The American experience suggests that advance directives may be very useful because they emphasise the patient's autonomy, reduce anxiety about unwanted aggressive therapy and are also of great assistance to the medical attendants. It is predicted that they will also reduce escalating healthcare costs because many patients are thought to want much less active intervention during a progressive illness than they actually receive. Problems occur because the patient, not unreasonably, is unable to imagine the full range of future events that are clinically possible and may alter their opinions during the evolution of their illness. It is likely that advance directives will play an increasingly important part in healthcare delivery, particularly with an ageing population, but there are many legal hurdles to be overcome at this time.

CLINICAL GOVERNANCE — AN INTRODUCTION

The immense range and complexity of possible surgical interventions means that adverse outcomes are inevitable and this is true no matter what type of surgery. Frequently performed procedures have usually been refined over a long period of time, so that the relative risk of complications is low although the actual number may be substantial because of the volume of patients involved. However, radical and innovative surgery is usually reserved for a highly selected patient group but the chance of problems may be higher, especially if a "learning curve" for either the surgeon or the procedure is involved. A number of studies have suggested that the potential scale of medical mishaps may be truly immense. For example, studies from the USA and Australia suggest that adverse events may occur in approximately 5–15% of inpatient episodes, with serious complications or death occurring in about 1%. Evidence from the UK suggests that nearly one million adverse events occur every year, leading to an additional £2 billion expenditure in resources and a litigation cost that may be between 5–10% of the total healthcare budget.

Studies on human error causing mistakes in healthcare have tended to be "person-centred", with an emphasis on the particular failings of the key practitioner, typically the doctor or nurse. These human failings include carelessness, incompetence, exhaustion or frank recklessness and clearly reflect the short-term "name and shame" management culture, which will see disciplinary action as the logical outcome. It is impossible to expect any healthcare worker to admit and frankly discuss a serious adverse event with the threat of personal or professional sanctions waiting in the shadows. There have been recent, misguided, attempts by the police in this country to seek criminal prosecutions for what are clearly mistakes of clinical judgement and this is probably the result of a lack of professional leadership. It is often argued that the medical profession is no different from other professions regulated by civil, rather than professional agencies. We think this is incorrect, for the reasons summarised above and, wherever possible, a doctor's work should be regulated by other members of the profession, rather than outsiders who do not understand what the profession involves and may have their own political or social agendas to fulfil.

The last 10 years have seen a welcome shift to the recognition of "system failure", with the realisation that a catastrophic outcome is usually the result of a number of sequential errors which, taken individually, would have had a barely perceptible impact. This understanding has come from the aviation industry, which has developed an anonymous reporting system and impersonal approach to error, which has been directly responsible for the current enviable safety record of air travel.

The lessons of "crew resource management" translate easily from the flight deck of a jumbo jet to the operating theatre. In both, a small number of people are involved in a complex yet repetitive process in which the importance of meticulous attention to detail becomes blunted by the very safety and predictability of the activity. Although unpredictable disaster can occur, it is not frequent and will need to be handled on its own merits, although some training for the unthinkable may be possible. The personal interactions of the flight crew or theatre team are open to the usual vagaries of all human relationships and the high workload which many surgeons seem actually to enjoy is also relevant. Experienced pilots have much to teach the doctors, nurses and assistants who work together in the operating theatre but the circumstances of the discussion have to be right. All members of the team, from the most senior to the most junior must be involved and efforts made to ensure that nobody feels intimidated to speak freely. A delicate touch is essential, so that everybody concerned can accept that individual or team failings are lessons to learn from and correct, rather than personal criticism.

Potentially, there is a huge amount of information to be gathered concerning clinical activities and adverse outcomes but there are real difficulties in collecting and processing this information. There is great variation among different countries in the balance between public and private healthcare, office or hospital-based procedures and government interest, so that no one solution is likely to be completely effective. A useful first step is to begin with confidential enquiries into areas of particular clinical concern; in the UK, maternal mortality in pregnancy and death in the postoperative period have been examined and important improvements in clinical guidelines and care outcomes have been the clear result. It is not easy to collect even the most basic data on clinical activity or simple outcome measures, and the provision of adequate resources is essential if the whole enterprise is not to be doomed to failure. Finally, everybody involved in healthcare provision must feel that they have ownership of the information and that the immense expenditure of time and effort involved will actually improve the outcomes for their patients.

The elements of effective clinical governance can therefore be simply summarised as:

- Adverse outcome analysis needs to focus on the multiple system failures which are usually present, rather then emphasising a judgmental approach which seeks to apportion blame to a particular individual.

- The resource implications of even the simplest information gathering must not be underestimated, but can be made more palatable to managers if they understand the benefits to patient care and reduction in litigation costs that will inevitably result.
- The most difficult part of the process is "closing the audit loop". It is not enough to decide where the focus of enquiry should be, to gather the information and to discuss it in an objective and transparent manner; there must be prompt action to remedy the problems, which are usually easy to identify, to avoid disappointment and disillusionment with the audit process.
- Surgical practice lends itself to some audit activities for which the information is relatively easy to collect and analyse in a productive manner. Comparative studies of morbidity, immediate and delayed mortality, postoperative complications and length of stay often indicate areas of best practice which deserve to be universally adopted. The usefulness of "routine practices" such as antibiotic prophylaxis, wound drainage and heparin for the prevention of venous thrombosis can easily be assessed in a simple controlled trial and the conclusions are particularly valuable because of their relevance to the individual unit that has carried out the study. Surgeons need to operate in teams, rather than in isolation and set aside time for regular interdisciplinary meetings with their colleagues in pathology and radiology. A simplistic approach to the publication of morbidity and mortality data must be avoided and a careful case-mix analysis is always necessary. There may be excellent reasons for actively seeking out the surgeon who has the highest mortality rate for a particular operation as it often means that he has a tertiary referral practice and colleagues send him only the most difficult cases that have already suffered complications from previous surgery.

LITIGATION ISSUES

Introduction

Modern surgical practice becomes even more successful such that a large section of the population now believe that for every disease there is a cure and soon death itself will no longer be a certainty. These unreasonable expectations have been fuelled by over-enthusiastic doctors who are less than objective in describing their successes or less than frank in listing their failures. Two particularly unattractive examples are the surgeon publicising his particular expertise with a new technique and the academic presenting the latest "research breakthrough" in the popular press rather than a peer-reviewed medical journal, sometimes for clear financial reasons.

The frequent occurrence of clinical negligence litigation should mean that accurate information is easily available for risk management purposes including the commonest reasons for litigation, the hospitals that have a bad overall record for litigation, and the individual practitioners who have recurrent problems. Such information would have great importance at the national, local and individual level but in the UK it is rather hard to obtain. Previously, the medical defence organisations had the greatest single experience of defending negligence claims, although this information was not widely available. In recent years, the NHS Litigation Authority has assumed responsibility for defending claims against hospitals, often in conjunction with the defence organisations, but the process has not been established long enough for the information to be usefully available. It would clearly be important for the national agency responsible for care standards to be able to target particular litigation black spots, but this state of affairs seems a long way away. In contrast, the very high level of medical litigation in the USA has produced detailed and useful information about the most litigation-prone procedures and for some specialities, audit information on the most litigation-prone practitioners. Therefore, many of the following comments are based on the American experience, which does not reflect current practice in many countries although it does show the likely future direction. The common issues in a number of surgical and related specialities are summarised below, followed by some general comments on the prevention and management of litigation when it occurs.

Radiology

We make no apology for the inclusion of this "support speciality" because it is the single most important source of information to guide the surgeon's actions and the rapid development of interventional radiology concerns almost all areas of surgical practice. Some common issues involve a missed diagnosis of cancer on the mammogram or chest X-ray and the complications of angiographic procedures using contrast. Mammography is now widely available and the vast majority of women undergoing this procedure will not be suffering from breast cancer. Multiple, benign breast lesions are usually present which, in a nervous society, may require a biopsy for exact diagnosis; it is estimated that the ratio of benign to malignant breast lesions diagnosed on biopsy in the USA may be at least 10–20 times greater than in the UK. This example provides one explanation for the fact that 10–15% of a doctor's income in the USA is spent on medical malpractice insurance.

When subtle chest X-ray abnormalities are being reviewed the conclusion can change in at least 10%, so that the supporting information provided by the clinician may be critically important, together with a willingness to reconsider the X-ray objectively if appropriate. The presence of an ageing population with an increased frequency of renal impairment due to renovascular disease has meant that the nephrotoxic potential of contrast agents is increasingly important. This particular group is likely to undergo repeated interventions for coronary or peripheral vascular disease and pre-procedure reno-protection with n-acetylcysteine and saline infusion must not be forgotten. Finally, the radiologist depends on an adequate technical standard for the films that he is reporting but this may often be impossible to obtain because of factors such as failure to co-operate, obesity or clinical circumstances. It is sensible for the reporting radiologist to note such problems and contact the clinician involved if the examination simply cannot be relied upon. The clinician responsible for the patient is sometimes irritated when suggestions or instructions about further imaging are made by his radiological colleague; by ignoring these suggestions the clinician runs the risk of missed or delayed diagnosis and subsequent litigation.

General Surgery

Currently, delayed diagnosis of breast cancer and complications of laparoscopic cholecystectomy are the two common issues in surgical litigation, although this will surely change with the advent of new therapies. Minimally invasive surgery is attractive to the patient because of the perceived benefits of avoidance of a surgical incision and more rapid recovery. The downside involves the potential for a set of complications different from those associated with an open operation, occasional prolonged anaesthesia and an inevitable conversion rate to open surgery. A particular type of manual dexterity and visuo-spatial co-ordination seems to be necessary for this work and the learning curve may be significant. There is also concern that an operator trained only in laparoscopic technique may not be able to deal with the inevitable complications that may occur, some of which may only become apparent after the patient has left the hospital and is admitted to another hospital where laparoscopic surgical experience is lacking. Bile duct strictures and ischaemic bowel damage with delayed perforation are two obvious examples.

In recent years, there has been increasing emphasis in the UK on the need for appropriate training and experience of the surgeon. It is no longer acceptable for a trainee to be left in charge of emergency surgery at night, where limited radiology and laboratory back-up may be available and the skills of a junior anaesthetist may be inadequate to deal with the acutely ill patient who requires surgery. It is inevitable that consultant-level seniors must be available to handle these complex patients, which account for a significant proportion of those whose deaths in the postoperative period could have been prevented. Although the implications for health care resource provision and surgical numbers are self-apparent in this country, at least, they have not yet been addressed.

Urology

Benign prostatic hypertrophy is inevitable in elderly men and trans-urethral resection of the prostate is the commonest operation performed in this particular age group, although some of the milder cases can be managed by medical means. The TURP syndrome should be a rare complication of the procedure, caused by absorption of glycine-containing irrigation fluid and resulting in severe hyponatraemia causing cardiac dysrhythmias, neurological damage and death. The risk factors include prolonged irrigation time with fluid at high pressure and an ill-judged decision to continue prostatic resection in the presence of heavy bleeding, when abandonment of the procedure would have been a safer option. In some patients "lower tract" symptoms are due to a neuropathic bladder rather than outlet obstruction and urodynamic studies are essential if postoperative urinary incontinence is to be avoided. This problem may also follow ill-advised resection of an excessive amount of prostatic tissue and some urologists would go so far as to take a cystoscopic picture of the external urinary sphincter at the end of the surgery to document that it has been left intact. Similarly, some gynaecologists advocate pre- and postoperative renal ultrasound examinations in patients undergoing a Caesarian section or hysterectomy to confirm that the ureters are intact; this represents the downside of defensive medicine, which may be deplorable but seems inevitable in the current climate.

Prostatic cancer has become a major issue as life expectancy increases and the controversy over the management of early disease has not yet been resolved. With options ranging from no treatment to radical prostatectomy, via hormonal manipulation and radiotherapy, the litigation potential seem to be immense and the lawyers may try to make the most of the lack of agreement about "best therapy". To an observer, the current mania for radical surgery as the only means of "curing" the disease seems ill-advised and recalls the huge number of jejuno-ileal bypass operations that were performed in the past as a safe and effective treatment for morbid obesity until the complications of the procedure became known.

Endoscopic procedures in urology have advanced rapidly so that open surgery can now be avoided in many cases of urinary calculi and urothelial tumour. Perforation and stricture of either urethra or ureter can occur and the occasional disaster of a forgotten ureteric stent may lead to encrustation and fracture when it is finally removed, sometimes requiring open surgery. A careful documentation of stent insertion and removal is clearly essential. Other recurring legal topics in urology include the management of a renal mass detected incidentally, testicular torsion, failed vasectomy and the management of erectile dysfunction.

Orthopaedic Surgery

Operations on the spine carry the risk of severe neurological damage and require the highest standards of surgical expertise, patient information and postoperative management if unreasonable litigation is to be avoided. Operations at the wrong level continue to occur and can be prevented. Joint replacements carry their own particular complications and the patient must understand the discussion about the type of prosthesis selected and its likely survival. Fractures usually occur in perfectly fit people with no previous history of joint problems and their expectation of a satisfactory postoperative result may be completely unrealistic; it is essential to give the patient all the necessary information as soon as possible after surgery, especially if other factors that may delay the recovery and outcome are present. Many negligence claims are either initiated or continued because of poor communication, with a perceived lack of interest and sympathy by the surgeon; time properly spent in consultation and advice is never wasted.

PREVENTION OF LITIGATION

The cornerstone of risk prevention in surgery, as in other medical specialities is, quite simply, good clinical practice. This means treating the patient courteously and respecting their autonomy, with the provision of sufficient objective information to allow them to reach the management decision that is best for them. This assumes that the doctor accepts the patient's decision, despite his own misgivings about it, except when issues of childhood or mental health are involved.

The "system failures" which ultimately lead to a disastrous outcome may have their beginnings in the very first consultation. This may be in a busy outpatient clinic with inadequate time to discuss the issues properly or a junior doctor may be called upon to provide a service that is beyond his training and experience. Blood test requests are lost, radiological procedures are delayed, operating dates need to be changed because of holidays and postoperative high dependency beds may not be available. If unexpected, life-threatening haemorrhage occurs at the time of surgery, the junior nurse may collect the wrong blood from the blood bank and the stressed anaesthetist may not perform the rigorous identification checks that would have prevented a mismatched blood transfusion. The surgeon has, in any case, operated on the wrong side because of an incorrectly labelled preoperative X-ray and the patient sustains a fractured femur when the operating table collapses. Finally, gentamicin is prescribed in full dose for a postoperative infection, without noticing that the patient was an elderly diabetic who had undergone a preoperative contrast procedure, and consequently acute renal failure and dialysis is then unavoidable.

Although this particular example is composite, all of the individual elements have occurred, and could have been prevented by a moment's forethought. Only rarely does an isolated, incompetent act by a surgeon result in a medical disaster. Good clinical practice also requires a high level of administrative support; X-ray and pathology reports must be promptly prepared and correctly dispatched, with an efficient mechanism in place to get them filed rapidly in the medical notes. Non-attendance for investigations must be noted and a recall system must be in place to ensure that patients do not default from follow-up. The doctor must write daily follow-on notes which are legible and signed, but need not need to be extensive if all is going well. Significant problems must be documented with a brief record of differential diagnosis and preferred management; in this country the doctor is not required to get it right on every occasion, but the logic and validity of the thought process which has led to the chosen line of management needs to be easily apparent. Ideally, medical notes should be written when the patient is seen, but if this is not possible then the retrospective nature of the note needs to be clearly recorded.

The principles of surgical audit have been outlined above and if properly applied, will reduce the level of litigation and also provide an important mechanism for continuing professional development. The audit process must have adequate time and resources set aside so that it can be effective and all the members of the team must be involved; often the most recent members will make the most innovative contributions because of their outside perspectives. Audit meetings must achieve a fine balance between a dispassionate and objective analysis of the subject and avoidance of personal criticism of a particular individual. Of course, serious issues of professional competence or technical ability may be highlighted by the audit process but are best addressed in a separate meeting between the clinical director and the doctor where a productive outcome is more likely to be achieved. To a physician, the requirement for a surgeon to maintain his technical skills and on-call capability as retirement is approaching seems both unrealistic and unreasonable; these senior doctors represent an important resource for their healthcare colleagues and need encouragement by sensitive discussion of their changing talents and contribution. We have to acknowledge that these principles represent no more than high ideals at the moment in the UK; risk management does not attract the attention it deserves, audit systems are poorly developed and fragmented and the "name and blame" culture is still favoured by the media and managers alike. Perhaps other countries whose healthcare systems are still in the rapid stage of development will be better placed to appreciate and apply the lessons learnt in the Western world.

WHEN LITIGATION OCCURS

A surgeon will usually be aware if an adverse outcome has occurred following surgery which is likely to lead either to a complaint or a lawsuit. It is right to express sympathy to a patient who has suffered a disastrous event and it is wrong to think that this will be taken as an admission of guilt, either by the patient or their lawyer at a later date. Under these circumstances, the relationship between the doctor and patient becomes more important than ever and the surgeon must continue to give sympathetic support and advice to the best of his ability. Occasionally, it may be a good idea to hand over the ongoing care of such a patient to a colleague.

A complaint about the management may be made to the hospital or surgeon directly or, more unusually, be initiated by a lawyer acting on the patient's behalf. The receipt of a formal complaint should not be regarded as a tiresome problem which will waste many hours of the surgeon's time, but as an opportunity to defuse a problem which may otherwise progress to a legal scenario, which be avoided if possible. The next step is usually a meeting between the patient and surgeon concerned, in the presence of representatives from the hospital. It is best if the patient can draw up a list of concerns before the meeting because this allows for a more structured discussion, facilitates dealing with the problems in a logical way, and is most likely to produce resolution. Most patient complaints following an adverse outcome are seeking an explanation, an apology and reassurance that another patient will not be similarly affected; financial reward is said to be an uncommon reason for proceeding to legal action except where care for an injured child is involved. Nevertheless, if a patient has clearly been harmed as a result of an error by the hospital or surgeon there is no reason why appropriate financial recompense cannot and should not be made; this can usually be done without a formal admission of liability and may prevent a long and arduous court case.

If a patient remains dissatisfied after the initial meeting, the next step is to commission a report by an independent medical expert, who is agreeable to both sides. If the matter cannot be resolved by the internal route an appeal to an independent government investigator (ombudsman) may be possible. If a complaint proceeds to the court it shifts to the hands of the lawyers; once here, events usually move very slowly. Expert testimony is produced for the patient and the doctor and the process is arduous for all concerned. The greatest stress is on the surgeon who has to cope with the weight of his usual clinical responsibilities, as well as deal with an allegation which may seriously damage his professional reputation or, indeed, make it impossible for him to earn a living. The surgeon may feel like a pariah amongs his professional colleagues and will, quite understandably, be reluctant to talk about the facts of the case and the stress that it is causing. His colleagues have an important part to play, particularly as litigation is now a fact of medical life and most practitioners are likely to be on the receiving end at least once in their professional career. For high-risk specialities such as obstetrics and gynaecology, plastic surgery and orthopaedic surgery litigation is so frequent that it may attract little attention.

CONCLUSION

As medicine has moved from being life-saving to life-enhancing, patient expectations have risen substantially and in many countries, nothing less than a perfect outcome is acceptable. However regrettable, defensive medicine has become a reality and many costly or unpleasant investigations are now ordered which are not always necessary. The surgeon perceives the rising tide of medical litigation as a personal threat and, in the USA, some specialities have become so high-risk that obtaining malpractice insurance is prohibitively expensive and trainees are increasingly hard to find.

The lawyers and patients would argue that a number of surgeons are technically incompetent and should not be allowed to continue in practice. By this view, the patient who has been damaged should receive financial compensation and the hospital where the surgeon worked will need to review its procedures to prevent the same mistake from recurring. The doctors feel that financial settlements and lawyers' fees are exorbitant and represent a source of easy money; patients and their lawyers do not understand why these surgeons were ever allowed to operate in the first place.

The divide between the two sides in medical litigation is clearly immense and the views are usually so strong that objective discussion and useful change is hard to achieve. Nevertheless, the cost in human terms to patients who have suffered an adverse event is immense, let alone the financial implications of medical mishaps and legal settlements. Clinical governance has immense potential for good but it needs to include patient education, clinical audit, professional development and risk management if it is to be effective. While all agree that something needs to be done — the only question is exactly what.

FURTHER READING

Law for Doctors: Principles and Practicalities
Branthwaite MA, Beresford, NW
2nd Edition, RSM Press, 2003.
A concise summary of relevant medical law with references to key cases and summaries of issues such as consent, confidentiality and legal procedure.

Medical Ethics and the Law — The Core Curriculum
Hope T, Savulescu J, Hendrick J
Churchill Livingstone, 2003.
An excellent and highly readable undergraduate text containing a detailed discussion of the major ethical issues; deserves to be read from cover to cover by all practising clinicians.

The Risk Management Handbook for Healthcare Professionals
Sanfilippo JS, Robinson CL
Parthenon Publishing Group, 2002.
A comprehensive description of the American approach to medical litigation, risk management and its prevention.
Readable and positively encouraging.

An Organisation With a Memory — Report of an Expert Group on Learning from Adverse Events in the NHS
The Stationery Office, London, 2000.
Unusually, a well written and thought-provoking review on developing proper risk management in the National Health Service which, sadly, has not yet been translated into action.

Useful Internet Resources

nuffieldbioethics.org
Online availability of the major reports from the Nuffield Bioethics Trust.

www.corec.org.uk
Provides access to the complex requirements of research ethics committees.

www.jmedethics.com
The website for the *Journal of Medical Ethics and Humanities* — stimulating and necessary reading for all interested in the subject.

www.medicolegaljournal.com
Online access to the *Journal of the Medico Legal Society* containing articles and lectures on a wide range of medico-legal topics.

INDEX